Animal Modeling in Cancer

Animal Modeling in Cancer

Editor

Vladimir Korinek

MDPI • Basel • Beijing • Wuhan • Barcelona • Belgrade • Manchester • Tokyo • Cluj • Tianjin

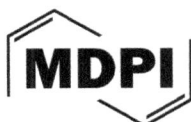

Editor
Vladimir Korinek
Institute of Molecular Genetics
of the Czech Academy of
Sciences
Czech Republic

Editorial Office
MDPI
St. Alban-Anlage 66
4052 Basel, Switzerland

This is a reprint of articles from the Special Issue published online in the open access journal *Actuators* (ISSN 2076-0825) (available at: https://www.mdpi.com/journal/genes/special_issues/ Anima_Modeling_Cancer).

For citation purposes, cite each article independently as indicated on the article page online and as indicated below:

LastName, A.A.; LastName, B.B.; LastName, C.C. Article Title. *Journal Name* **Year**, *Volume Number*, Page Range.

ISBN 978-3-0365-1276-1 (Hbk)
ISBN 978-3-0365-1277-8 (PDF)

Cover image courtesy of Lucie Janeckova.

© 2021 by the authors. Articles in this book are Open Access and distributed under the Creative Commons Attribution (CC BY) license, which allows users to download, copy and build upon published articles, as long as the author and publisher are properly credited, which ensures maximum dissemination and a wider impact of our publications.
The book as a whole is distributed by MDPI under the terms and conditions of the Creative Commons license CC BY-NC-ND.

Contents

About the Editor vii

Vladimir Korinek
Special Issue: Animal Modeling in Cancer
Reprinted from: *Genes* **2020**, *11*, 1009, doi:10.3390/genes11091009 1

Roger A. Moorehead
Rodent Models Assessing Mammary Tumor Prevention by Soy or Soy Isoflavones
Reprinted from: *Genes* **2019**, *10*, 566, doi:10.3390/genes10080566 5

Hala Skayneh, Batoul Jishi, Rita Hleihel, Maguy Hamieh, Nadine Darwiche, Ali Bazarbachi, Marwan El Sabban and Hiba El Hajj
A Critical Review of Animal Models Used in Acute Myeloid Leukemia Pathophysiology
Reprinted from: *Genes* **2019**, *10*, 614, doi:10.3390/genes10080614 19

Anna Michaelidesová, Jana Konířová, Petr Bartůněk and Martina Zíková
Effects of Radiation Therapy on Neural Stem Cells
Reprinted from: *Genes* **2019**, *10*, 640, doi:10.3390/genes10090640 55

Monika Stastna, Lucie Janeckova, Dusan Hrckulak, Vitezslav Kriz and Vladimir Korinek
Human Colorectal Cancer from the Perspective of Mouse Models
Reprinted from: *Genes* **2019**, *10*, 788, doi:10.3390/genes10100788 73

Lucie Lanikova, Olga Babosova and Josef T. Prchal
Experimental Modeling of Myeloproliferative Neoplasms
Reprinted from: *Genes* **2019**, *10*, 813, doi:10.3390/genes10100813 107

Nikol Baloghova, Tomas Lidak and Lukas Cermak
Ubiquitin Ligases Involved in the Regulation of Wnt, TGF-β, and Notch Signaling Pathways and Their Roles in Mouse Development and Homeostasis
Reprinted from: *Genes* **2019**, *10*, 815, doi:10.3390/genes10100815 121

Alyssa A. Leystra and Margie L. Clapper
Gut Microbiota Influences Experimental Outcomes in Mouse Models of Colorectal Cancer
Reprinted from: *Genes* **2019**, *10*, 900, doi:10.3390/genes10110900 165

Vratislav Horak, Anna Palanova, Jana Cizkova, Veronika Miltrova, Petr Vodicka and Helena Kupcova Skalnikova
Melanoma-Bearing Libechov Minipig (MeLiM): The Unique Swine Model of Hereditary Metastatic Melanoma
Reprinted from: *Genes* **2019**, *10*, 915, doi:10.3390/genes10110915 185

Kallayanee Chawengsaksophak
Cdx2 Animal Models Reveal Developmental Origins of Cancers
Reprinted from: *Genes* **2019**, *10*, 928, doi:10.3390/genes10110928 219

Martina Hason and Petr Bartůněk
Zebrafish Models of Cancer—New Insights on Modeling Human Cancer in a Non-Mammalian Vertebrate
Reprinted from: *Genes* **2019**, *10*, 935, doi:10.3390/genes10110935 235

About the Editor

Vladimir Korinek is head of the Laboratory of Cell and Development Biology at the Institute of Molecular Genetics of the Czech Academy of Sciences. Dr. Korinek serves as deputy director of the institute. Dr. Korinek is co-author of several seminal studies that describe the role of aberrant Wnt signaling in colorectal cancer and reveal the relation of the Wnt pathway to the physiology of intestinal stem cells. Dr. Korinek's current research is focused on gene targeting, genomic and bioinformatic approaches to studying the signaling mechanisms that influence the fate of normal and transformed adult stem cells in the gastrointestinal tract and hematopoietic system. Korinek's laboratory generated a collection of genetically modified mouse strains suitable for studying intestinal cancer. The laboratory established various techniques allowing phenotypic profiling of cancer cells isolated from gut tissues. The laboratory also developed its own (or participated in) high-throughput screens for small molecule Wnt pathway inhibitors. The screens resulted in identification of several chemical compounds potentially useful as anticancer drugs.

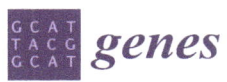 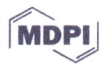

Editorial

Special Issue: Animal Modeling in Cancer

Vladimir Korinek

Institute of Molecular Genetics of the Czech Academy of Sciences, Videnska 1083, 142 20 Prague, Czech Republic; vladimir.korinek@img.cas.cz; Tel.: +420-241-063-146; Fax: +420-244-472-282

Received: 10 August 2020; Accepted: 25 August 2020; Published: 27 August 2020

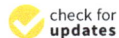

Abstract: Recent advances in high-throughput sequencing techniques have significantly accelerated the development of personalized diagnostic tools and cancer treatments. However, a comparative analysis of experimental animals that share similar genetic, physiological, and behavioral traits with humans remains the basis for understanding the pathological mechanisms associated with human diseases, including cancer. The generation and characterization of suitable animal models mimicking tumor growth and progression thus represents an important "component" of tumor biology research. The presented Special Issue contains ten review articles, which, based on data obtained from various animal models, summarize a number of aspects of the tumor formation process that include gastrointestinal neoplasia, breast cancer, hematological malignancies, melanoma, and brain tumors. This Special Issue nicely illustrates how the study of suitable living models uncovers not only the fundamental molecular and cellular bases of neoplastic growth, but might also indicate approaches to efficient cancer treatments.

Keywords: cancer; mouse models; non-mouse models; gene editing; stem cells; solid tumors; hematologic malignancies

---

The use of animal models to study the process of cell transformation and tumor formation has become a routine experimental approach. Initially, various types of neoplasms were induced in the experimental animal by exogenous substances or radiation. These techniques were extended by genetic models. Such models were first obtained by selecting "random" phenotypes, and later also by targeted genome modifications. Additionally, xenotransplantation techniques for implanting tumor cells or tumor tissue fragments directly into animals' bodies have been developed. Another technical improvement that accelerated and streamlined the preparation of animal models was based on the introduction of the method of conditional genetic modifications (especially the Cre/loxP system), which enabled tissue-specific and time-defined genetic changes. A breakthrough was brought by the introduction of programmable nuclease technology and the clustered regularly interspaced short palindromic repeats (CRISPR)/CAS9 system. The tumor process is associated with a number of genetic changes in the particular cell type, and these inventions have led to well-defined and sophisticated tumor models that resemble the complex pathological situations observed in human tumor tissue. This Special Issue has been dedicated to animal models used for cancer research and contains ten review articles. Not surprisingly, most of them are dedicated to rodents (especially mice and rats) as the main experimental model used in tumor biology.

Non-mammalian models are dominated by zebrafish (*Danio rerio*). The use of fish in biomedical research has its obvious advantages. These are, in particular, the relatively low costs of their breeding (related to a high reproductive capacity), extracorporeal development of embryos, and the possibility of performing genetic manipulations. The above advantages are somewhat complicated by the fact that during evolution, the zebrafish genome has undergone duplication, and its genes thus have more paralogs. The resulting redundancy or, conversely, species-specific variability of the original function of the studied gene might complicate the analysis and interpretation of the obtained results.

On the other hand, the natural transparency of zebrafish embryos and the existence of a mutant strain called *casper*, whose individuals are transparent even in adulthood, making it possible to monitor the growth and distribution of tumor cells directly in a living organism. Another complication is the relatively small amount of commercially available antibodies that recognize fish antigens. However, this disadvantage can be very well compensated for by the use of transgenic "reporter" strains, a large number of which are currently available. The above-mentioned features, together with the fact that the development of the hematopoietic system has cellular bases and regulatory mechanisms very similar to those described in mammals, make zebrafish a unique model for the study of hematooncological diseases. This is well illustrated by examples of myeloproliferative neoplasms (MPN) [1] and acute myeloid leukemias (AML) [2]. A comprehensive summary of zebrafish as a model in tumor biology with a detailed presentation of various types of studied neoplasms and techniques is given in a review article by M. Hason and P. Bartunek [3].

Carcinoma of the colon and rectum (colorectal cancer (CRC)) represents one of the most frequently diagnosed neoplasia in developed countries. Therefore, it is also not surprising that the two articles included in the Special Issue are dedicated to mouse models of intestinal cancer. The majority of CRCs progress through the conventional adenoma–carcinoma pathway. In recent years, there have been considerable efforts to unify the classification of colorectal tumors. These efforts have led to the establishment of the system of four consensus molecular subtypes (CMSs) defined by multiple characteristics that include gene expression profiles, microsatellite instability, genomic DNA methylation status, and differences in the status of the immune response and various signaling pathways. In their review, M. Stastna and colleagues have presented a broad spectrum of mouse intestinal cancer models that display pathological changes in Wnt, Hippo, p53, epidermal growth factor (EGF), and transforming growth factor β (TGFβ) signaling. They have also described microsatellite instability models and models of chemically induced tumorigenesis. Importantly, the authors reflect the categorization of human CRC into the CMS groups and indicate a possible assignment of the described mouse model to the CMS group [4]. The mammalian gut is a complex organ consisting not only of cells intrinsic for the organism, but also containing vast amounts of bacteria. Importantly, microbial colonization of the gut is essential for the development and function of the immune system, proper digestion and acquisition of nutrients, and vitamin production. In a well-structured and interesting comprehensive article, A.A. Leystra and M.L. Clapper present the topic of the influence of intestinal microbiome compositions on the phenotypes of mouse models with colon cancer. The article further summarizes the factors that significantly affect the composition of the intestinal microbiome in experimental mice. Importantly, the authors also propose strategies that might help to evaluate the effect(s) of the differing microbiome composition on the output of experiments related to intestinal tumorigenesis [5].

The issue of intestinal neoplasias is related to the article of K. Chawengsaksophak, which is fully dedicated to the role of the caudal type homeobox 2 (*Cdx2*) gene in esophageal and gastrointestinal cancer and leukemias, as shown by the analysis of mice and zebrafish models. Cdx2 is an important factor in defining the positional identity of cells. Pathological situations associated with tissue damage and its subsequent regeneration may cause changes to the cell identity called metaplasia, or an abnormal localization of otherwise morphologically and cytologically normal tissue. Importantly, metaplasias represent a significant factor in the development of cancer. An aberrant expression of the *Cdx2* gene induces a shift in cellular identity towards more posterior types and, in animal models, it results in an intestinal type of metaplasia of the esophageal epithelium (so-called Barrett's esophagus) and stomach. In contrast, a loss of the *Cdx2* gene in the colon induces neoplasias producing gastric markers. Finally, leukemia is one of the neoplasms for which Cdx2 (over)production is typical [6].

Two articles are dedicated to hematooncological models. L. Lanikova and colleagues thoroughly describe the genetic basis (the so-called mutation landscape) of MPN, which are represented by polycythemia vera, essential thrombocytosis and primary myelofibrosis. The authors introduce mouse and fish models with these disorders. They also provide examples of how the technology of induced pluripotent stem cells (iPSCs) has initiated a new era in human disease modeling. For example, iPS cells prepared from MPN allow for the reconstruction of the clonal hierarchy and investigation of the effects of oncogenic mutations at their endogenous settings [1]. The article by H. Skayneh and co-workers deals with zebrafish and rodent (rat, mouse) AML models. AML is a very common hematological neoplasia with a heterogeneous genetic basis, and suitable animal models are a key tool for the analysis of individual AML (sub)types. The authors also report the use of Drosophila as an invertebrate model to study the chromosomal translocation t (8:21) (q22; q22), which is very frequent in AML [2].

The article by V. Horak and colleagues focuses on animal models used in the study of melanoma. Melanoma is a very aggressive and deadly type of cancer, the incidence of which is increasing worldwide, especially in the Caucasian population. The introductory part comprehensively describes our current knowledge about the genetic changes and molecular mechanisms related to the origin and progression of the disease. A detailed description of animal models follows, which includes not only mouse models, but also dog and horse models, as well as three non-mammalian animal models (zebrafish, Xiphophorus and Drosophila). The most extensive part of the review is dedicated to the Melanoma-Bearing Libechov Minipig. The origin of this genetic model dates back to the late 1960s, and the knowledge about this model is thus very deep and extensive. The (mini)pig as a model for melanoma research has a number of advantages. The structure and distribution of melanocytes in the pig skin is more similar (unlike mouse skin) to the situation in the human skin. Moreover, the relatively long lifespan (12–18 years) allows the long-term monitoring of the experimental animals. Large animals also allow blood or tissue samples to be taken repeatedly during their life (and disease progression) of the experimental individuals [7].

Research over the last few decades has clearly shown that dysfunction of the evolutionarily conserved Wnt, Notch, and TGFβ signaling pathways may have critical consequences for cellular fate, often leading to cell transformation and tumorigenesis. The article by N. Baloghova and colleagues offers a new perspective on the regulation of these signaling pathways by the ubiquitin–proteasome (UPS) system. The authors summarized (in an "exhaustive" manner) the results obtained in the mouse models [8]. It should be emphasized that for therapy based on UPS function manipulation, a thorough understanding of the molecular mechanisms affecting the protein stability is essential. Additionally, a subsequent validation of this knowledge in living animal models is also required.

The last two review articles offer a somewhat different view of the use of animal models in tumor biology. R.A. Moorhead evaluates the possibility of whether the consumption of soy products or soy-derived isoflavones might prevent (or reduce) the risk of breast cancer. The author summarizes that while epidemiological studies conducted in Asian countries show that high levels of soy and soy product consumption are associated with a reduced risk of breast cancer, experiments using mouse or rat breast tumor models (with tumors induced by chemical carcinogens or ectopic oncogenes) have not been confirmatory [9]. Obviously, the negative outcomes of the experiments could be related to the overall experimental design; however, the main issue might be that rodents metabolize soy isoflavones differently than humans. The article by A. Michaelidesova and co-workers describes the basic characteristics of various types of brain tumors, radiotherapy techniques, and possible side effects of radiotherapy. For obvious reasons, it is difficult to study neurogenesis in the adult human brain, but postnatal neurogenesis has been studied in detail in rodents, as nicely summarized in this article—[10]. Here, again, it should be emphasized that the question of neurogenesis in the adult human brain is still controversial. Which brings me back to the idea that some caution is needed when generalizing the results obtained in animal models.

I thank all the authors and reviewers of the published articles and I wish the readers inspiring reading.

Funding: This research was funded by the Czech Science Foundation (grant number 18-26324S) and by the Academy of Sciences of the Czech Republic (RVO 68378050-KAV-NPUI).

Acknowledgments: We thank S. Takacova for critically reading the manuscript.

Conflicts of Interest: The author declares no conflict of interest.

References

1. Lanikova, L.; Babosova, O.; Prchal, J.T. Experimental modeling of myeloproliferative neoplasms. *Genes (Basel)* **2019**, *10*, 813. [CrossRef] [PubMed]
2. Skayneh, H.; Jishi, B.; Hleihel, R.; Hamieh, M.; Darwiche, N.; Bazarbachi, A.; El Sabban, M.; El Hajj, H. A critical review of animal models used in acute myeloid leukemia pathophysiology. *Genes (Basel)* **2019**, *10*, 614. [CrossRef] [PubMed]
3. Hason, M.; Bartunek, P. Zebrafish models of cancer-new insights on modeling human cancer in a non-mammalian vertebrate. *Genes (Basel)* **2019**, *10*, 935. [CrossRef] [PubMed]
4. Stastna, M.; Janeckova, L.; Hrckulak, D.; Kriz, V.; Korinek, V. Human colorectal cancer from the perspective of mouse models. *Genes (Basel)* **2019**, *10*, 788. [CrossRef] [PubMed]
5. Leystra, A.A.; Clapper, M.L. Gut microbiota influences experimental outcomes in mouse models of colorectal cancer. *Genes (Basel)* **2019**, *10*, 900. [CrossRef] [PubMed]
6. Chawengsaksophak, K. Cdx2 animal models reveal developmental origins of cancers. *Genes (Basel)* **2019**, *10*, 928. [CrossRef] [PubMed]
7. Horak, V.; Palanova, A.; Cizkova, J.; Miltrova, V.; Vodicka, P.; Skalníková, H.K. Melanoma-bearing libechov minipig (melim): The unique swine model of hereditary metastatic melanoma. *Genes (Basel)* **2019**, *10*, 915. [CrossRef] [PubMed]
8. Baloghova, N.; Lidak, T.; Cermak, L. Ubiquitin ligases involved in the regulation of wnt, tgf-beta, and notch signaling pathways and their roles in mouse development and homeostasis. *Genes (Basel)* **2019**, *10*, 815. [CrossRef] [PubMed]
9. Moorehead, R.A. Rodent models assessing mammary tumor prevention by soy or soy isoflavones. *Genes (Basel)* **2019**, *10*, 566. [CrossRef] [PubMed]
10. Michaelidesova, A.; Konirova, J.; Bartunek, P.; Zikova, M. Effects of radiation therapy on neural stem cells. *Genes (Basel)* **2019**, *10*, 640. [CrossRef] [PubMed]

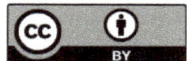

© 2020 by the author. Licensee MDPI, Basel, Switzerland. This article is an open access article distributed under the terms and conditions of the Creative Commons Attribution (CC BY) license (http://creativecommons.org/licenses/by/4.0/).

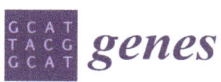

Review

Rodent Models Assessing Mammary Tumor Prevention by Soy or Soy Isoflavones

Roger A. Moorehead

Department of Biomedical Sciences, Ontario Veterinary College, University of Guelph, Guelph, ON N1G2W1, Canada; rmoorehe@uoguelph.ca

Received: 12 April 2019; Accepted: 9 July 2019; Published: 26 July 2019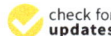

Abstract: While epidemiological studies performed in Asian countries generally show that high levels of dietary soy are associated with reduced breast cancer risk, studies in Western countries have typically failed to show this correlation. In an attempt to model the preventative actions of soy on mammary tumor development, rodent models have been employed. Thirty-four studies were identified that evaluated the impact of soy products or purified soy isoflavones on mammary tumor initiation (studies evaluating established mammary tumors or mammary tumor cell lines were not included) and these studies were separated into mammary tumors induced by chemical carcinogens or transgenic expression of oncogenes based on the timing of soy administration. Regardless of when soy-based diets or purified isoflavones were administered, no consistent protective effects were observed in either carcinogen-induced or oncogene-induced mammary tumors. While some studies demonstrated that soy or purified isoflavones could reduce mammary tumor incidence, other studies showed either no effect or tumor promoting effects of soy products or isoflavones. Most importantly, only five studies found a decrease in mammary tumor incidence and six studies observed a decrease in tumor multiplicity, two relevant measures of the tumor preventative effects of soy or isoflavones. The variable outcomes of the studies examined were not completely surprising given that few studies employed the same experimental design. Future studies should be carefully designed to more accurately emulate soy consumption observed in Asian cultures including lifetime exposure to less refined soy products and potentially the incorporation of multigenerational feeding studies.

Keywords: soy; isoflavones; mammary tumor prevention; rodent models; chemical carcinogens; transgenic mice

1. Introduction

It has been estimated that approximately 35% of human cancers are preventable through changes in lifestyle such as maintaining a healthy body weight, eliminating alcohol and tobacco, and adhering to cancer screening guidelines [1]. One lifestyle change that has been specifically associated with breast cancer is the consumption of high levels of dietary soy. Several epidemiologic studies found that women from cultures consuming high levels of dietary soy have an ~3-fold reduced risk of developing breast cancer compared to women that only consume small amounts of soy [2–6]. Several meta-analyses of the epidemiologic studies found that high consumption of soy reduced the risk of breast cancer in both pre- and post-menopausal women in studies performed on Asian populations but not on women from Western countries [6–8]. A 2019 meta-analysis found that individuals consuming high levels of isoflavones had similar breast cancer rates as those consuming low levels of isoflavones. When this meta-analysis only evaluated studies that reported the intake of soy foods, individuals consuming high levels of soy foods had a significant reduction in breast cancer risk compared to those in the low soy-food consumption group [9]. Therefore, although most studies suggest that consuming high levels of dietary soy may reduce the risk of developing breast cancer, there is no clear consensus.

However, some of this variation may stem from the population examined, types of soy products consumed (refined vs unrefined, fermented vs unfermented, and soy foods vs isoflavones), as well as the timing and duration of soy consumption. Ideally, randomized human prevention trials should be performed; however, these types of studies would take decades to complete, may raise ethical concerns of feeding developing fetuses or newborns specialized diets without their consent, and it would be difficult to maintain compliance to specific diets for such a long duration.

Since human randomized clinical trials are not feasible, animal models have been utilized with the most common being rodent models. Rodent mammary glands share features with the human breast including epithelial-lined ducts surrounded by myoepithelial cells, fibroblast and stroma [10]. In addition, both the mouse mammary gland and human breast respond to similar growth factors, cytokines and hormones during pubertal ductal development, alveologenesis and involution [10]. There are, however, differences in human and rodent mammary glands including the number of mammary glands, increased density of fibrous tissue in human breasts as well as more complex lobulo-alveolar structures in human breasts [11].

This review focuses on rodent models designed to assess the preventative actions of dietary soy products or purified isoflavones and includes papers published since 1995. For studies prior to 1995, please see the review by Barnes [12]. The efficacy of dietary soy or purified isoflavones in reducing breast cancer progression or tumor recurrence has been investigated but is beyond the scope of this review. While it is possible that soy isoflavones impact tumor cell progression or recurrence using similar mechanisms as those that prevent mammary tumor initiation, it is also possible that these tumor stages are regulated by distinct mechanisms and thus this review has focused on soy's impact on tumor initiation and not progression or recurrence.

2. Soy and Isoflavones

Soy products are derived from soybeans and contain a number of compounds including protease inhibitors, phytosterols, saponins, and phytoestrogens known as isoflavones. Most of the work has focused on the isoflavone component of soybeans and the main isoflavones are genistein, daidzein and glycitein [13]. Isoflavones have chemical structures similar to mammalian estrogens and thus can bind to estrogen receptor-α (ERα) and ERβ [14–16]. The affinity of isoflavones for ERα and ERβ is also different with isoflavones preferentially binding to ERβ [17–20]. However, soy isoflavones have relatively weak estrogenic activity compared to endogenous estrogens [21,22] and thus, it is thought that dietary isoflavones partially impede endogenous estrogen signaling [14,23,24]. Since elevated lifetime estrogen exposure is a breast cancer risk factor [25], soy isoflavones may reduce breast cancer risk by suppressing the effects of endogenous estrogen. In addition to altering estrogen signaling, soy isoflavones have been reported to decrease lipid peroxidation and oxidative DNA damage through their antioxidant properties [24,26–28], promote apoptosis [26,29], inhibit angiogenesis [27,30–32] and regulate DNA methylation [33]. It should be noted that most mechanistic studies of soy isoflavones are performed in vitro using isoflavone concentrations exceeding 25 micromolar, while circulating levels of isoflavones in rodents and humans consuming soy-rich diets are typically less than 1–5 micromolar [29,31,32,34–36]. Moreover, in vitro studies cannot account for modifications of isoflavones during normal metabolism that can influence the relative abundance of isoflavone metabolites and their bioactivity [37]. While most of the studies have focused on the isoflavone components of soy, other soybean components such as protease inhibitors, phytosterols and saponins that may also influence breast cancer risk [38–40].

Not all sources of dietary soy are equal. Asian cultures typically consume minimally processed soybeans and more fermented soy products such as miso or tempeh where isoflavones are primarily in their aglycone form (genistein, daidzein and glycitein) [41]. In contrast, Western societies typically consume non-fermented soy products such as soy milk or tofu which contains isoflavones primarily in their glucosides form (genistin, daidzin and glycitin). In addition, soy products in North America often undergo extensive extraction and purification processes producing a product known as isolated soy protein (ISP) or soy protein isolate, which lacks most of the carbohydrates and fiber, leaving a product that is approximately 90% protein. This processing also influences the levels of isoflavones [42–44] and removes a number of soy compounds including protease inhibitors, phytosterols and saponins that may alter the protective properties associated with soybeans [42].

3. Rodent Mammary Tumor Models

One of the first and most common rodent models used to evaluate the impact of soy isoflavones on mammary tumor develop is the administration of 7,12-Dimethylbenzathracene (DMBA) to rats. DMBA is typically given as a single dose to pubertal female rats through injection or oral gavage and tumor incidence is close to 100% with tumor onset ranging from 8–21 weeks, depending on the concentration of DMBA administered [45]. Mammary tumors induced by DBMA are typically minimally invasive but remain hormone-dependent and thus are reasonable models for estrogen dependent breast cancers [46]. Other chemical carcinogens have also been used including N-methyl-N-nitrosourea (NMU) and ethyl methanesulfonate (EMS), which are typically provided as a single administration to pubertal female rats and 2-amino-1-methyl-6-penylimidazo[4–b]pyridine (PhIP) is administered orally to rats four times per week for two weeks. Although chemically induced rat mammary tumor models share features with human breast cancer they frequently induce mutations in *Hras* [47–50], a phenomenon not frequently observed in human breast cancers. However, a more recent study evaluating genetic alterations induced by DMBA in mice frequently observed mutations in *Pi3kca* and *Pten*, two relevant human breast cancer genes [51]. Chemical carcinogens are used less frequently in mice as mice are more resistant to chemically induced mammary tumors than rats and require multiple doses of chemical carcinogens [51].

With the generation of genetically modified mice, alterations in specific oncogenes or tumor suppressor genes became possible. The most widely used transgenic mammary tumor model is MMTV-*neu* transgenic mice. MMTV-*neu* mice express elevated levels of *EbbB2* (rodent equivalent of human *HER-2*) in mammary epithelial cells as well as other epithelial cells where the mouse mammary tumor virus (MMTV) promoter is expressed [52–54]. MMTV-*neu* mice develop mammary tumors with a median onset of 5–10 months [55–57] and these tumors have characteristics similar to human HER2+ tumors [58]. Another MMTV driven transgene that induces mammary tumor development is *Wnt1*. MMTV-*Wnt1* transgenic mice develop mammary tumors expressing both luminal and myoepithelial genes and cluster most closely with normal human breast tissue [58]. One limitation with MMTV-driven transgenes is that the oncogene is expressed at low levels throughout the animal's lifespan. The MMTV promoter is responsive to steroid hormones [59–62] and thus its activity is highest during puberty and gestation with low levels of MMTV promoter activity prior to puberty. As it remains unclear when the initiating events for breast cancer occur, expression of an oncogene at all developmental stages may or may not accurately reflect oncogene expression in humans.

Two non-MMTV-driven transgenes have been used to study the impact of dietary soy on mammary tumor development: C(3)1/SV40 and Mt-*hGH*. C(3)1/SV40 transgenic mice express the simian virus 40 large T antigen driven by the rat prostatic steroid binding protein C3(1) 5′-flanking sequence. Female mice develop mammary tumors by 4 months of age and male mice develop prostate tumors by 1 year of age [63]. Mammary tumors from C(3)1/SV40 transgenic mice share characteristics with human basal-like tumors [58]. Mt-*hGH* transgenic mice express elevated levels of human growth hormone driven by a murine metallothionein promoter. These mice develop mammary tumors by 27–43 weeks of age [64]. Gene expression analysis has not been performed on these mammary tumors but the authors describe the tumors as malignant papillary adenocarcinomas [64].

In addition to the transgenic mice describe above, MTB-IGFIR transgenic mice [65] have also been used to investigate soy isoflavone's impact on mammary tumorigenesis [66]. MTB-IGFIR transgenic mice overexpress the human insulin-like growth factor receptor (IGF-IR) in mammary epithelial cells in a doxycycline-inducible manner [65]. Mammary tumors rapidly develop in 100% of the mice and these mammary tumors cluster most closely with human basal-like breast cancers [67]. The MTB-IGFIR transgenic mice overcome one of the limitations of constitutive transgenic models (i.e., MMTV-driven transgenes) in that the IGF-IR transgene is only expressed when doxycycline is present and thus transgene expression can be initiated in pubertal or adult mice [65,68].

4. Timing of Soy Exposure

A key difference in the studies evaluating the impact of soy isoflavones on mammary tumor development in rodent models is the timing of soy isoflavone administration. Most of the early studies and even some of the more recent studies initiate the feeding of soy diets or purified isoflavones in postnatal rodents. This experimental approach would presumably emulate the human situation where children or adolescents switch their diet to one containing high levels of soy. However, Asian cultures, where reduced breast cancer rates are observed, would presumably consume high levels of soy at all stages of life including during pregnancy and lactation as well as during childhood, adolescence and adulthood. Therefore, lifetime exposure (gestation, lactation and postnatal development) may more accurately model the isoflavone consumption of cultures with reduced breast cancer rates.

Given the potential importance of the timing of soy exposure this review has been organized into two main sections: mammary tumor development following postnatal soy/isoflavone exposure, and mammary tumor development following lifetime soy/isoflavone exposure. There were also four studies that investigated soy exposure only during the perinatal developmental window, which have been included in this review.

5. Mammary Tumor Development Following Postnatal Soy Isoflavone Administration

Twenty-three studies were identified that evaluated mammary tumorigenesis following the administration of soy-based diets or purified isoflavones during postnatal development; fourteen using chemical carcinogens in rats [69–82] and nine using transgenic mice [83–91]. For this review, postnatal administration was defined by the initiation of soy-based diets or isoflavones at weaning or later and the design of these studies and the main findings are summarized in Table 1. The impact of soy isoflavones on mammary tumor development were highly variable. This was not completely surprising given the differences in (1) the chemical carcinogen or oncogene used, (2) the source and concentration of soy products or purified isoflavones, and (3) the timing of soy/isoflavone administration. Within the 14 chemical carcinogen studies, 8 found that soy/isoflavones had some protective effect against mammary tumorigenesis (tumor incidence, latency, multiplicity or size) [70–74,76,79,82] but only 2 of these studies observed a truly protective effect against mammary tumor development as measured as a significant decrease in tumor incidence [71,72], while 3 studies demonstrated a significant reduction in tumor multiplicity [74,76,79]. Three of the studies using chemical carcinogens found that soy/isoflavones promoted mammary tumor incidence, multiplicity, or size [72,75,80].

The findings were also highly variable in the transgenic mouse models with four of the nine studies showing at least some protective effect against mammary tumorigenesis (tumor incidence, latency, multiplicity or size) [83,86–88], with two of these studies observing a significant decrease in tumor incidence [83,88]. Three of the studies found no effect [84,89,91] and three of the studies found that soy isoflavones promoted at least one mammary tumor property [83,85,90]. The transgenic data was more difficult to evaluate as often other characteristics (i.e., high fat diet, estrogen levels) and different concentrations of isoflavones were assessed in the same study. For example, the study by Zhang et al. [83] assessed the impact of soy on mammary tumor development in MMTV-*neu* mice with low (ovariectomized mice), normal or high (estradiol injection) levels of estrogen. In this study it was observed that diets high in soy increased tumor incidence in the low estrogen group, but the soy diet reduced tumor incidence in the high estrogen group (explaining why this study is referenced as soy-based diets having demonstrated both tumor protective and tumor promoting effects in the discussion above).

Table 1. Postnatal Soy/Isoflavone Administration.

Species	Isoflavone Diet/Timing	Tumor Inducer	Main Finding	Refs
rat	0.25 g/kg or 1 g/kg of daidzein or genistein separately or 1 g/kg of both daidzein and genistein, PND35-EOS	1 oral dose, 80 mg/kg body weight DMBA at PND50	No significant difference in tumor incidence or size compared to control diet	[69]
rat	500 ppm genistein in diet, PND15–30, PND15–30 and PND55-EOS or PND55-EOS	1 oral dose, 10 mg DMBA at PND48	Tumor onset delayed only in group fed genistein PND15–30 and PND55-EOS compared to control diet. No significant difference in tumor incidence	[70]
rat	2 mg/kg body weight, genistein orally, PND42-EOS	1 oral dose, 80 mg/kg body weight DMBA at PND55	Tumor incidence and size significantly reduced in genistein group compared to controls	[71]
rat	3.24 mg total isoflavones/g protein in diet of lean or obese rats, PND42-EOS	1 oral dose, 65 mg/kg body weight DMBA at PND50	Tumor incidence significantly reduced in lean soy fed rats vs lean casein fed rats yet tumor incidence significantly higher in obese soy-fed rats vs obese casein fed rats. No significant differences in tumor onset or multiplicity	[72]
rat	Genistein 20 mg/kg body weight, daidzein 20 mg/kg body weight or genistein + daidzein 20 mg/kg each), oral 1 week before DMBA-EOS	1 injection, 25 mg DMBA, exact age not defined	Genistein alone, daidzein alone and the combination significantly reduced tumor size compared to control mice. Tumor incidence appeared to be reduced, especially in combination group but no significance was indicated.	[73]
rat	Isoflavone-depleted soy peptide, PND28-PND56 and PND63-EOS	1 oral dose, 50 mg/kg body weight DMBA at PND56	Tumor latency was significantly increased, and tumor size and multiplicity were significantly decreased in isoflavone-deprived soy group vs control group	[74]
rat	Soy milk PND50-EOS	1 oral dose, 5 mg DMBA at PND49	Tumor incidence significantly higher in soy milk group compared to water group; no significant differences in tumor multiplicity or size	[75]
rat	20% soy protein, PND25-EOS	1 oral dose, 80 mg/kg body weight DMBA at PND50	Tumor onset significantly delayed, and tumor multiplicity significantly reduced in soy group vs control group but no difference in tumor incidence at study endpoint	[76]
rat	Soy-free diet with 0.35% or 0.7% (w/w) SOYSELECT (12% isoflavones and 35% saponins), PND21-EOS	1 oral dose, 80 mg/kg body weight DMBA at PND50	No significant differences observed at study endpoint	[77]
rat	0.03, 0.4 or 0.81 mg/g diet isoflavones, PND36-EOS	1 oral dose, 10 mg DMBA at PND50	No significant differences in tumor incidence, onset, multiplicity or burden	[78]
rat	200 mg/kg diet genistein, 200 mg/kg diet daidzein, 100 mg/kg diet each of genistein + daidzein, 160 g/kg diet SPI or 160 g/kg diet SPI depleted of isoflavones, PND43-EOS	1 oral dose, 15 mg DMBA at PND50	Tumor multiplicity significantly reduced in daidzein and both SPI diets; no significant difference in tumor incidence, mean latency or size in any of the diets	[79]
rat	1 mg/kg body weight genistein injected daily, PND45-EOS	1 injection, 40 mg/kg body weight NMU at PND45	Tumor multiplicity and size significantly elevated in genistein group vs control group	[80]
rat	0.03 or 1 mg/g of genistein in soy free diet or soy containing basal diet PND28-EOS	Oral, 10^{-3} M EMS in drinking water, PND28-PND112	no significance difference in tumor incidence, size or latency compared to control group	[81]
rat	100 g soymilk powder/kg diet alone or with 2 g/kg diet Lactobacillus casei in a high fat diet, PND35-EOS.	oral, 85 mg/kg PhIP, 4 x/week for 2 weeks, PND42-56	according to Table 2, no significant differences in tumor incidence, multiplicity or size in soymilk vs control, however Figure 1 indicates that tumor multiplicity significantly reduced at study endpoint. The combination of soymilk and Lactobacillus casei significantly reduced tumor multiplicity	[82]
mouse	Soybean diet (40% soybean meal), PND49-EOS	MMTV-neu, low estrogen (ovariectomy), normal estrogen (untreated), and high estrogen (estradiol injection)	Tumor incidence significantly increased in soy-fed, low estrogen group but tumor incidence significantly reduced in soy-fed, high estrogen group. No significant differences in tumor latency or size	[83]

Table 1. *Cont.*

Species	Isoflavone Diet/Timing	Tumor Inducer	Main Finding	Refs
mouse	21.7% soy protein isolate, PND60-EOS	MMTV-*neu* (did not consider ERΔ3/*neu* mice)	No significant effect on tumor incidence or latency in soy-fed MMTV-*neu* mice compared to MMTV-*neu* mice fed a control diet	[84]
mouse	0.004%, 0.02% or 0.06% wt/wt Prevastein (46.19% wt/wt isoflavones), PND25-EOS	MMTV-*neu* fed a Western diet (high fat, moderate fiber, low calcium)	Significant increase in tumor multiplicity and size in highest isoflavone group compared to control group; no differences in medium or low isoflavone group and no significant differences in tumor incidence between any of the groups	[85]
mouse	Purina 5001 (soy diet), PND28-EOS	MMTV-*neu* implanted with 0.5 mg, 60-day constant release estrogen pellet	Tumor onset significantly delayed in soy group for both placebo and estrogen pellet mice vs control mice; no significance different in tumor incidence was reported	[86]
mouse	250 mg/kg genistein, 250 mg/kg daidzein, NovaSoy, PND56-EOS	MMTV-*neu*, 1 pregnancy and 2 weeks of lactation	Tumor latency delayed in all isoflavone groups, tumor growth, incidence, multiplicity and size not affected	[87]
mouse	Supro 670 with low or high isoflavone (0.2 and 1.81 mg isoflavone/g protein isolate), PND28-EOS	MMTV-*neu* on high fat diet	No significant difference in tumor incidence, onset, multiplicity or size	[91]
mouse	430 mg isoflavones/kg diet, PND21-EOS	MMTV-*Wnt1*	Tumor incidence and latency reduced in isoflavone group	[88]
mouse	250 mg/kg genistein, PND28-EOS	C(3)1-SV40	No effect on tumor incidence or growth rate	[89]
mouse	32 mg/kg or 972 mg/kg isoflavones, PND22-EOS	MT-*hGH*	Tumor latency reduced, and tumor size increased in high isoflavone group	[90]

PND = post-natal day; EOS = end of study; DMBA = 7,12-Dimethylbenzathracene; NMU = *N*-methyl-*N*-nitrosourea; PhIP = 2-amino-1-methyl-6-phenylimidazo[4,5-*b*]pyridine.

Genistein is the most studied individual soy isoflavone as it is the predominant isoflavone in soy and it can bind to estrogen receptors [92]. When evaluating only those studies that utilized purified genistein, eight studies [69–71,73,79–81,87,89] examined the impact of postnatal genistein administration on mammary tumor development with six of these studies performed on rats [69–71,73,79–81] and two in mice [87,89]. Three of the studies evaluating genistein in rats demonstrated some protective effect such as increased tumor latency or decreased tumor size [70,71,73]. Only one study demonstrated a significant decrease in tumor incidence [71]; however, a second study found a decrease in tumor multiplicity [74]. Of the two studies evaluating postnatal genistein administration in transgenic mice, one study observed an increase in tumor latency but no significant effect on tumor size, incidence or multiplicity [87], while the second study found no significant differences in tumor incidence or growth rate [89].

6. Mammary Tumor Development Following Lifetime Soy Isoflavone Administration

Fewer studies have evaluated the benefits of lifetime soy isoflavone exposure in rodent models of mammary tumor development and these studies are summarized in Table 2. Lifetime soy/isoflavone exposure was defined as soy/isoflavone administration during gestation, lactation and postnatal development. Only two studies using chemical induction of mammary tumors were found and both utilized NMU. While one study demonstrated a significant reduction in tumor incidence and prolonged tumor latency [93], the other study found no significant difference in tumor incidence [94].

Table 2. Lifetime Soy/Isoflavone Administration.

Species	Isoflavone Diet/Timing	Tumor Inducer	Main Finding	Refs
rat	ISP, gestation day 4-EOS[1]	1 injection of 50 mg/kg body weight NMU at PND50	Tumor incidence reduced, and latency increased in SPI group; tumor multiplicity not affected	[93]
rats	ISP, gestation day 4-EOS	1 injection of 50 mg/kg body weight NMU at PND51	No significant differences in tumor incidence or multiplicity	[94]
mice	90 mg/kg Prevastein (46.19% wt/wt isoflavones) 2 weeks prior to mating-EOS	MMTV-*neu* on high fat diet with either corn oil or fish oil	Decreased tumor incidence and increased tumor latency in isoflavone group with corn oil but no significant differences in group with fish oil	[96]
mice	Soy containing 4RF21, breeding-weaning and then 4RF21, SPI or isoflavone poor concentrate, PND21-EOS	MMTV-*neu*	No difference in tumor incidence	[95]
mice	20% ISP, breeding-EOS	MTB-IGFIR (IGF-IR induced at PND45 or PND100)	Tumor onset reduced, and incidence increased in ISP group	[66]

[1] EOS = end of study; PND = post-natal days; ISP = isolated soy protein; NMU = *N*-methyl-*N*-nitrosourea.

There were also three studies using transgenic mice. One study using MMTV-*neu* mice found that mice fed a diet containing the isoflavone-enriched product, Prevastein, had reduced tumor incidence and prolonged tumor latency in the group that were fed a high-fat diet based on corn oil, but not in the group with a diet based on fish oil. Meanwhile, the other study found no impact on tumor incidence in MMTV-*neu* transgenic mice fed a high soy diet compared to controls [95]. In the study using MTB-IGFIR mice, tumor incidence was increased and tumor latency was decreased in MTB-IGFIR mice fed a diet containing 20% ISP compared to casein-fed MTB-IGFIR mice [66].

7. Mammary Tumor Development Following Perinatal Soy Isoflavone Administration

For this review, perinatal exposure was defined by soy or isoflavone administration between conception and weaning. Using this definition, there were six studies identified, four of which used chemical carcinogens in rats [94,97–99] and two studies that used MMTV-*neu* transgenic mice [91,96]. These studies are summarized in Table 3. None of the studies demonstrated a decrease in tumor incidence in soy/isoflavone treated rodents; however, three of the studies using chemical carcinogens found a decrease in tumor multiplicity [94,98,99]. One study using MMTV-*neu* transgenic mice found no significant difference in the tumor incidence or onset in Prevastein-treated mice compared to control mice [96] while the other study found that tumor multiplicity and size increased in the medium- and high-Prevastein groups compared to controls [91].

Table 3. Perinatal Soy/Isoflavone Administration.

Species	Isoflavone Diet/Timing	Tumor Inducer	Main Finding	Refs
rat	250 mg daidzein/kg diet 2 week prior to mating-weaning	1 oral dose, 40 mg DMBA at PND50	No significant differences in tumor onset or incidence	[97]
rat	25 or 250 mg genistein/kg diet conception-weaning	1 oral dose, 80 mg/kg DMBA at PND50	Tumor multiplicity reduced in isoflavone group	[98]
rat	20 ug genistein injected on PND7, 10, 14, 17 and 20	1 injection, 10 mg DMBA at PND45	No significant effect on tumor latency or incidence but multiplicity and growth rate significantly lower in genistein group vs control group	[99]
rats	SPI, gestation day 4-EOS	1 injection of 50 mg/kg body weight NMU at PND51	No significant differences in tumor incidence but multiplicity significantly reduced	[94]
mice	0, 18, 90 or 270 mg/kg Prevastein (46.19% wt/wt isoflavones), conception-weaning	MMTV-neu on normal or high fat diet	No significant difference in tumor incidence but tumor multiplicity and size significantly increased in medium and high isoflavone group	[91]
mice	90 mg/kg Prevastein (46.19% wt/wt isoflavones) 2 weeks prior to mating-weaning	MMTV-*neu* on high fat diet with either corn oil of fish oil	No differences in tumor incidence or onset	[96]

8. Conclusions and Future Considerations

The most appropriate measure of reduced breast cancer risk would be a reduction in tumor incidence (number of animals that develop mammary tumors) in rodents fed diets containing soy or isoflavones compared to rodents fed control diets. Of the 34 studies evaluated, only 5 demonstrated a significant reduction in tumor incidence in response to diets enriched with soy products or purified isoflavones. Tumor multiplicity was reduced in soy-fed mice in an additional 6 studies and thus 11 of 34 studies demonstrated that soy products or purified isoflavones reduced either the percentage of rodents that developed mammary tumors or the number of tumors that developed in each animal. When focusing on the studies that evaluated the administration of the purified soy isoflavone genistein, 4 of the 8 studies demonstrated that postnatal genistein reduced at least one tumor characteristic, with only 2 of these studies demonstrating a decrease in tumor incidence or multiplicity. Given that less than a third of the studies demonstrated a decrease in tumor incidence or multiplicity suggests that the current studies have failed to demonstrate a consistent, protective effect of soy isoflavones in preventing mammary tumor development.

Before concluding that either rodent models are unsuitable for breast cancer prevention studies or high levels of dietary soy do not reduce breast cancer risk, further research should be encouraged. However, a number of factors require careful consideration, including (i) the type of soy (unrefined/refined, fermented/unfermented, or purified isoflavones), (ii) the experimental model (mice, rats or another model such as primates), and (iii) when to initiate soy-based diets and how long these diets should be continued. Future studies should emulate the human data that most clearly implicates that the consumption of dietary soy reduces breast cancer risk, and these are the epidemiologic studies showing that lifetime/multigenerational exposure to diets containing unrefined, fermented soy products by some Asian cultures reduces breast cancer risk. Therefore, diets containing high levels of unrefined and possibly fermented soy products should be tested. The unrefined soy products would maintain most of the soybean components such as protease inhibitors, phytosterols and saponins that are typically lost during the refinement process. With respect to timing, lifetime exposure to soy-based diets should be the minimum and multigenerational exposure should be evaluated. No study investigating mammary tumor development following multigeneration soy exposure could be found, and it is possible that soy induces epigenetic alterations in the gametes of animals with lifetime soy exposure that then impacts the gene expression and tumor sensitivity of their offspring.

The most relevant animal model is more debatable. Although non-human primates likely represent the best model, large dietary studies in non-human primates genetically altered to express relevant human oncogenes or lacking key tumor suppressor genes are not feasible and would raise ethical concerns. Therefore, genetically altered mice or rats expressing inducible, tissue-specific oncogenes or inducible, tissue-specific knockouts utilizing known human tumor suppressor genes probably represent the most appropriate model since this system (i) uses known oncogenes and tumor suppressor genes and thus the mechanisms of tumor initiation will be more relevant to human breast cancer, (ii) permits oncogene expression or tumor suppressor gene ablation in postnatal animals which presumably emulates the timing of spontaneous activation of an oncogene or loss of a tumor suppressor gene in humans, and (iii) several inducible mouse models are currently available and their genetic similarity to different human breast cancer subtypes is often known.

However, a main concern with rodent models is that rodents and humans metabolize soy isoflavones differently [100,101]. These alterations in metabolism influence the amount of isoflavones present in their aglycone form and the amount of daidzein that is converted to equol [101]. Only approximately 30% of the western population produces equol [102] as a product of isoflavone metabolism while equol production has been reported in 50–60% of Asian adults [103–106]. One hundred percent of mice and rats produce equol [101]. Soy metabolism is further complicated by the fact that diets high in soy can alter the composition of the gut microbiome [107] and thus influence circulating isoflavone levels. Isoflavone levels in tissue has been poorly studied. Chang et al. (2000, genistein) evaluated the levels of genistein in rats and found genistein in a number of tissue including the mammary gland and tissue typically contain a higher percentage of the aglycone form of genistein than the plasma [98,108]. Only a small number of studies have evaluated isoflavone levels in human breast tissue, and the limited data suggests that isoflavones or particular metabolites do not preferentially accumulate in breast tissue [41]. Given the differences in isoflavone metabolism, future animal studies should measure plasma and tissue isoflavone levels so isoflavone levels and composition in animal models can be compared to those achievable in humans.

Funding: This research was funded by a grant from the Canadian Cancer Society Research Institute, grant number 702774" and a grant from the Canadian Institutes of Health Research, grant number OCP-137736.

Conflicts of Interest: The authors declare no conflict of interest.

References

1. Danaei, G.; Vander Hoorn, S.; Lopez, A.D.; Murray, C.J.; Ezzati, M.; Comparative Risk Assessment collaborating, g. Causes of cancer in the world: Comparative risk assessment of nine behavioural and environmental risk factors. *Lancet* **2005**, *366*, 1784–1793. [CrossRef]
2. Wu, A.H.; Lee, E.; Vigen, C. Soy isoflavones and breast cancer. *Am. Soc. Clin. Oncol. Educ. Book* **2013**, *2013*, 102–106. [CrossRef]
3. Qin, L.Q.; Xu, J.Y.; Wang, P.Y.; Hoshi, K. Soyfood intake in the prevention of breast cancer risk in women: A meta-analysis of observational epidemiological studies. *J. Nutr. Sci. Vitamin* **2006**, *52*, 428–436. [CrossRef]
4. Trock, B.J.; Hilakivi-Clarke, L.; Clarke, R. Meta-analysis of soy intake and breast cancer risk. *J. Natl. Cancer Inst.* **2006**, *98*, 459–471. [CrossRef] [PubMed]
5. Enderlin, C.A.; Coleman, E.A.; Stewart, C.B.; Hakkak, R. Dietary soy intake and breast cancer risk. *Oncol. Nurs. Forum* **2009**, *36*, 531–539. [CrossRef]
6. Dong, J.Y.; Qin, L.Q. Soy isoflavones consumption and risk of breast cancer incidence or recurrence: A meta-analysis of prospective studies. *Breast Cancer Res. Treat.* **2011**, *125*, 315–323. [CrossRef] [PubMed]
7. Chen, M.; Rao, Y.; Zheng, Y.; Wei, S.; Li, Y.; Guo, T.; Yin, P. Association between soy isoflavone intake and breast cancer risk for pre- and post-menopausal women: A meta-analysis of epidemiological studies. *PLoS ONE* **2014**, *9*, e89288. [CrossRef]
8. Xie, Q.; Chen, M.L.; Qin, Y.; Zhang, Q.Y.; Xu, H.X.; Zhou, Y.; Mi, M.T.; Zhu, J.D. Isoflavone consumption and risk of breast cancer: A dose-response meta-analysis of observational studies. *Asia Pac. J. Clin. Nutr.* **2013**, *22*, 118–127. [CrossRef]

9. Zhao, T.T.; Jin, F.; Li, J.G.; Xu, Y.Y.; Dong, H.T.; Liu, Q.; Xing, P.; Zhu, G.L.; Xu, H.; Miao, Z.F. Dietary isoflavones or isoflavone-rich food intake and breast cancer risk: A meta-analysis of prospective cohort studies. *Clin. Nutr.* **2019**, *38*, 136–145. [CrossRef]
10. McNally, S.; Stein, T. Overview of Mammary Gland Development: A Comparison of Mouse and Human. *Methods Mol. Biol.* **2017**, *1501*, 1–17. [CrossRef]
11. Cardiff, R.D.; Wellings, S.R. The comparative pathology of human and mouse mammary glands. *J. Mammary Gland Biol. Neoplasia* **1999**, *4*, 105–122. [CrossRef]
12. Barnes, S. Effect of genistein on in vitro and in vivo models of cancer. *J. Nutr.* **1995**, *125*, 777S–783S. [CrossRef]
13. Messina, M.; Wu, A.H. Perspectives on the soy-breast cancer relation. *Am. J. Clin. Nutr.* **2009**, *89*, 1673S–1679S. [CrossRef]
14. Murkies, A.L.; Wilcox, G.; Davis, S.R. Clinical review 92: Phytoestrogens. *J. Clin. Endocrinol. Metab.* **1998**, *83*, 297–303. [CrossRef]
15. Price, K.R.; Fenwick, G.R. Naturally occurring oestrogens in foods—a review. *Food Addit. Contam.* **1985**, *2*, 73–106. [CrossRef]
16. Krizova, L.; Dadakova, K.; Kasparovska, J.; Kasparovsky, T. Isoflavones. *Molecules* **2019**, *24*, 1076. [CrossRef]
17. An, J.; Tzagarakis-Foster, C.; Scharschmidt, T.C.; Lomri, N.; Leitman, D.C. Estrogen receptor β-selective transcriptional activity and recruitment of coregulators by phytoestrogens. *J. Biol. Chem.* **2001**, *276*, 17808–17814. [CrossRef]
18. Margeat, E.; Bourdoncle, A.; Margueron, R.; Poujol, N.; Cavailles, V.; Royer, C. Ligands differentially modulate the protein interactions of the human estrogen receptors α and β. *J. Mol. Biol.* **2003**, *326*, 77–92. [CrossRef]
19. Kostelac, D.; Rechkemmer, G.; Briviba, K. Phytoestrogens modulate binding response of estrogen receptors α and β to the estrogen response element. *J. Agric. Food Chem.* **2003**, *51*, 7632–7635. [CrossRef]
20. Rietjens, I.; Louisse, J.; Beekmann, K. The potential health effects of dietary phytoestrogens. *Br. J. Pharmacol.* **2017**, *174*, 1263–1280. [CrossRef]
21. Vitale, D.C.; Piazza, C.; Melilli, B.; Drago, F.; Salomone, S. Isoflavones: Estrogenic activity, biological effect and bioavailability. *Eur. J. Drug Metab. Pharmacokinet.* **2013**, *38*, 15–25. [CrossRef]
22. Morito, K.; Hirose, T.; Kinjo, J.; Hirakawa, T.; Okawa, M.; Nohara, T.; Ogawa, S.; Inoue, S.; Muramatsu, M.; Masamune, Y. Interaction of phytoestrogens with estrogen receptors alpha and beta. *Biol. Pharm. Bull.* **2001**, *24*, 351–356. [CrossRef]
23. Mazur, W.; Adlercreutz, H. Overview of naturally occurring endocrine-active substances in the human diet in relation to human health. *Nutrition* **2000**, *16*, 654–658. [CrossRef]
24. Omoni, A.O.; Aluko, R.E. Soybean foods and their benefits: Potential mechanisms of action. *Nutr. Rev.* **2005**, *63*, 272–283. [CrossRef]
25. Lippman, M.E.; Krueger, K.A.; Eckert, S.; Sashegyi, A.; Walls, E.L.; Jamal, S.; Cauley, J.A.; Cummings, S.R. Indicators of lifetime estrogen exposure: Effect on breast cancer incidence and interaction with raloxifene therapy in the multiple outcomes of raloxifene evaluation study participants. *J. Clin. Oncol.* **2001**, *19*, 3111–3116. [CrossRef]
26. Messina, M.; McCaskill-Stevens, W.; Lampe, J.W. Addressing the soy and breast cancer relationship: Review, commentary, and workshop proceedings. *J. Natl. Cancer Inst.* **2006**, *98*, 1275–1284. [CrossRef]
27. Setchell, K.D. Phytoestrogens: The biochemistry, physiology, and implications for human health of soy isoflavones. *Am. J. Clin. Nutr.* **1998**, *68*, 1333S–1346S. [CrossRef]
28. Kladna, A.; Berczynski, P.; Kruk, I.; Piechowska, T.; Aboul-Enein, H.Y. Studies on the antioxidant properties of some phytoestrogens. *Luminescence* **2016**, *31*, 1201–1206. [CrossRef]
29. Chae, H.S.; Xu, R.; Won, J.Y.; Chin, Y.W.; Yim, H. Molecular Targets of Genistein and Its Related Flavonoids to Exert Anticancer Effects. *Int. J. Mol. Sci.* **2019**, *20*, 2420. [CrossRef]
30. Fotsis, T.; Pepper, M.S.; Montesano, R.; Aktas, E.; Breit, S.; Schweigerer, L.; Rasku, S.; Wahala, K.; Adlercreutz, H. Phytoestrogens and inhibition of angiogenesis. *Baillieres Clin. Endocrinol. Metab.* **1998**, *12*, 649–666. [CrossRef]
31. Mukund, V.; Saddala, M.S.; Farran, B.; Mannavarapu, M.; Alam, A.; Nagaraju, G.P. Molecular docking studies of angiogenesis target protein HIF-1alpha and genistein in breast cancer. *Gene* **2019**, *701*, 169–172. [CrossRef]
32. Berndt, S.; Issa, M.E.; Carpentier, G.; Cuendet, M. A Bivalent Role of Genistein in Sprouting Angiogenesis. *Planta Med.* **2018**, *84*, 653–661. [CrossRef]
33. Lecomte, S.; Demay, F.; Ferriere, F.; Pakdel, F. Phytochemicals Targeting Estrogen Receptors: Beneficial Rather Than Adverse Effects? *Int. J. Mol. Sci.* **2017**, *18*, 1381. [CrossRef]

34. Setchell, K.D.; Brown, N.M.; Zhao, X.; Lindley, S.L.; Heubi, J.E.; King, E.C.; Messina, M.J. Soy isoflavone phase II metabolism differs between rodents and humans: Implications for the effect on breast cancer risk. *Am. J. Clin. Nutr.* **2011**, *94*, 1284–1294. [CrossRef]
35. van der Velpen, V.; Hollman, P.C.; van Nielen, M.; Schouten, E.G.; Mensink, M.; Van't Veer, P.; Geelen, A. Large inter-individual variation in isoflavone plasma concentration limits use of isoflavone intake data for risk assessment. *Eur. J. Clin. Nutr.* **2014**, *68*, 1141–1147. [CrossRef]
36. Chang, Y.; Choue, R. Plasma pharmacokinetics and urinary excretion of isoflavones after ingestion of soy products with different aglycone/glucoside ratios in South Korean women. *Nutr. Res. Pract.* **2013**, *7*, 393–399. [CrossRef]
37. Peiroten, A.; Bravo, D.; Landete, J.M. Bacterial metabolism as responsible of beneficial effects of phytoestrogens on human health. *Crit. Rev. Food Sci. Nutr.* **2019**, *4*, 1–16. [CrossRef]
38. Rowlands, J.C.; Berhow, M.A.; Badger, T.M. Estrogenic and antiproliferative properties of soy sapogenols in human breast cancer cells in vitro. *Food Chem. Toxicol.* **2002**, *40*, 1767–1774. [CrossRef]
39. Hsieh, C.C.; Hernandez-Ledesma, B.; Jeong, H.J.; Park, J.H.; de Lumen, B.O. Complementary roles in cancer prevention: Protease inhibitor makes the cancer preventive peptide lunasin bioavailable. *PLoS ONE* **2010**, *5*, e8890. [CrossRef]
40. Chatterjee, C.; Gleddie, S.; Xiao, C.W. Soybean Bioactive Peptides and Their Functional Properties. *Nutrients* **2018**, *10*, 1211. [CrossRef]
41. Huser, S.; Guth, S.; Joost, H.G.; Soukup, S.T.; Kohrle, J.; Kreienbrock, L.; Diel, P.; Lachenmeier, D.W.; Eisenbrand, G.; Vollmer, G.; et al. Effects of isoflavones on breast tissue and the thyroid hormone system in humans: A comprehensive safety evaluation. *Arch. Toxicol.* **2018**, *92*, 2703–2748. [CrossRef]
42. Barnes, S. The biochemistry, chemistry and physiology of the isoflavones in soybeans and their food products. *Lymphat. Res. Biol.* **2010**, *8*, 89–98. [CrossRef]
43. Setchell, K.D.; Cole, S.J. Variations in isoflavone levels in soy foods and soy protein isolates and issues related to isoflavone databases and food labeling. *J. Agric. Food Chem.* **2003**, *51*, 4146–4155. [CrossRef]
44. Fang, N.; Yu, S.; Badger, T.M. Comprehensive phytochemical profile of soy protein isolate. *J. Agric. Food Chem.* **2004**, *52*, 4012–4020. [CrossRef]
45. Rogers, A.E.; Lee, S.Y. Chemically-induced mammary gland tumors in rats: Modulation by dietary fat. *Prog. Clin. Biol. Res.* **1986**, *222*, 255–282.
46. Russo, J.; Gusterson, B.A.; Rogers, A.E.; Russo, I.H.; Wellings, S.R.; van Zwieten, M.J. Comparative study of human and rat mammary tumorigenesis. *Lab. Invest* **1990**, *62*, 244–278.
47. Sukumar, S.; Notario, V.; Martin-Zanca, D.; Barbacid, M. Induction of mammary carcinomas in rats by nitroso-methylurea involves malignant activation of H-ras-1 locus by single point mutations. *Nature* **1983**, *306*, 658–661. [CrossRef]
48. Zarbl, H.; Sukumar, S.; Arthur, A.L.; Martin-Zanca, D.; Barbacid, M. Activation of H-ras-1 oncogenes by chemical carcinogens. *Basic Life Sci.* **1986**, *38*, 385–397.
49. Zarbl, H.; Sukumar, S.; Arthur, A.V.; Martin-Zanca, D.; Barbacid, M. Direct mutagenesis of Ha-ras-1 oncogenes by N-nitroso-N-methylurea during initiation of mammary carcinogenesis in rats. *Nature* **1985**, *315*, 382–385. [CrossRef]
50. Dandekar, S.; Sukumar, S.; Zarbl, H.; Young, L.J.; Cardiff, R.D. Specific activation of the cellular Harvey-ras oncogene in dimethylbenzanthracene-induced mouse mammary tumors. *Mol. Cell Biol.* **1986**, *6*, 4104–4108. [CrossRef]
51. Abba, M.C.; Zhong, Y.; Lee, J.; Kil, H.; Lu, Y.; Takata, Y.; Simper, M.S.; Gaddis, S.; Shen, J.; Aldaz, C.M. DMBA induced mouse mammary tumors display high incidence of activating Pik3caH1047 and loss of function Pten mutations. *Oncotarget* **2016**, *7*, 64289–64299. [CrossRef]
52. Choi, Y.W.; Henrard, D.; Lee, I.; Ross, S.R. The mouse mammary tumor virus long terminal repeat directs expression in epithelial and lymphoid cells of different tissues in transgenic mice. *J. Virol.* **1987**, *61*, 3013–3019.
53. Wagner, K.U.; McAllister, K.; Ward, T.; Davis, B.; Wiseman, R.; Hennighausen, L. Spatial and temporal expression of the Cre gene under the control of the MMTV-LTR in different lines of transgenic mice. *Transgenic Res.* **2001**, *10*, 545–553. [CrossRef]
54. Yang, G.; Park, S.; Cao, G.; Goltsov, A.; Ren, C.; Truong, L.D.; Demayo, F.; Thompson, T.C. MMTV promoter-regulated caveolin-1 overexpression yields defective parenchymal epithelia in multiple exocrine organs of transgenic mice. *Exp. Mol. Pathol.* **2010**, *89*, 9–19. [CrossRef]

55. Muller, W.J.; Sinn, E.; Pattengale, P.K.; Wallace, R.; Leder, P. Single-step induction of mammary adenocarcinoma in transgenic mice bearing the activated *c-neu* oncogene. *Cell* **1988**, *54*, 105–115. [CrossRef]
56. Bouchard, L.; Lamarre, L.; Tremblay, P.J.; Jolicoeur, P. Stochastic appearance of mammary tumors in transgenic mice carrying the MMTV/c-neu oncogene. *Cell* **1989**, *57*, 931–936. [CrossRef]
57. Guy, C.T.; Cardiff, R.D.; Muller, W.J. Activated neu induces rapid tumor progression. *J. Biol. Chem.* **1996**, *271*, 7673–7678. [CrossRef]
58. Herschkowitz, J.I.; Simin, K.; Weigman, V.J.; Mikaelian, I.; Usary, J.; Hu, Z.; Rasmussen, K.E.; Jones, L.P.; Assefnia, S.; Chandrasekharan, S.; et al. Identification of conserved gene expression features between murine mammary carcinoma models and human breast tumors. *Genome Biol.* **2007**, *8*, R76. [CrossRef]
59. Truss, M.; Bartsch, J.; Mows, C.; Chavez, S.; Beato, M. Chromatin structure of the MMTV promoter and its changes during hormonal induction. *Cell Mol. Neurobiol.* **1996**, *16*, 85–101. [CrossRef]
60. Cato, A.C.; Henderson, D.; Ponta, H. The hormone response element of the mouse mammary tumour virus DNA mediates the progestin and androgen induction of transcription in the proviral long terminal repeat region. *EMBO J.* **1987**, *6*, 363–368. [CrossRef]
61. Ham, J.; Thomson, A.; Needham, M.; Webb, P.; Parker, M. Characterization of response elements for androgens, glucocorticoids and progestins in mouse mammary tumour virus. *Nucleic Acids Res.* **1988**, *16*, 5263–5276. [CrossRef]
62. Truss, M.; Chalepakis, G.; Beato, M. Interplay of steroid hormone receptors and transcription factors on the mouse mammary tumor virus promoter. *J. Steroid Biochem. Mol. Biol.* **1992**, *43*, 365–378. [CrossRef]
63. Maroulakou, I.G.; Anver, M.; Garrett, L.; Green, J.E. Prostate and mammary adenocarcinoma in transgenic mice carrying a rat C3(1) simian virus 40 large tumor antigen fusion gene. *Proc. Natl. Acad. Sci. USA* **1994**, *91*, 11236–11240. [CrossRef]
64. Tornell, J.; Rymo, L.; Isaksson, O.G. Induction of mammary adenocarcinomas in metallothionein promoter-human growth hormone transgenic mice. *Int. J. Cancer* **1991**, *49*, 114–117. [CrossRef]
65. Jones, R.A.; Campbell, C.I.; Gunther, E.J.; Chodosh, L.A.; Petrik, J.J.; Khokha, R.; Moorehead, R.A. Transgenic overexpression of IGF-IR disrupts mammary ductal morphogenesis and induces tumor formation. *Oncogene* **2007**, *26*, 1636–1644. [CrossRef]
66. Watson, K.L.; Stalker, L.; Jones, R.A.; Moorehead, R.A. High levels of dietary soy decrease mammary tumor latency and increase incidence in MTB-IGFIR transgenic mice. *BMC Cancer* **2015**, *15*, 37. [CrossRef]
67. Franks, S.E.; Campbell, C.I.; Barnett, E.F.; Siwicky, M.D.; Livingstone, J.; Cory, S.; Moorehead, R.A. Transgenic IGF-IR overexpression induces mammary tumors with basal-like characteristics while IGF-IR independent mammary tumors express a claudin-low gene signature. *Oncogene* **2012**, *31*, 3298–3309. [CrossRef]
68. Jones, R.A.; Watson, K.L.; Campbell, C.I.; Moorehead, R.A. IGF-IR mediated mammary tumorigenesis is enhanced during pubertal development. *PLoS ONE* **2014**, *9*, e108781. [CrossRef]
69. Manjanatha, M.G.; Shelton, S.; Bishop, M.E.; Lyn-Cook, L.E.; Aidoo, A. Dietary effects of soy isoflavones daidzein and genistein on 7,12-dimethylbenz[a]anthracene-induced mammary mutagenesis and carcinogenesis in ovariectomized Big Blue transgenic rats. *Carcinogenesis* **2006**, *27*, 2555–2564. [CrossRef]
70. Zhang, X.; Cook, K.L.; Warri, A.; Cruz, I.M.; Rosim, M.; Riskin, J.; Helferich, W.; Doerge, D.; Clarke, R.; Hilakivi-Clarke, L. Lifetime Genistein Intake Increases the Response of Mammary Tumors to Tamoxifen in Rats. *Clin. Cancer Res.* **2017**, *23*, 814–824. [CrossRef]
71. Sahin, K.; Tuzcu, M.; Sahin, N.; Akdemir, F.; Ozercan, I.; Bayraktar, S.; Kucuk, O. Inhibitory effects of combination of lycopene and genistein on 7,12- dimethyl benz(a)anthracene-induced breast cancer in rats. *Nutr. Cancer* **2011**, *63*, 1279–1286. [CrossRef]
72. Hakkak, R.; Shaaf, S.; Jo, C.H.; Macleod, S.; Korourian, S. Effects of high-isoflavone soy diet vs. casein protein diet and obesity on DMBA-induced mammary tumor development. *Oncol. Letters* **2011**, *2*, 29–36. [CrossRef]
73. Pugalendhi, P.; Manoharan, S. Chemopreventive potential of genistein and daidzein in combination during 7,12-dimethylbenz[a]anthracene (DMBA) induced mammary carcinogenesis in Sprague-Dawley rats. *Pak. J. Biol. Sci.* **2010**, *13*, 279–286. [CrossRef]
74. Park, K.; Choi, K.; Kim, H.; Kim, K.; Lee, M.H.; Lee, J.H.; Kim Rim, J.C. Isoflavone-deprived soy peptide suppresses mammary tumorigenesis by inducing apoptosis. *Exp. Mol. Med.* **2009**, *41*, 371–381. [CrossRef]
75. Qin, L.Q.; Xu, J.Y.; Tezuka, H.; Wang, P.Y.; Hoshi, K. Commercial soy milk enhances the development of 7,12-dimethylbenz(a)anthracene-induced mammary tumors in rats. *In Vivo* **2007**, *21*, 667–671.

76. Mukhopadhyay, S.; Ballard, B.R.; Mukherjee, S.; Kabir, S.M.; Das, S.K. Beneficial effects of soy protein in the initiation and progression against dimethylbenz [a] anthracene-induced breast tumors in female rats. *Mol. Cell Biochem.* **2006**, *290*, 169–176. [CrossRef]
77. Gallo, D.; Giacomelli, S.; Cantelmo, F.; Zannoni, G.F.; Ferrandina, G.; Fruscella, E.; Riva, A.; Morazzoni, P.; Bombardelli, E.; Mancuso, S.; et al. Chemoprevention of DMBA-induced mammary cancer in rats by dietary soy. *Breast Cancer Res. Treat.* **2001**, *69*, 153–164. [CrossRef]
78. Appelt, L.C.; Reicks, M.M. Soy induces phase II enzymes but does not inhibit dimethylbenz[a]anthracene-induced carcinogenesis in female rats. *J. Nutr.* **1999**, *129*, 1820–1826. [CrossRef]
79. Constantinou, A.I.; Lantvit, D.; Hawthorne, M.; Xu, X.; van Breemen, R.B.; Pezzuto, J.M. Chemopreventive effects of soy protein and purified soy isoflavones on DMBA-induced mammary tumors in female Sprague-Dawley rats. *Nutr. Cancer* **2001**, *41*, 75–81. [CrossRef]
80. Kijkuokool, P.; Parhar, I.S.; Malaivijitnond, S. Genistein enhances N-nitrosomethylurea-induced rat mammary tumorigenesis. *Cancer Lett.* **2006**, *242*, 53–59. [CrossRef]
81. Ono, M.; Koga, T.; Ueo, H.; Nakano, S. Effects of dietary genistein on hormone-dependent rat mammary carcinogenesis induced by ethyl methanesulphonate. *Nutr. Cancer* **2012**, *64*, 1204–1210. [CrossRef]
82. Kaga, C.; Takagi, A.; Kano, M.; Kado, S.; Kato, I.; Sakai, M.; Miyazaki, K.; Nanno, M.; Ishikawa, F.; Ohashi, Y.; et al. Lactobacillus casei Shirota enhances the preventive efficacy of soymilk in chemically induced breast cancer. *Cancer Sci.* **2013**, *104*, 1508–1514. [CrossRef]
83. Zhang, G.P.; Han, D.; Liu, G.; Gao, S.G.; Cai, X.Q.; Duan, R.H.; Feng, X.S. Effects of soy isoflavone and endogenous oestrogen on breast cancer in MMTV-erbB2 transgenic mice. *J. Int. Med. Res.* **2012**, *40*, 2073–2082. [CrossRef]
84. Davis, V.L.; Shaikh, F.; Gallagher, K.M.; Villegas, M.; Rea, S.L.; Cline, J.M.; Hughes, C.L. Inhibition of Neu-induced mammary carcinogenesis in transgenic mice expressing ERDelta3, a dominant negative estrogen receptor alpha variant. *Horm. Cancer* **2012**, *3*, 227–239. [CrossRef]
85. Thomsen, A.R.; Mortensen, A.; Breinholt, V.M.; Lindecrona, R.H.; Penalvo, J.L.; Sorensen, I.K. Influence of Prevastein, an isoflavone-rich soy product, on mammary gland development and tumorigenesis in Tg.NK (MMTV/c-neu) mice. *Nutr. Cancer* **2005**, *52*, 176–188. [CrossRef]
86. Yang, X.; Edgerton, S.M.; Kosanke, S.D.; Mason, T.L.; Alvarez, K.M.; Liu, N.; Chatterton, R.T.; Liu, B.; Wang, Q.; Kim, A.; et al. Hormonal and dietary modulation of mammary carcinogenesis in mouse mammary tumor virus-c-erbB-2 transgenic mice. *Cancer Res.* **2003**, *63*, 2425–2433.
87. Jin, Z.; MacDonald, R.S. Soy isoflavones increase latency of spontaneous mammary tumors in mice. *J. Nutr.* **2002**, *132*, 3186–3190. [CrossRef]
88. Rahal, O.M.; Machado, H.L.; Montales, M.T.; Pabona, J.M.; Heard, M.E.; Nagarajan, S.; Simmen, R.C. Dietary suppression of the mammary CD29(hi)CD24(+) epithelial subpopulation and its cytokine/chemokine transcriptional signatures modifies mammary tumor risk in MMTV-Wnt1 transgenic mice. *Stem Cell Res.* **2013**, *11*, 1149–1162. [CrossRef]
89. Paul, B.; Li, Y.; Tollefsbol, T.O. The Effects of Combinatorial Genistein and Sulforaphane in Breast Tumor Inhibition: Role in Epigenetic Regulation. *Int. J. Mol. Sci.* **2018**, *19*, 1754. [CrossRef]
90. Hickey, J.; Bartke, A.; Winters, T.; Henry, N.; Banz, W. Effects of soy protein and soy phytochemicals on mammary tumor development in female transgenic mice overexpressing human pituitary growth hormone. *J. Med. Food* **2005**, *8*, 556–559. [CrossRef]
91. Luijten, M.; Thomsen, A.R.; van den Berg, J.A.; Wester, P.W.; Verhoef, A.; Nagelkerke, N.J.; Adlercreutz, H.; van Kranen, H.J.; Piersma, A.H.; Sorensen, I.K.; et al. Effects of soy-derived isoflavones and a high-fat diet on spontaneous mammary tumor development in Tg.NK (MMTV/c-neu) mice. *Nutr. Cancer* **2004**, *50*, 46–54. [CrossRef]
92. Lamartiniere, C.A.; Cotroneo, M.S.; Fritz, W.A.; Wang, J.; Mentor-Marcel, R.; Elgavish, A. Genistein chemoprevention: Timing and mechanisms of action in murine mammary and prostate. *J. Nutr.* **2002**, *132*, 552S–558S. [CrossRef]
93. Simmen, R.C.; Eason, R.R.; Till, S.R.; Chatman, L., Jr.; Velarde, M.C.; Geng, Y.; Korourian, S.; Badger, T.M. Inhibition of NMU-induced mammary tumorigenesis by dietary soy. *Cancer Lett.* **2005**, *224*, 45–52. [CrossRef]

94. Su, Y.; Eason, R.R.; Geng, Y.; Till, S.R.; Badger, T.M.; Simmen, R.C. In utero exposure to maternal diets containing soy protein isolate, but not genistein alone, protects young adult rat offspring from NMU-induced mammary tumorigenesis. *Carcinogenesis* **2007**, *28*, 1046–1051. [CrossRef]
95. Chiesa, G.; Rigamonti, E.; Lovati, M.R.; Disconzi, E.; Soldati, S.; Sacco, M.G.; Cato, E.M.; Patton, V.; Scanziani, E.; Vezzoni, P.; et al. Reduced mammary tumor progression in a transgenic mouse model fed an isoflavone-poor soy protein concentrate. *Mol. Nutr. Food Res.* **2008**, *52*, 1121–1129. [CrossRef]
96. Luijten, M.; Verhoef, A.; Dormans, J.A.; Beems, R.B.; Cremers, H.W.; Nagelkerke, N.J.; Adlercreutz, H.; Penalvo, J.L.; Piersma, A.H. Modulation of mammary tumor development in Tg.NK (MMTV/c-neu) mice by dietary fatty acids and life stage-specific exposure to phytoestrogens. *Reprod. Toxicol.* **2007**, *23*, 407–413. [CrossRef]
97. Lamartiniere, C.A.; Wang, J.; Smith-Johnson, M.; Eltoum, I.E. Daidzein: Bioavailability, potential for reproductive toxicity, and breast cancer chemoprevention in female rats. *Toxicol. Sci.* **2002**, *65*, 228–238. [CrossRef]
98. Fritz, W.A.; Coward, L.; Wang, J.; Lamartiniere, C.A. Dietary genistein: Perinatal mammary cancer prevention, bioavailability and toxicity testing in the rat. *Carcinogenesis* **1998**, *19*, 2151–2158. [CrossRef]
99. Hilakivi-Clarke, L.; Onojafe, I.; Raygada, M.; Cho, E.; Skaar, T.; Russo, I.; Clarke, R. Prepubertal exposure to zearalenone or genistein reduces mammary tumorigenesis. *Br. J. Cancer* **1999**, *80*, 1682–1688. [CrossRef]
100. Mortensen, A.; Kulling, S.E.; Schwartz, H.; Rowland, I.; Ruefer, C.E.; Rimbach, G.; Cassidy, A.; Magee, P.; Millar, J.; Hall, W.L.; et al. Analytical and compositional aspects of isoflavones in food and their biological effects. *Mol. Nutr. Food Res.* **2009**, *53* (Suppl. 2), S266–S309. [CrossRef]
101. Soukup, S.T.; Helppi, J.; Muller, D.R.; Zierau, O.; Watzl, B.; Vollmer, G.; Diel, P.; Bub, A.; Kulling, S.E. Phase II metabolism of the soy isoflavones genistein and daidzein in humans, rats and mice: A cross-species and sex comparison. *Arch. Toxicol.* **2016**, *90*, 1335–1347. [CrossRef]
102. Rafii, F. The role of colonic bacteria in the metabolism of the natural isoflavone daidzin to equol. *Metabolites* **2015**, *5*, 56–73. [CrossRef]
103. Watanabe, S.; Yamaguchi, M.; Sobue, T.; Takahashi, T.; Miura, T.; Arai, Y.; Mazur, W.; Wahala, K.; Adlercreutz, H. Pharmacokinetics of soybean isoflavones in plasma, urine and feces of men after ingestion of 60 g baked soybean powder (kinako). *J. Nutr.* **1998**, *128*, 1710–1715. [CrossRef]
104. Arai, Y.; Watanabe, S.; Kimira, M.; Shimoi, K.; Mochizuki, R.; Kinae, N. Dietary intakes of flavonols, flavones and isoflavones by Japanese women and the inverse correlation between quercetin intake and plasma LDL cholesterol concentration. *J. Nutr.* **2000**, *130*, 2243–2250. [CrossRef]
105. Akaza, H.; Miyanaga, N.; Takashima, N.; Naito, S.; Hirao, Y.; Tsukamoto, T.; Fujioka, T.; Mori, M.; Kim, W.J.; Song, J.M.; et al. Comparisons of percent equol producers between prostate cancer patients and controls: Case-controlled studies of isoflavones in Japanese, Korean and American residents. *Jpn. J. Clin. Oncol.* **2004**, *34*, 86–89. [CrossRef]
106. Song, K.B.; Atkinson, C.; Frankenfeld, C.L.; Jokela, T.; Wahala, K.; Thomas, W.K.; Lampe, J.W. Prevalence of daidzein-metabolizing phenotypes differs between Caucasian and Korean American women and girls. *J. Nutr.* **2006**, *136*, 1347–1351. [CrossRef]
107. Brink, L.; Chintapalli, S.; Mercer, K.; Piccolo, B.; Adams, S.; Bowlin, A.; Matazel, K.; Shankar, K.; Badger, T.; Andres, A.; et al. Early Postnatal Diet Differentially Affects the Fecal Microbiome and Metabolome (FS04-02-19). *Curr. Dev. Nutr.* **2019**, *3* (Suppl. 1). [CrossRef]
108. Chang, H.C.; Churchwell, M.I.; Delclos, K.B.; Newbold, R.R.; Doerge, D.R. Mass spectrometric determination of genistein tissue distribution in diet-exposed Sprague-Dawley rats. *J. Nutr.* **2000**, *130*, 1963–1970. [CrossRef]

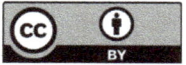

© 2019 by the author. Licensee MDPI, Basel, Switzerland. This article is an open access article distributed under the terms and conditions of the Creative Commons Attribution (CC BY) license (http://creativecommons.org/licenses/by/4.0/).

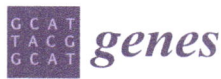

Review

A Critical Review of Animal Models Used in Acute Myeloid Leukemia Pathophysiology

Hala Skayneh [1,†], Batoul Jishi [2,†], Rita Hleihel [3], Maguy Hamieh [1,3], Nadine Darwiche [4], Ali Bazarbachi [2,3], Marwan El Sabban [2,*,‡] and Hiba El Hajj [1,3,*,‡]

1. Department of Experimental Pathology, Microbiology and Immunology, Faculty of Medicine, American University of Beirut, Beirut 1107 2020, Lebanon
2. Department of Anatomy, Cell Biology and Physiological Sciences, Faculty of Medicine, American University of Beirut, Beirut 1107 2020, Lebanon
3. Department of Internal Medicine, Faculty of Medicine, American University of Beirut, Beirut 1107 2020, Lebanon
4. Department of Biochemistry and Molecular Genetics, Faculty of Medicine, American University of Beirut, Beirut 1107 2020, Lebanon
* Correspondence: me00@aub.edu.lb (M.E.S.); he21@aub.edu.lb (H.E.H.)
† H.S. and B.J. contributed equally to this study.
‡ H.E.H and M.E.S contributed equally to this study.

Received: 5 July 2019; Accepted: 1 August 2019; Published: 13 August 2019

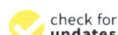

Abstract: Acute myeloid leukemia (AML) is one of the most frequent, complex, and heterogeneous hematological malignancies. AML prognosis largely depends on acquired cytogenetic, epigenetic, and molecular abnormalities. Despite the improvement in understanding the biology of AML, survival rates remain quite low. Animal models offer a valuable tool to recapitulate different AML subtypes, and to assess the potential role of novel and known mutations in disease progression. This review provides a comprehensive and critical overview of select available AML animal models. These include the non-mammalian *Zebrafish* and *Drosophila* models as well as the mammalian rodent systems, comprising rats and mice. The suitability of each animal model, its contribution to the advancement of knowledge in AML pathophysiology and treatment, as well as its advantages and limitations are discussed. Despite some limitations, animal models represent a powerful approach to assess toxicity, and permit the design of new therapeutic strategies.

Keywords: Zebrafish; Drosophila; rats; mice; NPM-1; FLT3 ITD; ETO-1; IDH1/2

1. Introduction

Acute myeloid leukemia (AML) is an aggressive and heterogeneous hematological group of neoplasms characterized by increased proliferation of myeloid progenitor cells and a reduced capacity to differentiate. This results in the accumulation of myeloblasts in the bone marrow (BM), which negatively impacts hematopoiesis and leads to BM failure [1]. AML is one of the most common acute leukemia in adults [2]. Its incidence rate is 2.5 per 100,000 cases/year and the median overall survival (OS) is approximately nine months [3]. AML treatment and prognosis largely depend on the patients' age [4–6]. AML was historically divided into eight major groups according to cell morphology and immune phenotype (M0 to M7) [7]. This classification has been revised several iterations since then [8–12]. Exome sequencing in AML patients led to the current classification through identification of more than 20 driver recurrent mutations [13]. These mainly include *Nucleophosmin-1* (*NPM1*), *DNA methyltransferase 3A* (*DNMT3A*), *Fms-like tyrosine kinase-3* (*FLT3*), *isocitrate dehydrogenase* (*IDH*), *Ten–Eleven Translocation 2* (*TET-2*), *Runt-related transcription factor* (*RUNX-1*), *CCAAT enhancer binding protein α* (*CEBPA*), *additional sex comb-like 1* (*ASXL1*), *mixed lineage leukemia* (*MLL*), tumor protein *p53*

(*TP53*), *c-KIT* [14]. These mutations dictate the response to treatment, rates of complete remission, disease-free survival, overall survival, and classify AML into three prognostic risk factors (favorable, intermediate, and adverse) (Table 1).

Animal models provide an excellent tool to understand the biology of pathological mechanisms involved in human diseases. Diverse animal species were used to answer pivotal questions related to disease progression, genetic mutations, immunity, and response to treatment. Among these models, Zebrafish was exploited to generate different mutations mimicking several subtypes of human AML.

Table 1. 2017 European LeukemiaNet (ELN) prognostic groups according to genetic abnormalities of acute myeloid leukemia (AML) [12].

Prognostic Group	Genetic Mutations and Abnormalities
Favorable	• t(8;21)/RUNX1-RUNX1T1 • inv(16) or t(16;16)/*CBFB-MYH11* • Mutated *NPM1* without *FLT3*-ITD • or with *FLT3*-ITD ^{low} * • Biallelic mutated *CEBPA*
Intermediate	• Mutated *NPM1* and *FLT3*-ITD ^{high} * • Wild-type *NPM1* without *FLT3*-ITD or with *FLT3*-ITD ^{low} * • t(9;11)/*MLLT3-KMT2A* • Cytogenetic abnormalities not classified as favorable or adverse
Adverse	• t(6;9)/ DEK-NUP214 • t(v;11q23.3)/*KMT2A* rearranged • t(9;22)/*BCR-ABL1* • inv(3) or t(3;3)/*GATA2,MECOM(EVI1)* • Complex karyotype • Monosomal karyotype • Wild-type *NPM1* and *FLT3*-ITD ^{high} * • Mutated *RUNX1* † • Mutated *ASXL1* † • Mutated *TP53*

* ^{Low}, low allelic ratio (<0.5); ^{high}, high allelic ratio (>0.5); † these mutations should not be used as an adverse prognostic marker if they co-occur with favorable-risk AML subtypes.

2. Zebrafish: Characteristics and Relevance to Human Blood Malignancies

Danio rerio, commonly known as Zebrafish, shares genetic and molecular mechanisms of hematopoiesis with humans [15]. This model offers many advantages, including low-cost, optically transparent embryos, high fecundity, rapid embryogenesis, and short gestation time. The genome editing in zebrafish was known since 1970s, when the first transgenic zebrafish was generated by inserting naked linear DNA [16]. Since then, the genetic manipulation of this model evolved to include clustered regularly interspaced short palindromic repeats (CRISPR) technology [17], which renders zebrafish an attractive model for studying specific gene involvement and for drug screening in blood malignancies [18–20].

During normal zebrafish hematopoiesis, both the primitive and definitive waves arise from the mesoderm germ layer under the control of the Transforming Growth Factor beta (TGF-β) superfamily proteins, known as bone morphogenic proteins (BMP such as bmp2b and bmp7) [21–23]. The generated transient primitive erythroid and myeloid cells are essential for the embryonic development, while the hematopoietic stem cells (HSCs) and progenitor cells (HSPCs) produce blood lineages in the adult fish [24]. In the below section, we will provide an overview of AML models of Zebrafish (summarized in Table 2).

2.1. AML Models of Zebrafish

2.1.1. Spi-1: MYST3/NCOA2-EGFP

MYST3 (MOZ) is a member of the MOZ, YBF2, SAS2, TIP60 (MYST) family of histone acetyl-transferases (HAT), while NCOA2 (TIF2) is a member of the p160 HAT family [25–28]. The first AML model in Zebrafish was created by expressing the fusion protein, MYST3/NCOA2 (MOZ/TIF2). This fusion targets hematopoietic cells under the control of *spi-1 (pu.1)*, an early myeloid promoter [29]. pu.1 is an ETS-domain transcription factor expressed in both immature lymphoid/hematopoietic cells and myeloid cells during zebrafish hematopoiesis [30]. Cells expressing pu.1 differentiate into myeloid progeny, whereas cells with low pu.1 expression shift to the erythroid fate [31]. After an extended latent period, a small percentage of transgenic fish developed AML [29]. These animals presented with an extensive invasion of kidneys by myeloid blast cells, proving the oncogenic potency of *MYST3/NCOA2* fusion gene [29]. Although this model is useful as a chemical library screen, especially for compounds that target epigenetic regulation of gene expression [29], the long latency and low incidence waned the enthusiasm for its use.

2.1.2. hsp70: AML1-ETO

A chromosomal translocation between chromosomes 8 and 21 (t(8;21)(q22;q22)) occurs in 12–15% of AML patients [32]. This chromosomal rearrangement yields a fusion transcription factor encoding AML1 (RUNX1) linked to ETO, forming the AML1-ETO fusion product [33–35]. This translocation was introduced under the control of the heat shock promoter *hsp70* in zebrafish embryos (*hsp70: AML1-ETO*). Transgenic Zebrafish recapitulated the human AML features, at both the cytological and transcriptional levels [36]. The expression of this fusion protein led to the accumulation of non-circulating hematopoietic cells, whereby the intermediate cell mass was enriched with myeloperoxidase positive neutrophils and morphologically immature hematopoietic blasts [36]. The disruption of definitive hematopoiesis led to switching the cells fate from the erythroid to the myeloid lineage [36]. Overexpression of the transcription factor reversed the observed phenotypes, implicating scl, as major player downstream of AML1-ETO [36]. This model enabled the screening of a small molecule library and discovery of compounds that antagonize the activity of AML1-ETO in the hematopoietic progenitor cells (HPCs) [36]. Inhibition of COX-2 and β-catenin signaling antagonized AML1-ETOs effects on HPCs differentiation and may have implications in human AML [37].

2.1.3. MYCN: HSE: EGFP

MYCN (N-myc) proto-oncogene is upregulated in many types of hematological malignancies [38,39] including 20 to 40% of pediatric AML patients [40]. To unravel the molecular and transcriptional networks by which MYCN induces malignancy, Shen et al. established a transgenic embryonic zebrafish model, Tg (*MYCN: HSE: EGFP*), expressing the murine MYCN under a heat shock promoter [41]. MYCN overexpression induced immature myeloid blast cell expansion and reprogrammed the hematopoietic cell fate through MYCN downstream-regulated gene 1b (ndrg1b) and other lineage-specific hematopoietic transcription factors regulation [41]. The primitive hematopoiesis was enhanced through scl and lmo2 upregulation. Furthermore, erythroid differentiation was blocked through downregulation of gata1, while myelopoiesis was promoted by pu.1 overexpression [41]. This model presents a high AML incidence (~75% of transgenic zebrafish) and a rapid onset occurrence, providing a platform for whole-organism chemical suppressor screens, to identify compounds that can reverse MYCN function in vivo [41].

2.1.4. FLT3-ITD and NPM1c+ Models in Zebrafish

FLT3-ITD and NPM1 are two major players in defining the prognosis and response to treatment in AML patients. FLT3 is a tyrosine kinase receptor that plays a major role in hematopoiesis through the regulation of proliferation, differentiation, and apoptosis of HPCs [42]. It is highly expressed on leukemic blasts of 70–100% of AML patients [43,44]. Several mutations occur in the FLT3 receptor, the most common of which leads to an internal tandem duplication (ITD) [45]. FLT3-ITD occurs in 20% of AML patients and is strongly associated with poor prognosis [46,47]. NPM1, a shuttling protein between the nucleoplasm and the cytoplasm, plays several roles, notably ribosomal biogenesis [48,49]. NPM1 is mutated (NPM1c+) in around 30% of AML patients with normal karyotype [50]. NPM1c+ is continuously translocated to the cytoplasm contributing to leukemogenesis [50].

FLT3-ITD plays a role in embryonic primitive and definitive hematopoiesis in zebrafish. Transgenic zebrafish embryos with human FLT3-ITD showed expansion and clustering of myeloid cells [51]. Thus far, the impact of FLT3-ITD on adult zebrafish remains underexplored.

Bolli et al. generated a transgenic zebrafish model expressing NPM1c+, which perturbed primitive hematopoiesis by promoting the early expansion of pu.1+ myeloid cells [52]. This phenotype was even more pronounced in a p53-deficient background [52]. An increase in the number of gata1+/lmo2 indicating expansion of erythro-myeloid progenitors (EMPs) was also observed. These EMPs highly expressed both c-myb and CD41 but not RUNX1, suggesting a disruption of definitive hematopoiesis where these cells could be the main target of NPM1c+. This model provides a tractable in vivo system for the study of the mechanisms through which hematopoietic development is perturbed in the presence of NPM1c+ [52].

Transgenic zebrafish models expressing either human FLT3-ITD or NPM1 proteins under the control of *pu.1* promoter were also generated [53]. For that purpose, *spi-1*: FLT3-ITD-2A-EGFP/CG2 expressing mutant FTL3-ITD and *spi-1*: NPM1-Mut-PA/CG2 expressing mutant NPM1 constructs were designed. This double mutant transgenic fish (FLT3-ITD/NPM1.Mut) exhibited an accelerated rate of myeloid leukemogenesis [53]. By the age of six months, around 66% of the transgenic fish produced significantly increased precursor cells in the kidney marrow along with dedifferentiated myeloid blasts [53].

2.1.5. Spi-1: CREB-EGFP

The cAMP response element binding protein (CREB) plays a major role in hematopoiesis through the regulation of proliferation and differentiation of myeloid progenitor cells [54]. Overexpression of CREB is associated with immortalization, growth factor-independent proliferation and blast-like phenotype in BM progenitor cells [55]. CREB is highly expressed in BM samples of both adult and pediatric AML patients [56]. Tregnago et al. generated a transgenic zebrafish model (*spi-1: CREB-EGFP*) expressing the *CREB* gene downstream *pu.1* promoter in the myeloid cell lineage. CREB overexpression resulted in upregulation of erythroid and myeloid genes, altering primitive hematopoiesis. Among adult transgenic zebrafish, 80% of the fish developed AML after 9–14 months through the blockage of myeloid differentiation [57]. These fish showed aberrant expression of a set of 20 genes in common with pediatric AML. The most intriguing is the CCAAT-enhancer-binding-protein-δ (C/EBPδ) that acts downstream CREB. It resulted in impaired myeloid differentiation that could be reversed through inhibition of the CREB-C/EBPδ axis. These findings are complementary with the data obtained by screening for CREB and C/EBPδ in pediatric AML patients, offering an opportunity to test for novel therapeutics through this model [57].

2.1.6. Spi-1: SOX4-EGFP

SOX4 is a transcription factor belonging to the SOX (Sry-related high-mobility groupbox) family [58]. In AML patients, SOX4 overexpression results in poor prognosis and short overall survival [59]. SOX4 was reported to contribute to the leukemic phenotype of C/EBPα mutant AML in murine models as well as in human AML. C/EBPα protein typically inhibits the self-renewal of leukemic cells and restores cellular differentiation. SOX4 overexpression results in C/EBPα inactivation, enabling leukemic cells proliferation and AML development [60,61].

Lu et al. generated a transgenic zebrafish model Tg (spi-1:SOX4-EGFP) expressing SOX4 protein downstream the spi-1 myeloid promoter. Early developmental stages of transgenic zebrafish did not reveal a difference of expression of SOX4. However, by the age of five months, Tg (spi-1:SOX4-EGFP) zebrafish kidneys started showing mild vacuoles in the renal tubule which evolved into effacement, distorted structure, and increased infiltration of myeloid cells by the ages of 9 and 12 months. A higher number of myeloid progenitor cells and excess blast cells with focal aggregation were observed in the kidney marrow blood cells of 9-, 12-, and 15-months old fish but not younger ones, highlighting that myeloid transformation is age-dependent [59].

2.1.7. IDH 1/2 Mutation

Mutations identified in a family of enzymes involved in the citric acid cycle, isocitrate dehydrogenases 1/2 (IDH1/2), account for 16% of AML patients [62]. These mutations substitute arginine residue almost exclusively at codon 132 in IDH1 (IDH1-R132H) and codons 140 and 172 in IDH2 [62]. To study the involvement of IDH in AML, zidh1 was either suppressed or deleted and resulted in the blockage of differentiation and accumulation of early myeloid progenitor cells, while decreasing macrophage and natural killer progenitor cells [63]. The importance of IDH1 mutation was asserted when plasmids of IDH1-R132H were injected into zebrafish embryos [63]. An increase in 2-hydroxyglutarate (2-HG) level, a reduction of 5-Hydroxymethylcytotsine (5-hmC), and an expansion of myelopoiesis were obtained in these embryos. A human IDH1-R132H–specific inhibitor significantly ameliorated both hematopoietic and 2-HG responses in human but not zebrafish IDH1 mutant expression [63]. This result is not surprising and highlights some of the drawbacks using Zebrafish as a model for human diseases. On the other hand, studies on zidh2 were restricted to the regulation of embryonic hematopoiesis in zebrafish but with no relevance to the human AML [63].

Even with the drawbacks of not possessing many mammalian-like organs, zebrafish still provides an excellent, affordable, and rapid platform for evaluating several aspects of AML. The variations in the biological microenvironment might impede drug delivery and performance in humans. Additionally, zebrafish are ectothermic (cold-blooded), so their physiology is not identical to humans, which might affect enzyme kinetics and metabolism. The genetic diversity detected between individual zebrafish belonging to the same strain confounds data and could be misleading [64]. The sparsity of reagents to study zebrafish at the molecular level is contrasted by the abundance of mouse-specific reagents.

3. Rodent Models

Due to the complexity and heterogeneity of AML in humans, rodent models have been instrumental in providing a platform for answering pivotal questions related to AML pathogenesis, disease progression, and developing new effective therapeutic approaches. Among these models, rats and mice represent the closest accepted mammalian models to AML.

3.1. Rats

Several transplantable leukemia rat models were established using carcinogens, radiations, and pollutants [65–67].

Transplantable Rat Models

Acute Myeloid Leukemia/ Chronic Meylogenous Leukemia (AML/CML) leukemia: Repeated intravenous injections of 7, 12-dimethylbenz (a) anthracene (DMBA) into WOP/H-Onc strain or Wistar/H-Onc strain, induced leukemia in 10% of the rats in 5–9 months. This leukemia has myeloid characteristics as revealed by hematological and histological examination, as well as infiltration of myeloid blasts into several organs (BM, liver, spleen, and lymph nodes). This myeloid nature showed similarities with both human CML (as demonstrated by high peroxidase and Sudan black B positive cells and reduction in alkaline phosphatase positivity) and human AML (non-specific esterase activity, highly reduced in the peripheral blood but slightly reduced in BM). These findings do not support the use of these rats as an exclusive AML model [68].

Brown Norwegian Myelogenous Leukemia (BNML): The transplantable promyelocytic leukemia in BN rat (BNML) was first described in 1971. This slow growing leukemia shares many common characteristics with AML, including the disappearance of normal hematopoiesis [69]. Similarities in in vitro colony forming assays between AML patients and BNML rats validated it as a model for AML [70,71]. Several therapeutic modalities were optimized using this model; these include the combination of anthracyclines, [72,73] Ara-C [74,75], 4′-(9-acridinylamino) methanesulfon-m-anisidide (AMSA) [76], and other therapeutics [77–79]. One of the most significant advantages in the BNML model is its contribution to the improvement of minimal residual disease (MRD) detection by karyotyping [80] and multidimensional flow cytometry [81,82].

3.2. Mice

Mice offer an invaluable model due to their small size, cost-effectiveness, and easy maintenance, availability of research tools, and ease of manipulation to produce and recapitulate several human diseases, including cancer. Since hematopoiesis in mice has been well characterized, they provide a reasonably reproducible model to study AML pathogenesis and potential therapies. Murine AML models include induced, transgenic animals, and humanized mouse models (Table 3) among others.

3.2.1. Chemically-Induced Model

AML models were generated using the L1210 and p388 cell lines, isolated from DBA/2 mice chemically exposed to the carcinogen 3-methylcholantrene [83]. These models were transplantable and provided a platform for testing chemotherapeutic drugs, studying their kinetics, and evaluating their anti-leukemic effectiveness [84]. The L1210 model was used to screen anthracyclines [85] and antimetabolites [86,87] including Cytarabine [88]. The p388 model was used to investigate the efficacy of natural products as topoisomerase II inhibitors [89]. These models allowed significant improvement in the treatment of AML, including the currently used Cytarabine [90]. The main limitation of using these animal models is the induction of more lymphoid than myeloid leukemia, and the needed prolonged exposure to those carcinogens to develop leukemia [91].

3.2.2. Radiation-Induced Model

The correlation between radiation and leukemia was established in patients exposed to x-rays, and survivors of nuclear attacks. Among this cohort of subjects, children presented mostly with ALL, whereas adults were more prone to CML and AML [92–95]. All established radiation-induced AML models carry deletions on chromosome 2, where the hematopoietic transcription factor *Sfpi1/pu.1* is located [96].

RF Model

The RF strain was developed by Furth in 1933 at the Rockefeller Institute [97]. In this model, myeloid leukemia was developed following exposure to fission neutron irradiation or gamma irradiation [98]. In the RF model, a single dose of ionizing radiation-induced myeloid leukemogenesis in 4–6 months, with symptoms reminiscent to human AML [99]. Flt3-ITD mutations were identified in 10% of RF mice [100], which correlates with the occurrence of this mutation in human AML [101].

SJL/J Model

This model is characterized by high spontaneous frequency of reticulum cell neoplasm type B at an early age [102]. The radiation-induced AML in this model is similar to the secondary human AML occurring after irradiation of Hodgkin disease patients [103]. The efficient development of AML required the addition of promoting factors, such as corticosteroids and growth factors, colony stimulating factor CSF-1, known to be high in AML patients [104].

C3H/He and CBA Models (CBA/Ca, CBA/Cne, and CBA/H)

These models were generated in 1920, by cross-breeding Bragg albino with DBA mice. While C3H/He was specifically selected for the high incidence of mammary tumors [105], CBA was selected for a lower incidence of mammary tumors. The C3H/He was detected 24 h after irradiation in BM cells; this indicates that chromosomal 2 alteration is responsible for the initiation of myeloid leukemogenesis [106]. CBA showed chromosome 2 and 4 aberrations [107,108]. Moreover, an 8% decrease in DNA methylation was observed after exposure to radiation. This hypomethylation played a role in leukemogenesis [109]. The CBA model is considered the most favorable model in radiation-induced AML because of low spontaneous leukemia incidence (0.1 to 1%), high incidence of AML after exposure to radiation or benzene, with lower latency, compared to other models, and more importantly, it mimics human AML at the cytological, histopathological, and molecular levels.

3.2.3. Virally Induced Leukemia Models

Murine leukemia viruses (MuLV) induce non-B and non-T cell leukemia in mice [110,111] and are considered among the simplest retroviruses that shed light on the pathogenesis of leukemia [112,113]. A model was created by injecting cell-free filtrates, including replication-deficient spleen focus forming virus (SFFV) and a replication-competent Friend MuLV [114,115]. It was noticed that the same infection of MuLV induces several subtypes of AML (Table 4), resembling French–American–British (FAB) classification of human AML [116]. Furthermore, MuLV-induced AML led to the discovery of several genes with a significant role in the regulation of growth, death, lineage determination, and development of hematopoietic precursor cells [117]. MuLV induced AML is considered a critical landmark for understanding the pathogenesis of human AML, since it unraveled relevant unknown oncogenes to leukemogenesis (Table 4).

3.2.4. Transposon Models

Sleeping Beauty (SB) transposon is an insertional mutagenesis system, allowing overexpression or inactivation of specific genes depending on the transposon orientation and integration site [118,119]. SB consists of a mobilized piece of DNA, transposon, and a transposase enzyme [120]. In a transgenic animal with a humanized NPM1c+ knock-in allele, this system enhanced the incidence and onset of AML in NPM1c+ mice [121]. An advantage of this model was the identification of mutations in leukemia genes [121].

3.2.5. Transgenic Models: Single Mutation

PML-RARα t(15;17)

Acute promyelocytic leukemia (APL) is a subtype of AML, characterized by t(15;17) chromosomal translocation, resulting in the promyelocytic leukemia-retinoic acid receptor α (PML-RARα) fusion protein [122,123]. PML-RARα was expressed in three mouse models under the myeloid regulatory promoters. Under the CD11b promoter, transgenic mice showed abnormal myelopoiesis and increased radiation sensitivity, however, did not develop any leukemia [124]. Mice expressing the transgene under the human cathepsin G (HCG) and human MRP8 (hMRP8) promoters [124–126] developed APL phenotypes after a long period of latency [125,126]. These two models recapitulated the remissions seen after all trans-retinoic acid (ATRA) treatment in human APL [125,126].

AML1-Eight-Twenty One Oncoprotein

AML1-Eight-Twenty One oncoprotein (ETO) chimeric product, encoded by the t(8;21), occurs in around 12–15% of AML [32]. Knock-in mice expressing AML1-ETO is embryonic lethal due to the complete absence of liver-derived definitive hematopoiesis [127,128]. Embryonic livers contained dysplastic multilineage hematopoietic progenitors that had an abnormally high self-renewal capacity in vitro, a phenotype typical of leukemic cells [129]. To bypass the embryonic lethality, inducible transgenic models were generated. These mice expressed AML1-ETO in their BM progenitor cells [130,131]. Although abnormal maturation and proliferation of progenitor cells were observed, mice failed to develop leukemia [130,131]. Expression of AML1-ETO under the control of *hMRP8* promoter was unable to develop AML until their exposure to a robust DNA-alkylating mutagen, *N*-ethyl-*N*-nitrosourea [132]. To further enhance AML development, this mouse model was modified by either the expression of other factors or mutations in tyrosine kinases such as c-KIT, FLT3-ITD, or the TEL- platelet-derived growth factor receptor β (PDGFbR) [133,134].

CBFB-MYH11

The beta subunit of the core binding complex (CBFB) is a heterodimeric core-binding transcription factor, with a critical role in hematopoiesis [135]. CBF products, due to chromosomal translocations, account for approximately 25% of pediatric and 15% of adult AML patients [136]. The translocation Inv(16) (p13;q22) is a result of the binding of CBFB subunit to the tail region of the smooth muscle myosin heavy chain (*SMMHC*) gene, MYH11 [137]. The resulting fusion protein (CBFB-MYH11) competes with the binding of CBF to target genes, disrupting transcriptional regulation, thus contributing to leukemic transformation [137]. Similar to embryos with homozygous mutations in AML1 [128], knock-in embryonic mice ($Cbfb^{+/Cbfb-MYH11}$) lacked definitive hematopoiesis and died during gestation [138]. Chemically or retrovirally induced mutations in heterozygous CBFB-MYH11 adults led to AML development [138,139]. A conditional knock-in mouse model expressing *CBFB-MYH11* fusion protein in adult mice ($Cbfb^{+/56M}$) was also generated [140] and led to AML development in 90% of the mice within five months [140].

Mutant Nucleophosmin-1 (NPM1c+)

Mutations in the *Nucleophosmin-1 (NPM1)* gene represent one of the most frequent genetic aberrations in AML [141] and account for 30% of AML patients [50]. Transgenic mice harboring the *NPM1c+* mutation developed myeloproliferation in BM and spleen, supporting a role of NPM1c+ in AML [142]. Chou et al. generated a knock-in transgenic mouse model by inserting the most frequent mutation, TCTG called mutation A, in the C-terminus of wt-NPM1 [143]. Mice homozygous for the transgene encountered embryonic lethality, whereas one-third of the heterozygotes (*Npm1wt/c+*) developed the fetal myeloproliferative disease but not AML [143]. Conditional expression of *NPM1c+* with further genetic manipulations resulted in two models [121,144]. In one model, one-third of the transgenic mice developed leukemia after a long period of latency associated with AML features [144]. In the other model, the expression of humanized NPM1c+ in the hematopoietic stem cells caused *HOX* overexpression, enhanced self-renewal, and expanded myelopoiesis [121].

Fms-Related Tyrosine Kinase 3 Internal Tandem Repeats

The second most common genetic aberrations in de novo AML patients occur in the fms-related tyrosine kinase 3 internal tandem repeats (*FLT3-ITD*) gene on chromosome 13. These associate with poor prognosis and short overall survival (OS) [145]. A transgenic mouse model expressing FLT3-ITD under the *vav* hematopoietic promoter was created [146]. The majority of transgenic mice developed a myeloproliferative syndrome (MPS) characterized by megakaryocytic hyperplasia and thrombocytosis but not AML [146]. In FLT3-ITD knock-in mice, loss of FLT3 wild-type allele contributed to myeloid expansion and aggressiveness of the MPS disease [147]. Several other models expressing this mutation also revealed MPS but not AML [148,149].

Mixed Lineage Leukemia (MLL)

The translocation t(9;11)(p22;q23) produces the fusion product MLL-AF9 [150,151]. In one model, embryonic stem cells were generated from an in-frame fusion of AF9 with exon 8 of mouse MLL [152]. Other models conditionally expressed MLL-AF9 [153]. These models developed only

AML despite the widespread activity of the MLL promoter [152,153]. Conditional expression of MLL-AF9 in long-term hematopoietic stem cells (LT-HSC) produced aggressive AML with extensive tissue infiltration, chemo-resistance, and expressed genes related to epithelial-mesenchymal transition in solid cancers [154]. MLL early introduction results in abnormalities of myeloid cell proliferation and differentiation [155]. Moreover, HOXa9 was found to be essential for the MLL-dependent leukemogenesis in vivo [156].

The translocation t(4;11)(q21;q23) produces the fusion product MLL-AF4. This translocation is associated with pro-B-ALL and rarely AML [157]. Although several models have been established for this translocation, only few models resulted in AML. MLL-*AF4* models generated using both a knock-in [158] and *Cre*-inducible invertor model [159] produced large B-cell lymphoma rather than the immature acute leukemia observed in humans [158,159]. The MLL-AF4 expression in hematopoietic precursors, during mouse embryonic development, developed long latency B-cell lymphoma [159,160]. Furthermore, MLL-AF4 knock-in followed by in vitro inducible transduction generated mice with both AML and pre-B-ALL as well as a few MLLs [161].

Leukemia with the t(11;19)(q23;p13.3) translocation express MLL-ENL fusion proteins capable of malignant transformation of myeloid and/or lymphoid progenitor(s). Immortalized cells containing MLL-ENL proviral DNA or enriched primary hematopoietic stem cells transduced with MLL-ENL induced myeloid leukemia in syngeneic and SCID recipients [162]. Using an in vitro B-cell differentiation system, retroviral transduction of *MLL-ENL* generated a leukemia reminiscent of human MLL-ENL ALL [163]. Other models expressed MLL-ENL-ERTm, the ligand-binding domain of the estrogen receptor modified to specifically recognize synthetic but not endogenous estrogens, using retroviral transduction approach [164]. Several other models were generated encountering more mutation along with MLL-ENL [165,166].

IDH 1/2

A conditional knock-in mouse model was created by inserting the mutated human IDH1 (R132H) into the endogenous murine *idh1* locus. IDH1 (R132H) was expressed in all hematopoietic cells under the *vav* promoter (vav-KI mice) or specifically in cells of the myeloid lineage (LysM-KI mice) [167]. Transgenic mice showed increased number of early hematopoietic progenitors and developed splenomegaly and anemia with extramedullary hematopoiesis, characteristics of a dysfunctional BM niche, along with partial blockage in myeloid differentiation [167]. Moreover, LysM-KI cells have hypermethylated histones and changes to DNA methylation similar to those observed in human *IDH1*- or *IDH2*-mutant AML, demonstrating the induction of leukemic DNA methylation signature in the mouse model [167].

3.2.6. Transgenic Models: Compound Transgenic Mouse Models

K-RAS-G12D + PML-RARα

4% and 10% of APL patients with PML-RARα fusion had oncogenic *N-RAS* and *K-RAS* mutations, respectively [168,169]. The conditional expression of oncogenic K-RAS and PML-RARα in mice induced a rapid-onset and highly penetrant, lethal APL-like disease [170].

These mice may be used to test for the therapeutic efficacy of inhibitors of RAS post-translational modifications and RAS downstream signaling [170].

N-RASD12 + BCL-2

N-RAS, a protein belonging to the family of RAS GTP-ases, is mutated in patients at risk of leukemic transformation after chemotherapy and/or radiotherapy [171]. *N-RAS* mutation at codon 12 is the most frequent abnormality in myelodysplastic syndromes (MDS), associated with AML transformation and poor OS [172]. B-cell lymphoma 2 (BCL-2) protein is an apoptosis regulatory protein. BCL-2 is overexpressed in AML patients [173], which blocks the differentiation of myeloid progenitors [174]. Both mutants have been previously identified as risk factors for AML in MDS patients [172].

Two murine models of initiation and progression of human MDS/AML were generated [175]. The transplantable model expressing hBCL-2 in a primitive compartment by mouse mammary tumor virus–long terminal repeat *(MMTVtTA /TBCL-2/NRASD12)* represents human MDS, whereas the constitutive *MRP8 [BCL-2/NRASD12]* model is closer to AML [175]. Both models showed expanded leukemic stem cell (Lin$^-$/Sca-1$^+$/c-Kit$^+$) populations. hBCL-2 is observed in the increased RAS-GTP complex within the expanded Sca-1$^+$ compartment [175]. The difference of hBCL-2 oncogenic compartmentalization associates with the pro-apoptotic mechanisms in MDS and the anti-apoptotic in AML mice [175]. Downregulation of hBCL-2 in MDS mice partially reversed the phenotype and prolonged survival; however BM blasts and tissue infiltration persisted [175]. This model revealed that the two candidate oncogenes *BCL-2* and mutant *N-RAS* can cooperate to give rise to malignant disease with a penetrance of around 80% and a latency period of 3 to 6 months [175].

Mixed Lineage Leukemia-Partial Tandem Duplication + FLT3-ITD

Mixed lineage leukemia-partial tandem duplication *(MLL-PTD)* is expressed in 5 to 7% of cytogenetically normal (CN)-AML patients [176,177]. Approximately 25% of these patients have constitutive activation of FLT3-ITD, conferring a poor prognosis [178]. To recapitulate the *Mll$^{PTD/WT}$:flt3$^{ITD/WT}$* AML found in humans, a double knock-in mouse model was generated by expressing these two mutated genes under their respective endogenous promoters [179]. After a period of latency, this model developed AML with a short life span, extensive extramedullary involvement, and increased aggressiveness [179]. Reminiscent of this subtype of AML in humans, these transgenic mice have normal chromosomal structures, reduced *MLL-WT* expression, loss of *FLT3-WT*, and increased total *FLT3* expression [179–182]. Moreover, increased *HOXA9* transcript levels were observed, rendering this model valuable for the assessment of epigenetic modifying agents combined with tyrosine kinase inhibitors [179].

NUP98-HOXD13 + FLT3-ITD

The chromosomal translocation t(2;11)(q31;p15) leads to the fusion of Nucleoporin *(NUP98)*, a structural component of the nuclear pore complex, to the homeobox protein NHD13 (HOXD13), inducing leukemogenesis [183]. *NUP98-HOX* fusions are observed in human and murine MDS [184]. Clinical and experimental evidence demonstrated that high rate of FLT3-ITD mutations was observed in patients with NUP98 translocations [185]. High-level transcriptional expression of *NUP98-HOX* correlated with higher transcript levels of *FLT3* and an increased incidence of FLT3 activating mutations [185]. A novel model combining an FLT3-ITD mutation with NHD13 (HOXD13) was generated using their respective endogenous promoters [186]. Initially, these transgenic mice developed leukemia with both primitive myeloid and lymphoid origin. Later, strictly myeloid leukemia with minimal differentiation were monitored [186]. Indeed, *NHD13* transgene enhanced the overexpression of the *HOX* genes, *HOXA7*, *HOXA9*, *HOXB4*, *HOXB6*, *HOXB7*, *HOXC4*, and *HOXC6* [186], shown to play an important role in HSC self-renewal and are upregulated in acute leukemia [187–189]. Nevertheless, mice encountered a spontaneous loss of heterozygosity with a high frequency, resulting in the loss of WT *FLT3* allele, [186], a characteristic of patients with FLT3-ITD mutations [180]. These transgenic mice provide a model to study the molecular pathways underlying MDS-related AML [186].

NPM1c+/FLT3

NPM1c+ and FLT3-ITD double mutations are found in about 40% of AML patients [190]. A compound transgenic mouse model with a double mutation in NPM1 and FLT3 was generated by crossing conditional *Npm1$^{flox-cA/+}$* with constitutive *Flt3$^{ITD/+}$* mice [191]. Inducing recombination of *Npm1$^{flox-cA}$* in hematopoietic stem cells was accomplished by crossing the double heterozygous mice into *Mx1-Cre* transgenic mice [191]. Double mutant mice developed AML and died by the age of 31–68 days. Peripheral blood showed increased leukocyte counts, reduced numbers of circulating

B and T lymphocytes along with a marked population of immature blasts, while BM cells exhibited increased self-renewal potential [191]. Solid organs were infiltrated with abnormal myeloid cells inducing splenomegaly and hepatomegaly by the time of death, highlighting the role of this double mutation in leukemogenesis [191].

N-RAS-G12D + CBFB-MYH11

A knock-in mice ($Nras^{LSL-G12D}$; $Cbfb^{56M}$) with an allelic expression of oncogenic N-RAS^{G12D} and CBFB-MYH11 developed leukemia in a cell-autonomous manner, with a short median latency and high leukemia-initiating cell activity [192]. Mice displayed an increased survival of pre-leukemic short-term HSCs and myeloid progenitor cells with a sustained blocked differentiation induced by the fusion protein [192]. $Nras^{LSL-G12D}$; $Cbfb^{56M}$ leukemic cells were sensitive to pharmacologic inhibition of the MEK/ERK signaling pathway [192], highlighting the importance of this pathway in AML and proposing MEK inhibitors as potential therapeutic agents in inv16/ N-RAS^{G12D} AML [192].

NPM1c + N-RAS-G12D

One of the most common mutations with NPM1c+ is the *N-RAS* mutation occurring *in* 20% of NPM1c+ AML patients [190]. *NPM1* and *N-RAS* double mutant transgenic mice ($Npm1^{cA/+}$; $Nras^{G12D/+}$) developed high penetrance, enhanced self-renewal capacity in hematopoietic progenitors, and AML-like myeloid differentiation bias [193]. At the genomic level, frequent amplification of the mutant *N-RAS-G12D* allele was observed, along with other somatic mutations in AML driver genes [193]. Within the *HOX* genes, which were overexpressed, *HOXa* genes and downstream targets were crucial for the survival of the double-mutant mice [193].

WT1-R394W + FLT3-ITD

Wilms tumor 1 (WT1) is a zinc finger transcriptional regulator of target genes implicated in cell differentiation and quiescence [194]. Mutations in *WT1* occur in 10–15% of CN-AML, and it is frequently associated with mutations in several genes [194,195]. *FLT3-ITD* and *WT1* mutations, when present concomitantly, identify a group of AML patients that fail to respond to the standard induction chemotherapy, which results in poor OS [195,196]. Double mutant mice $Flt3^{+/ITD}/Wt1^{+/R394W}$ displayed manifestations of shortened survival, myeloid expansion in the BM, anemia, and erythroid dysplasia [197]. Although this model did not appear sufficient to consistently recapitulate human AML, it demonstrated that the combined mutations resulted in a more aggressive disease than either mutant genotype [197].

3.2.7. Humanized Models

Humanized mouse models, injected with AML cell lines or patient-derived AML blasts, offered a faster approach and were instrumental in studying different aspects of AML. Several models were attempted to study AML in Nude mice with little success [198,199]. This section will focus on promising models for AML studies.

SCID Mice

The severe combined immuno-deficient (*SCID*) mice lacking B and T cell immunity [200], represent essential humanized AML mouse models [201]. Indeed, patient-derived AML cells engraftment enabled the identification of leukemia-initiating cells (LIC), expressing CD34$^+$ CD38$^−$ surface markers, recapitulating the human HSCs signature [202]. Engraftment of AMLs from different FAB classes into *SCID* mice reflected their intrinsic biologic behavior, suggesting a clinical correlation to the growth and dissemination of these leukemic subtypes [203]. However, lack of species cross-reactivity of cytokines and the innate host immunity against human AML cells resulted in poor engraftment of the BM [204]. In an attempt to overcome these limitations, exogenous human cytokines and growth factors were provided, which resulted in better engraftment of human cells [202,204–206]. One limitation of this model is the "leakiness" of the *SCID* mutation occurring in around 10% of the mice [207]. These mice present functional B and T cells, enhanced natural killer (NK) cell activity, and complement activation decreasing the engraftment efficiency [208]. An attempt to bypass this problem uses radiation and/or anti-asialo-GM1 antibody pretreatment. Unfortunately, it reduced the survival of the host, rendering this model unsuitable for human xenograft [209,210].

NOD/SCID Mice

To further improve tumor engraftment, a non-obese diabetic (NOD/*SCID*) model exhibiting further impairment of NK activity, reduced mature macrophage, and total lack of B and T cells was generated [211]. This model yielded higher engraftment rates with fewer human AML cells, yet with preserved morphological, phenotypical, and genotypical characteristics of the AML donors [212–215]. This model was used successfully in the screening for new therapeutics in AML [216]. In addition, human AML cells engraftment enabled the fractionation of LICs (CD34$^+$ CD38$^-$) into CD34$^+$/CD71$^-$/HLA-DR [217], CD34 Thy1 hematopoietic stem cells [218] and CD34/CD117 (or ckit) [219] subpopulations. Nevertheless, the NOD/*SCID* model presents the limitation by which higher engraftment rates required the supplementation of human cytokines or transplantation of growth-factor producing cells [220,221]. Moreover, long term engraftments (more than 8.5 months) were disabled due to the development of thymic lymphomas and restoration of NK cells activity during this period [211]. A variant with NOD/*SCID* background is the NSS model (N/S-S/GM/3) expressing Steel factor (SF), granulocyte macrophage-colony-stimulating factor (GM-CSF) and interleukin-3 (IL-3) human growth factors was generated [222]. NSS displayed enhanced engraftment of pre-leukemic myeloid cell cultures, as well as primary human AML samples, suggesting that the NSS mouse is a better host for at least a subset of AML samples [223].

NSG Mice

NOD/*SCID* mice were further immunosuppressed to generate the NOD/*SCID* b2-microglobulin null mice with a complete abolishment of the NK cell activity [224]. Importantly, a NOD/*SCID* IL2-R$\gamma^{-/-}$ or NSG model was generated by deletion or truncation of the gamma chain of IL-2R [225]. In addition to all the abnormalities of their predecessors, NSG mice possess a defective production of IL-2, IL-4, IL-7, IL-9, IL-15, and IL-21 as well as a severe impairment of the dendritic cell (DC) and their capacity to produce interferon γ (IFN-γ) upon stimulation [225,226]. Engraftment of newborn NSG mice with human CD34$^+$ HSCs leads to the generation of a complete hematopoietic system, including red blood cells and platelets [226]. Studies revealed a significantly higher potential of AML cells engraftment in adult NSG mice in comparison to previous immunodeficient hosts [227,228]. Attempts to create different subtypes of AML were successful in NSGs [228]. NSG mice xenotransplanted with five well-characterized AML cell lines established AML models of particular relevance and significance to drug-sensitivity studies [228]. These models were exploited to study the in vivo potency of an Imidazoquinoxalines immunomodulatory drug, EAPB0503, and showed its specific activity in NPM1c+ AML subtype [229]. The usability of NSG model allowed the evaluation of the effect of a synthetic retinoid ST1926, or its encapsulated form in nanoparticles (ST1926-NP). El-Houjeiri et al. demonstrated that ST1926-NP is more potent in NSG injected with THP-1 cells [230]. MOLM-13-injected NSG mice showed strong efficacy to chemotherapy (cytarabine, 50 mg/kg) and 5+3 regimen of daunorubicin (1.5 mg/kg) [231]. These models enabled the in vivo tracking of UCB-NK cells, demonstrating their capability to migrate to BM and inhibit progression of human leukemia cells. Administering a low dose of human IL-15 enhanced survival of these mice, emphasizing the role of innate immunity in AML outcome [232]. In that sense, utilization of NSG model enabled the assessment of the combination of HSPC-NK cell adoptive transfer with the hypomethylating agents (HMAs), azacitidine (AZA), and decitabine (DAC). Cany et al. signified that the therapeutic combination exerted a significant delay in AML progression in these mice [233].

Table 2. A summary of generated AML Zebrafish models and their contribution to the understanding of the disease.

Zebrafish Model	Zebrafish Manipulation	Model Features and Major Findings	References
spi-1: MYST3/NCOA2-EGFP	Transgenic expression of human MYST3/NCOA2 fusion under the spi-1/pu.1 promoter	First AML model in zebrafish. 1.1% of transgenic fishes expressing the transgene developed AML after long latency	[29]
hsp70: AML1-ETO	Transgenic expression of human AML1-ETO fusion under hsp70 promoter	A phenotype similar to human AML. Disruption of definitive hematopoiesis: the switch of cell fates from erythroid to myeloid through gata1 downregulation and pu.1 overexpression. AML1-ETOs effects on HPCs differentiation was mediated through Cycloxygenase-2 (COX-2) and β-catenin signaling pathways	[36,37]
mRNA: NPMc+	mRNAs injection into 1-cell-stage embryos followed by morpholinos (MOs) targeting npm1a and npm1b	Perturbation of primitive and definitive hematopoiesis. Alterations in the expression of major transcription factors (pu.1+, mpx+, csf1r+, c-myb, CD41, RUNX1)	[52]
HSE-MYCN-EGFP	Induction of murine N-myc gene through heat-shock promoter	AML development with high incidence and rapid onset. Enhancement of primitive hematopoiesis through alteration of transcription factors (pu.1, gata1, scl, lmo2, p27kip and p21cip1). Activation of major cancer signaling pathways	[41]
IDH1/2 mutants	Knockdown of zebrafish idh1 and idh2 (zidh1 and zidh2) by morpholino knockdown and Transcription activator-like effector nuclease (TALEN-)mediated mutagenesis	zidh1 suppression/deletion is correlated with a blockade of differentiation of the myeloid lineage. zidh1 effects definitive hematopoiesis exclusively. zidh2 affects primitive hematopoiesis exclusively	[63]
	Transgenic expression of human IDH1 mutation	Embryos recapitulated the features of human AML	
FLT3-ITD-2A-EGFP spi-1; NPM1-Mut-PA spi-1;	Transgenic expression of human FLT3-ITD or/and NPM1 mutations under the spi-1 promoter	Myeloproliferative neoplasm (MPN) development as a result of a single mutation. 66.6% of double mutant transgenic fish showed increased precursor cells in the kidney marrow along with dedifferentiated myeloid blasts.	[53]
spi-1: CREB-EGFP	Expression of CREB-EGFP under spi-1 promoter in myeloid lineage	Alteration of primitive hematopoiesis in embryos. AML development in 79% of adult fishes by 9–14 months. Aberrant expression of 20 genes diagnosed in pediatric AML.	[57]
Spi-1: SOX4-EGFP	Expression of SOX4 protein downstream the spi-1 promoter	Increase in the number of myeloid progenitor cells and blast cells in the kidney marrow. Distortion of the kidney structure	[59]

Table 3. A summary of generated AML mice models and their contribution to the understanding of the disease.

Mouse Model		Manipulation	Outcomes and Major Findings	References
Chemically-Induced Model		Transplantable AML models were generated using the L1210 and p388 cell lines, isolated from DBA/2 mice chemically exposed to the carcinogen 3-methylcholantrene	Provide a platform for testing chemotherapeutic drugs, studying their kinetics, and evaluating their anti-leukemic effectiveness (mainly Cytarabine)	[83,84,90]
Radiation- Induced Model	RF model	Myeloid leukemia was developed following exposure to fission neutron irradiation or γ irradiation	FLT3-ITD mutations were identified in 10% of RF-AML mice which correlates with the occurrence of mutation of human AML	[98,100,101]
	SJL/J model	The radiation induced AML (RI-AML) in this model, is similar to the secondary human AML occurring after irradiation of Hodgkin disease patients	The efficient development of AML in this model was achieved by adding promoting factors, corticosteroids and growth factors like colony stimulating factor CSF-1, known to be high in AML patients	[103,104]
	C3H/He and CBA models (CBA/Ca, CBA/Cne, and CBA/H)	These models were generated by cross breeding Bragg albino with DBA mice	CBA model is considered the most favorable model in RI-AML. High incidence of AML after exposure to radiation or benzene with lower latency compared to other models. Mimics human AML at the cytological, histopathological, and molecular levels.	[107,108,234]
Virally-induced leukemia models MuLV		Murine leukemia viruses (MuLV) induce non-B and non-T cell leukemia in mice	Same infection of MuLV induces several subtypes of AML that resembles FAB classification. Identifies unknown oncogenes contributing to leukemogenesis.	[112,113,116, 117] + Table 2
Transposon models		Sleeping Beauty (SB) transposon is another insertional mutagenesis system, allowing overexpression or inactivation of specific genes depending on the transposon orientation and integration site	Identification of mutations in leukemia genes, which provided new pathogenetic insights and potential therapeutic targets in NPM1c+ AML.	[118,119,121]

Table 3. Cont.

	Mouse Model		Manipulation	Outcomes and Major Findings	References
Trans-genic models	Single mutation	Promyelocytic Leukemia protein (PML)-RARα t(15;17)	Expressing PML-RARα under CD11b promoter	Abnormal myelopoiesis and increased radiation sensitivity No AML development	[124]
			Expressing PML-RARα under human cathepsin G (HCG) promoter	APL phenotype after long latency period Remission seen after All Trans Retinoic Acid (ATRA) treatment in APL	[125]
			Expressing PML-RARα under human MRP8 (hMRP8) promoter	APL phenotype after long latency period Remission seen after ATRA treatment in APL	[126]
		AML1- Eight-Twenty One oncoprotein (ETO)	Knock-in of AML1-ETO into mouse embryos (AML1-ETO/+)	Absence of liver-derived definitive hematopoiesis Embryonic lethality	[127,128]
			Expressing AML1-ETO in adult bone marrow progenitor cells	Abnormal maturation and proliferation of progenitor cells No AML development	[130,131]
			Expressing AML1-ETO under human MRP8 (hMRP8) promoter	AML development after exposure to N-ethyl-N-nitrosourea	[132]
		CBFB-MYH11	Knock-in embryonic mice (Cbfb+/Cbfb-MYH11)	Lack of definitive hematopoiesis Embryonic lethality	[138]
			Chemical/ retroviral mutagens on heterozygous CBFB-MYH11 adults	AML development	[138,139]
			Conditional knock-in adult mice (Cbfb+/56M)	AML development in 90% of mice after 5 months	[140]
		Mutant Nucleophosmin-1 (NPM1c+)	Knock-in mice expressing NPM1 with mutation A (NPM1c+)	Homozygotes encountered embryonic lethality 1/3 of the heterozygotes (Npm1ca/c+) developed fetal myeloproliferative disease but not AML	[143]

Table 3. Cont.

Mouse Model	Manipulation	Outcomes and Major Findings	References
	Expression of NPM1 with mutation A (NPM1c+) under the pCAG promoter	1/3 of the transgenic mice developed leukemia after a long period of latency	[144]
	Expression of humanized NPM1c+ in the hematopoietic stem cells	HOX overexpression Enhanced self-renewal Expanded myelopoiesis	[121]
Fms-related tyrosine kinase 3 internal tandem repeats (FLT3-ITD)	Expressing FLT3-ITD under the vav hematopoietic promoter	Myeloproliferative syndrome (MPS) Megakaryocytic hyperplasia and thrombocytosis No AML development	[146]
	FLT3-ITD knock-in mice with lost FLT3 wild-type allele	Myeloid expansion and aggressiveness of the MPS disease No AML development	[147]
Mixed Lineage Leukemia (MLL)	Embryonic stem cell formed by in-frame fusion of AF9 with exon 8 of mouse MLL	AML development	[152]
	Conditional expression of MLL-AF9 using programmed interchromosomal recombination	AML development	[153]
	Conditional expression of MLL-AF9 in LT-HSC	Aggressive AML Extensive tissue infiltration Chemoresistance Expression of genes related to epithelial-mesenchymal transition (EMT) in solid cancers	[154]
	Early introduction of MLL	Abnormalities of myeloid cell proliferation and differentiation	[155]
IDH 1/2	Expressing IDH1/2 under the vav promoter (Vav-KI mice) or specifically in cells of the myeloid lineage (LysM-KI mice)	Increased number of early hematopoietic progenitors Splenomegaly Anemia Extramedullary hematopoiesis, characteristics of a dysfunctional BM niche and partial blockage in myeloid differentiation Induction of leukemic DNA methylation signature in mouse model	[167]

Table 3. Cont.

Mouse Model		Manipulation	Outcomes and Major Findings	References
Compound mutations	K-RAS-G12D + PML-RARα	Constitutive expression of K-RAS and PML-RARα	Rapid-onset and highly penetrant, lethal APL-like disease	[170]
	N-RAS12D + BCL-2	*MMTVtTA/TBCL-2/NRASD12* Expression of hBCL2 in a primitive compartment by mouse mammary tumor virus–long terminal repeat	MDS development Expanded leukemic stem cell (Lin⁻/Sca-1⁺/c-Kit⁺) populations Increased apoptosis Malignant disease with a penetrance of around 80% and a latency period of 3 to 6 months	[175]
		MRP8 [BCL-2/NRASD12] Constitutive expression of *BCL-2* under human *MRP8* promoter	AML development Expanded leukemic stem cell (Lin⁻/Sca-1⁺/c-Kit⁺) populations No apoptotic cells Malignant disease with a penetrance of around 80% and a latency period of 3 to 6 months	[175]
	MLL-PTD + FLT3-ITD	Expressing MLL-PTD and FLT3-ITD under their respective endogenous promoters	Latent AML with a short life span, extensive extramedullary involvement and increased aggressiveness Normal chromosomal structures Reduced *MLL-WT* expression Loss of *FLT3-WT* and increased total *FLT3* expression Increased *HOXA9* transcript levels	[179]
	NUP98-HOXD13 + FLT3-ITD	Expressing FLT3-ITD and NHD13 (HOXD13) under their respective endogenous promoters	Myeloid leukemia with minimal differentiation Overexpression of several *HOX* genes Spontaneous loss of heterozygosity with a high frequency, resulting in the loss of WT *FLT3* allele	[186]
	NPM1c+ - FLT3	Crossing conditional $Npm1^{flox-cA/+}$ with constitutive $Flt3^{ITD/+}$ mice	AML development Lethality by the age of 31-68 days Modified blood cell counts Immature blasts in BM Myeloid cells infiltration into organs Splenomegaly and hepatomegaly	[191]

Table 3. Cont.

Mouse Model		Manipulation	Outcomes and Major Findings	References
	N-RAS-G12D + CBFB-MYH11	Allelic expression of oncogenic N-RAS^{G12D} and CBFB-MYH11	Leukemia development in a cell-autonomous manner with a short median latency High leukemia-initiating cell activity Increased survival of pre-leukemic short-term HSCs and myeloid progenitor cells with blocked differentiation Leukemic cells were sensitive to MEK/ERK inhibitors	[192]
	NPM1c + N-RAS-G12D	Conditional expression of NPM1c+ and N-RAS-G12D	AML-like myeloid differentiation bias Hematopoietic progenitors with high penetrance and enhanced self-renewal capacity Frequent amplification of the mutant N-RAS-G12D allele Somatic mutations in AML driver genes Overexpression of HOX genes	[193]
	WT1-R394W + FLT3-ITD	Crossing Flt3$^{+/ITD}$ mice with Wt1$^{+/R394W}$ mice	MDS/MPN development Shortened survival Myeloid expansion in the BM, Anemia Erythroid dysplasia	[197]
Xenograft/humanized models	SCID mice	Autosomal recessive mutation	Lack of B and T cells Retained innate immunity and cytokines Identification of leukemia initiating cells (LIC) Poor engraftment of human AML cells in the BM	[200]
	NOD/SCID mice	NOD/SCID model: Express additional mutations	Impairment of NK activity Reduced mature macrophages Total lack of B and T cells Fractionation of LIC into subpopulations	[211]
		NSS model (N/S/GM/3); variant of NOD/SCID mice expressing SF, GM-CSF and IL-3	Better host for a subset of AML	[222,223]
	NSG mice	Deletion or truncation of the γ chain of IL-2R	Defective production of major interleukins and IFN-γ Impairment of dendritic cells Complete abolishment of the NK cell activity Higher engraftment capacity of human AML cells than previous models	[224]

Table 4. Murine leukemia virus (MuLV) induced AML models: Major gene discoveries and their involvement in different French–American–British (FAB) AML subtypes.

MuLV Virus	Mouse Strain	AML Subtype	FAB Classification	Major Gene Discoveries	References
CasBrM-MuLV	NFS	Granulocytic	M1 or M2	*His-1*	[235,236]
CasBrE MuLV	NIH Swiss	Myeloid	M1 or M2	*Fli-1*	[237–239]
Endogenous ecotropic MuLV	AKXD-23	Granulocytic	M1 or M2	*Evi-1*	[240,241]
Friend-MuLV	C57BL/6	Granulocytic	M1 or M2	*Ccnd1*	[237,242,243]
Friend-MuLV	DBA/2	Myeloblastic	M1 or M2	*Evi-1, & c-myb*	[244–246]
M-MuLV	BALB/c	Promonocytic	M5	*c-myb*	[246,247]
B ecotropic MuLV	BXH-2	Myelomonocytic	M4	*c-myb, HOXa7, HOXa9, Meis1, CBFa1, SOX4, Hhex, Rarg, Sharp1, Ccnd3, Cdc25l, RASGRP, Clabp, Hmgcr, Nf1, & Il17r*	[248–255]

4. Drosophila Melanogaster

AML1-ETO

The chromosomal translocation t(8;21)(q22;q22) is frequent and common in AML. It represents up to 40% of AML subtype M2 of the FAB classification [256]. The fusion gene resulting in this translocation encodes for the chimeric protein AML1-ETO, which contains the N-terminus of AML1 (including its DNA binding domain) and most of the ETO protein [33,257], and inhibits the expression of AML1 target genes leading to leukemogenesis [258]. The detailed molecular mechanism governing this interference is poorly understood, which enticed the generation of several animal models to understand its mode of action. AML1-ETO alone is not sufficient to induce leukemia unless accompanied by secondary mutations [130,131,259]. The simplicity of genetics and ease of manipulation in *Drosophila* presents it as an attractive model to study this complex translocation. In addition, *Drosophila* hematopoiesis is comparable to that of mammals [260]. Two AML1-ETO models of genetically engineered *Drosophila* were generated. In the first model, AML1-ETO is a constitutive transcriptional repressor of AML1 target genes. In the second model, AML1-ETO dominantly interferes with AML1 activity by potentially competing for a common co-factor [261]. The transcription factor Lozenge (Lz) that is similar to human AML1 protein is necessary for the development of crystal cells, one of the major *Drosophila* blood cells, during hematopoiesis [262]. Using these models and by comparison with loss-of-function phenotypes of Lz, AML-1-ETO was shown to act as a constitutive transcriptional repressor [261]. Osman et al. reported that AML1-ETO inhibits the differentiation of crystal cell lineage, and induces an increase in the number of circulating LZ+ progenitors. Moreover, large scale RNA interference screen for suppressors of AML1-ETO in vivo showed that *calpainB* is required for AML1-ETO-induced leukemia in *Drosophila*. Surprisingly, calpainB inhibition in Kasumi-1 cells (AML patient cell line carrying t(8;21) translocation) leads to AML1-ETO degradation and impairs their clonogenic potential [263]. Another study identified pontin/RUVBL1as a suppressor of AML1-ETO. Indeed, PONTIN knock-down inhibits the proliferation of t(8;21) positive cells, and that PONTIN is essential for Kasumi-1 clonogenic potential and cell cycle progression [264]. Thus, AML1-ETO can be recapitulated in Drosophila blood for investigating its mechanism and identifying potential targeted therapeutics for this AML subtype.

Despite advances in our understanding of many molecular mechanisms, in vitro research falls short in determining overall effect of treatment modalities or drug discovery. AML is an intricate disease where culture consisting of a single cell line system, can never recapitulate the complexity of the disease. In the difficulty of obtaining primate models of AML, small rodents, zebrafish, and Drosophila with well characterized genetic background and relative ease of manipulation, are the backbone of current work where leukemic cells are interfaced with the host immunity, metabolic environment and importance of the niche ation. Not one model is sufficient to address all posed questions. However, collectively, these models have expanded our knowledge and understanding of several pathways and important players in AML pathogenesis.

Author Contributions: All authors listed have made a substantial, direct and intellectual contribution to the work, and approved it for publication. H.S., B.J., R.H., M.H. writing—original draft preparation, N.D., A.B. writing—review and editing, M.E.S. and H.E.H. supervision, review and editing.

Funding: This research received no external funding.

Conflicts of Interest: The authors declare no conflict of interest.

References

1. Lowenberg, B.; Downing, J.R.; Burnett, A. Acute myeloid leukemia. *N. Engl. J. Med.* **1999**, *341*, 1051–1062. [CrossRef] [PubMed]
2. Yamamoto, J.F.; Goodman, M.T. Patterns of leukemia incidence in the United States by subtype and demographic characteristics, 1997–2002. *Cancer Causes Control* **2008**, *19*, 379–390. [CrossRef] [PubMed]

3. Maynadie, M.; Girodon, F.; Manivet-Janoray, I.; Mounier, M.; Mugneret, F.; Bailly, F.; Favre, B.; Caillot, D.; Petrella, T.; Flesch, M.; et al. Twenty-five years of epidemiological recording on myeloid malignancies: Data from the specialized registry of hematologic malignancies of Cote d'Or (Burgundy, France). *Haematologica* **2011**, *96*, 55–61. [CrossRef] [PubMed]
4. Dohner, H.; Weisdorf, D.J.; Bloomfield, C.D. Acute Myeloid Leukemia. *N. Engl. J. Med.* **2015**, *373*, 1136–1152. [CrossRef] [PubMed]
5. Deschler, B.; Lübbert, M. Acute myeloid leukemia: Epidemiology and etiology. *Cancer* **2006**, *107*, 2099–2107. [CrossRef] [PubMed]
6. Lowenberg, B.; Suciu, S.; Archimbaud, E.; Haak, H.; Stryckmans, P.; de Cataldo, R.; Dekker, A.W.; Berneman, Z.N.; Thyss, A.; van der Lelie, J.; et al. Mitoxantrone versus daunorubicin in induction-consolidation chemotherapy—The value of low-dose cytarabine for maintenance of remission, and an assessment of prognostic factors in acute myeloid leukemia in the elderly: Final report. European Organization for the Research and Treatment of Cancer and the Dutch-Belgian Hemato-Oncology Cooperative Hovon Group. *J. Clin. Oncol.* **1998**, *16*, 872–881. [PubMed]
7. Bennett, J.M.; Catovsky, D.; Daniel, M.-T.; Flandrin, G.; Galton, D.A.G.; Gralnick, H.R.; Sultan, C. Proposals for the Classification of the Acute Leukaemias French-American-British (FAB) Co-operative Group. *Br. J. Haematol.* **1976**, *33*, 451–458. [CrossRef] [PubMed]
8. Vardiman, J.W.; Harris, N.L.; Brunning, R.D. The World Health Organization (WHO) classification of the myeloid neoplasms. *Blood* **2002**, *100*, 2292–2302. [CrossRef]
9. Vardiman, J.W.; Thiele, J.; Arber, D.A.; Brunning, R.D.; Borowitz, M.J.; Porwit, A.; Harris, N.L.; Le Beau, M.M.; Hellström-Lindberg, E.; Tefferi, A.; et al. The 2008 revision of the World Health Organization (WHO) classification of myeloid neoplasms and acute leukemia: Rationale and important changes. *Blood* **2009**, *114*, 937–951. [CrossRef]
10. Arber, D.A.; Orazi, A.; Hasserjian, R.; Thiele, J.; Borowitz, M.J.; Le Beau, M.M.; Bloomfield, C.D.; Cazzola, M.; Vardiman, J.W. The 2016 revision to the World Health Organization classification of myeloid neoplasms and acute leukemia. *Blood* **2016**, *127*, 2391–2405. [CrossRef]
11. Dohner, H.; Estey, E.H.; Amadori, S.; Appelbaum, F.R.; Buchner, T.; Burnett, A.K.; Dombret, H.; Fenaux, P.; Grimwade, D.; Larson, R.A.; et al. Diagnosis and management of acute myeloid leukemia in adults: Recommendations from an international expert panel, on behalf of the European LeukemiaNet. *Blood* **2010**, *115*, 453–474. [CrossRef] [PubMed]
12. Dohner, H.; Estey, E.; Grimwade, D.; Amadori, S.; Appelbaum, F.R.; Buchner, T.; Dombret, H.; Ebert, B.L.; Fenaux, P.; Larson, R.A.; et al. Diagnosis and management of AML in adults: 2017 ELN recommendations from an international expert panel. *Blood* **2017**, *129*, 424–447. [CrossRef] [PubMed]
13. Weinstein, J.N.; Collisson, E.A.; Mills, G.B.; Shaw, K.M.; Ozenberger, B.A.; Ellrott, K.; Shmulevich, I.; Sander, C.; Stuart, J.M. The Cancer Genome Atlas Pan-Cancer Analysis Project. *Nat. Genet.* **2013**, *45*, 1113–1120. [CrossRef] [PubMed]
14. Ley, T.J.; Miller, C.; Ding, L.; Raphael, B.J.; Mungall, A.J.; Robertson, A.; Hoadley, K.; Triche, T.J., Jr.; Laird, P.W.; Baty, J.D.; et al. Genomic and epigenomic landscapes of adult de novo acute myeloid leukemia. *N. Engl. J. Med.* **2013**, *368*, 2059–2074. [PubMed]
15. Howe, K.; Clark, M.D.; Torroja, C.F.; Torrance, J.; Berthelot, C.; Muffato, M.; Collins, J.E.; Humphray, S.; McLaren, K.; Matthews, L.; et al. The zebrafish reference genome sequence and its relationship to the human genome. *Nature* **2013**, *496*, 498–503. [CrossRef]
16. Stuart, G.W.; McMurray, J.V.; Westerfield, M. Replication, integration and stable germ-line transmission of foreign sequences injected into early zebrafish embryos. *Development* **1988**, *103*, 403–412. [PubMed]
17. Hwang, W.Y.; Fu, Y.; Reyon, D.; Maeder, M.L.; Tsai, S.Q.; Sander, J.D.; Peterson, R.T.; Yeh, J.R.; Joung, J.K. Efficient genome editing in zebrafish using a CRISPR-Cas system. *Nat. Biotechnol.* **2013**, *31*, 227–229. [CrossRef]
18. Rasighaemi, P.; Basheer, F.; Liongue, C.; Ward, A.C. Zebrafish as a model for leukemia and other hematopoietic disorders. *J. Hematol. Oncol.* **2015**, *8*, 35. [CrossRef]
19. Macrae, C.A.; Peterson, R.T. Zebrafish as tools for drug discovery. *Nat. Rev. Drug Discov.* **2015**, *14*, 721–731. [CrossRef]

20. Pruvot, B.; Jacquel, A.; Droin, N.; Auberger, P.; Bouscary, D.; Tamburini, J.; Muller, M.; Fontenay, M.; Chluba, J.; Solary, E. Leukemic cell xenograft in zebrafish embryo for investigating drug efficacy. *Haematologica* **2011**, *96*, 612–616. [CrossRef]
21. Dick, A.; Hild, M.; Bauer, H.; Imai, Y.; Maifeld, H.; Schier, A.F.; Talbot, W.S.; Bouwmeester, T.; Hammerschmidt, M. Essential role of Bmp7 (snailhouse) and its prodomain in dorsoventral patterning of the zebrafish embryo. *Development* **2000**, *127*, 343–354. [PubMed]
22. Schmid, B.; Fürthauer, M.; Connors, S.A.; Trout, J.; Thisse, B.; Thisse, C.; Mullins, M.C. Equivalent genetic roles for bmp7/snailhouse and bmp2b/swirl in dorsoventral pattern formation. *Development* **2000**, *127*, 957–967. [PubMed]
23. Kishimoto, Y.; Lee, K.H.; Zon, L.; Hammerschmidt, M.; Schulte-Merker, S. The molecular nature of zebrafish swirl: BMP2 function is essential during early dorsoventral patterning. *Development* **1997**, *124*, 4457–4466. [PubMed]
24. Paik, E.J.; Zon, L.I. Hematopoietic development in the zebrafish. *Int. J. Dev. Boil.* **2010**, *54*, 1127–1137. [CrossRef] [PubMed]
25. Carapeti, M.; Aguiar, R.C.; Goldman, J.M.; Cross, N.C. A novel fusion between MOZ and the nuclear receptor coactivator TIF2 in acute myeloid leukemia. *Blood* **1998**, *91*, 3127–3133.
26. Coulthard, S.; Chase, A.; Watmore, A.; Swirsky, D.M.; Orchard, K.; Vora, A.; Goldman, J.M. Two cases of inv(8)(p11q13) in AML with erythrophagocytosis: A new cytogenetic variant. *Br. J. Haematol.* **1998**, *100*, 561–563. [CrossRef] [PubMed]
27. Aguiar, R.C.; Chase, A.; Coulthard, S.; Macdonald, D.H.; Carapeti, M.; Reiter, A.; Sohal, J.; Lennard, A.; Goldman, J.M.; Cross, N.C. Abnormalities of chromosome band 8p11 in leukemia: Two clinical syndromes can be distinguished on the basis of MOZ involvement. *Blood* **1997**, *90*, 3130–3135.
28. Liang, J.; Prouty, L.; Williams, B.J.; Dayton, M.A.; Blanchard, K.L. Acute mixed lineage leukemia with an inv(8)(p11q13) resulting in fusion of the genes for MOZ and TIF2. *Blood* **1998**, *92*, 2118–2122.
29. Zhuravleva, J.; Paggetti, J.; Martin, L.; Hammann, A.; Solary, E.; Bastie, J.-N.; Delva, L. MOZ/TIF2-induced acute myeloid leukaemia in transgenic fish. *Br. J. Haematol.* **2008**, *143*, 378–382. [CrossRef]
30. Hsu, K.; Traver, D.; Kutok, J.L.; Hagen, A.; Liu, T.-X.; Paw, B.H.; Rhodes, J.; Berman, J.N.; Zon, L.I.; Kanki, J.P.; et al. The pu.1 promoter drives myeloid gene expression in zebrafish. *Blood* **2004**, *104*, 1291–1297. [CrossRef]
31. Voso, M.T.; Burn, T.C.; Wulf, G.; Lim, B.; Leone, G.; Tenen, D.G. Inhibition of hematopoiesis by competitive binding of transcription factor PU. *Proc. Natl. Acad. Sci. USA* **1994**, *91*, 7932–7936. [CrossRef] [PubMed]
32. Rowley, J.D. Identificaton of a translocation with quinacrine fluorescence in a patient with acute leukemia. *Ann. Genet.* **1973**, *16*, 109–112. [PubMed]
33. Erickson, P.; Gao, J.; Chang, K.S.; Look, T.; Whisenant, E.; Raimondi, S.; Lasher, R.; Trujillo, J.; Rowley, J.; Drabkin, H. Identification of breakpoints in t(8;21) acute myelogenous leukemia and isolation of a fusion transcript, AML1/ETO, with similarity to Drosophila segmentation gene, runt. *Blood* **1992**, *80*, 1825–1831. [PubMed]
34. Miyoshi, H.; Shimizu, K.; Kozu, T.; Maseki, N.; Kaneko, Y.; Ohki, M. t(8;21) breakpoints on chromosome 21 in acute myeloid leukemia are clustered within a limited region of a single gene, AML1. *Proc. Natl. Acad. Sci. USA* **1991**, *88*, 10431–10434. [CrossRef] [PubMed]
35. Nisson, P.E.; Watkins, P.C.; Sacchi, N. Transcriptionally active chimeric gene derived from the fusion of the AML1 gene and a novel gene on chromosome 8 in t(8;21) leukemic cells. *Cancer Genet. Cytogenet.* **1992**, *63*, 81–88. [CrossRef]
36. Yeh, J.R.; Munson, K.M.; Chao, Y.L.; Peterson, Q.P.; Macrae, C.A.; Peterson, R.T. AML1-ETO reprograms hematopoietic cell fate by downregulating scl expression. *Development* **2008**, *135*, 401–410. [CrossRef] [PubMed]
37. Yeh, J.-R.J.; Munson, K.M.; Elagib, K.E.; Goldfarb, A.N.; Sweetser, D.A.; Peterson, R.T. Discovering chemical modifiers of oncogene-regulated hematopoietic differentiation. *Nat. Methods* **2009**, *5*, 236–243. [CrossRef] [PubMed]
38. Hirvonen, H.; Hukkanen, V.; Salmi, T.T.; Mäkelä, T.P.; Pelliniemi, T.T.; Knuutila, S.; Alitalo, R. Expression of L-myc and N-myc proto-oncogenes in human leukemias and leukemia cell lines. *Blood* **1991**, *78*, 3012–3020. [PubMed]

39. Hirvonen, H.; Hukkanen, V.; Salmi, T.T.; Pelliniemi, T.T.; Alitalo, R. L-myc and N-myc in hematopoietic malignancies. *Leuk Lymphoma* **1993**, *11*, 197–205. [CrossRef] [PubMed]
40. Ross, M.E.; Mahfouz, R.; Onciu, M.; Liu, H.-C.; Zhou, X.; Song, G.; Shurtleff, S.A.; Pounds, S.; Cheng, C.; Ma, J.; et al. Gene expression profiling of pediatric acute myelogenous leukemia. *Blood* **2004**, *104*, 3679–3687. [CrossRef] [PubMed]
41. Shen, L.J.; Chen, F.Y.; Zhang, Y.; Cao, L.F.; Kuang, Y.; Zhong, M.; Wang, T.; Zhong, H. MYCN transgenic zebrafish model with the characterization of acute myeloid leukemia and altered hematopoiesis. *PLoS ONE* **2013**, *8*, e59070. [CrossRef] [PubMed]
42. Mackarehtschian, K.; Hardin, J.D.; Moore, K.A.; Boast, S.; Goff, S.P.; Lemischka, I.R. Targeted disruption of the flk2/flt3 gene leads to deficiencies in primitive hematopoietic progenitors. *Immunity* **1995**, *3*, 147–161. [CrossRef]
43. Carow, C.E.; Levenstein, M.; Kaufmann, S.H.; Chen, J.; Amin, S.; Rockwell, P.; Witte, L.; Borowitz, M.J.; Civin, C.I.; Small, D. Expression of the hematopoietic growth factor receptor FLT3 (STK-1/Flk2) in human leukemias. *Blood* **1996**, *87*, 1089–1096. [PubMed]
44. Rosnet, O.; Bühring, H.J.; Marchetto, S.; Rappold, I.; Lavagna, C.; Sainty, D.; Arnoulet, C.; Chabannon, C.; Kanz, L.; Hannum, C.; et al. Human FLT3/FLK2 receptor tyrosine kinase is expressed at the surface of normal and malignant hematopoietic cells. *Leukemia* **1996**, *10*, 238–248. [PubMed]
45. Kiyoi, H.; Ohno, R.; Ueda, R.; Saito, H.; Naoe, T. Mechanism of constitutive activation of FLT3 with internal tandem duplication in the juxtamembrane domain. *Oncogene* **2002**, *21*, 2555–2563. [CrossRef] [PubMed]
46. Horiike, S.; Yokota, S.; Nakao, M.; Iwai, T.; Sasai, Y.; Kaneko, H.; Taniwaki, M.; Kashima, K.; Fujii, H.; Abe, T.; et al. Tandem duplications of the FLT3 receptor gene are associated with leukemic transformation of myelodysplasia. *Leukemia* **1997**, *11*, 1442–1446. [CrossRef] [PubMed]
47. Kiyoi, H.; Naoe, T.; Nakano, Y.; Yokota, S.; Minami, S.; Miyawaki, S.; Asou, N.; Kuriyama, K.; Jinnai, I.; Shimazaki, C.; et al. Prognostic implication of FLT3 and N-RAS gene mutations in acute myeloid leukemia. *Blood* **1999**, *93*, 3074–3080.
48. Yu, Y.; Maggi, L.B.; Brady, S.N.; Apicelli, A.J.; Dai, M.-S.; Lu, H.; Weber, J.D. Nucleophosmin Is Essential for Ribosomal Protein L5 Nuclear Export. *Mol. Cell. Boil.* **2006**, *26*, 3798–3809. [CrossRef]
49. Savkur, R. Preferential cleavage in pre-ribosomal RNA byprotein B23 endoribonuclease. *Nucleic Acids Res.* **1998**, *26*, 4508–4515. [CrossRef]
50. Falini, B.; Mecucci, C.; Tiacci, E.; Alcalay, M.; Rosati, R.; Pasqualucci, L.; La Starza, R.; Diverio, D.; Colombo, E.; Santucci, A.; et al. Cytoplasmic nucleophosmin in acute myelogenous leukemia with a normal karyotype. *N. Engl. J. Med.* **2005**, *352*, 254–266. [CrossRef]
51. He, B.-L.; Shi, X.; Man, C.H.; Ma, A.C.H.; Ekker, S.C.; Chow, H.C.H.; So, C.W.E.; Choi, W.W.L.; Zhang, W.; Zhang, Y.; et al. Functions of flt3 in zebrafish hematopoiesis and its relevance to human acute myeloid leukemia. *Blood* **2014**, *123*, 2518–2529. [CrossRef] [PubMed]
52. Bolli, N.; Payne, E.M.; Grabher, C.; Lee, J.S.; Johnston, A.B.; Falini, B.; Kanki, J.P.; Look, A.T. Expression of the cytoplasmic NPM1 mutant (NPMc+) causes the expansion of hematopoietic cells in zebrafish. *Blood* **2010**, *115*, 3329–3340. [CrossRef] [PubMed]
53. Lu, J.-W.; Hou, H.-A.; Hsieh, M.-S.; Tien, H.-F.; Lin, L.-I. Overexpression of FLT3-ITD driven by spi-1 results in expanded myelopoiesis with leukemic phenotype in zebrafish. *Leukemia* **2016**, *30*, 2098–2101. [CrossRef] [PubMed]
54. Cheng, J.C.; Kinjo, K.; Judelson, D.R.; Chang, J.; Wu, W.S.; Schmid, I.; Shankar, D.B.; Kasahara, N.; Stripecke, R.; Bhatia, R.; et al. CREB is a critical regulator of normal hematopoiesis and leukemogenesis. *Blood* **2008**, *111*, 1182–1192. [CrossRef] [PubMed]
55. Kinjo, K.; Sandoval, S.; Sakamoto, K.M.; Shankar, D.B. The Role of CREB as a Proto-oncogene in Hematopoiesis. *Cell Cycle* **2005**, *4*, 1134–1135. [CrossRef] [PubMed]
56. Crans, H.N.; Sakamoto, K.M. Transcription factors and translocations in lymphoid and myeloid leukemia. *Leukemia* **2001**, *15*, 313–331. [CrossRef] [PubMed]
57. Tregnago, C.; Manara, E.; Zampini, M.; Bisio, V.; Borga, C.; Bresolin, S.; Aveic, S.; Germano, G.; Basso, G.; Pigazzi, M. CREB engages C/EBPdelta to initiate leukemogenesis. *Leukemia* **2016**, *30*, 1887–1896. [CrossRef]
58. Gubbay, J.; Collignon, J.; Koopman, P.; Capel, B.; Economou, A.; Münsterberg, A.; Vivian, N.; Goodfellow, P.; Lovell-Badge, R. A gene mapping to the sex-determining region of the mouse Y chromosome is a member of a novel family of embryonically expressed genes. *Nature* **1990**, *346*, 245–250. [CrossRef]

59. Lu, J.W.; Hsieh, M.S.; Hou, H.A.; Chen, C.Y.; Tien, H.F.; Lin, L.I. Overexpression of SOX4 correlates with poor prognosis of acute myeloid leukemia and is leukemogenic in zebrafish. *Blood Cancer J.* **2017**, *7*, e593. [CrossRef]
60. Zhang, H.; Alberich-Jorda, M.; Amabile, G.; Yang, H.; Staber, P.B.; Di Ruscio, A.; Welner, R.S.; Ebralidze, A.; Zhang, J.; Levantini, E.; et al. Sox4 is a key oncogenic target in C/EBPalpha mutant acute myeloid leukemia. *Cancer Cell* **2013**, *24*, 575–588. [CrossRef]
61. Fung, T.K.; Leung, A.Y.; So, C.W. Sox4you: A new player in C/EBPalpha leukemia. *Cancer Cell* **2013**, *24*, 557–559. [CrossRef] [PubMed]
62. Paschka, P.; Schlenk, R.F.; Gaidzik, V.I.; Habdank, M.; Krönke, J.; Bullinger, L.; Späth, D.; Kayser, S.; Zucknick, M.; Götze, K.; et al. IDH1 and IDH2 Mutations Are Frequent Genetic Alterations in Acute Myeloid Leukemia and Confer Adverse Prognosis in Cytogenetically Normal Acute Myeloid Leukemia with NPM1 Mutation Without FLT3 Internal Tandem Duplication. *J. Clin. Oncol.* **2010**, *28*, 3636–3643. [CrossRef] [PubMed]
63. Shi, X.; He, B.-L.; Ma, A.C.H.; Guo, Y.; Chi, Y.; Man, C.H.; Zhang, W.; Zhang, Y.; Wen, Z.; Cheng, T.; et al. Functions of idh1 and its mutation in the regulation of developmental hematopoiesis in zebrafish. *Blood* **2015**, *125*, 2974–2984. [CrossRef] [PubMed]
64. Guryev, V.; Koudijs, M.J.; Berezikov, E.; Johnson, S.L.; Plasterk, R.H.; van Eeden, F.J.; Cuppen, E. Genetic variation in the zebrafish. *Genome Res.* **2006**, *16*, 491–497. [CrossRef] [PubMed]
65. Svejda, J.; Kossey, P.; Hlavayova, E.; Svec, F. Histological picture of the transplantable rat leukaemia induced by x-irradiation and methylcholanthrene. *Neoplasma* **1958**, *5*, 123–131. [PubMed]
66. Huggins, C.B.; Sugiyama, T. Induction of leukemia in rat by pulse doses of 7,12-dimethylbenz(a)anthracene. *Proc. Natl. Acad. Sci. USA* **1966**, *55*, 74–81. [CrossRef] [PubMed]
67. Huggins, C.B.; Grand, L.; Ueda, N. Specific induction of erythroleukemia and myelogenous leukemia in Sprague-Dawley rats. *Proc. Natl. Acad. Sci. USA* **1982**, *79*, 5411–5414. [CrossRef] [PubMed]
68. Somfai, S.; Szentirmay, Z.; Gál, F. Transplantable Myeloid Rat Leukaemia Induced by 7,12-Dimethylbenz(a)anthracene. *Acta Haematol.* **1973**, *49*, 281–290.
69. Bekkum, D.W.; van Hagenbeek, A. Relevance of the BN leukemia as a model for human acute myeloid leukemia. *Blood Cells Mol. Dis.* **1977**, *3*, 565–579.
70. Van Bekkum, D.W.; Van Oosterom, P.; Dicke, K.A. In vitro colony formation of transplantable rat leukemias in comparison with human acute myeloid leukemia. *Cancer Res.* **1976**, *36*, 941–946.
71. Hagenbeek, A.; van Bekkum, D.W. Comparitive evaluation of the L5222 and the BNML rat leukaemia models and their relavance to human acute leukaemia. *Leuk. Res.* **1977**, *1*, 75–256. [CrossRef]
72. Nooter, K.; Sonneveld, P.; Deurloo, J.; Oostrum, R.; Schultz, F.; Martens, A.; Hagenbeek, A. Repeated daunomycin administration in rats. *Cancer Chemother. Pharmacol.* **1984**, *12*, 187–189. [CrossRef] [PubMed]
73. Sonneveld, P.; Van Bekkum, D.W. Different distribution of adriamycin in normal and leukaemic rats. *Br. J. Cancer* **1981**, *43*, 464–470. [CrossRef] [PubMed]
74. Colly, L.P.; Van Bekkum, D.W.; Hagenbeek, A. Enhanced tumor load reduction after chemotherapy induced recruitment and synchronization in a slowly growing rat leukemia model (BNML) for human acute myelocytic leukemia. *Leuk. Res.* **1984**, *8*, 953–963. [CrossRef]
75. Aglietta, M.; Sonneveld, P. The relevance of cell kinetics for optimal scheduling of 1-beta-D-arabinofuranosyl cytosine and methotrexate in a slow growing acute myeloid leukemia (BNML). *Cancer Chemother. Pharmacol.* **1978**, *1*, 219–223. [CrossRef] [PubMed]
76. Hagenbeek, A.; Martens, A.C. AMSA: In vivo log cell kill for leukemic clonogenic cells versus toxicity for normal hemopoietic stem cells in a rat model for human acute myelocytic leukemia (BNML). *Eur. J. Cancer Clin. Oncol.* **1986**, *22*, 1255–1258. [CrossRef]
77. Ermens, A.A.; Kroes, A.C.; Lindemans, J.; Abels, J. 5-Fluorouracil treatment of rat leukemia and a reappraisal of its application in human leukemia. *Anticancer Res.* **1986**, *6*, 797–800. [PubMed]
78. Kroes, A.C.M.; Lindemans, J.; Schoester, M.; Abels, J. Enhanced therapeutic effect of methotrexate in experimental rat leukemia after inactivation of cobalamin (vitamin B12) by nitrous oxide. *Cancer Chemother. Pharmacol.* **1986**, *17*, 114–120. [CrossRef] [PubMed]
79. Sonneveld, P.; Holcenberg, J.; Van Bekkum, D. Effect of succinylated Acinetobacter glutaminase-asparaginase treatment on an acute myeloid leukemia in the rat (BNML). *Eur. J. Cancer (1965)* **1979**, *15*, 1061–1063. [CrossRef]

80. Arkesteijn, G.J.A.; Martens, A.C.M.; Jonker, R.R.; Hagemeijer, A.; Hagenbeek, A. Bivariate flow karyotyping of acute myelocytic leukemia in the BNML rat model. *Cytometry* **1987**, *8*, 618–624. [CrossRef]
81. Martens, A.C.M.; Hagenbeek, A. Detection of minimal disease in acute leukemia using flow cytometry: Studies in a rat model for human acute leukemia. *Cytometry* **1985**, *6*, 342–347. [CrossRef] [PubMed]
82. Martens, A.C.M.; Van Bekkum, D.W.; Hagenbeek, A. Minimal residual disease in leukemia: Studies in an animal model for acute myelocytic leukemia (bnml). *Stem Cells* **1990**, *8*, 27–38. [CrossRef] [PubMed]
83. Law, L.W.; Taormina, V.; Boyle, P.J. Response of acute lymphocytic leukemias to the purine antagonist 6-mercaptopurine. *Ann. N. Y. Acad. Sci.* **1954**, *60*, 244–250. [CrossRef] [PubMed]
84. Skipper, H.E.; Perry, S. Kinetics of normal and leukemic leukocyte populations and relevance to chemotherapy. *Cancer Res.* **1970**, *30*, 1883–1897. [PubMed]
85. Casazza, A.M.; Pratesi, G.; Giuliani, F.; Di Marco, A. Antileukemic Activity of 4-Demethoxydaunorubicin in Mice. *Tumori J.* **1980**, *66*, 549–564. [CrossRef]
86. Law, L.W.; Dunn, T.B.; Boyle, P.J.; Miller, J.H. Observations on the Effect of a Folic-Acid Antagonist on Transplantable Lymphoid Leukemias in Mice. *J. Natl. Cancer Inst.* **1949**, *10*, 179–192.
87. Kline, I.; Venditti, J.M.; Mead, J.A.; Tyrer, D.D.; Goldin, A. The antileukemic effectiveness of 5-fluorouracil and methotrexate in the combination chemotherapy of advanced leukemia L1210 in mice. *Cancer Res.* **1966**, *26*, 848–852. [PubMed]
88. Kline, I.; Venditti, J.M.; Tyrer, D.D.; Mantel, N.; Goldin, A. Chemotherapy of leukemia L1210 in mice with 1-beta-D-arabinofuranosylcytosine hydrochloride. II. Effectiveness against intracerebrally and subcutaneously inoculated leukemic cells. *Cancer Res.* **1966**, *26*, 1930–1937. [PubMed]
89. Jensen, P.B.; Roed, H.; Skovsgaard, T.; Friche, E.; Spang-Thomsen, M. Antitumor activity of the two epipodophyllotoxin derivatives VP-16 and VM-26 in preclinical systems: A comparison of in vitro and in vivo drug evaluation. *Cancer Chemother. Pharmacol.* **1990**, *27*, 194–198. [CrossRef] [PubMed]
90. Skipper, H.E.; Schabel, F.M.; Wilcox, W.S. Experimental evaluation of potential anticancer agents. XXI. Scheduling of arabinosylcytosine to take advantage of its S-phase specificity against leukemia cells. *Cancer Chemother. Rep.* **1967**, *51*, 125–165. [PubMed]
91. Kawasaki, Y.; Hirabayashi, Y.; Kaneko, T.; Kanno, J.; Kodama, Y.; Matsushima, Y.; Ogawa, Y.; Saitoh, M.; Sekita, K.; Uchida, O.; et al. Benzene-Induced Hematopoietic Neoplasms Including Myeloid Leukemia in Trp53-Deficient C57BL/6 and C3H/He Mice. *Toxicol. Sci.* **2009**, *110*, 293–306. [CrossRef] [PubMed]
92. Preston, D.L.; Kusumi, S.; Tomonaga, M.; Izumi, S.; Ron, E.; Kuramoto, A.; Kamada, N.; Dohy, H.; Matsuo, T.; Matsui, T.; et al. Cancer incidence in atomic bomb survivors. Part III. Leukemia, lymphoma and multiple myeloma, 1950–1987. *Radiat. Res.* **1994**, *137* (Suppl. 2), S68–S97. [CrossRef] [PubMed]
93. Weiss, H.A.; Boice, J.D.; Muirhead, C.R.; Little, M.P.; Darby, S.C.; Day, N.E. Risks of Leukemia in Japanese Atomic Bomb Survivors, in Women Treated for Cervical Cancer, and in Patients Treated for Ankylosing Spondylitis. *Radiat. Res.* **1999**, *152*, 280.
94. Tomonaga, M. Leukaemia in Nagasaki atomic bomb survivors from 1945 through 1959. *Bull. World Health Organ.* **1962**, *26*, 619–631. [PubMed]
95. Finch, S.C. Radiation-induced leukemia: Lessons from history. *Best Pract. Res. Clin. Haematol.* **2007**, *20*, 109–118. [CrossRef] [PubMed]
96. Silver, A.; Moody, J.; Dunford, R.; Clark, D.; Ganz, S.; Bulman, R.; Bouffler, S.; Finnon, P.; Meijne, E.; Huiskamp, R.; et al. Molecular mapping of chromosome 2 deletions in murine radiation-induced AML localizes a putative tumor suppressor gene to a 1.0 cM region homologous to human chromosome segment 11p11–12. *Genes Chromosome Cancer* **1999**, *24*, 95–104. [CrossRef]
97. Furth, J.; Seibold, H.R.; Rathbone, R.R. Experimental studies on lymphomatosis. *Am. J. Cancer* **1933**, *19*, 521–604.
98. Ullrich, R.L.; Preston, R.J. Myeloid leukemia in male RFM mice following irradiation with fission spectrum neutrons or gamma rays. *Radiat. Res.* **1987**, *109*, 165–170. [CrossRef]
99. Wolman, S.R.; McMorrow, L.E.; Cohen, M.W. Animal model of human disease: Myelogenous leukemia in the RF mouse. *Am. J. Pathol.* **1982**, *107*, 280–284.
100. Finnon, R.; Brown, N.; Moody, J.; Badie, C.; Olme, C.-H.; Huiskamp, R.; Meijne, E.; Sutmuller, M.; Rosemann, M.; Bouffler, S.D. Flt3-ITD mutations in a mouse model of radiation-induced acute myeloid leukaemia. *Leukemia* **2012**, *26*, 1445–1446. [CrossRef]

101. Small, D. FLT3 mutations: Biology and treatment. *Hematol. Am. Soc. Hematol. Educ. Program* **2006**, 178–184. [CrossRef] [PubMed]
102. Dunn, T.B. Normal and Pathologic Anatomy of the Reticular Tissue in Laboratory Mice, With a Classification and Discussion of Neoplasms. *J. Natl. Cancer Inst.* **1954**, *14*, 1281–1433. [PubMed]
103. Pedersen-Bjergaard, J.; Philip, P.; Pedersen, N.T.; Hou-Jensen, K.; Svejgaard, A.; Jensen, G.; Nissen, N.I. Acute nonlymphocytic leukemia, preleukemia, and acute myeloproliferative syndrome secondary to treatment of other malignant diseases. II. Bone marrow cytology, cytogenetics, results of HLA typing, response to antileukemic chemotherapy, and survival in a total series of 55 patients. *Cancer* **1984**, *54*, 452–462. [PubMed]
104. Haran-Ghera, N.; Krautghamer, R.; Lapidot, T.; Peled, A.; Dominguez, M.G.; Stanley, E.R. Increased circulating colony-stimulating factor-1 (CSF-1) in SJL/J mice with radiation-induced acute myeloid leukemia (AML) is associated with autocrine regulation of AML cells by CSF-1. *Blood* **1997**, *89*, 2537–2545. [PubMed]
105. Chia, R.; Achilli, F.; Festing, M.F.W.; Fisher, E.M.C. The origins and uses of mouse outbred stocks. *Nat. Genet.* **2005**, *37*, 1181–1186. [CrossRef] [PubMed]
106. Ban, N.; Kai, M.; Kusama, T. Chromosome Aberrations in Bone Marrow Cells of C3H/He Mice at an Early Stage after Whole-Body Irradiation. *J. Radiat. Res.* **1997**, *38*, 219–231. [CrossRef] [PubMed]
107. Rithidech, K.; Dunn, J.J.; Bond, V.P.; Gordon, C.R.; Cronkite, E.P. Characterization of genetic instability in radiation- and benzene-induced murine acute leukemia. *Mutat. Res. Mol. Mech. Mutagen.* **1999**, *428*, 33–39. [CrossRef]
108. Cleary, H. Allelic loss on chromosome 4 (Lyr2/TLSR5) is associated with myeloid, B-lympho-myeloid, and lymphoid (B and T) mouse radiation-induced leukemias. *Blood* **2001**, *98*, 1549–1554. [CrossRef]
109. Giotopoulos, G.; McCormick, C.; Cole, C.; Zanker, A.; Jawad, M.; Brown, R.; Plumb, M. DNA methylation during mouse hemopoietic differentiation and radiation-induced leukemia. *Exp. Hematol.* **2006**, *34*, 1462–1470. [CrossRef]
110. Siegler, R.; Rich, M.A. Pathogenesis of Virus-Induced Myeloid Leukemia in Mice. *J. Natl. Cancer Inst.* **1967**, *38*, 31–50.
111. McGarry, M.P.; Steeves, R.A.; Eckner, R.J.; Mirand, E.A.; Trudel, P.J. Isolation of a myelogenous leukemia-inducing virus from mice infected with the friend virus complex. *Int. J. Cancer* **1974**, *13*, 867–878. [CrossRef] [PubMed]
112. Rein, A. Murine Leukemia Viruses: Objects and Organisms. *Adv. Virol.* **2011**, *2011*, 1–14. [CrossRef] [PubMed]
113. Gross, L. Development and serial cellfree passage of a highly potent strain of mouse leukemia virus. *Proc. Soc. Exp. Biol. Med.* **1957**, *94*, 767–771. [CrossRef] [PubMed]
114. Linemeyer, D.L.; Menke, J.G.; Ruscetti, S.K.; Evans, L.H.; Scolnick, E.M. Envelope gene sequences which encode the gp52 protein of spleen focus-forming virus are required for the induction of erythroid cell proliferation. *J. Virol.* **1982**, *43*, 223–233. [PubMed]
115. Ruscetti, S.; Wolff, L. Malignant transformation of erythroid cells in vivo by introduction of a nonreplicating retrovirus vector. *Science* **1985**, *228*, 1549–1552.
116. Perkins, A.S. The Pathology of Murine Myelogenous Leukemias. *Curr. Top. Microbiol. Immunol.* **1989**, *149*, 3–21.
117. Largaespada, D.A. Genetic heterogeneity in acute myeloid leukemia: Maximizing information flow from MuLV mutagenesis studies. *Leukemia* **2000**, *14*, 1174–1184. [CrossRef]
118. Dupuy, A.J. Transposon-based screens for cancer gene discovery in mouse models. *Semin. Cancer Biol.* **2010**, *20*, 261–268. [CrossRef]
119. Largaespada, D.A. Transposon-mediated mutagenesis of somatic cells in the mouse for cancer gene identification. *Methods* **2009**, *49*, 282–286. [CrossRef]
120. Collier, L.S.; Adams, D.J.; Hackett, C.S.; Bendzick, L.E.; Akagi, K.; Davies, M.N.; Diers, M.D.; Rodriguez, F.J.; Bender, A.M.; Tieu, C.; et al. Whole-body Sleeping Beauty mutagenesis can cause penetrant leukemia/lymphoma and rare high-grade glioma without associated embryonic lethality. *Cancer Res.* **2009**, *69*, 8429–8437. [CrossRef]
121. Vassiliou, G.S.; Cooper, J.L.; Rad, R.; Li, J.; Rice, S.; Uren, A.; Rad, L.; Ellis, P.; Andrews, R.; Banerjee, R.; et al. Mutant nucleophosmin and cooperating pathways drive leukemia initiation and progression in mice. *Nat. Genet.* **2011**, *43*, 470–475. [PubMed]

122. Kakizuka, A.; Miller, W.H.; Umesono, K.; Warrell, R.P.; Frankel, S.R.; Murty, V.V.; Dmitrovsky, E.; Evans, R.M. Chromosomal translocation t(15;17) in human acute promyelocytic leukemia fuses RAR alpha with a novel putative transcription factor, PML. *Cell* **1991**, *66*, 663–674. [CrossRef]
123. De Thé, H.; Lavau, C.; Marchio, A.; Chomienne, C.; Degos, L.; Dejean, A. The PML-RAR alpha fusion mRNA generated by the t(15;17) translocation in acute promyelocytic leukemia encodes a functionally altered RAR. *Cell* **1991**, *66*, 675–684. [CrossRef]
124. Early, E.; Moore, M.A.; Kakizuka, A.; Nason-Burchenal, K.; Martin, P.; Evans, R.M.; Dmitrovsky, E. Transgenic expression of PML/RARalpha impairs myelopoiesis. *Proc. Natl. Acad. Sci. USA* **1996**, *93*, 7900–7904. [CrossRef] [PubMed]
125. Grisolano, J.L.; Wesselschmidt, R.L.; Pelicci, P.G.; Ley, T.J. Altered myeloid development and acute leukemia in transgenic mice expressing PML-RAR alpha under control of cathepsin G regulatory sequences. *Blood* **1997**, *89*, 376–387. [PubMed]
126. Brown, D.; Kogan, S.; Lagasse, E.; Weissman, I.; Alcalay, M.; Pelicci, P.G.; Atwater, S.; Bishop, J.M. A PMLRARalpha transgene initiates murine acute promyelocytic leukemia. *Proc. Natl. Acad. Sci. USA* **1997**, *94*, 2551–2556. [CrossRef] [PubMed]
127. Wang, Q.; Stacy, T.; Binder, M.; Marin-Padilla, M.; Sharpe, A.H.; Speck, N.A. Disruption of the Cbfa2 gene causes necrosis and hemorrhaging in the central nervous system and blocks definitive hematopoiesis. *Proc. Natl. Acad. Sci. USA* **1996**, *93*, 3444–3449. [CrossRef]
128. Okuda, T.; Van Deursen, J.; Hiebert, S.W.; Grosveld, G.; Downing, J.R. AML1, the Target of Multiple Chromosomal Translocations in Human Leukemia, Is Essential for Normal Fetal Liver Hematopoiesis. *Cell* **1996**, *84*, 321–330. [CrossRef]
129. Okuda, T.; Cai, Z.; Yang, S.; Lenny, N.; Lyu, C.J.; Van Deursen, J.M.; Harada, H.; Downing, J.R. Expression of a knocked-in AML1-ETO leukemia gene inhibits the establishment of normal definitive hematopoiesis and directly generates dysplastic hematopoietic progenitors. *Blood* **1998**, *91*, 3134–3143.
130. Rhoades, K.L.; Hetherington, C.J.; Harakawa, N.; Yergeau, D.A.; Zhou, L.; Liu, L.Q.; Little, M.T.; Tenen, D.G.; Zhang, D.E. Analysis of the role of AML1-ETO in leukemogenesis, using an inducible transgenic mouse model. *Blood* **2000**, *96*, 2108–2115.
131. Higuchi, M.; O'Brien, D.; Kumaravelu, P.; Lenny, N.; Yeoh, E.-J.; Downing, J.R. Expression of a conditional AML1-ETO oncogene bypasses embryonic lethality and establishes a murine model of human t(8;21) acute myeloid leukemia. *Cancer Cell* **2002**, *1*, 63–74. [CrossRef]
132. Yuan, Y.; Zhou, L.; Miyamoto, T.; Iwasaki, H.; Harakawa, N.; Hetherington, C.J.; Burel, S.A.; Lagasse, E.; Weissman, I.L.; Akashi, K.; et al. AML1-ETO expression is directly involved in the development of acute myeloid leukemia in the presence of additional mutations. *Proc. Natl. Acad. Sci. USA* **2001**, *98*, 10398–10403. [CrossRef] [PubMed]
133. Nick, H.J.; Kim, H.G.; Chang, C.W.; Harris, K.W.; Reddy, V.; Klug, C.A. Distinct classes of c-Kit-activating mutations differ in their ability to promote RUNX1-ETO-associated acute myeloid leukemia. *Blood* **2012**, *119*, 1522–1531. [CrossRef]
134. Schessl, C.; Rawat, V.P.; Cusan, M.; Deshpande, A.; Kohl, T.M.; Rosten, P.M.; Spiekermann, K.; Humphries, R.K.; Schnittger, S.; Kern, W.; et al. The AML1-ETO fusion gene and the FLT3 length mutation collaborate in inducing acute leukemia in mice. *J. Clin. Investig.* **2005**, *115*, 2159–2168. [CrossRef] [PubMed]
135. Wang, S.; Wang, Q.; Crute, B.E.; Melnikova, I.N.; Keller, S.R.; Speck, N.A. Cloning and characterization of subunits of the T-cell receptor and murine leukemia virus enhancer core-binding factor. *Mol. Cell. Boil.* **1993**, *13*, 3324–3339. [CrossRef] [PubMed]
136. Schoch, C.; Kern, W.; Schnittger, S.; Büchner, T.; Hiddemann, W.; Haferlach, T. The influence of age on prognosis of de novo acute myeloid leukemia differs according to cytogenetic subgroups. *Haematologica* **2004**, *89*, 1082–1090. [PubMed]
137. Liu, P.; Tarlé, S.; Hajra, A.; Claxton, D.; Marlton, P.; Freedman, M.; Siciliano, M.; Collins, F. Fusion between transcription factor CBF beta/PEBP2 beta and a myosin heavy chain in acute myeloid leukemia. *Science* **1993**, *261*, 1041–1044. [CrossRef] [PubMed]
138. Castilla, L.H.; Garrett, L.; Adya, N.; Orlic, D.; Dutra, A.; Anderson, S.; Owens, J.; Eckhaus, M.; Bodine, D.; Liu, P.P. The fusion gene Cbfb-MYH11 blocks myeloid differentiation and predisposes mice to acute myelomonocytic leukaemia. *Nat. Genet.* **1999**, *23*, 144–146. [CrossRef] [PubMed]

139. Castilla, L.H.; Perrat, P.; Martinez, N.J.; Landrette, S.F.; Keys, R.; Oikemus, S.; Flanegan, J.; Heilman, S.; Garrett, L.; Dutra, A.; et al. Identification of genes that synergize with Cbfb-MYH11 in the pathogenesis of acute myeloid leukemia. *Proc. Natl. Acad. Sci. USA* **2004**, *101*, 4924–4929. [CrossRef]
140. Kuo, Y.H.; Landrette, S.F.; Heilman, S.A.; Perrat, P.N.; Garrett, L.; Liu, P.P.; Le Beau, M.M.; Kogan, S.C.; Castilla, L.H. Cbf beta-SMMHC induces distinct abnormal myeloid progenitors able to develop acute myeloid leukemia. *Cancer Cell* **2006**, *9*, 57–68. [CrossRef]
141. Verhaak, R.G.W. Mutations in nucleophosmin (NPM1) in acute myeloid leukemia (AML): Association with other gene abnormalities and previously established gene expression signatures and their favorable prognostic significance. *Blood* **2005**, *106*, 3747–3754. [CrossRef] [PubMed]
142. Cheng, K.; Sportoletti, P.; Ito, K.; Clohessy, J.G.; Teruya-Feldstein, J.; Kutok, J.L.; Pandolfi, P.P. The cytoplasmic NPM mutant induces myeloproliferation in a transgenic mouse model. *Blood* **2010**, *115*, 3341–3345. [CrossRef] [PubMed]
143. Chou, S.H.; Ko, B.S.; Chiou, J.S.; Hsu, Y.C.; Tsai, M.H.; Chiu, Y.C.; Yu, I.S.; Lin, S.W.; Hou, H.A.; Kuo, Y.Y.; et al. A knock-in Npm1 mutation in mice results in myeloproliferation and implies a perturbation in hematopoietic microenvironment. *PLoS ONE* **2012**, *7*, e49769. [CrossRef] [PubMed]
144. Mallardo, M.; Caronno, A.; Pruneri, G.; Raviele, P.R.; Viale, A.; Pelicci, P.G.; Colombo, E. NPMc+ and FLT3_ITD mutations cooperate in inducing acute leukaemia in a novel mouse model. *Leukemia* **2013**, *27*, 2248–2251. [CrossRef] [PubMed]
145. Gilliland, D.G.; Griffin, J.D. The roles of FLT3 in hematopoiesis and leukemia. *Blood* **2002**, *100*, 1532–1542. [CrossRef] [PubMed]
146. Lee, B.H.; Williams, I.R.; Anastasiadou, E.; Boulton, C.L.; Joseph, S.W.; Amaral, S.M.; Curley, D.P.; Duclos, N.; Huntly, B.J.P.; Fabbro, D.; et al. FLT3 internal tandem duplication mutations induce myeloproliferative or lymphoid disease in a transgenic mouse model. *Oncogene* **2005**, *24*, 7882–7892. [CrossRef] [PubMed]
147. Li, L.; Bailey, E.; Greenblatt, S.; Huso, D.; Small, D. Loss of the wild-type allele contributes to myeloid expansion and disease aggressiveness in FLT3/ITD knockin mice. *Blood* **2011**, *118*, 4935–4945. [CrossRef] [PubMed]
148. Lee, B.H.; Tothova, Z.; Levine, R.L.; Anderson, K.; Buza-Vidas, N.; Cullen, D.E.; McDowell, E.P.; Adelsperger, J.; Fröhling, S.; Huntly, B.J.; et al. FLT3 mutations confer enhanced proliferation and survival properties to multipotent progenitors in a murine model of chronic myelomonocytic leukemia. *Cancer Cell* **2007**, *12*, 367–380. [CrossRef]
149. Kharazi, S.; Mead, A.J.; Mansour, A.; Hultquist, A.; Böiers, C.; Luc, S.; Buza-Vidas, N.; Ma, Z.; Ferry, H.; Atkinson, D.; et al. Impact of gene dosage, loss of wild-type allele, and FLT3 ligand on Flt3-ITD-induced myeloproliferation. *Blood* **2011**, *118*, 3613–3621. [CrossRef]
150. Iida, S.; Seto, M.; Yamamoto, K.; Komatsu, H.; Tojo, A.; Asano, S.; Kamada, N.; Ariyoshi, Y.; Takahashi, T.; Ueda, R. MLLT3 gene on 9p22 involved in t(9;11) leukemia encodes a serine/proline rich protein homologous to MLLT1 on 19p13. *Oncogene* **1993**, *8*, 3085–3092.
151. Nakamura, T.; Alder, H.; Gu, Y.; Prasad, R.; Canaani, O.; Kamada, N.; Gale, R.P.; Lange, B.; Crist, W.M.; Nowell, P.C.; et al. Genes on chromosomes 4, 9, and 19 involved in 11q23 abnormalities in acute leukemia share sequence homology and/or common motifs. *Proc. Natl. Acad. Sci. USA* **1993**, *90*, 4631–4635. [CrossRef] [PubMed]
152. Corral, J.; Lavenir, I.; Impey, H.; Warren, A.J.; Forster, A.; Larson, T.A.; Bell, S.; McKenzie, A.N.; King, G.; Rabbitts, T.H. An Mll–AF9 Fusion Gene Made by Homologous Recombination Causes Acute Leukemia in Chimeric Mice: A Method to Create Fusion Oncogenes. *Cell* **1996**, *85*, 853–861. [CrossRef]
153. Collins, E.C.; Pannell, R.; Simpson, E.M.; Forster, A.; Rabbitts, T.H. Inter-chromosomal recombination of Mll and Af9 genes mediated by cre-loxP in mouse development. *EMBO Rep.* **2000**, *1*, 127–132. [CrossRef] [PubMed]
154. Stavropoulou, V.; Kaspar, S.; Brault, L.; Sanders, M.A.; Juge, S.; Morettini, S.; Tzankov, A.; Iacovino, M.; Lau, I.-J.; Milne, T.A.; et al. MLL-AF9 Expression in Hematopoietic Stem Cells Drives a Highly Invasive AML Expressing EMT-Related Genes Linked to Poor Outcome. *Cancer Cell* **2016**, *30*, 43–58. [CrossRef]
155. Johnson, J.J.; Chen, W.; Hudson, W.; Yao, Q.; Taylor, M.; Rabbitts, T.H.; Kersey, J.H. Prenatal and postnatal myeloid cells demonstrate stepwise progression in the pathogenesis of MLL fusion gene leukemia. *Blood* **2003**, *101*, 3229–3235. [CrossRef] [PubMed]

156. Ayton, P.M.; Cleary, M.L. Transformation of myeloid progenitors by MLL oncoproteins is dependent on Hoxa7 and Hoxa9. *Genome Res.* **2003**, *17*, 2298–2307. [CrossRef] [PubMed]
157. Meyer, C.; Hofmann, J.; Burmeister, T.; Gröger, D.; Park, T.S.; Emerenciano, M.; Pombo-De-Oliveira, M.D.S.; Renneville, A.; Villarese, P.; MacIntyre, E.; et al. The MLL recombinome of acute leukemias in 2013. *Leukemia* **2013**, *27*, 2165–2176. [CrossRef] [PubMed]
158. Chen, W.; Li, Q.; Hudson, W.A.; Kumar, A.; Kirchhof, N.; Kersey, J.H. A murine Mll-AF4 knock-in model results in lymphoid and myeloid deregulation and hematologic malignancy. *Blood* **2006**, *108*, 669–677. [CrossRef] [PubMed]
159. Metzler, M.; Förster, A.; Pannell, R.; Arends, M.J.; Daser, A.; Lobato, M.N.; Rabbitts, T.H. A conditional model of MLL-AF4 B-cell tumourigenesis using invertor technology. *Oncogene* **2006**, *25*, 3093–3103. [CrossRef]
160. Barrett, N.A.; Malouf, C.; Kapeni, C.; Bacon, W.A.; Giotopoulos, G.; Jacobsen, S.E.W.; Huntly, B.J.; Ottersbach, K. Mll-AF4 Confers Enhanced Self-Renewal and Lymphoid Potential during a Restricted Window in Development. *Cell Rep.* **2016**, *16*, 1039–1054. [CrossRef]
161. Krivtsov, A.V.; Feng, Z.; Lemieux, M.E.; Faber, J.; Vempati, S.; Sinha, A.U.; Xia, X.; Jesneck, J.; Bracken, A.P.; Silverman, L.B.; et al. H3K79 methylation profiles define murine and human MLL-AF4 leukemias. *Cancer Cell* **2008**, *14*, 355–368. [CrossRef] [PubMed]
162. Lavau, C.; Szilvassy, S.J.; Slany, R.; Cleary, M.L. Immortalization and leukemic transformation of a myelomonocytic precursor by retrovirally transduced HRX-ENL. *EMBO J.* **1997**, *16*, 4226–4237. [CrossRef] [PubMed]
163. Zeisig, B.B.; García-Cuéllar, M.P.; Winkler, T.H.; Slany, R.K. The Oncoprotein MLL–ENL disturbs hematopoietic lineage determination and transforms a biphenotypic lymphoid/myeloid cell. *Oncogene* **2003**, *22*, 1629–1637. [CrossRef] [PubMed]
164. Zeisig, B.B.; Milne, T.; García-Cuéllar, M.-P.; Schreiner, S.; Martin, M.-E.; Fuchs, U.; Borkhardt, A.; Chanda, S.K.; Walker, J.; Soden, R.; et al. Hoxa9 and Meis1 are key targets for MLL-ENL-mediated cellular immortalization. *Mol. Cell. Boil.* **2004**, *24*, 617–628. [CrossRef] [PubMed]
165. Kennedy, J.A.; Hope, K.J.; Dick, J.E.; Barabé, F. Modeling the Initiation and Progression of Human Acute Leukemia in Mice. *Science* **2007**, *316*, 600–604.
166. Ugale, A.; Säwén, P.; Dudenhöffer-Pfeifer, M.; Wahlestedt, M.; Norddahl, G.L.; Bryder, D. MLL-ENL-mediated leukemia initiation at the interface of lymphoid commitment. *Oncogene* **2017**, *36*, 3207–3212. [CrossRef] [PubMed]
167. Sasaki, M.; Knobbe, C.B.; Munger, J.C.; Lind, E.F.; Brenner, D.; Brüstle, A.; Harris, I.S.; Holmes, R.; Wakeham, A.; Haight, J.; et al. IDH1(R132H) mutation increases murine haematopoietic progenitors and alters epigenetics. *Nature* **2012**, *488*, 656–659. [CrossRef]
168. Callens, C.; Chevret, S.; Cayuela, J.M.; Cassinat, B.; Raffoux, E.; de Botton, S.; Thomas, X.; Guerci, A.; Fegueux, N.; Pigneux, A.; et al. Prognostic implication of FLT3 and Ras gene mutations in patients with acute promyelocytic leukemia (APL): A retrospective study from the European APL Group. *Leukemia* **2005**, *19*, 1153–1160. [CrossRef]
169. Bowen, D.T.; Frew, M.E.; Hills, R.; Gale, R.E.; Wheatley, K.; Groves, M.J.; Langabeer, S.E.; Kottaridis, P.D.; Moorman, A.V.; Burnett, A.K.; et al. RAS mutation in acute myeloid leukemia is associated with distinct cytogenetic subgroups but does not influence outcome in patients younger than 60 years. *Blood* **2005**, *106*, 2113–2119. [CrossRef]
170. Chan, I.T.; Kutok, J.L.; Williams, I.R.; Cohen, S.; Moore, S.; Shigematsu, H.; Ley, T.J.; Akashi, K.; Le Beau, M.M.; Gilliland, D.G. Oncogenic K-ras cooperates with PML-RAR alpha to induce an acute promyelocytic leukemia-like disease. *Blood* **2006**, *108*, 1708–1715. [CrossRef]
171. Taylor, C.; McGlynn, H.; Carter, G.; Baker, A.H.; Warren, N.; Ridge, S.A.; Owen, G.; Thompson, E.; Thompson, P.W.; Jacobs, A. RAS and FMS mutations following cytotoxic therapy for childhood acute lymphoblastic leukaemia. *Leukemia* **1995**, *9*, 466–470. [PubMed]
172. Padua, R.A.; Guinn, B.-A.; Al-Sabah, A.I.; Smith, M.; Taylor, C.; Pettersson, T.; Ridge, S.; Carter, G.; White, D.; Oscier, D.; et al. RAS, FMS and p53 mutations and poor clinical outcome in myelodysplasias: A 10-year follow-up. *Leukemia* **1998**, *12*, 887–892. [CrossRef] [PubMed]
173. Karakas, T.; Maurer, U.; Weidmann, E.; Miething, C.C.; Hoelzer, D.; Bergmann, L. High expression of bcl-2 mRNA as a determinant of poor prognosis in acute myeloid leukemia. *Ann. Oncol.* **1998**, *9*, 159–165. [CrossRef] [PubMed]

174. Benito, A.; Grillot, D.; Nuñez, G.; Fernández-Luna, J.L. Regulation and function of Bcl-2 during differentiation-induced cell death in HL-60 promyelocytic cells. *Am. J. Pathol.* **1995**, *146*, 481–490. [PubMed]
175. Omidvar, N.; Kogan, S.; Beurlet, S.; Le Pogam, C.; Janin, A.; West, R.; Noguera, M.-E.; Reboul, M.; Soulié, A.; Leboeuf, C.; et al. BCL-2 and Mutant NRAS Interact Physically and Functionally in a Mouse Model of Progressive Myelodysplasia. *Cancer Res.* **2007**, *67*, 11657–11667. [CrossRef] [PubMed]
176. Steudel, C.; Wermke, M.; Schaich, M.; Schakel, U.; Illmer, T.; Ehninger, G.; Thiede, C. Comparative analysis of MLL partial tandem duplication and FLT3 internal tandem duplication mutations in 956 adult patients with acute myeloid leukemia. *Genes Chromosomes Cancer* **2003**, *37*, 237–251. [CrossRef] [PubMed]
177. Shih, L.Y.; Liang, D.C.; Fu, J.F.; Wu, J.H.; Wang, P.N.; Lin, T.L.; Dunn, P.; Kuo, M.C.; Tang, T.C.; Lin, T.H.; et al. Characterization of fusion partner genes in 114 patients with de novo acute myeloid leukemia and MLL rearrangement. *Leukemia* **2006**, *20*, 218–223. [CrossRef]
178. Whitman, S.P.; Ruppert, A.S.; Marcucci, G.; Mrózek, K.; Paschka, P.; Langer, C.; Baldus, C.D.; Wen, J.; Vukosavljevic, T.; Powell, B.L.; et al. Long-term disease-free survivors with cytogenetically normal acute myeloid leukemia and MLL partial tandem duplication: A Cancer and Leukemia Group B study. *Blood* **2007**, *109*, 5164–5167. [CrossRef]
179. Zorko, N.A.; Bernot, K.M.; Whitman, S.P.; Siebenaler, R.F.; Ahmed, E.H.; Marcucci, G.G.; Yanes, D.A.; McConnell, K.K.; Mao, C.; Kalu, C.; et al. Mll partial tandem duplication and Flt3 internal tandem duplication in a double knock-in mouse recapitulates features of counterpart human acute myeloid leukemias. *Blood* **2012**, *120*, 1130–1136. [CrossRef]
180. Whitman, S.P.; Archer, K.J.; Feng, L.; Baldus, C.; Becknell, B.; Carlson, B.D.; Carroll, A.J.; Mrózek, K.; Vardiman, J.W.; George, S.L.; et al. Absence of the wild-type allele predicts poor prognosis in adult de novo acute myeloid leukemia with normal cytogenetics and the internal tandem duplication of FLT3: A cancer and leukemia group B study. *Cancer Res.* **2001**, *61*, 7233–7239.
181. Whitman, S.P.; Liu, S.; Vukosavljevic, T.; Rush, L.J.; Yu, L.; Liu, C.; Klisovic, M.I.; Maharry, K.; Guimond, M.; Strout, M.P.; et al. The MLL partial tandem duplication: Evidence for recessive gain-of-function in acute myeloid leukemia identifies a novel patient subgroup for molecular-targeted therapy. *Blood* **2005**, *106*, 345–352. [CrossRef] [PubMed]
182. Döhner, K.; Tobis, K.; Ulrich, R.; Fröhling, S.; Benner, A.; Schlenk, R.F. Prognostic Significance of Partial Tandem Duplications of the MLL Gene in Adult Patients 16 to 60 Years Old With Acute Myeloid Leukemia and Normal Cytogenetics: A Study of the Acute Myeloid Leukemia Study Group Ulm. *J. Clin. Oncol.* **2002**, *20*, 3254–3261. [CrossRef] [PubMed]
183. Raza-Egilmez, S.Z.; Jani-Sait, S.N.; Grossi, M.; Higgins, M.J.; Shows, T.B.; Aplan, P.D. NUP98-HOXD13 gene fusion in therapy-related acute myelogenous leukemia. *Cancer Res.* **1998**, *58*, 4269–4273. [PubMed]
184. Slape, C.; Lin, Y.W.; Hartung, H.; Zhang, Z.; Wolff, L.; Aplan, P.D. NUP98-HOX translocations lead to myelodysplastic syndrome in mice and men. Journal of the National Cancer Institute. *Monographs* **2008**, 64–68. [CrossRef] [PubMed]
185. Palmqvist, L.; Argiropoulos, B.; Pineault, N.; Abramovich, C.; Sly, L.M.; Krystal, G.; Wan, A.; Humphries, R.K. The Flt3 receptor tyrosine kinase collaborates with NUP98-HOX fusions in acute myeloid leukemia. *Blood* **2006**, *108*, 1030–1036. [CrossRef] [PubMed]
186. Greenblatt, S.; Li, L.; Slape, C.; Nguyen, B.; Novak, R.; Duffield, A.; Huso, D.; Desiderio, S.; Borowitz, M.J.; Aplan, P.; et al. Knock-in of a FLT3/ITD mutation cooperates with a NUP98-HOXD13 fusion to generate acute myeloid leukemia in a mouse model. *Blood* **2012**, *119*, 2883–2894. [CrossRef]
187. Giampaolo, A.; Felli, N.; Diverio, D.; Morsilli, O.; Samoggia, P.; Breccia, M.; Coco, F.L.; Peschle, C.; Testa, U. Expression pattern of HOXB6 homeobox gene in myelomonocytic differentiation and acute myeloid leukemia. *Leukemia* **2002**, *16*, 1293–1301. [CrossRef]
188. Amsellem, S.; Pflumio, F.; Bardinet, D.; Izac, B.; Charneau, P.; Roméo, P.-H.; Dubart-Kupperschmitt, A.; Fichelson, S. Ex vivo expansion of human hematopoietic stem cells by direct delivery of the HOXB4 homeoprotein. *Nat. Med.* **2003**, *9*, 1423–1427. [CrossRef]
189. Soulier, J.; Clappier, E.; Cayuela, J.-M.; Regnault, A.; García-Peydró, M.; Dombret, H.; Baruchel, A.; Toribio, M.-L.; Sigaux, F. HOXA genes are included in genetic and biologic networks defining human acute T-cell leukemia (T-ALL). *Blood* **2005**, *106*, 274–286. [CrossRef]

190. Papaemmanuil, E.; Gerstung, M.; Bullinger, L.; Gaidzik, V.I.; Paschka, P.; Roberts, N.D.; Potter, N.E.; Heuser, M.; Thol, F.; Bolli, N.; et al. Genomic Classification and Prognosis in Acute Myeloid Leukemia. *N. Engl. J. Med.* **2016**, *374*, 2209–2221. [CrossRef]
191. Mupo, A.; Celani, L.; Dovey, O.; Cooper, J.L.; Grove, C.; Rad, R.; Sportoletti, P.; Falini, B.; Bradley, A.; Vassiliou, G.S. A powerful molecular synergy between mutant Nucleophosmin and Flt3-ITD drives acute myeloid leukemia in mice. *Leukemia* **2013**, *27*, 1917–1920. [CrossRef] [PubMed]
192. Xue, L.; Pulikkan, J.A.; Valk, P.J.; Castilla, L.H. NrasG12D oncoprotein inhibits apoptosis of preleukemic cells expressing Cbfbeta-SMMHC via activation of MEK/ERK axis. *Blood* **2014**, *124*, 426–436. [CrossRef] [PubMed]
193. Dovey, O.M.; Cooper, J.L.; Mupo, A.; Grove, C.S.; Lynn, C.; Conte, N.; Andrews, R.M.; Pacharne, S.; Tzelepis, K.; Vijayabaskar, M.S.; et al. Molecular synergy underlies the co-occurrence patterns and phenotype of NPM1-mutant acute myeloid leukemia. *Blood* **2017**, *130*, 1911–1922. [CrossRef] [PubMed]
194. Ellisen, L.W.; Carlesso, N.; Cheng, T.; Scadden, D.T.; Haber, D.A. The Wilms tumor suppressor WT1 directs stage-specific quiescence and differentiation of human hematopoietic progenitor cells. *EMBO J.* **2001**, *20*, 1897–1909. [CrossRef] [PubMed]
195. Summers, K.; Stevens, J.; Kakkas, I.; Smith, M.; Smith, L.L.; MacDougall, F.; Cavenagh, J.; Bonnet, D.; Young, B.D.; Lister, T.A.; et al. Wilms' tumour 1 mutations are associated with FLT3-ITD and failure of standard induction chemotherapy in patients with normal karyotype AML. *Leukemia* **2007**, *21*, 550–551. [CrossRef] [PubMed]
196. Hou, H.-A.; Huang, T.-C.; Lin, L.-I.; Liu, C.-Y.; Chen, C.-Y.; Chou, W.-C.; Tang, J.-L.; Tseng, M.-H.; Huang, C.-F.; Chiang, Y.-C.; et al. WT1 mutation in 470 adult patients with acute myeloid leukemia: Stability during disease evolution and implication of its incorporation into a survival scoring system. *Blood* **2010**, *115*, 5222–5231. [CrossRef]
197. Annesley, C.E.; Rabik, C.; Duffield, A.S.; Rau, R.E.; Magoon, D.; Li, L.; Huff, V.; Small, D.; Loeb, D.M.; Brown, P. Knock-in of the Wt1 R394W mutation causes MDS and cooperates with Flt3/ITD to drive aggressive myeloid neoplasms in mice. *Oncotarget* **2018**, *9*, 35313–35326. [CrossRef]
198. Nara, N.; Miyamoto, T. Direct and serial transplantation of human acute myeloid leukaemia into nude mice. *Br. J. Cancer* **1982**, *45*, 778–782. [CrossRef]
199. Caretto, P.; Forni, M.; d'Orazi, G.; Scarpa, S.; Feraiorni, P.; Jemma, C.; Modesti, A.; Ferrarini, M.; Roncella, S.; Foa, R.; et al. Xenotransplantation in immunosuppressed nude mice of human solid tumors and acute leukemias directly from patients or in vitro cell lines. *Res. Clin. Lab.* **1989**, *19*, 231–243.
200. Bosma, G.C.; Custer, R.P.; Bosma, M.J. A severe combined immunodeficiency mutation in the mouse. *Nature* **1983**, *301*, 527–530. [CrossRef]
201. De Lord, C.; Clutterbuck, R.; Titley, J.; Ormerod, M.; Gordon-Smith, T.; Millar, J.; Powles, R. Growth of primary human acute leukemia in severe combined immunodeficient mice. *Exp. Hematol.* **1991**, *19*, 991–993.
202. Lapidot, T.; Sirard, C.; Vormoor, J.; Murdoch, B.; Hoang, T.; Caceres-Cortes, J.; Minden, M.; Paterson, B.; Caligiuri, M.A.; Dick, J.E. A cell initiating human acute myeloid leukaemia after transplantation into SCID mice. *Nature* **1994**, *367*, 645–648. [CrossRef] [PubMed]
203. Yan, Y.; Salomon, O.; McGuirk, J.; Dennig, D.; Fernandez, J.; Jagiello, C.; Nguyen, H.; Collins, N.; Steinherz, P.; O'Reilly, R.J. Growth pattern and clinical correlation of subcutaneously inoculated human primary acute leukemias in severe combined immunodeficiency mice. *Blood* **1996**, *88*, 3137–3146.
204. Lapidot, T.; Pflumio, F.; Doedens, M.; Murdoch, B.; Williams, D.; Dick, J. Cytokine stimulation of multilineage hematopoiesis from immature human cells engrafted in SCID mice. *Science* **1992**, *255*, 1137–1141. [CrossRef] [PubMed]
205. Goan, S.R.; Fichtner, I.; Just, U.; Karawajew, L.; Schultze, W.; Krause, K.P.; Von Harsdorf, S.; Von Schilling, C.; Herrmann, F. The severe combined immunodeficient-human peripheral blood stem cell (SCID-huPBSC) mouse: A xenotransplant model for huPBSC-initiated hematopoiesis. *Blood* **1995**, *86*, 89–100. [PubMed]
206. Cashman, J.D.; Lapidot, T.; Wang, J.C.; Doedens, M.; Shultz, L.D.; Lansdorp, P.; Dick, J.E.; Eaves, C.J. Kinetic evidence of the regeneration of multilineage hematopoiesis from primitive cells in normal human bone marrow transplanted into immunodeficient mice. *Blood* **1997**, *89*, 4307–4316.
207. Nonoyama, S.; Smith, F.O.; Bernstein, I.D.; Ochs, H.D. Strain-dependent leakiness of mice with severe combined immune deficiency. *J. Immunol.* **1993**, *150*, 3817–3824.
208. Carroll, A.M.; Hardy, R.R.; Bosma, M.J. Occurrence of mature B (IgM+, B220+) and T (CD3+) lymphocytes in scid mice. *J. Immunol.* **1989**, *143*, 1087–1093.

209. Kudo, T.; Saijyo, S.; Saeki, H.; Sato, N.; Tachibana, T.; Habu, S. Production of a Human Monoclonal Antibody to a Synthetic Peptide by Active In Vivo Immunization Using a SCID Mouse Grafted with Human Lymphocytes. *Tohoku J. Exp. Med.* **1993**, *171*, 327–338. [CrossRef]
210. Shpitz, B.; Chambers, C.A.; Singhal, A.B.; Hozumi, N.; Fernandes, B.J.; Roifman, C.M.; Weiner, L.M.; Roder, J.C.; Gallinger, S. High level functional engraftment of severe combined immunodeficient mice with human peripheral blood lymphocytes following pretreatment with radiation and anti-asialo GM. *J. Immunol. Methods* **1994**, *169*, 1–15. [CrossRef]
211. Shultz, L.D.; Schweitzer, P.A.; Christianson, S.W.; Gott, B.; Schweitzer, I.B.; Tennent, B.; McKenna, S.; Mobraaten, L.; Rajan, T.V.; Greiner, D.L. Multiple defects in innate and adaptive immunologic function in NOD/LtSz-scid mice. *J. Immunol.* **1995**, *154*, 180–191. [PubMed]
212. Bonnet, D.; Dick, J.E. Human acute myeloid leukemia is organized as a hierarchy that originates from a primitive hematopoietic cell. *Nat. Med.* **1997**, *3*, 730–737. [CrossRef] [PubMed]
213. Ailles, L.E.; Gerhard, B.; Kawagoe, H.; Hogge, D.E. Growth characteristics of acute myelogenous leukemia progenitors that initiate malignant hematopoiesis in nonobese diabetic/severe combined immunodeficient mice. *Blood* **1999**, *94*, 1761–1772. [PubMed]
214. Lumkul, R.; Gorin, N.-C.; Malehorn, M.T.; Hoehn, G.T.; Zheng, R.; Baldwin, B.; Small, D.; Gore, S.; Smith, D.; Meltzer, P.S.; et al. Human AML cells in NOD/SCID mice: Engraftment potential and gene expression. *Leukemia* **2002**, *16*, 1818–1826. [CrossRef] [PubMed]
215. Marx, J. Cancer research. Mutant stem cells may seed cancer. *Science* **2003**, *301*, 1308–1310. [CrossRef] [PubMed]
216. Ye, P.; Zhao, L.; McGirr, C.; Gonda, T.J. MYB down-regulation enhances sensitivity of U937 myeloid leukemia cells to the histone deacetylase inhibitor LBH589 in vitro and in vivo. *Cancer Lett.* **2014**, *343*, 98–106. [CrossRef] [PubMed]
217. Blair, A.; Hogge, D.E.; Sutherland, H.J. Most acute myeloid leukemia progenitor cells with long-term proliferative ability in vitro and in vivo have the phenotype CD34(+)/CD71(-)/HLA-DR. *Blood* **1998**, *92*, 4325–4335.
218. Blair, A.; Hogge, D.E.; Ailles, L.E.; Lansdorp, P.M.; Sutherland, H.J. Lack of expression of Thy-1 (CD90) on acute myeloid leukemia cells with long-term proliferative ability in vitro and in vivo. *Blood* **1997**, *89*, 3104–3112.
219. Blair, A.; Sutherland, H.J. Primitive acute myeloid leukemia cells with long-term proliferative ability in vitro and in vivo lack surface expression of c-kit (CD117). *Exp. Hematol.* **2000**, *28*, 660–671. [CrossRef]
220. Ahmed, F.; Ings, S.J.; Pizzey, A.R.; Blundell, M.P.; Thrasher, A.J.; Ye, H.T.; Fahey, A.; Linch, D.C.; Yong, K.L. Impaired bone marrow homing of cytokine-activated CD34+ cells in the NOD/SCID model. *Blood* **2004**, *103*, 2079–2087. [CrossRef]
221. Bonnet, D.; Bhatia, M.; Wang, J.C.Y.; Kapp, U.; Dick, J.E. Cytokine treatment or accessory cells are required to initiate engraftment of purified primitive human hematopoietic cells transplanted at limiting doses into NOD/SCID mice. *Bone Marrow Transplant.* **1999**, *23*, 203–209. [CrossRef] [PubMed]
222. Feuring-Buske, M.; Gerhard, B.; Cashman, J.; Humphries, R.K.; Eaves, C.J.; Hogge, D.E.; Humphries, R. Improved engraftment of human acute myeloid leukemia progenitor cells in beta 2-microglobulin-deficient NOD/SCID mice and in NOD/SCID mice transgenic for human growth factors. *Leukemia* **2003**, *17*, 760–763. [CrossRef] [PubMed]
223. Wunderlich, M.; Chou, F.-S.; Link, K.I.; Mizukawa, B.; Perry, R.L.; Carroll, M.; Mulloy, J.C. AML xenograft efficiency is significantly improved in NOD/SCID-IL2RG mice constitutively expressing human SCF, GM-CSF and IL-3. *Leukemia* **2010**, *24*, 1785–1788. [CrossRef] [PubMed]
224. Koller, B.H.; Smithies, O. Inactivating the beta 2-microglobulin locus in mouse embryonic stem cells by homologous recombination. *Proc. Natl. Acad. Sci. USA* **1989**, *86*, 8932–8935. [CrossRef] [PubMed]
225. Ito, M.; Hiramatsu, H.; Kobayashi, K.; Suzue, K.; Kawahata, M.; Hioki, K.; Ueyama, Y.; Koyanagi, Y.; Sugamura, K.; Tsuji, K.; et al. NOD/SCID/gamma(c)(null) mouse: An excellent recipient mouse model for engraftment of human cells. *Blood* **2002**, *100*, 3175–3182. [CrossRef] [PubMed]
226. Ishikawa, F.; Yasukawa, M.; Lyons, B.; Yoshida, S.; Miyamoto, T.; Yoshimoto, G.; Watanabe, T.; Akashi, K.; Shultz, L.D.; Harada, M. Development of functional human blood and immune systems in NOD/SCID/IL2 receptor {gamma} chain(null) mice. *Blood* **2005**, *106*, 1565–1573. [CrossRef] [PubMed]

227. Agliano, A.; Martin-Padura, I.; Mancuso, P.; Marighetti, P.; Rabascio, C.; Pruneri, G.; Shultz, L.D.; Bertolini, F. Human acute leukemia cells injected in NOD/LtSz-scid/IL-2Rgamma null mice generate a faster and more efficient disease compared to other NOD/scid-related strains. *Int. J. Cancer* **2008**, *123*, 2222–2227. [CrossRef] [PubMed]
228. Saland, E.; Boutzen, H.; Castellano, R.; Pouyet, L.; Griessinger, E.; Larrue, C.; de Toni, F.; Scotland, S.; David, M.; Danet-Desnoyers, G.; et al. A robust and rapid xenograft model to assess efficacy of chemotherapeutic agents for human acute myeloid leukemia. *Blood Cancer J.* **2015**, *5*, e297. [CrossRef]
229. Nabbouh, A.I.; Hleihel, R.S.; Saliba, J.L.; Karam, M.M.; Hamie, M.H.; Wu, H.-C.J.H.-C.J.M.; Berthier, C.P.; Tawil, N.M.; Bonnet, P.-A.A.; Deleuze-Masquefa, C.; et al. Imidazoquinoxaline derivative EAPB0503: A promising drug targeting mutant nucleophosmin 1 in acute myeloid leukemia. *Cancer* **2017**, *123*, 1662–1673. [CrossRef]
230. El-Houjeiri, L.; Saad, W.; Hayar, B.; Aouad, P.; Tawil, N.; Abdel-Samad, R.; Hleihel, R.; Hamie, M.; Mancinelli, A.; Pisano, C.; et al. Antitumor Effect of the Atypical Retinoid ST1926 in Acute Myeloid Leukemia and Nanoparticle Formulation Prolongs Lifespan and Reduces Tumor Burden of Xenograft Mice. *Mol. Cancer Ther.* **2017**, *16*, 2047–2057. [CrossRef]
231. Mu, H.; Konopleva, M.; Jacamo, R.; Carter, B.Z.; McQueen, T.; Andreeff, M. Comparison of Induction Chemotherapy in NSG and NOD- Rag1 ^{null} IL2rg ^{null} Mouse Models of FLT3 Mutant AML. *Blood* **2017**, *130*, 2692.
232. Cany, J.; van der Waart, A.B.; Tordoir, M.; Franssen, G.M.; Hangalapura, B.N.; de Vries, J.; Boerman, O.; Schaap, N.; van der Voort, R.; Spanholtz, J.; et al. Natural killer cells generated from cord blood hematopoietic progenitor cells efficiently target bone marrow-residing human leukemia cells in NOD/SCID/IL2Rg(null) mice. *PLoS ONE* **2013**, *8*, e64384.
233. Cany, J.; Roeven, M.W.H.; Hoogstad-van Evert, J.S.; Hobo, W.; Maas, F.; Franco Fernandez, R.; Blijlevens, N.M.A.; van der Velden, W.J.; Huls, G.; Jansen, J.H.; et al. Decitabine enhances targeting of AML cells by CD34(+) progenitor-derived NK cells in NOD/SCID/IL2Rg(null) mice. *Blood* **2018**, *131*, 202–214. [CrossRef] [PubMed]
234. Hayata, I.; Ishihara, T.; Hirashima, K.; Sado, T.; Yamagiwa, J. Partial deletion of chromosome No. 2 in myelocytic leukemias of irradiated C3H/He and RFM mice. *J. Natl. Cancer Inst.* **1979**, *63*, 843–848. [CrossRef]
235. Fredrickson, T.N.; Langdon, W.Y.; Hoffman, P.M.; Hartley, J.W.; Morse, H.C., 3rd. Histologic and cell surface antigen studies of hematopoietic tumors induced by Cas-Br-M murine leukemia virus. *J. Natl. Cancer Inst.* **1984**, *72*, 447–454. [PubMed]
236. Askew, D.S.; Bartholomew, C.; Buchberg, A.M.; Valentine, M.B.; Jenkins, N.A.; Copeland, N.G.; Ihle, J.N. His-1 and His-2: Identification and chromosomal mapping of two commonly rearranged sites of viral integration in a myeloid leukemia. *Oncogene* **1991**, *6*, 2041–2047. [PubMed]
237. Rassart, E.; Houde, J.; Denicourt, C.; Ru, M.; Barat, C.; Edouard, E.; Poliquin, L.; Bergeron, D. Molecular Analysis and Characterization of Two Myeloid Leukemia Inducing Murine Retroviruses. *Curr. Top. Microbiol. Immunol.* **1996**, *211*, 201–210. [PubMed]
238. Bergeron, D.; Poliquin, L.; Houde, J.; Barbeau, B.; Rassart, E. Analysis of proviruses integrated in Fli-1 and Evi-1 regions in Cas-Br-E MuLV-induced non-T-, non-B-cell leukemias. *Virology* **1992**, *191*, 661–669. [CrossRef]
239. Bergeron, D.; Poliquin, L.; Kozak, C.A.; Rassart, E. Identification of a common viral integration region in Cas-Br-E murine leukemia virus-induced non-T-, non-B-cell lymphomas. *J. Virol.* **1991**, *65*, 7–15.
240. Mucenski, M.L.; Taylor, B.A.; Jenkins, N.A.; Copeland, N.G. AKXD recombinant inbred strains: Models for studying the molecular genetic basis of murine lymphomas. *Mol. Cell. Boil.* **1986**, *6*, 4236–4243. [CrossRef]
241. Mucenski, M.L.; Taylor, B.A.; Ihle, J.N.; Hartley, J.W.; Morse, H.C., 3rd; Jenkins, N.A.; Copeland, N.G. Identification of a common ecotropic viral integration site, Evi-1, in the DNA of AKXD murine myeloid tumors. *Mol. Cell. Biol.* **1988**, *8*, 301–308. [CrossRef] [PubMed]
242. Fredrickson, T.N.; Silver, J.E. Susceptibility to Friend helper virus leukemias in CXB recombinant inbred mice. *J. Exp. Med.* **1983**, *158*, 1693–1702.

243. Silver, J.; Buckler, C.E. A preferred region for integration of Friend murine leukemia virus in hematopoietic neoplasms is closely linked to the Int-2 oncogene. *J. Virol.* **1986**, *60*, 1156–1158. [PubMed]
244. Chesebro, B.; Portis, J.L.; Wehrly, K.; Nishio, J. Effect of murine host genotype on MCF virus expression, latency, and leukemia cell type of leukemias induced by Friend murine leukemia helper virus. *Virology* **1983**, *128*, 221–233. [CrossRef]
245. Bordereaux, D.; Fichelson, S.; Sola, B.; Tambourin, P.E.; Gisselbrecht, S. Frequent involvement of the fim-3 region in Friend murine leukemia virus-induced mouse myeloblastic leukemias. *J. Virol.* **1987**, *61*, 4043–4045. [PubMed]
246. Nazarov, V.; Wolff, L. Novel integration sites at the distal 3' end of the c-myb locus in retrovirus-induced promonocytic leukemias. *J. Virol.* **1995**, *69*, 3885–3888. [PubMed]
247. Shen-Ong, G.L.; Wolff, L. Moloney murine leukemia virus-induced myeloid tumors in adult BALB/c mice: Requirement of c-myb activation but lack of v-abl involvement. *J. Virol.* **1987**, *61*, 3721–3725. [PubMed]
248. Bedigian, H.G.; Johnson, D.A.; Jenkins, N.A.; Copeland, N.G.; Evans, R. Spontaneous and induced leukemias of myeloid origin in recombinant inbred BXH mice. *J. Virol.* **1984**, *51*, 586–594. [PubMed]
249. Copeland, N.G.; Buchberg, A.M.; Gilbert, D.J.; Jenkins, N.A. Recombinant Inbred Mouse Strains: Models for Studying the Molecular Genetic Basis of Myeloid Tumorigenesis. *Curr. Top. Microbiol. Immunol.* **1989**, *149*, 45–57.
250. Nakamura, T.; Largaespada, D.A.; Shaughnessy, J.D.; Jenkins, N.A.; Copeland, N.G. Cooperative activation of Hoxa and Pbx1-related genes in murine myeloid leukaemias. *Nat. Genet.* **1996**, *12*, 149–153. [CrossRef]
251. Moskow, J.J.; Bullrich, F.; Huebner, K.; Daar, I.O.; Buchberg, A.M. Meis1, a PBX1-related homeobox gene involved in myeloid leukemia in BXH-2 mice. *Mol. Cell. Boil.* **1995**, *15*, 5434–5443. [CrossRef] [PubMed]
252. Li, J.; Shen, H.; Himmel, K.L.; Dupuy, A.J.; Largaespada, D.A.; Nakamura, T.; Shaughnessy, J.D.; Jenkins, N.A.; Copeland, N.G. Leukaemia disease genes: Large-scale cloning and pathway predictions. *Nat. Genet.* **1999**, *23*, 348–353. [CrossRef] [PubMed]
253. Buchberg, A.M.; Bedigian, H.G.; Jenkins, N.A.; Copeland, N.G. Evi-2, a common integration site involved in murine myeloid leukemogenesis. *Mol. Cell. Boil.* **1990**, *10*, 4658–4666. [CrossRef] [PubMed]
254. Largaespada, D.A.; Brannan, C.I.; Jenkins, N.A.; Copeland, N.G. Nf1 deficiency causes Ras-mediated granulocyte/macrophage colony stimulating factor hypersensitivity and chronic myeloid leukaemia. *Nat. Genet.* **1996**, *12*, 137–143. [CrossRef] [PubMed]
255. Tian, E.; Sawyer, J.R.; Largaespada, D.A.; Jenkins, N.A.; Copeland, N.G.; Shaughnessy, J.D. Evi27 encodes a novel membrane protein with homology to the IL17 receptor. *Oncogene* **2000**, *19*, 2098–2109. [CrossRef]
256. Peterson, L.F.; Zhang, D.-E. The 8;21 translocation in leukemogenesis. *Oncogene* **2004**, *23*, 4255–4262. [CrossRef] [PubMed]
257. Kozu, T.; Miyoshi, H.; Shimizu, K.; Maseki, N.; Kaneko, Y.; Asou, H.; Kamada, N.; Ohki, M. Junctions of the AML1/MTG8(ETO) fusion are constant in t(8;21) acute myeloid leukemia detected by reverse transcription polymerase chain reaction. *Blood* **1993**, *82*, 1270–1276.
258. Tonks, A.; Pearn, L.; Musson, M.; Gilkes, A.; Mills, K.I.; Burnett, A.K.; Darley, R.L. Transcriptional dysregulation mediated by RUNX1-RUNX1T1 in normal human progenitor cells and in acute myeloid leukaemia. *Leukemia* **2007**, *21*, 2495–2505. [CrossRef]
259. De Guzman, C.G.; Warren, A.J.; Zhang, Z.; Gartland, L.; Erickson, P.; Drabkin, H.; Hiebert, S.W.; Klug, C.A. Hematopoietic Stem Cell Expansion and Distinct Myeloid Developmental Abnormalities in a Murine Model of the AML1-ETO Translocation. *Mol. Cell. Boil.* **2002**, *22*, 5506–5517. [CrossRef]
260. Crozatier, M.; Meister, M. Drosophila haematopoiesis. *Cell. Microbiol.* **2007**, *9*, 1117–1126. [CrossRef]
261. Wildonger, J. The t(8;21) translocation converts AML1 into a constitutive transcriptional repressor. *Development* **2005**, *132*, 2263–2272. [CrossRef] [PubMed]
262. Lebestky, T. Specification of Drosophila Hematopoietic Lineage by Conserved Transcription Factors. *Science* **2000**, *288*, 146–149. [CrossRef] [PubMed]

263. Osman, D.; Gobert, V.; Ponthan, F.; Heidenreich, O.; Haenlin, M.; Waltzer, L. A Drosophila model identifies calpains as modulators of the human leukemogenic fusion protein AML1-ETO. *Proc. Natl. Acad. Sci. USA* **2009**, *106*, 12043–12048. [CrossRef] [PubMed]
264. Breig, O.; Bras, S.; Martinez Soria, N.; Osman, D.; Heidenreich, O.; Haenlin, M.; Waltzer, L. Pontin is a critical regulator for AML1-ETO-induced leukemia. *Leukemia* **2014**, *28*, 1271–1279. [CrossRef] [PubMed]

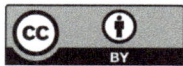

© 2019 by the authors. Licensee MDPI, Basel, Switzerland. This article is an open access article distributed under the terms and conditions of the Creative Commons Attribution (CC BY) license (http://creativecommons.org/licenses/by/4.0/).

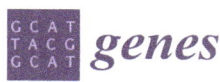

Review

Effects of Radiation Therapy on Neural Stem Cells

Anna Michaelidesová [1,2], Jana Konířová [1,2], Petr Bartůněk [1] and Martina Zíková [1,*]

[1] Laboratory of Cell Differentiation, Institute of Molecular Genetics of the Czech Academy of Sciences, v. v. i., Vídeňská 1083, 142 20 Prague 4, Czech Republic
[2] Department of Radiation Dosimetry, Nuclear Physics Institute of the Czech Academy of Sciences, v. v. i., Na Truhlářce 39/64, 180 00 Prague 8, Czech Republic
[*] Correspondence: mzikova@img.cas.cz; Tel.: +420-241063113

Received: 13 June 2019; Accepted: 22 August 2019; Published: 24 August 2019

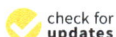

Abstract: Brain and nervous system cancers in children represent the second most common neoplasia after leukemia. Radiotherapy plays a significant role in cancer treatment; however, the use of such therapy is not without devastating side effects. The impact of radiation-induced damage to the brain is multifactorial, but the damage to neural stem cell populations seems to play a key role. The brain contains pools of regenerative neural stem cells that reside in specialized neurogenic niches and can generate new neurons. In this review, we describe the advances in radiotherapy techniques that protect neural stem cell compartments, and subsequently limit and prevent the occurrence and development of side effects. We also summarize the current knowledge about neural stem cells and the molecular mechanisms underlying changes in neural stem cell niches after brain radiotherapy. Strategies used to minimize radiation-related damages, as well as new challenges in the treatment of brain tumors are also discussed.

Keywords: neural stem cells; brain and nervous system cancers; neurogenic niches; radiotherapy; sparing of neurogenic regions

1. Introduction

During 2018, 17 million new cancer cases and 9.6 million cancer-associated deaths were reported worldwide [1]. According to the International Agency for Research on Cancer, the worldwide estimated incidence of brain and nervous system cancers in 2018 for both sexes and all ages was 3.5 per 100,000 population, being the 18th most common cancer site [2]. The incidence of brain and nervous system cancers for both sexes and ages from 0 to 19 years old was 1.2 per 100,000, making it the second most common cancer site after leukemia for this age group [2].

Primary brain tumors can be divided into several categories, such as tumors of neuroepithelial tissue (e.g., astrocytoma, glioblastoma), ependymal, choroid plexus, pineal parenchymal, embryonal (medulloblastoma), meningeal tumors, and primary central nervous system (CNS) lymphomas [3]. The most commonly diagnosed CNS tumors, occurring as much as 10 times more frequently than primary malignant brain tumors, are intracranial or brain metastases (BM) [4,5]. Brain metastases are mostly connected to lung, breast, colon, and skin (melanoma) primary cancers [4–7]; they occur in approximately 30% of all cancer patients [8], and most of the BM patients develop multiple intracranial BMs [9]. They are mostly located at the gray–white matter, with 80% occurrence in the cerebral hemispheres, 15% in the cerebellum, and 5% in the brainstem [9].

There are several options for cancer treatment including surgery, chemotherapy, immunotherapy, hormonotherapy, radiotherapy, and others. Selection of the most appropriate treatment strategy depends on several parameters, such as the cancer site/type and stage [10]. In general, radiotherapy seems to be an appropriate treatment in more than 50% of all cancer patients [11] and it is, next to surgery, the standard treatment strategy for most primary CNS malignancies and BMs [7,12].

Chemotherapeutic treatment of CNS tumors is hampered by the blood–brain barrier (BBB), which protects the brain from exposure to toxins, and, thus– blocks the entry of many water-soluble drugs from the blood into the brain parenchyma [7,13]. One of the most studied proteins that play a significant role in the BBB is efflux transporter permeability glycoprotein, also known as ATP-binding cassette sub-family B member 1 (ABCB1) [12]. It was shown that inhibition of this protein in in vivo models increases the brain penetration of several chemotherapeutic agents [14–17]. Unfortunately, clinical trials using permeability glycoprotein inhibitors showed unacceptable toxicities and were terminated early [18]. More recently, inhibition of a related protein, breast cancer resistance protein ABCG2, was found to increase the permeability of BBB in the mouse [19], thus identifying an alternative molecular target for potential adjuvant therapy. Radiotherapy can also disrupt the BBB, increasing the penetration of chemotherapeutic agents to the brain [13,20–22]. Due to this effect of radiotherapy, it is often beneficial to use a combination of radiotherapy and chemotherapy, known as chemoradiotherapy [23,24].

Brain radiotherapy improves the lives of cancer patients and concurrently, advances in these techniques allow a significant increase in the proportion of patient survivors. However, the use of these therapies is not without devastating side effects that impact the patients' autonomy, as well as their social and professional life. Although the effect of radiation-induced damage to the brain is multifactorial, injury to the neural stem cell (NSC) compartments and damage to NSC populations is hypothesized to be central to the pathogenesis of radiation-induced cognitive decline. Sensitivity of NSC compartments to radiation has been extensively studied using rodent models, also permitting the study of possible links between cancer therapy and the onset of cognitive deficits.

2. Radiotherapy Techniques

2.1. Techniques for Delivering Radiation Therapy

The main aim of radiotherapy is to destroy cancer cells while causing minimal damage to the surrounding healthy tissues. Indeed, this is not always possible, and in some cases even not applicable, for example during total body or whole brain irradiation.

Radiotherapy can be divided into external and internal. In external radiotherapy, ionizing radiation is delivered to the patient's body using external beams consisting of either photons, electrons, neutrons, protons, or other ions (e.g., carbons). Internal radiotherapy can be divided into brachytherapy and nuclear medicine. In brachytherapy, small sources of ionizing radiation are delivered inside or to the proximity of the tumor [25], and, in the case of nuclear medicine, radiopharmaceutical agents are delivered into the patient's body using specialized molecular vehicles [26].

The therapeutic dose is mostly delivered to the patients in several doses (so-called fractionation). This means that the patient is not irradiated in one session, but the dose is delivered in parts. It was shown that the time needed for the repair of cancer cells is longer than in case of normal (healthy) cells. This means that by using multiple optimally spaced irradiation sessions, normal cells will have time to repair and the cancer cells will be preferentially eliminated [27]. Another factor that makes fractionation beneficial is the cell cycle dependency of cellular radiosensitivity. In an asynchronous cell population, cells in M phase will be more likely killed by radiation than cells in G_1 or S phase. Thus, irradiating cancer cells in more than one session increases the probability of their elimination [28].

In general, irradiation limited to cancer cells only is impossible. The radiation is usually directed to a restricted body volume (defined by the physician), which is selected based on the tumor histology and location. Most used for external radiotherapy are photon beams (X-rays). These X-rays are generated inside a clinical linear accelerator (LINAC). A wide X-ray beam is then extracted from the LINAC for patient irradiations. The LINACs are able to rotate around the patient and are equipped with collimators that reduce the size of the photon beam to a square region that through an additional collimation system, mostly a Multi-leaf collimator (MLC), can be adjusted to copy the treatment volume shape.

In most cases, the treatment dose is not delivered from one direction only, but sophisticated treatment planning systems are used for the calculation of the most appropriate dose distributions. The treatment plan is always constructed based on the actual patient's anatomy obtained mostly by computed tomography. Recently, a large percentage of treatment plans are prepared using the approach of intensity-modulated radiotherapy (IMRT), where the dose is delivered using non-uniform beams by the use of MLC from multiple directions. This approach enables the physician to achieve delivery of the full treatment dose only within the designated treatment volume, with maximal sparing of the healthy tissues [29].

2.2. Brain Radiotherapy

In case of brain tumors, the whole brain, or only parts of it, can be irradiated [30]. Whole brain radiation therapy (WBRT) has been routinely used since the 1960s in cases of multiple BMs [31,32]. As the incidence of BM in NSC regions was found to be low, sparing of the neurogenic compartments could help reducing the neurocognitive decline observed after WBRT [31]. The neurogenic niches can be spared using the above-mentioned IMRT techniques based on photons or alternatively, delivering protons using the pencil-beam scanning (PBS) mode [33]. In PBS, it is possible to irradiate the patient's volume using a thin pencil beam, which is redirected using magnets to smaller sub-volumes of the total volume to facilitate more conformal irradiation while sparing healthy tissues.

Although shown to prolong a patient's life, WBRT is also associated with several side effects such as hair loss, skin irritation, nausea, hearing loss, cerebral edema, radionecrosis, neurological deterioration, cognitive and endocrine dysfunctions, and dementia [32,34]. Less side effects were observed when using stereotactic radiosurgery (SR). During SR, a high dose is delivered using multiple focused beams to the brain regions where metastases are located. This can be achieved by the use of modified LINACs, i.e., use of stereotactic tubes or microMLC in order to restrict the beam size to a smaller area, multiple ^{60}Co sources from several directions (Gammaknife), or robotic LINAC (Cyberknife). Stereotactic radiosurgery is in general less invasive and is mostly executed in one session due to the possibility to irradiate small tissue volumes and minimally affect the healthy tissues [32]. In many cases, SR can be used instead of surgery in combination with WBRT [35], or as an adjuvant therapeutic strategy after resection of the metastases [8]. In addition to these external beam techniques, radioactive sources can be implanted into the tumor cavity during surgery (intracranial brachytherapy) [8,25]. These radioactive implants can be placed into the patient permanently or temporarily. As temporary implants necessitate an additional surgery, permanent implants are more preferred [8].

In external radiotherapy and brachytherapy, cancer cells cannot be irradiated selectively, but always a targeted volume is irradiated, which contains healthy cells as well. However, nuclear medicine offers the possibility to treat cancer using targeted radiotherapy. During targeted radiotherapy, molecular vehicles are used to selectively deliver a radionuclide to malignant cell populations [26]. For example, glioblastoma multiforme cells highly express G protein-coupled receptor neurokinin 1, so a modified substance P as its ligand (^{213}Bi-DOTA-Substance P, where ^{213}Bi is a short-range alpha particle emitter) can be used for targeting neurokinin type 1 receptor-producing cells [36]. The used radionuclides mostly emit electrons with a range of a few millimeters, or they can emit alpha particles with a range of only a few cell diameters [26]. The low range of these beta and alpha emitters, respectively, reduces irradiation of the healthy tissues and thus the unwanted side effects of radiotherapy.

2.3. Side Effects of Radiation Therapy

The unwanted side effects of radiation therapy can be divided into three categories: acute, subacute, and late [37]. Acute effects are mostly caused by BBB disruption leading to cerebral edema, and they may be improved using corticosteroid medications [38–40]. These effects occur during the first few weeks of radiotherapy and are characterized by drowsiness, headache, fever, nausea, and vomiting [39,40]. Subacute effects occur one to six months post-irradiation, and they include several symptoms such as headache, somnolence, weakness, anorexia, and aggravation of preexisting deficits [39,40]. Late effects are mostly irreversible, and they appear more than six months after the treatment and are associated with white matter damage caused by vascular injuries, demyelination, or radiation-induced necrosis [39–41]. These effects can be mild, such as tiredness, or significant, such as memory loss, dementia [39], leukoencephalopathy [42], and secondary-induced brain tumors (meningioma, glioma, sarcoma) [40]. Importantly, late effects are even more severe for pediatric patients; childhood cancer survivors are increasingly predisposed to cognitive deficits [33,43]. It was observed that long-term survivors of brain cancer irradiations in childhood suffer losses in intelligence quotient, learning disabilities, hormonal deficits, growth and psychomotor retardation [38]. Some of these pathological states are associated with the radiation damage to the neurogenic niche, which is involved in memory formation, spatial processing, and mood regulation [44].

3. Neural Stem Cells

The adult brain has long been considered limited in its regenerative capacity; it was believed that neurogenesis ceased after development. However, over 50 years ago, this concept was changed after neurogenesis in the adult mammalian brain was discovered [45]. Since then, enormous progress has been made in the understanding of this process. Neural stem cells are undifferentiated cells that are defined by their replicative potential and their ability to differentiate into multiple neuronal and glial cell types, as well as their capacity for long-term self-renewal. The adult brain contains two NSC pools located in the sub-ventricular zone of the lateral ventricles (V-SVZ) [46] and the dentate gyrus of the hippocampus [47]. Both NSC pools produce new neurons that can integrate into functional circuits [48,49]. Although high proliferative capacity is a feature of the 'stemness", another unique characteristic of NSCs is their ability to stay dormant for long periods, providing a reserve pool of cells available for tissue regeneration throughout life [50]. As radiotherapy exerts its effect on dividing cells, leading them to stop proliferation, the cognitive decline in patients indicates a dysfunction in mitotically active NSCs.

Most of the findings on NSC behavior derive from studies in rodent models, and the knowledge about NSCs in human brain is still very limited. Whether neurogenesis in humans exists has been investigated using various approaches, such as BrdU incorporation [51] and carbon dating [52], and has brought conclusive evidence about the presence of adult neurogenesis in the human brain. However, two recently published reports with opposite conclusions have reopened discussion concerning the existence of human adult hippocampal neurogenesis. Sorrells et al. [53] reported that there is no evidence of hippocampal neurogenesis in humans after adolescence, while Boldrini et al. [54] demonstrated the opposite by showing that adult neurogenesis persists during life, although with a small decrease with aging. Comparative analyses of adult neurogenesis have uncovered a large variance in this phenomenon among different species [55]. The neurogenesis in the V-SZV niche differs between humans and mice, based on the cell types that form this area [56]. Also, newly formed neural progenitors in this zone have distinct fates, becoming medium spiny neurons in human striatum [57], instead of forming olfactory interneurons as in mice [58].

Studies in the adult mouse brain demonstrated that NSCs are not homogenous cells, but rather a combination of distinct subpopulations recognizable mainly by their state of quiescence or activation. Neural stem cells display regional heterogeneity, which is acquired from their embryonic origin and niche patterning. Neural stem cells in the adult V-SZV niche originate from a subpopulation of embryonic radial glial cells, which became specified during development and maintain their quiescence until reactivation in adulthood [59]. Current progress in single-cell transcriptomics provides extremely useful information about the different states of NSCs and suggests a high degree of transcriptional dynamics throughout these states. Multiple molecular markers are currently used to distinguish particular NSC subsets, which in combination with the use of transgenic mice, flow cytometry, and single-cell RNA sequencing, reveal the complexity within the NSC population. Purification of V-SZV NSCs revealed four types of cells: dormant NSCs, quiescent NSCs (qNSCs), activated NSCs (aNSCs), and progenitor cells (NPCs). Most NSCs are qNSCs that express glial fibrillary acidic protein (GFAP) and prominin-1 (PROM1) markers. These cells give rise to activated, cycling and epidermal growth factor receptor (EGFR)-positive aNSCs, which differentiate into highly proliferative NPCs and finally to neuroblasts [60–63] (Figure 1).

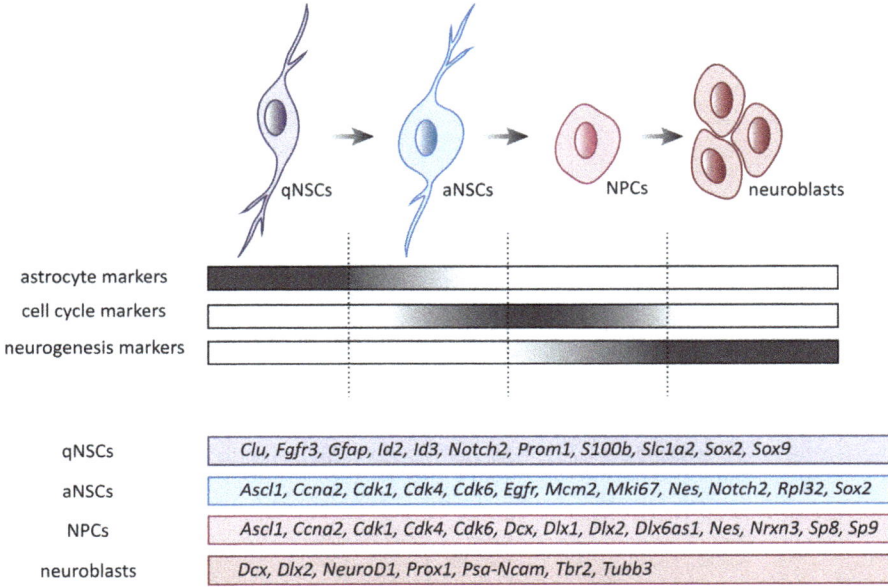

Figure 1. Cell subtypes involved in progression from quiescent neural stem cells (qNSCs) to neuroblasts. Schematic representation of lineage progression. QNSCs give rise to activated neural stem cells (aNSCs), which differentiate into highly proliferative progenitor cells (NPCs) and finally to neuroblasts. Expression of key genes related to particular cell subtypes is depicted. *Ascl1*, achaete-scute family bHLH transcription factor 1; *Ccna2*, cyclin A2; *Cdk1*, cyclin dependent kinase 1; *Cdk4*, cyclin dependent kinase 4; *Cdk6*, cyclin dependent kinase 6; *Clu*, clusterin; Dcx, doublecortin; *Dlx1*, distal-less homeobox 1; *Dlx2*, distal-less homeobox 2; *Dlx6as1*, distal-less homeobox 6, opposite strand 1; *Egfr*, epidermal growth factor receptor; *Gfap*, glial fibrillary acidic protein; *Id2*, inhibitor of DNA binding 2; *Id3*, inhibitor of DNA binding 3; *Mcm2*, minichromosome maintenance complex component 2; *Mki67*, antigen identified by monoclonal antibody Ki-67; *Nes*, nestin; *NeuroD1*, neurogenic differentiation 1; *Notch2*, notch 2; *Nrxn3*, neurexin 3; *Prom1*, prominin-1; *Prox1*, prospero homeobox 1; *Psa-Ncam*, polysialylated neural cell adhesion molecule; *Rpl32*, ribosomal protein L32; *S100b*, S100 protein, beta polypeptide, neural; *Slc1a2*, solute carrier family 1 (glial high affinity glutamate transporter), member 2; *Sox2*, SRY (sex determining region Y)-box 2; *Sox9*, SRY (sex determining region Y)-box 9; *Sp8*, trans-acting transcription factor 8; *Sp9*, trans-acting transcription factor 9; *Tbr2*, eomesodermin; *Tubb3*, tubulin, beta 3 class III.

Moreover, additional subpopulations in intermediate states have recently been discovered. Pseudotemporal ordering, based on single-cell transcription profiling data, revealed three subpopulations of aNSCs, which exhibit differential expression of specific genes, placing these subpopulations in a continuum between quiescence and activation [64]. In addition, single-cell RNA sequencing in dentate gyrus revealed that hippocampal NSCs also exhibit molecular heterogeneity [65].

The adult mouse brain contains two neurogenic niches located in V-SVZ and the dentate gyrus of the hippocampus. The neurogenic niche is a microenvironment supporting and nourishing NSCs through the secretion of local factors, nutrients and oxygen necessary for their maintenance. Local stimuli from the niche, as well as circulating blood factors can affect the NSC state and differentiation potential, and in consequence, neurogenesis in adult brain [66] (Figure 2).

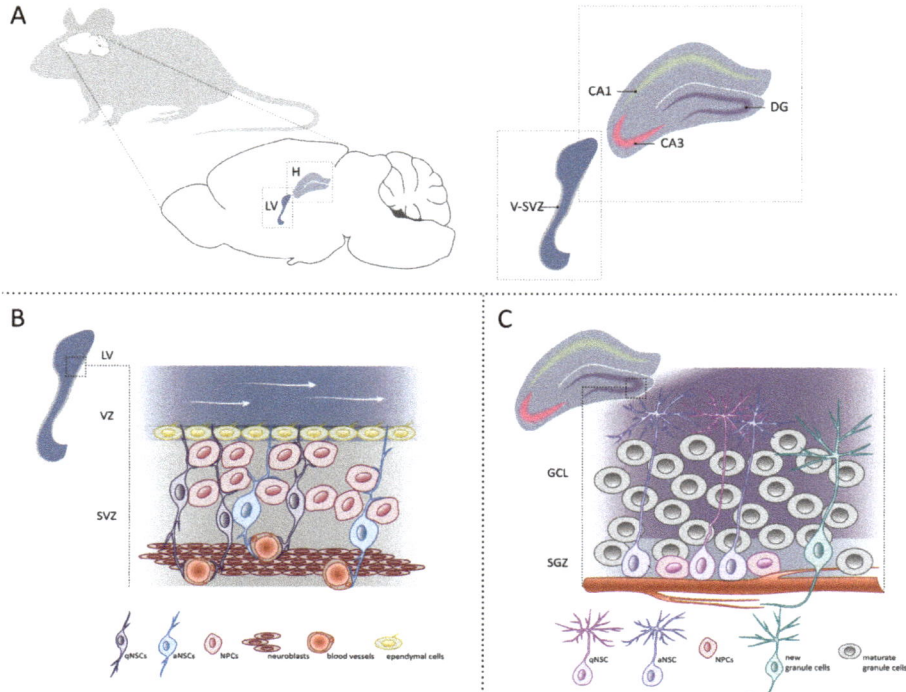

Figure 2. Neurogenesis in adult mouse brain. (**A**) Sagittal view of adult mouse brain focusing on two neurogenic niches where NSCs reside—the ventricular-subventricular zone (V-SVZ) of the lateral ventricle (LV) and dentate gyrus (DG) of the hippocampus (H). Cornu Ammonis 1 (CA1) and Cornu Ammonis 3 (CA3) subfields of the hippocampus are depicted. (**B**) Schematic representation of the organization and composition of the adult mouse V-SVZ niche. qNSCs share many characteristics with aNSCs, including contact with blood vessels. White arrows show the flow of the cerebrospinal fluid. (**C**) Schematic representation of the cell types present in the mouse subgranular zone (SGZ) and granule cell layer (GCL) in the dentate gyrus of the hippocampus.

Adult NSCs also receive feedback signals from cells at later stages in the lineage. For instance, neuroblasts secrete non-synaptic γ-aminobutyric acid (GABA) that binds to GABA type A receptor (GABA$_A$R) expressed by qNSCs and inhibits their proliferation [67,68]. Interestingly, it was also shown that adult neurogenesis could be modulated depending on hunger or satiety, via hypothalamic control. The hypothalamus, a brain area regulating physiological states, provides long-range signals to the V-SZV niche and promotes proliferation of specific NSC populations [69].

4. Molecular Mechanism Underlying Brain Radiotherapy

The cytotoxicity caused by radiation is mainly the result of DNA damage. Radiation induces several forms of DNA damage, which include single-strand breaks, double-strand breaks, sugar and base modification, and DNA-protein crosslinking [70]. Among these, double-strand breaks are the dominant form of damage caused by ionizing radiation that when unrepaired can lead to lethality of cells [71]. In response to DNA damage, cell cycle checkpoints become activated to block cell cycle progression, allowing cells to repair the damage [72]. Depending on the phase of the cell cycle at which cells are damaged, the cells can be blocked at either the G_1/S or G_2/M checkpoints. If the damage is irreversible, apoptosis, programmed cell death, is triggered to eliminate the injured cells. Apoptosis after irradiation has been described in both neurogenic niches of experimental animals. Radiotherapy kills proliferating cells in V-SVZ of the brain in young adult rats [73]; similarly, apoptosis occurs in dentate gyrus of the adult rat hippocampus [74,75].

Radiation therapy reduces adult neurogenesis through two mechanisms. Ionizing radiation, by inducing acute apoptosis in dividing cells, reduces the pool of mitotic NSCs, mainly aNSCs and NPCs, and consequently reduces generation of new neurons [76,77]. However, at moderate doses of irradiation, proliferation in the V-SZV niche restarts 2–3 days after exposure by recruiting qNSCs [73,78]. Similar effects of irradiation on neurogenesis recovery have been reported in the hippocampus following moderate dose exposure [79]. A key feature of NSCs is their proliferative capacity that ensures regeneration of damaged tissue through the activation of qNSCs [61,78]. A vast majority of slowly dividing qNSCs survive a moderate dose of radiation exposure and enter the cell cycle to regenerate the irradiated neurogenic niche [78]. Transcriptomic analysis of qNSCs sorted from the V-SVZ zone of 2-month-old mice revealed that genes upregulated after whole-brain irradiation are mainly associated with cell cycle, DNA/RNA processes, translation, and ribosomal activity [80]. This illustrates the transcriptomic shift of irradiated qNSCs towards cell cycle entry. Interestingly, gene set enrichment analysis also showed enrichment in genes associated with the tricarboxylic acid cycle and respiratory electron transport, indicating that the cell cycle entry of qNSCs after radiation was accompanied by a shift toward an oxidative metabolism. Furthermore, it was shown that the $GABA_AR$ signaling regulates qNSC cell cycle entry by using specific $GABA_AR$ agonists/antagonists and that the radiation-induced depletion of neuroblasts, the major GABA source, provokes qNSCs to exit quiescence in the irradiated V-SVZ [78].

Radiation exposure of neonatal brain has been shown not only to diminish the cognitive function, but also to enhance carcinogenesis. The analysis shows that juvenile mouse V-SZV has a larger number of proliferating progenitors than the adult brain [81,82]. However, the neonatal progenitor cells have diminished ability to undergo proliferative arrest compared to adult progenitors and recover the proliferative capacity more rapidly. Thus, neuroblasts in neonates are derived from irradiated proliferating cells, and this may influence the level of genomic DNA alterations they contain and consequently their ability to become carcinogenic [81].

Another mechanism that affects neurogenesis after radiation exposure are changes within the NSC microenvironment. The exposure to high doses causes permanent inhibition of proliferation and neurogenesis in the neurogenic niche [83], which is a direct consequence of the changes in the NSC niche [84,85]. Even if qNSCs survive irradiation and, thus, are potentially able to reconstitute neurogenesis, such regeneration may be counteracted by sustained inflammation and vascular damage in the stem cell niche. Radiation may also lead to premature differentiation of neural precursors and adoption of glial fate [84,86,87]. After high doses of radiation, the neurogenic niche is chronically altered and generates a hostile environment. Experiments demonstrated that irradiated neuronal precursors are able to differentiate in vitro, but transplanted non-irradiated precursors cells are unable to differentiate in an irradiated hippocampus [84]. This illustrates that the alteration of neurogenesis that occurs following irradiation is largely due to modifications of the neurogenic niche. In irradiated mice, a marked increase in transforming growth factor β1 (TGF-β1) production by endothelial cells in the stem cell niche was observed. The increased synthesis of TGF-β1 by brain endothelial cells provokes qNSC dormancy and increases susceptibility of proliferative NSCs to apoptosis [85]. In co-cultures, irradiated brain endothelial cells induce apoptosis of NSCs via TGF-β/Smad3 signaling. Interestingly, the inhibition of TGF-β signaling improves neurogenesis in irradiated mice by preventing apoptosis of neural progenitors and by inducing proliferation of NSCs, and, consequently, restores production of new neurons [85].

Although radiation kills proliferating cells in both neurogenic niches, differential recovery of NSCs in V-SVZ and dentate gyrus of the hippocampus after moderate doses has been reported in the brains of young rats. While an initial response to radiation injury is similar in both neurogenic niches, the long-term effect on NSCs and neurogenesis in these two areas differs significantly. The dentate gyrus of the hippocampus is severely affected in the long term, whereas V-SVZ appears to recover with time [88].

Cranial irradiation not only affects the NSC populations, but also causes vascular damage. Irradiation disrupts the vasculature of the niche, reduces the microvessel area, the number of microvessels and the number of microvessel branching points in the hippocampus of young mice [89]. Proliferative neural precursor cells tend to be clustered around vessels [90]. This association is lost in the irradiated hippocampus, where the distance between microvessels and the resident NSC population is increased [84,91].

A microglial inflammatory response accompanied by an abnormal increase of cytokines occurs in NSC niches after brain radiation exposure and, in consequence, negatively affects neurogenesis and cognition. Microglia do not originate from NSCs, but differentiate through the monocyte lineage from hematopoietic stem cells and act as the resident macrophages of the central nervous system. Rola et al. [92] observed that after irradiation, reduced neurogenesis within the dentate gyrus of young mice occurs in conjunction with a chronic inflammatory reaction. An increase in the number of microglia present in the brain is correlated with increased radiation doses [93]. Whole-brain irradiation induces regionally specific pro-inflammatory environments with elevated expression of cytokines, including tumor necrosis factor α, interleukin 1 β and monocyte chemotactic protein 1 [94] (Figure 3).

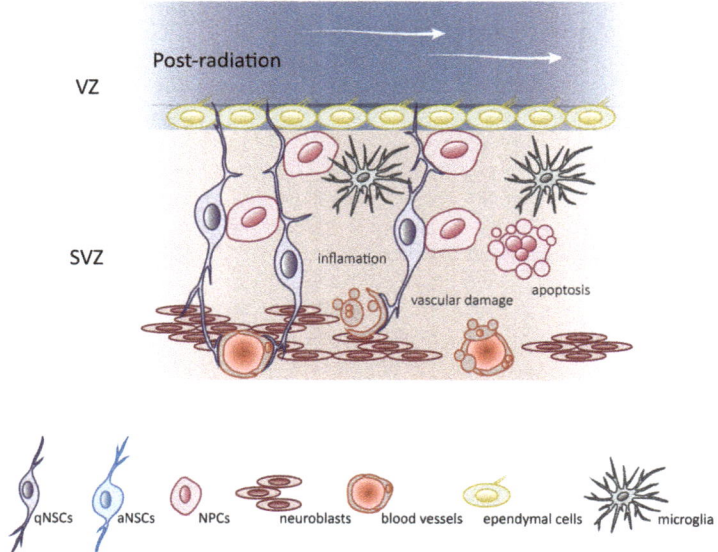

Figure 3. Radiation disrupts the V-SVZ niche. Schematic representation of mice V-SVZ niche after radiation. Following radiation, the V-SVZ niche shows a depletion of proliferating aNSCs, NPCs, and neuroblasts, a vascular damage and an increase in the number of microglia. Compare with schematic representation of mice V-SVZ niche in a pre-radiation condition (Figure 2B).

5. Strategies to Minimize Radiation-Related Damages in the Neurogenic Niche

The high-precision technologies that individualize target volume and dose of radiation therapy are increasingly used to limit injury to neurogenic niches. These techniques have been described above; we mention for example SR that is increasingly used technique with mild toxicity to patients [95]. Similarly, PBT offers the potential to minimize late-onset damages [96]; maximal sparing of the healthy tissues also ensures the using of IMRT technology [29].

Much effort is currently dedicated to find pre-irradiation treatments that may prevent the negative effects of radiation on the niche and NSCs. This is particularly important in the course of irradiation of the juvenile brain, where the consequences are more severe in comparison to irradiation of the adult brain. Lithium was shown to reduce damage and enhance neurogenesis, and has been explored as a pre-treatment option. Pre-irradiation administration of lithium resulted in reduced apoptosis and microglial activation [97,98]. Lithium increases proliferation of hippocampal NSCs and rescues radiation-induced cell cycle arrest in vitro. Treatment with 3mM LiCl was sufficient to increase NSCs in S phase, boost neurosphere growth, and reduce DNA damage [99]. It was shown that much of the lithium effect in hippocampal progenitors is attributable to the activation of Wnt canonical pathway by inhibition of glycogen synthase kinase 3 [100]. Another neuroprotective agent that can be a useful supplement to hippocampal sparing is natural polyphenol resveratrol. Resveratrol was shown to inhibit radiation-induced apoptosis in the hippocampus [101] and has a neuroprotective effect on irradiated NSCs in hippocampal slice cultures [102]. The resveratrol's neuroprotective effect was dependent on its ability to selectively induce expression of mitochondrial superoxide dismutase, enzyme whose function is to clear mitochondrial reactive oxygen species and, as a result, to reduce oxidative stress and damage [103]. Several studies demonstrated that melatonin, a regulator of circadian rhythm produced in the pineal gland, appeared to ameliorate radiation-induced injury in various organs of rats [104]. Melatonin is known to be an effective antioxidant that scavenges free radicals produced by radiation before they induce DNA damage, and it also stimulates activities of antioxidant enzymes [105]. It was shown that melatonin has a protective effect on NSCs against lipopolysaccharide-induced inflammation [106], decreases apoptosis, and upregulates neural stem cell marker nestin in the V-SZV zone of irradiated rats [107].

Neuroinflammation is a significant component of the brain's response to radiation. Interleukin 6, a mediator of the inflammatory response produced by microglia, was found to block neuronal differentiation of hippocampal NSCs, and administering a common nonsteroidal anti-inflammatory drug indomethacin to irradiated rats partly restored neurogenesis [108]. Jenrow et al. [109] administered pro-inflammatory cytokine production inhibitor MW-151 following irradiation and demonstrated a treatment-induced increase in migratory neuroblasts within the dentate gyrus of the hippocampus of adult rats. The peroxisomal proliferator-activated receptors (PPARs) are ligand-activated transcription factors [110], which have been shown to confer neuroprotection in a variety of models [111]. Administration of PPARα agonist fenofibrate preserved hippocampal neurogenesis and prevented radiation-induced cognitive impairment [112,113]; the application of pioglitazone, the PPARγ agonist, significantly recovered cognitive impairment in irradiated rats [114]. Furthermore, radiation-induced impairment of hippocampal neurogenesis in rats was mitigated by using combined administration of avorvastatin and angiotensin converting enzyme inhibitor ramipril [115].

The effect of selective inhibition of autophagy on NSCs in the dentate gyrus after cerebral irradiation was studied using mice with neural-specific deletion of autophagy related 7 gene, which is involved in autophagy induction and autophagosome formation. Selective inhibition of autophagy reduced radiation-induced cell death and caspase-dependent apoptosis in the dentate gyrus and cerebellum; moreover, the levels of pro-inflammatory cytokines decreased [116]. These results suggest that autophagy might be another potential target for preventing radiotherapy-induced cell death and its associated long-term effects.

A new strategy that could be used to prevent radiation-induced injury is stem cell therapy. As cranial irradiation induces progressive depletion of NSCs, the use of NSCs replacement constitutes a novel alternative to combat radiation-induced cognitive decline. Studies demonstrated that irradiated rats engrafted with human NSCs (hNSCs) showed less decline in cognition when compared to irradiated animals. Transplantation promotes not only early, but also long-term recovery of the irradiated brain [117,118]. However, there are concerns regarding stem cell use due to the possibility of teratoma formation and immune rejection, which subsequently requires immunosuppression [119]. The hNSC-derived microvesicles then provide attractive alternatives to stem cells, avoiding teratoma formation in the brain and minimizing the host graft rejection. It was shown that cranial grafting of microvesicles secreted from hNSCs attenuates neuroinflammation and preserves the structural integrity of the irradiated microenviroment and consequently improves cognition of irradiated rats [120]. The supplementation of whole brain irradiated mice with fetal mouse NSCs, injected via the tail vein, led to exogenous NSCs differentiation into neuronal and glial lineages but moreover, NSCs also differentiated into brain endothelial cells, which was accompanied by the restoration of cerebral blood flow [121]. Radiation-related symptoms cannot be attributed only to the disruption of neurogenesis. Brain irradiation damages brain white matter and causes demyelination and oligodendrocytes have been investigated to be a target of high-dose radiation [122]. Oligodendrocyte progenitors, derived from human pluripotent stem cells and grafted to rat's forebrain, were able to remyelinate the irradiated brain and to rescue animal's cognitive deficits. Additional recovery from motor deficits requires concomitant oligodendrocyte progenitors transplantation into the cerebellum [123]. The effects of intranasal administration of human mesenchymal stem cells (hMSCs), as a neuroprotective strategy for cranial irradiation, was investigated by Soria et al. [124]. The transplantation of hMSCs alters the gene expression profile of irradiated brain, modulates genetic pathways associated with inflammation, immune system and cell motility, and reduces oxidative damage and neuronal loss in brains of irradiated mice. The authors demonstrated that intranasally delivered hMSCs promote radiation-induced brain injury repair and improved neurological function, and suggest the therapeutic use of hMSCs as a non-invasive approach to prevent neurological complications of radiotherapy.

Additional strategies that promise to support the treatment of brain tumors are metabolic therapies, such as caloric restriction, intermittent fasting or a ketogenic diet [125]. Current treatment of primary brain cancers utilizes a multifactorial approach involving maximal safe resection, followed by radiotherapy and simultaneous chemotherapy [126]. Under normal physiological conditions, brain cells obtain energy from either glucose or ketones. Tumor cells rely preferentially on anaerobic glycolysis rather than on respiration, a phenomenon known as the Warburg effect [127]. High glucose levels accelerate brain tumor growth and angiogenesis while preventing apoptosis [128]. A strong dependence on glucose renders cancer cells vulnerable to therapy that targets glucose metabolism. The restricted diet is, thus, well suited as a non-toxic metabolic therapy for the treatment of malignant brain cancers as demonstrated in many case reports [129–131]. Moreover, it has been demonstrated that chemotherapy and high-dose radiation, used in the treatment of brain tumors, creates a tumor microenviroment that is rich in glucose and glutamine and this can further contribute to tumor progression [132]. In the tumor microenviroment, the neoplastic cell populations are associated with macrophages/monocytes cells. These associated cell populations contribute to tumor progression through the release of pro-inflammatory and pro-angiogenic factors [132–134]. Nevertheless, several studies in rodents demonstrated that caloric restriction not only leads to reduced tumor growth but also mitigates inflammation, improves macrophages function [135], and lowers cytokines expression [136].

6. Concluding Remarks

Whether hippocampal neurogenesis persists throughout life in the human brain is not fully resolved. It was believed that the human hippocampus continues to generate new neurons, but a report by Sorrells et al. [53] concluded that neurogenesis does not continue in the human adult hippocampus, or is extremely rare. Moreover, this study also reminds us that simple translation of results from animal studies to humans may be problematic. On the contrary, persistent hippocampal neurogenesis was demonstrated in aging brains and detected in patients with mild cognitive impairments and Alzheimer's disease [137,138]. Importantly, a study by Tobin et al. [137] also provided evidence that the extent of neurogenesis, particularly the number of newly forming neurons, is associated with better cognitive diagnosis. Nevertheless, they also showed that the number of neuroblasts greatly varied between individuals. The evidence for adult neurogenesis in the human brain comes from studies using thymidine analogs that are incorporated into the DNA of dividing cells, and from studies that only used immunohistochemistry to detect cell proliferation markers in human postmortem brains. It should be emphasized that there are many potential technical obstacle to studying post mortem brain tissues. One of them is the post mortem brain interval which can have deleterious effect on brain antigenicity and should be taken into consideration during tissue selection for analysis. Another important limitation that applies to studies of human neurogenesis are fixation time and tissue processing, the limitation of antibodies and marker specificity and interpersonal variability of marker expression. To finally resolve if neurogenesis persists in the human adult brain will need a more complete analysis by using for example, single-cell RNA sequencing, standardization of methodologies and the creation of an open-access brain bank from a large cohort of patients [139,140].

The human brain tumors classification is currently based mainly on microscopic morphology and immunochemistry; nevertheless, many tumors are characterized by a distinct molecular signature which enables their genomic classification. For instance, medulloblastomas comprise an explicit subgroup with distinct molecular characteristics [141,142] and provide a clear example of how a detailed understanding of genomics can guide the treatment procedure. Evidence that medulloblastomas, which display active Wnt-signaling pathway, lacks the blood–brain barrier and, therefore, are highly vulnerable to chemotherapy [143] led to a series of studies testing reduced-intensity radiotherapy in patients with this disease subtype [144]. This also shows that although recent technical advances in radiotherapy allow localized and concentrated treatment, reducing of radiotherapy for some types of brain tumors is one of the main challenges [144,145].

Although it is difficult to examine adult neurogenesis in humans, postnatal neurogenesis has been well studied in rodents. Animal studies have shown that proliferative and migratory capacities of neural precursors are disrupted by irradiation, however depletion of neuroblasts provokes qNSCs to exit quiescence and activate. The mechanisms that could explain reduction of neurogenesis and the resultant negative long-term side effects of radiation therapy, is the premature exhaustion of a finite NSC pool that is a detrimental consequence of aberrant NSCs activation [146] together with the chronic alteration of the neurogenic microenviroment. Nevertheless, radiotherapy is still the standard treatment strategy for most human brain tumors, which by increasing the radiation dose can lead to improved tumor outcomes. This ambiguity of radiation treatment is necessary to keep in mind when treating brain tumors. Determining the subcategories of individual tumors and following the expression of biomarkers in time will help in deciding which patients will benefit from radiation treatment.

Author Contributions: A.M., J.K., and M.Z. prepared the manuscript. M.Z. and P.B. reviewed and edited manuscript. All authors discussed and reviewed the manuscript.

Funding: This work was supported by the Ministry of Education, Youth and Sports (project LO1419).

Acknowledgments: We thank Trevor Allan Epp and Šárka Takáčová for proofreading the manuscript and Ivana Dobiášovská for preparation of illustrations.

Conflicts of Interest: The authors declare no competing interests.

References

1. Worldwide Cancer Statistics. Available online: https://www.cancerresearchuk.org/health-professional/cancer-statistics/worldwide-cancer (accessed on 26 April 2019).
2. Cancer Today. Available online: http://gco.iarc.fr/today/home (accessed on 26 April 2019).
3. Behin, A.; Hoang-Xuan, K.; Carpentier, A.F.; Delattre, J.Y. Primary brain tumours in adults. *Lancet* **2003**, *361*, 323–331. [CrossRef]
4. Ostrom, Q.T.; Wright, C.H.; Barnholtz-Sloan, J.S. Brain metastases: Epidemiology. *Handb. Clin. Neurol.* **2018**, *149*, 27–42. [PubMed]
5. Villano, J.L.; Durbin, E.B.; Normandeau, C.; Thakkar, J.P.; Moirangthem, V.; Davis, F.G. Incidence of brain metastasis at initial presentation of lung cancer. *Neuro-Oncology* **2015**, *17*, 122–128. [CrossRef] [PubMed]
6. Feng, W.; Zhang, P.; Zheng, X.; Chen, M.; Mao, W.M. Incidence and treatment of brain metastasis in patients with esophageal carcinoma. *World J. Gastroenterol.* **2015**, *21*, 5805–5812. [CrossRef] [PubMed]
7. Deeken, J.F.; Löscher, W. The Blood-Brain Barrier and Cancer: Transporters, Treatment, and Trojan Horses. *Clin. Cancer Res.* **2007**, *13*, 1663–1674. [CrossRef] [PubMed]

8. Mahase, S.S.; Navrazhina, K.; Schwartz, T.H.; Parashar, B.; Wernicke, A.G. Intraoperative brachytherapy for resected brain metastases. *Brachytherapy* **2019**, *18*, 258–270. [CrossRef] [PubMed]
9. Delattre, J.Y.; Krol, G.; Thaler, H.T.; Posner, J.B. Distribution of Brain Metastases. *Arch. Neurol.* **1988**, *45*, 741–744. [CrossRef] [PubMed]
10. Siegel, R.; DeSantis, C.; Virgo, K.; Stein, K.; Mariotto, A.; Smith, T.; Cooper, D.; Gansler, T.; Lerro, C.; Fedewa, S.; et al. Cancer treatment and survivorship statistics. *CA Cancer J. Clin.* **2012**, *62*, 220–241. [CrossRef]
11. Delaney, G.; Jacob, S.; Featherstone, C.; Barton, M. The role of radiotherapy in cancer treatment—Estimating optimal utilization from a review of evidence-based clinical guidelines. *Cancer* **2005**, *104*, 1129–1137. [CrossRef]
12. Gerstner, E.R.; Fine, R.L. Increased Permeability of the Blood-Brain Barrier to Chemotherapy in Metastatic Brain Tumors: Establishing a Treatment Paradigm. *J. Clin. Oncol.* **2007**, *25*, 2306–2312. [CrossRef]
13. Van Vulpen, M.; Kal, H.B.; Taphoorn, M.J.B.; El-Sharouni, S.Y. Changes in blood-brain barrier permeability induced by radiotherapy: Implications for timing of chemotherapy? *Oncol. Rep.* **2002**, *9*, 683–688. [CrossRef]
14. Miller, D.S. Regulation of P-glycoprotein and other ABC drug transporters at the blood-brain barrier. *Trends Pharmacol. Sci.* **2010**, *31*, 246–254. [CrossRef]
15. Elsinga, P.; Hendrikse, N.; Bart, J.; Vaalburg, W.; Waarde, A. PET Studies on P-Glycoprotein Function in the Blood-Brain Barrier: How it Affects Uptake and Binding of Drugs within the CNS. *Curr. Pharm. Des.* **2004**, *10*, 1493–1503. [CrossRef]
16. Kemper, E.M.; Van Zandbergen, A.E.; Cleypool, C.; Mos, H.A.; Boogerd, W.; Beijnen, J.H.; Van Tellingen, O. Increased penetration of paclitaxel into the brain by inhibition of P-Glycoprotein. *Clin. Cancer Res.* **2003**, *9*, 2849–2855.
17. Drion, N.; Lemaire, M.; Lefauconnier, J.M.; Scherrmann, J.M. Role of P-glycoprotein in the blood-brain transport of colchicine and vinblastine. *J. Neurochem.* **1996**, *67*, 1688–1693. [CrossRef]
18. Chung, F.S.; Santiago, J.S.; Jesus, M.F.; Trinidad, C.V.; See, M.F. Disrupting P-glycoprotein function in clinical settings: What can we learn from the fundamental aspects of this transporter? *Am. J. Cancer Res.* **2016**, *6*, 1583–1598.
19. Traxl, A.; Mairinger, S.; Filip, T.; Sauberer, M.; Stanek, J.; Poschner, S.; Jager, W.; Zoufal, V.; Novarino, G.; Tournier, N.; et al. Inhibition of ABCB1 and ABCG2 at the Mouse Blood Brain-Barrier with Marketed Drugs to Improve Brain Delivery of the Model ABCB1/ABCG2 Substrate [C-11] erlotinib. *Mol. Pharm.* **2019**, *16*, 1282–1293. [CrossRef]
20. Rubin, P.; Gash, D.; Hansen, J.; Nelson, D.; Williams, J. Disruption of the blood-brain barrier as the primary effect of CNS irradiation. *Radiother. Oncol.* **1994**, *31*, 51–60. [CrossRef]
21. Jahnke, K.; Doolittle, N.D.; Muldoon, L.L.; Neuwelt, E.A. Implications of the blood–brain barrier in primary central nervous system lymphoma. *Neurosurg. Focus* **2006**, *21*, 1–11. [CrossRef]
22. Fauquette, W.; Amourette, C.; Dehouck, M.P.; Diserbo, M. Radiation-induced blood–brain barrier damages: An in vitro study. *Brain Res.* **2012**, *1433*, 114–126. [CrossRef]
23. Qin, D.; Ou, G.; Mo, H.; Song, Y.; Kang, G.; Hu, Y.; Gu, X. Improved efficacy of chemotherapy for glioblastoma by radiation-induced opening of blood-brain barrier: Clinical results. *Int. J. Radiat. Oncol.* **2001**, *51*, 959–962. [CrossRef]
24. Qin, D.; Ma, J.; Xiao, J.; Tang, Z. Effect of brain irradiation on blood-CSF barrier permeability of chemotherapeutic agents. *Am. J. Clin. Oncol.* **1997**, *20*, 263–265. [CrossRef]
25. Vitaz, T.W.; Warnke, P.C.; Tabar, V.; Gutin, P.H. Brachytherapy for brain tumors. *J. Neurooncol.* **2005**, *73*, 71–86. [CrossRef]
26. Zalutsky, M.R. Targeted radiotherapy of brain tumours. *Br. J. Cancer* **2004**, *90*, 1469–1473. [CrossRef]
27. Mitchell, G. The Rationale for Fractionation in Radiotherapy. *Clin. J. Oncol. Nurs.* **2013**, *17*, 412–417. [CrossRef]
28. Withers, H.R. The Four R's of Radiotherapy. In *Advances in Radiation Biology*; Lett, J.T., Adler, H., Zelle, M., Eds.; Elsevier: Amsterdam, The Netherlands, 1975; Volume 5, pp. 241–271.
29. Hermanto, U.; Frija, E.K.; Lii, M.J.; Chang, E.L.; Mahajan, A.; Woo, S.Y. Intensity-modulated radiotherapy (IMRT) and conventional three-dimensional conformal radiotherapy for high-grade gliomas: Does IMRT increase the integral dose to normal brain? *Int. J. Radiat. Oncol.* **2007**, *67*, 1135–1144. [CrossRef]
30. Leibel, S.A.; Sheline, G.E. Radiation therapy for neoplasms of the brain. *J. Neurosurg.* **1987**, *66*, 1–22. [CrossRef]

31. Oskan, F.; Ganswindt, U.; Schwarz, S.; Manapov, F.; Belka, C.; Niyazi, M. Hippocampus sparing in whole-brain radiotherapy. *Strahlenther. Onkol.* **2014**, *190*, 337–341. [CrossRef]
32. Stafinski, T.; Jhangri, G.S.; Yan, E.; Menon, D. Effectiveness of stereotactic radiosurgery alone or in combination with whole brain radiotherapy compared to conventional surgery and/or whole brain radiotherapy for the treatment of one or more brain metastases: A systematic review and meta-analysis. *Cancer Treat. Rev.* **2006**, *32*, 203–213. [CrossRef]
33. Blomstrand, M.; Brodin, N.P.; Rosenschold, P.M.A.; Vogelius, I.R.; Merino, G.S.; Kiil-Berthlesen, A.; Blomgren, K.; Lannering, B.; Bentzen, S.M.; Björk-Eriksson, T. Estimated clinical benefit of protecting neurogenesis in the developing brain during radiation therapy for pediatric medulloblastoma. *Neuro-Oncology* **2012**, *14*, 882–889. [CrossRef]
34. Marsh, J.C.; Ziel, G.E.; Diaz, A.Z.; Wendt, J.A.; Gobole, R.; Turian, J.V. Integral dose delivered to normal brain with conventional intensity-modulated radiotherapy (IMRT) and helical tomotherapy IMRT during partial brain radiotherapy for high-grade gliomas with and without selective sparing of the hippocampus, limbic circuit and neural stem cell compartment. *J. Med. Imaging Radiat. Oncol.* **2013**, *57*, 378–383.
35. Muacevic, A.; Wowra, B.; Siefert, A.; Tonn, J.C.; Steiger, H.J.; Kreth, F.W. Microsurgery plus whole brain irradiation versus Gamma Knife surgery alone for treatment of single metastases to the brain: A randomized controlled multicentre phase III trial. *J. Neurooncol.* **2008**, *87*, 299–307. [CrossRef]
36. Krolicki, L.; Bruchertseifer, F.; Kunikowska, J.; Koziara, H.; Krolicki, B.; Jakucinski, M.; Pawlak, D.; Apostolidis, C.; Mirzadeh, S.; Rola, R.; et al. Safety and efficacy of targeted alpha therapy with Bi-213-DOTA-substance P in recurrent glioblastoma. *Eur. J. Nucl. Med. Mol. Imaging* **2019**, *46*, 614–622. [CrossRef]
37. Sheline, G.E.; Wara, W.M.; Smith, V. Therapeutic irradiation and brain injury. *Int. J. Radiat. Oncol.* **1980**, *6*, 1215–1228. [CrossRef]
38. Perry, A.; Schmidt, R.E. Cancer therapy-associated CNS neuropathology: An update and review of the literature. *Acta Neuropathol.* **2006**, *111*, 197–212. [CrossRef]
39. Patel, R.R.; Mehta, M. Targeted Therapy for Brain Metastases: Improving the Therapeutic Ratio. *Clin. Cancer Res.* **2007**, *13*, 1675–1683. [CrossRef]
40. Soussain, C.; Ricard, D.; Fike, J.R.; Mazeron, J.J.; Psimaras, D.; Delattre, J.Y. CNS complications of radiotherapy and chemotherapy. *Lancet* **2009**, *374*, 1639–1651. [CrossRef]
41. Freund, D.; Zhang, R.; Sanders, M.; Newhauser, W. Predictive Risk of Radiation Induced Cerebral Necrosis in Pediatric Brain Cancer Patients after VMAT versus Proton Therapy. *Cancers* **2015**, *7*, 617–630. [CrossRef]
42. Dietrich, J.; Monje, M.; Wefel, J.; Meyers, C. Clinical Patterns and Biological Correlates of Cognitive Dysfunction Associated with Cancer Therapy. *Oncologist* **2008**, *13*, 1285–1295. [CrossRef]
43. Padovani, L.; Andre, N.; Constine, L.S.; Muracciole, X. Neurocognitive function after radiotherapy for paediatric brain tumours. *Nat. Rev. Neurol.* **2012**, *8*, 578–588. [CrossRef]
44. Pereira Dias, G.; Hollywood, R.; Bevilaqua, M.C.; da Luz, A.C.; Hindges, R.; Nardi, A.E.; Thuret, S. Consequences of cancer treatments on adult hippocampal neurogenesis: Implications for cognitive function and depressive symptoms. *Neuro-Oncology* **2014**, *16*, 476–492. [CrossRef]
45. Altman, J. Autoradiographic study of degenerative and regenerative proliferation of neuroglia cells with tritiated thymidine. *Exp. Neurol.* **1962**, *5*, 302–318. [CrossRef]
46. Doetsch, F.; García-Verdugo, J.M.; Alvarez-Buylla, A. Cellular Composition and Three-Dimensional Organization of the Subventricular Germinal Zone in the Adult Mammalian Brain. *J. Neurosci.* **1997**, *17*, 5046–5061. [CrossRef]
47. Kuhn, H.; Dickinson-Anson, H.; Gage, F. Neurogenesis in the dentate gyrus of the adult rat: Age-related decrease of neuronal progenitor proliferation. *J. Neurosci.* **1996**, *16*, 2027–2033. [CrossRef]
48. Zhao, C.; Deng, W.; Gage, F.H. Mechanisms and Functional Implications of Adult Neurogenesis. *Cell* **2008**, *132*, 645–660. [CrossRef]
49. Bonaguidi, M.A.; Stadel, R.P.; Berg, D.A.; Sun, J.; Ming, G.L.; Song, H. Diversity of Neural Precursors in the Adult Mammalian Brain. *Cold Spring Harb. Perspect. Biol.* **2016**, *8*, a018838. [CrossRef]
50. Li, L.; Clevers, H. Coexistence of Quiescent and Active Adult Stem Cells in Mammals. *Science* **2010**, *327*, 542–545. [CrossRef]
51. Eriksson, P.S.; Perfilieva, E.; Björk-Eriksson, T.; Alborn, A.M.; Nordborg, C.; Peterson, D.A.; Gage, F.H. Neurogenesis in the adult human hippocampus. *Nat. Med.* **1998**, *4*, 1313–1317. [CrossRef]

52. Spalding, K.L.; Bergmann, O.; Alkass, K.; Bernard, S.; Salehpour, M.; Huttner, H.B.; Boström, E.; Westerlund, I.; Vial, C.; Buchholz, B.A.; et al. Dynamics of hippocampal neurogenesis in adult humans. *Cell* **2013**, *153*, 1219–1227. [CrossRef]
53. Sorrells, S.F.; Paredes, M.F.; Cebrian-Silla, A.; Sandoval, K.; Qi, D.; Kelley, K.W.; James, D.; Mayer, S.; Chang, J.; Auguste, K.I.; et al. Human hippocampal neurogenesis drops sharply in children to undetectable levels in adults. *Nature* **2018**, *555*, 377–381. [CrossRef]
54. Boldrini, M.; Fulmore, C.A.; Tartt, A.N.; Simeon, L.R.; Pavlova, I.; Poposka, V.; Rosoklija, G.B.; Stankov, A.; Arango, V.; Dwork, A.J.; et al. Human Hippocampal Neurogenesis Persists throughout Aging. *Cell Stem Cell* **2018**, *22*, 589–599. [CrossRef]
55. Lindsey, B.W.; Tropepe, V. A comparative framework for understanding the biological principles of adult neurogenesis. *Prog. Neurobiol.* **2006**, *80*, 281–307. [CrossRef]
56. Quinones-Hinojosa, A.; Sanai, N.; Soriano-Navarro, M.; Gonzalez-Perez, O.; Mirzadeh, Z.; Gil-Perotin, S.; Romero-Rodriguez, R.; Berger, M.S.; Garcia-Verdugo, J.M.; Alvarez-Buylla, A. Cellular composition and cytoarchitecture of the adult human subventricular zone: A niche of neural stem cells. *J. Comp. Neurol.* **2006**, *494*, 415–434. [CrossRef]
57. Ernst, A.; Alkass, K.; Bernard, S.; Salehpour, M.; Perl, S.; Tisdale, J.; Possnert, G.; Druid, H.; Frisén, J. Neurogenesis in the Striatum of the Adult Human Brain. *Cell* **2014**, *156*, 1072–1083. [CrossRef]
58. Ming, G.L.; Song, H. Adult Neurogenesis in the Mammalian Brain: Significant Answers and Significant Questions. *Neuron* **2011**, *70*, 687–702. [CrossRef]
59. Fuentealba, L.C.; Rompani, S.B.; Parraguez, J.I.; Obernier, K.; Romero, R.; Cepko, C.L.; Alvarez-Buylla, A. Embryonic origin of postnatal neural stem cells. *Cell* **2015**, *161*, 1644–1655. [CrossRef]
60. Llorens-Bobadilla, E.; Zhao, S.; Baser, A.; Saiz-Castro, G.; Zwadlo, K.; Martin-Villalba, A. Single-Cell Transcriptomics Reveals a Population of Dormant Neural Stem Cells that Become Activated upon Brain Injury. *Cell Stem Cell* **2015**, *17*, 329–340. [CrossRef]
61. Codega, P.; Silva-Vargas, V.; Paul, A.; Maldonado-Soto, A.R.; DeLeo, A.M.; Pastrana, E.; Doetsch, F. Prospective Identification and Purification of Quiescent Adult Neural Stem Cells from Their In Vivo Niche. *Neuron* **2014**, *82*, 545–559. [CrossRef]
62. Obernier, K.; Alvarez-Buylla, A. Neural stem cells: Origin, heterogeneity and regulation in the adult mammalian brain. *Development* **2019**, *146*, 156059. [CrossRef]
63. Chaker, Z.; Codega, P.; Doetsch, F. A mosaic world: Puzzles revealed by adult neural stem cell heterogeneity. *Wiley Interdiscip. Rev. Dev. Biol.* **2016**, *5*, 640–658. [CrossRef]
64. Dulken, B.W.; Leeman, D.S.; Boutet, S.C.; Hebestreit, K.; Brunet, A. Single cell transcriptomic analysis defines heterogeneity and transcriptional dynamics in the adult neural stem cell lineage. *Cell Rep.* **2017**, *18*, 777–790. [CrossRef]
65. Artegiani, B.; Lyubimova, A.; Muraro, M.; Van Es, J.H.; Van Oudenaarden, A.; Clevers, H. A Single-Cell RNA Sequencing Study Reveals Cellular and Molecular Dynamics of the Hippocampal Neurogenic Niche. *Cell Rep.* **2017**, *21*, 3271–3284. [CrossRef]
66. Lim, D.A.; Alvarez-Buylla, A. The Adult Ventricular–Subventricular Zone (V-SVZ) and Olfactory Bulb (OB) Neurogenesis. *Cold Spring Harb. Perspect. Biol.* **2016**, *8*, a018820. [CrossRef]
67. Alfonso, J.; Le Magueresse, C.; Zuccotti, A.; Khodosevich, K.; Monyer, H. Diazepam Binding Inhibitor Promotes Progenitor Proliferation in the Postnatal SVZ by Reducing GABA Signaling. *Cell Stem Cell* **2012**, *10*, 76–87. [CrossRef]
68. Liu, X.X.; Wang, Q.; Haydar, T.F.; Bordey, A. Nonsynaptic GABA signaling in postnatal subventricular zone controls proliferation of GFAP-expressing progenitors. *Nat. Neurosci.* **2005**, *8*, 1179–1187. [CrossRef]
69. Paul, A.; Chaker, Z.; Doetsch, F. Hypothalamic regulation of regionally distinct adult neural stem cells and neurogenesis. *Science* **2017**, *356*, 1383–1386. [CrossRef]
70. Yu, H. Typical Cell Signaling Response to Ionizing Radiation: DNA Damage and Extranuclear Damage. *Chin. J. Cancer Res.* **2012**, *24*, 83–89. [CrossRef]
71. Ward, J.F. DNA Damage as the Cause of Ionizing Radiation-Induced Gene Activation. *Radiat. Res.* **1994**, *138*, S85–S88. [CrossRef]
72. Sancar, A.; Lindsey-Boltz, L.A.; Ünsal-Kaçmaz, K.; Linn, S. Molecular Mechanisms of Mammalian DNA Repair and the DNA Damage Checkpoints. *Annu. Rev. Biochem.* **2004**, *73*, 39–85. [CrossRef]

73. Bellinzona, M.; Gobbel, G.T.; Shinohara, C.; Fike, J.R. Apoptosis is induced in the subependyma of young adult rats by ionizing irradiation. *Neurosci. Lett.* **1996**, *208*, 163–166. [CrossRef]
74. Peißner, W.; Kocher, M.; Treuer, H.; Gillardon, F. Ionizing radiation-induced apoptosis of proliferating stem cells in the dentate gyrus of the adult rat hippocampus. *Mol. Brain Res.* **1999**, *71*, 61–68. [CrossRef]
75. Tada, E.; Parent, J.; Lowenstein, D.; Fike, J. X-irradiation causes a prolonged reduction in cell proliferation in the dentate gyrus of adult rats. *Neuroscience* **2000**, *99*, 33–41. [CrossRef]
76. Mizumatsu, S.; Monje, M.L.; Morhardt, D.R.; Rola, R.; Palmer, T.D.; Fike, J.R. Extreme sensitivity of adult neurogenesis to low doses of X-irradiation. *Cancer Res.* **2003**, *63*, 4021–4027.
77. Achanta, P.; Capilla-Gonzalez, V.; Purger, D.; Reyes, J.; Sailor, K.; Song, H.; Garcia-Verdugo, J.M.; Gonzalez-Perez, O.; Ford, E.; Quinones-Hinojosa, A. Subventricular zone localized irradiation affects the generation of proliferating neural precursor cells and the migration of neuroblasts. *Stem Cells* **2012**, *30*, 2548–2560. [CrossRef]
78. Daynac, M.; Chicheportiche, A.; Pineda, J.R.; Gauthier, L.R.; Boussin, F.D.; Mouthon, M.A. Quiescent neural stem cells exit dormancy upon alteration of GABA(A)R signaling following radiation damage. *Stem Cell Res.* **2013**, *11*, 516–528. [CrossRef]
79. Ben Abdallah, N.M.B.; Slomianka, L.; Lipp, H.P. Reversible effect of X-irradiation on proliferation, neurogenesis, and cell death in the dentate gyrus of adult mice. *Hippocampus* **2007**, *17*, 1230–1240. [CrossRef]
80. Morizur, L.; Chicheportiche, A.; Gauthier, L.R.; Daynac, M.; Boussin, F.D.; Mouthon, M.A. Distinct Molecular Signatures of Quiescent and Activated Adult Neural Stem Cells Reveal Specific Interactions with Their Microenvironment. *Stem Cell Rep.* **2018**, *11*, 565–577. [CrossRef]
81. Barazzuol, L.; Ju, L.; Jeggo, P.A. A coordinated DNA damage response promotes adult quiescent neural stem cell activation. *PLoS Biol.* **2017**, *15*, e2001264. [CrossRef]
82. Maslov, A.Y.; Barone, T.A.; Plunkett, R.J.; Pruitt, S.C. Neural Stem Cell Detection, Characterization, and Age-Related Changes in the Subventricular Zone of Mice. *J. Neurosci.* **2004**, *24*, 1726–1733. [CrossRef]
83. Lazarini, F.; Mouthon, M.A.; Gheusi, G.; De Chaumont, F.; Olivo-Marin, J.C.; Lamarque, S.; Abrous, D.N.; Boussin, F.D.; Lledo, P.M. Cellular and Behavioral Effects of Cranial Irradiation of the Subventricular Zone in Adult Mice. *PLoS ONE* **2009**, *4*, e7017. [CrossRef]
84. Monje, M.L.; Mizumatsu, S.; Fike, J.R.; Palmer, T.D. Irradiation induces neural precursor-cell dysfunction. *Nat. Med.* **2002**, *8*, 955–962. [CrossRef]
85. Pineda, J.R.; Daynac, M.; Chicheportiche, A.; Cebrian-Silla, A.; Felice, K.S.; Garcia-Verdugo, J.M.; Boussin, F.D.; Mouthon, M.A. Vascular-derived TGF-β increases in the stem cell niche and perturbs neurogenesis during aging and following irradiation in the adult mouse brain. *EMBO Mol. Med.* **2013**, *5*, 548–562. [CrossRef]
86. Schneider, L.; Pellegatta, S.; Favaro, R.; Pisati, F.; Roncaglia, P.; Testa, G.; Nicolis, S.K.; Finocchiaro, G.; Di Fagagna, F.D. DNA Damage in Mammalian Neural Stem Cells Leads to Astrocytic Differentiation Mediated by BMP2 Signaling through JAK-STAT. *Stem Cell Rep.* **2013**, *1*, 123–138. [CrossRef]
87. Konirova, J.; Cupal, L.; Jarosova, S.; Michaelidesova, A.; Vachelova, J.; Davidkova, M.; Bartunek, P.; Zikova, M. Differentiation Induction as a Response to Irradiation in Neural Stem Cells In Vitro. *Cancers* **2019**, *11*, 913. [CrossRef]
88. Hellström, N.A.; Blomgren, K.; Kuhn, H.G.; Björk-Eriksson, T.; Björk-Eriksson, T. Differential Recovery of Neural Stem Cells in the Subventricular Zone and Dentate Gyrus After Ionizing Radiation. *Stem Cells* **2009**, *27*, 634–641. [CrossRef]
89. Boström, M.; Kalm, M.; Karlsson, N.; Erkenstam, N.H.; Blomgren, K. Irradiation to the young mouse brain caused long-term, progressive depletion of neurogenesis but did not disrupt the neurovascular niche. *Br. J. Pharmacol.* **2013**, *33*, 935–943. [CrossRef]
90. Palmer, T.D.; Willhoite, A.R.; Gage, F.H. Vascular niche for adult hippocampal neurogenesis. *J. Comp. Neurol.* **2000**, *425*, 479–494. [CrossRef]
91. Boström, M.; Erkenstam, N.H.; Kaluza, D.; Jakobsson, L.; Kalm, M.; Blomgren, K. The hippocampal neurovascular niche during normal development and after irradiation to the juvenile mouse brain. *Int. J. Radiat. Biol.* **2014**, *90*, 778–789. [CrossRef]
92. Rola, R.; Raber, J.; Rizk, A.; Otsuka, S.; Vandenberg, S.R.; Morhardt, D.R.; Fike, J.R.; Rizk-Jackson, A. Radiation-induced impairment of hippocampal neurogenesis is associated with cognitive deficits in young mice. *Exp. Neurol.* **2004**, *188*, 316–330. [CrossRef]

93. Chiang, C.S.; McBride, W.; Withers, H. Radiation-induced astrocytic and microglial responses in mouse brain. *Radiother. Oncol.* **1993**, *29*, 60–68. [CrossRef]
94. Lee, W.H.; Sonntag, W.E.; Mitschelen, M.; Yan, H.; Lee, Y.W. Irradiation induces regionally specific alterations in pro-inflammatory environments in rat brain. *Int. J. Radiat. Biol.* **2010**, *86*, 132–144. [CrossRef]
95. Gilbo, P.; Zhang, I.; Knisely, J. Stereotactic radiosurgery of the brain: A review of common indications. *Chin. Clin. Oncol.* **2017**, *6* (Suppl. S2), 14. [CrossRef]
96. Ladra, M.M.; Macdonald, S.M.; Terezakis, S.A. Proton therapy for central nervous system tumors in children. *Pediatr. Blood Cancer* **2018**, *65*, e27046. [CrossRef]
97. Huo, K.; Sun, Y.; Li, H.; Du, X.; Wang, X.; Karlsson, N.; Zhu, C.; Blomgren, K. Lithium reduced neural progenitor apoptosis in the hippocampus and ameliorated functional deficits after irradiation to the immature mouse brain. *Mol. Cell. Neurosci.* **2012**, *51*, 32–42. [CrossRef]
98. Malaterre, J.; McPherson, C.S.; Denoyer, D.; Lai, E.; Hagekyriakou, J.; Lightowler, S.; Shudo, K.; Ernst, M.; Ashley, D.M.; Short, J.L.; et al. Enhanced Lithium-Induced Brain Recovery Following Cranial Irradiation Is Not Impeded by Inflammation. *Stem Cell Transl. Med.* **2012**, *1*, 469–479. [CrossRef]
99. Zanni, G.; Di Martino, E.; Omelyanenko, A.; Andäng, M.; Delle, U.; Elmroth, K.; Blomgren, K. Lithium increases proliferation of hippocampal neural stem/progenitor cells and rescues irradiation-induced cell cycle arrest in vitro. *Oncotarget* **2015**, *6*, 37083–37097. [CrossRef]
100. Wexler, E.M.; Geschwind, D.H.; Palmer, T.D. Lithium regulates adult hippocampal progenitor development through canonical Wnt pathway activation. *Mol. Psychiatry* **2008**, *13*, 285–292. [CrossRef]
101. Li, J.; Feng, L.; Xing, Y.; Wang, Y.; Du, L.; Xu, C.; Cao, J.; Wang, Q.; Fan, S.; Liu, Q.; et al. Radioprotective and Antioxidant Effect of Resveratrol in Hippocampus by Activating Sirt. *Int. J. Mol. Sci.* **2014**, *15*, 5928–5939. [CrossRef]
102. Prager, I.; Patties, I.; Himmelbach, K.; Kendzia, E.; Merz, F.; Müller, K.; Kortmann, R.D.; Glasow, A. Dose-dependent short-and long-term effects of ionizing irradiation on neural stem cells in murine hippocampal tissue cultures: Neuroprotective potential of resveratrol. *Brain Behav.* **2016**, *6*, e00548. [CrossRef]
103. Fukui, M.; Choi, H.J.; Zhu, B.T. Mechanism for the Protective Effect of Resveratrol against Oxidative Stress-Induced Neuronal Death. *Free Radic. Biol. Med.* **2010**, *49*, 800–813. [CrossRef]
104. Şener, G.; Jahovic, N.; Tosun, O.; Atasoy, B.M.; Yeğen, B.C. Melatonin ameliorates ionizing radiation-induced oxidative organ damage in rats. *Life Sci.* **2003**, *74*, 563–572. [CrossRef]
105. Reiter, R.J.; Tan, D.X.; Manchester, L.C.; Qi, W. Biochemical Reactivity of Melatonin with Reactive Oxygen and Nitrogen Species: A Review of the Evidence. *Cell Biophys.* **2001**, *34*, 237–256. [CrossRef]
106. Song, J.; Kang, S.M.; Lee, K.M.; Lee, J.E. The Protective Effect of Melatonin on Neural Stem Cell against LPS-Induced Inflammation. *BioMed Res. Int.* **2015**, *2015*, 854359. [CrossRef]
107. Naseri, S.; Moghahi, S.M.H.N.; Mokhtari, T.; Roghani, M.; Shirazi, A.R.; Malek, F.; Rastegar, T. Radio-Protective Effects of Melatonin on Subventricular Zone in Irradiated Rat: Decrease in Apoptosis and Upregulation of Nestin. *J. Mol. Neurosci.* **2017**, *63*, 198–205. [CrossRef]
108. Monje, M.L.; Toda, H.; Palmer, T.D. Inflammatory Blockade Restores Adult Hippocampal Neurogenesis. *Science* **2003**, *302*, 1760–1765. [CrossRef]
109. Jenrow, K.A.; Brown, S.L.; Lapanowski, K.; Naei, H.; Kolozsvary, A.; Kim, J.H. Selective Inhibition of Microglia-Mediated Neuroinflammation Mitigates Radiation-Induced Cognitive Impairment. *Radiat. Res.* **2013**, *179*, 549–556. [CrossRef]
110. Willson, T.M.; Brown, P.J.; Sternbach, D.D.; Henke, B.R. The PPARs: From Orphan Receptors to Drug Discovery. *J. Med. Chem.* **2000**, *43*, 527–550. [CrossRef]
111. Bordet, R.; Ouk, T.; Petrault, O.; Gélé, P.; Gautier, S.; Laprais, M.; Deplanque, D.; Duriez, P.; Staels, B.; Fruchart, J.; et al. PPAR: A new pharmacological target for neuroprotection in stroke and neurodegenerative diseases. *Biochem. Soc. Trans.* **2006**, *34*, 1341–1346. [CrossRef]
112. Ramanan, S.; Kooshki, M.; Zhao, W.; Hsu, F.C.; Riddle, D.R.; Robbins, M.E. The PPARalpha agonist fenofibrate preserves hippocampal neurogenesis and inhibits microglial activation after whole-brain irradiation. *Int. J. Radiat. Oncol. Biol. Phys.* **2009**, *75*, 870–877. [CrossRef]

113. Greene-Schloesser, D.; Payne, V.; Peiffer, A.M.; Hsu, F.C.; Riddle, D.R.; Zhao, W.; Chan, M.D.; Metheny-Barlow, L.; Robbins, M.E. The peroxisomal proliferator-activated receptor (PPAR) alpha agonist, fenofibrate, prevents fractionated whole-brain irradiation-induced cognitive impairment. *Radiat. Res.* **2014**, *181*, 33–44. [CrossRef]
114. Zhao, W.; Payne, V.; Tommasi, E.; Diz, D.I.; Hsu, F.C.; Robbins, M.E. Administration of the peroxisomal proliferator-activated receptor gamma agonist pioglitazone during fractionated brain irradiation prevents radiation-induced cognitive impairment. *Int. J. Radiat. Oncol. Biol. Phys.* **2007**, *67*, 6–9. [CrossRef]
115. Jenrow, K.A.; Liu, J.; Brown, S.L.; Kolozsvary, A.; Lapanowski, K.; Kim, J.H. Combined atorvastatin and ramipril mitigate radiation-induced impairment of dentate gyrus neurogenesis. *J. Neurooncol.* **2011**, *101*, 449–456. [CrossRef]
116. Wang, Y.; Zhou, K.; Li, T.; Xu, Y.; Xie, C.; Sun, Y.; Zhang, Y.; Rodriguez, J.; Blomgren, K.; Zhu, C. Inhibition of autophagy prevents irradiation-induced neural stem and progenitor cell death in the juvenile mouse brain. *Cell Death Dis.* **2017**, *8*, e2694. [CrossRef]
117. Acharya, M.M.; Christie, L.A.; Lan, M.L.; Giedzinski, E.; Fike, J.R.; Rosi, S.; Limoli, C.L. Human Neural Stem Cell Transplantation Ameliorates Radiation-Induced Cognitive Dysfunction. *Cancer Res.* **2011**, *71*, 4834–4845. [CrossRef]
118. Acharya, M.M.; Rosi, S.; Jopson, T.; Limoli, C.L. Human Neural Stem Cell Transplantation Provides Long-Term Restoration of Neuronal Plasticity in the Irradiated Hippocampus. *Cell Transplant.* **2015**, *24*, 691–702. [CrossRef]
119. Ramos-Zuñiga, R.; Gonzalez-Perez, O.; Macías-Ornelas, A.; Capilla-Gonzalez, V.; Quiñones-Hinojosa, A. Ethical Implications in the Use of Embryonic and Adult Neural Stem Cells. *Stem Cells Int.* **2012**, *2012*, 470949. [CrossRef]
120. Baulch, J.E.; Acharya, M.M.; Allen, B.D.; Ru, N.; Chmielewski, N.N.; Martirosian, V.; Giedzinski, E.; Syage, A.; Park, A.L.; Benke, S.N.; et al. Cranial grafting of stem cell-derived microvesicles improves cognition and reduces neuropathology in the irradiated brain. *Proc. Natl. Acad. Sci. USA* **2016**, *113*, 4836–4841. [CrossRef]
121. Joo, K.M.; Jin, J.; Kang, B.G.; Lee, S.J.; Kim, K.H.; Yang, H.; Lee, Y.A.; Cho, Y.J.; Im, Y.S.; Lee, D.S.; et al. Trans-Differentiation of Neural Stem Cells: A Therapeutic Mechanism Against the Radiation Induced Brain Damage. *PLoS ONE* **2012**, *7*, e25936. [CrossRef]
122. Sano, K.; Morii, K.; Sato, M.; Mori, H.; Tanaka, R. Radiation-induced Diffuse Brain Injury in the Neonatal Rat Model. Radiation-induced Apoptosis of Oligodendrocytes. *Neurol. Med. Chir.* **2000**, *40*, 495–500. [CrossRef]
123. Piao, J.; Major, T.; Auyeung, G.; Policarpio, E.; Menon, J.; Droms, L.; Gutin, P.; Uryu, K.; Tchieu, J.; Soulet, D.; et al. Human Embryonic Stem Cell-Derived Oligodendrocyte Progenitors Remyelinate the Brain and Rescue Behavioral Deficits following Radiation. *Cell Stem Cell* **2015**, *16*, 198–210. [CrossRef]
124. Soria, B.; Martin-Montalvo, A.; Aguilera, Y.; Mellado-Damas, N.; López-Beas, J.; Herrera-Herrera, I.; López, E.; Barcia, J.A.; Alvarez-Dolado, M.; Hmadcha, A.; et al. Human Mesenchymal Stem Cells Prevent Neurological Complications of Radiotherapy. *Front. Cell. Neurosci.* **2019**, *13*, 204. [CrossRef]
125. Simone, B.A.; Champ, C.E.; Rosenberg, A.L.; Berger, A.C.; Monti, D.A.; Dicker, A.P.; Simone, N.L. Selectively starving cancer cells through dietary manipulation: Methods and clinical implications. *Future Oncol.* **2013**, *9*, 959–976. [CrossRef]
126. Alifieris, C.; Trafalis, D.T. Glioblastoma multiforme: Pathogenesis and treatment. *Pharmacol. Ther.* **2015**, *152*, 63–82. [CrossRef]
127. Weinhouse, S.; Warburg, O.; Burk, D.; Schade, A.L. On Respiratory Impairment in Cancer Cells. *Science* **1956**, *124*, 267–272. [CrossRef]
128. Marsh, J.; Mukherjee, P.; Seyfried, T. Akt-Dependent Proapoptotic Effects of Dietary Restriction on Late-Stage Management of a Phosphatase and Tensin Homologue/Tuberous Sclerosis Complex 2-Deficient Mouse Astrocytoma. *Clin. Cancer Res.* **2008**, *14*, 7751–7762. [CrossRef]
129. Zuccoli, G.; Marcello, N.; Pisanello, A.; Servadei, F.; Vaccaro, S.; Mukherjee, P.; Seyfried, T.N. Metabolic management of glioblastoma multiforme using standard therapy together with a restricted ketogenic diet: Case Report. *Nutr. Metab.* **2010**, *7*, 33. [CrossRef]
130. Schwartz, K.; Chang, H.T.; Nikolai, M.; Pernicone, J.; Rhee, S.; Olson, K.; Kurniali, P.C.; Hord, N.G.; Noel, M. Treatment of glioma patients with ketogenic diets: Report of two cases treated with an IRB-approved energy-restricted ketogenic diet protocol and review of the literature. *Cancer Metab.* **2015**, *3*, 3. [CrossRef]

131. Elsakka, A.M.A.; Bary, M.A.; Abdelzaher, E.; Elnaggar, M.; Kalamian, M.; Mukherjee, P.; Seyfried, T.N. Management of Glioblastoma Multiforme in a Patient Treated with Ketogenic Metabolic Therapy and Modified Standard of Care: A 24-Month Follow-Up. *Front. Nutr.* **2018**, *5*, 20. [CrossRef]
132. Seyfried, T.N.; Flores, R.; Poff, A.M.; D'Agostino, D.P.; Mukherjee, P. Metabolic therapy: A new paradigm for managing malignant brain cancer. *Cancer Lett.* **2015**, *356*, 289–300. [CrossRef]
133. Nishie, A.; Ono, M.; Shono, T.; Fukushi, J.; Otsubo, M.; Onoue, H.; Ito, Y.; Inamura, T.; Ikezaki, K.; Fukui, M.; et al. Macrophage infiltration and heme oxygenase-1 expression correlate with angiogenesis in human gliomas. *Clin. Cancer Res.* **1999**, *5*, 1107–1113.
134. Lewis, C.; Murdoch, C. Macrophage responses to hypoxia: Implications for tumor progression and anti-cancer therapies. *Am. J. Pathol.* **2005**, *167*, 627–635. [CrossRef]
135. Dong, W.; Selgrade, M.K.; Gilmour, M.I.; Lange, R.W.; Park, P.; Luster, M.I.; Kari, F.W. Altered Alveolar Macrophage Function in Calorie-restricted Rats. *Am. J. Respir. Cell Mol. Biol.* **1998**, *19*, 462–469. [CrossRef]
136. Apple, D.M.; Mahesula, S.; Fonseca, R.S.; Zhu, C.; Kokovay, E. Calorie restriction protects neural stem cells from age-related deficits in the subventricular zone. *Aging* **2019**, *11*, 115–126. [CrossRef]
137. Tobin, M.K.; Musaraca, K.; Disouky, A.; Shetti, A.; Bheri, A.; Honer, W.G.; Kim, N.; Dawe, R.J.; Bennett, D.A.; Arfanakis, K.; et al. Human Hippocampal Neurogenesis Persists in Aged Adults and Alzheimer's Disease Patients. *Cell Stem Cell* **2019**, *24*, 974–982. [CrossRef]
138. Moreno-Jiménez, E.P.; Flor-García, M.; Terreros-Roncal, J.; Rábano, A.; Cafini, F.; Pallas-Bazarra, N.; Ávila, J.; Llorens-Martín, M. Adult hippocampal neurogenesis is abundant in neurologically healthy subjects and drops sharply in patients with Alzheimer's disease. *Nat. Med.* **2019**, *25*, 554–560. [CrossRef]
139. Kempermann, G.; Gage, F.H.; Aigner, L.; Song, H.; Curtis, M.A.; Thuret, S.; Kuhn, H.G.; Jessberger, S.; Frankland, P.W.; Cameron, H.A.; et al. Human adult neurogenesis: Evidence and remaining questions. *Cell Stem Cell* **2018**, *23*, 25–30. [CrossRef]
140. Gage, F.H. Adult neurogenesis in mammals. *Science* **2019**, *364*, 827–828. [CrossRef]
141. Northcott, P.A.; Buchhalter, I.; Morrissy, A.S.; Hovestadt, V.; Weischenfeldt, J.; Ehrenberger, T.; Groebner, S.; Segura-Wang, M.; Zichner, T.; Rudneva, V.A.; et al. The whole-genome landscape of medulloblastoma subtypes. *Nature* **2017**, *547*, 311–317. [CrossRef]
142. Archer, T.C.; Ehrenberger, T.; Mundt, F.; Gold, M.P.; Krug, K.; Mah, C.K.; Mahoney, E.L.; Daniel, C.J.; Lenail, A.; Ramamoorthy, D.; et al. Proteomics, Post-translational Modifications, and Integrative Analyses Reveal Molecular Heterogeneity within Medulloblastoma Subgroups. *Cancer Cell* **2018**, *34*, 396–410. [CrossRef]
143. Phoenix, T.N.; Patmore, D.M.; Boop, S.; Boulos, N.; Jacus, M.O.; Patel, Y.T.; Roussel, M.F.; Finkelstein, D.; Goumnerova, L.; Perreault, S.; et al. Medulloblastoma genotype dictates blood brain barrier phenotype. *Cancer Cell* **2016**, *29*, 508–522. [CrossRef]
144. Aldape, K.; Brindle, K.M.; Chesler, L.; Chopra, R.; Gajjar, A.; Gilbert, M.R.; Gottardo, N.; Gutmann, D.H.; Hargrave, D.; Holland, E.C.; et al. Challenges to curing primary brain tumours. *Nat. Rev. Clin. Oncol.* **2019**, *16*, 509–520. [CrossRef]
145. Krishnatry, R.; Zhukova, N.; Stucklin, A.S.G.; Pole, J.D.; Mistry, M.; Fried, I.; Ramaswamy, V.; Bartels, U.; Huang, A.; Laperriere, N.; et al. Clinical and treatment factors determining long-term outcomes for adult survivors of childhood low-grade glioma: A population-based study. *Cancer* **2016**, *122*, 1261–1269. [CrossRef]
146. Pilz, G.A.; Bottes, S.; Betizeau, M.; Jörg, D.J.; Carta, S.; Simons, B.D.; Helmchen, F.; Jessberger, S. Live imaging of neurogenesis in the adult mouse hippocampus. *Science* **2018**, *359*, 658–662. [CrossRef]

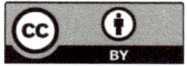

© 2019 by the authors. Licensee MDPI, Basel, Switzerland. This article is an open access article distributed under the terms and conditions of the Creative Commons Attribution (CC BY) license (http://creativecommons.org/licenses/by/4.0/).

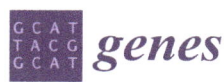 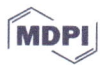

Review

Human Colorectal Cancer from the Perspective of Mouse Models

Monika Stastna, Lucie Janeckova, Dusan Hrckulak, Vitezslav Kriz and Vladimir Korinek *

Institute of Molecular Genetics of the Czech Academy of Sciences, Videnska 1083, 142 20 Prague, Czech Republic; monika.stastna@img.cas.cz (M.S.); lucie.janeckova@img.cas.cz (L.J.); dusan.hrckulak@img.cas.cz (D.H.); vitezslav.kriz@img.cas.cz (V.K.)
* Correspondence: korinek@img.cas.cz; Tel.: +420-241-063-146; Fax: +420-244-472-282

Received: 20 August 2019; Accepted: 8 October 2019; Published: 11 October 2019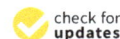

Abstract: Colorectal cancer (CRC) is a heterogeneous disease that includes both hereditary and sporadic types of tumors. Tumor initiation and growth is driven by mutational or epigenetic changes that alter the function or expression of multiple genes. The genes predominantly encode components of various intracellular signaling cascades. In this review, we present mouse intestinal cancer models that include alterations in the Wnt, Hippo, p53, epidermal growth factor (EGF), and transforming growth factor β (TGFβ) pathways; models of impaired DNA mismatch repair and chemically induced tumorigenesis are included. Based on their molecular biology characteristics and mutational and epigenetic status, human colorectal carcinomas were divided into four so-called consensus molecular subtype (CMS) groups. It was shown subsequently that the CMS classification system could be applied to various cell lines derived from intestinal tumors and tumor-derived organoids. Although the CMS system facilitates characterization of human CRC, individual mouse models were not assigned to some of the CMS groups. Thus, we also indicate the possible assignment of described animal models to the CMS group. This might be helpful for selection of a suitable mouse strain to study a particular type of CRC.

Keywords: carcinoma; consensus molecular subtypes; intestine; oncogenes; signaling cascades; tumor suppressors; tumorigenesis

1. Introduction

Cancer of the colon and rectum (colorectal cancer (CRC)) is one of the most commonly diagnosed cancer types in Western countries. In the United States (US), the lifetime risk of CRC is 5%, and the death rate of diagnosed patients exceeds 30% [1]. Approximately 85% of colorectal tumors arise sporadically, and 15% are underlined by hereditary predispositions (reviewed in Reference [2]). The early stages of colorectal tumors are predominantly associated with mutations in the tumor suppressor adenomatous polyposis coli (*APC*) [3], resulting in aberrant activation of the Wnt signaling pathway. A subsequent mutation usually affects the Kirsten rat sarcoma viral oncogene homolog (*KRAS*) gene, which further enhances Wnt signaling and thereby facilitates the adenoma growth [4,5]. In addition, mutations inactivating tumor protein 53 (encoded by the *TP53* gene) and some of the SMAD (an acronym of *Caenorhabditis elegans sma* and *Drosophila melanogaster* mothers against decapentaplegic genes) family member genes accumulate in the cancer cell; these mutations further promote progression of premalignant intestinal polyps toward carcinomas [6–8].

Colitis-associated colorectal cancer (CAC) arises as a result of chronic inflammation in the intestine and accounts for 1–2% of all CRCs (reviewed in Reference [9]). CAC tumors are situated within the colon in the areas of active inflammation and develop similarly to CRC via accumulation of numerous mutations in intestinal epithelial cells (reviewed in Reference [10]). However, while sporadic

CRC is underlined by *APC* disruption, the earliest mutation event in CAC mainly affects the *TP53* gene [11]. Nevertheless, as in case of sporadic CRC, early activation of Wnt signaling is critical for the colitis-to-cancer transition [12]. *TP53* mutations were found in up to 89% of CAC patients [13], while other mutations present in sporadic CRC were less frequent, e.g., the *APC* gene alterations were found in less than 30% of CAC specimens [14]. In addition, *KRAS* mutations were detected in approximately 30–40% of both sporadic CRC and CAC [13,15,16]. CAC differs from sporadic CRC not only in the order of acquired mutations, but also by the type of mutations in individual genes. For example, in sporadic CRC, mutations in the *TP53* gene mainly impair the protein ability to bind DNA; however, in CAC such mutations are less frequent. In contrast, several "gain of function" (GOF) alterations of the *TP53* gene that increase tumor invasiveness, attenuate apoptosis, and increase genomic instability were predominantly found in CAC [13,17].

The classification of colorectal tumors underwent significant changes over the last few years. The original approach of CRC classification was based on gene expression analysis, which, however, often showed considerable differences depending on the dataset used and experimental approach employed by individual research groups. To unify the classification of intestinal tumors, Guinney and colleagues performed a large-scale data analysis by linking six previously published CRC subtyping algorithms [18–23]. The analysis resulted in the system of four consensus molecular subtypes (CMSs). Individual CMSs were defined not only by gene expression, but also by other characteristics such as mutation counts, somatic copy number alterations (SCNAs), i.e., gain or loss in copies of genomic DNA, microsatellite instability (MSI), cytosine-phosphate diester-guanine nucleotide (CpG) island methylator phenotype (CIMP), and differences in the immune response and activation status of various signaling pathways. The authors created a "gold standard" of CRC classification, where each CMS group is defined by certain biological properties, gene expression profiles, and clinical course [24]. According to this classification, most intestinal tumors (78% of 4151 tumors analyzed) may be assigned to one of the four CMS groups: CMS1 (also named "MSI immune"; 14% cases), CMS2 ("canonical"; 37%), CMS3 ("metabolic"; 13%), and CMS4 ("mesenchymal"; 23%) (Table 1). Tumors from the CMS1 group differed markedly from all other groups by high mutation counts and low SCNA counts, pronounced MSI, and wide-spread DNA hypermethylation. They overexpressed proteins involved in DNA damage repair and frequently carried mutations in the B-Raf proto-oncogene (*BRAF*); however, mutations in *APC*, *TP53*, and *KRAS* often occurred as well. The tumors also exhibited strong immune cell infiltration and activation, they predominantly occurred in the right colon, and patients had a low survival rate after relapse. In contrast, tumors from other groups had elevated SCNA counts, possibly related to high chromosomal instability (CIN). CMS2 group tumors displayed more frequent gains in the copy number of oncogenes and losses in tumor suppressor genes in comparison to other groups displaying CIN, i.e., CMS3 and CMS4 groups. The CMS2 tumors also exhibited elevated epithelial differentiation and hyperactivation of the Wnt pathway and increased Myc-dependent transcription. On the other hand, gene signatures indicating epithelial–mesenchymal transition (EMT) and matrix remodeling were underrepresented. Moreover, CMS2 group patients had tumors distributed within the left colon and rectum and better survival rates than those in other groups. Although tumors from the CMS3 group displayed high CIN in comparison to the CMS2 and CMS4 groups, they showed less SCNA counts and higher CIMP, and they were "hypermutated". CMS3 group tumors displayed the highest incidence of *KRAS* mutations, which are possibly linked to metabolic deregulation found in this type of CRC. Finally, CMS4 group tumors had typically high SCNA counts, hyperactivated transforming growth factor β (TGFβ) signaling, and increased expression of genes involved in EMT, angiogenesis, and matrix remodeling. Interestingly, CMS4 group tumors as the only group showed a gene expression profile indicating infiltration by both mesenchymal and immune cells. Patients from the CMS4 tumor group had the worst overall and relapse-free survival rates of all CMS groups [24]. Whereas the CMS classification is mainly based on analysis of sporadic CRC, the question arises with regard to how to assign CAC malignancies to the system. Since the initial mutation in CAC affects the *TP53* gene, CAC tumors could be included in the CMS2 or CMS4. However, CMS2 group tumors displayed decreased immune infiltration, which does not correspond to elevated pro-inflammatory nuclear factor kappa-light-chain-enhancer of activated B cells (NF-κB) signaling in CAC. On the other hand, tumors from the CMS1 group showed high immune infiltration and, in addition, CMS4 group neoplasms exhibited robust complement activation that was reported to contribute to CAC in the mouse model [25]. In conclusion, CAC characteristics do not completely fall into any particular CMS group. Moreover, although CAC tumors share multiple mutations with CRCs, the mutations are accumulated in a different order and the tumors develop in a specific microenvironment caused by chronic inflammation. Thus, CAC lies beyond the categorization developed for CRC.

Table 1. Biological characteristics of consensus molecular subtype (CMS) groups of colorectal tumors.

CMS1 MSI Immune 14%	CMS2 Canonical 37%	CMS3 Metabolic 13%	CMS4 Mesenchymal 23%
MSI high	MSI negative	Mixed MSI status	MSI low
CIMP high	CIMP negative	CIMP low	CIMP negative
SCNA low	SCNA high	SCNA moderate	SCNA high
BRAF mutations	TP53 mutations	KRAS mutations	TP53 mutations
	epithelial signature	epithelial signature	mesenchymal signature
	Wnt and Myc target genes upregulation	enhanced metabolism	EMT activation and matrix remodeling
immune infiltration			stromal infiltration TGFβ signaling activation
worse survival after relaps			worse relaps-free and overall survival

BRAF, B-Raf proto-oncogene; CIMP, cytosine-phosphate diester-guanine nucleotide (CpG) island methylator phenotype; EMT, epithelial–mesenchymal transition; KRAS, Kirsten rat sarcoma viral oncogene homolog; MSI, microsatellite instability; SCNA, somatic copy number alterations; TP53, tumor protein 53 (adopted from Reference [24]).

The conclusions of the Guinney et al. study were used by Linnekamp and co-workers, who tested different CRC cell lines and, based on their properties, categorized them into the individual CMS groups [26]. Using different gene expression datasets from publicly available databases, 43 CRC cell lines were classified into individual CMS groups. Although the assignment into a particular CMS group often varied depending on the dataset used, 66% of the CRC cell lines showed consistent assignment to a specific CMS group across the datasets tested. The study also included mutational changes in CRC cell lines and alterations in the status of five major pathways that are frequently deregulated in CRC. The Wnt, p53, and receptor tyrosine kinase (RTK)/Ras pathways displayed similar alterations in CRC cells as in patient samples, whereas phosphatidylinositol-3-kinase (PI3K) and TGFβ pathways were mutated in CRC-derived cell lines with significantly lower frequencies than in tumor specimens. Furthermore, 18 cell lines were grown as xenografts and, even after multiple transfer, the cells maintained the original gene expression profiles. Moreover, cells isolated from 33 CRC patients were cultured in vitro as organoids. Interestingly, according to gene expression, organoids might also be classified into the four CMS groups. Importantly, with one exception, organoids retained the same expression patterns observed in the original tumor specimens [26]. Studies of CRC specimens, CRC-derived cell lines, and organoids brought considerable simplification, clarification, and unification of CRC characterization. However, elucidation of the molecular mechanisms involved in tumor initiation and progression requires analysis in living organisms. Although several recent articles provided an overview of mouse models suitable for studying CRC [27,28], individual mouse models and strains remain to be assigned to the particular CMS group. Since CRC is a highly heterogeneous disease and the individual tumor subtypes display various characteristics, it is important to select the right preclinical model to best mimic the human disease and thereby reduce misleading conclusions. Therefore, in the following chapters, mouse models that are broadly used to study mutations frequently observed in human CRC are discussed, and the possible assignment of a specific cancer model to some of the CMS group(s) is suggested. We anticipate that many of the mouse models do not easily align with the established CMS classification. Nevertheless, for each CMS group, mouse strains that best fit the group characteristics are summarized in Table 2. Finally, the best studied so-called canonical branches of the particular signaling pathways are discussed throughout the review. These pathways are believed to function in an analogous manner in both human and mouse. Nonetheless, species-specific differences are indicated when appropriate.

Table 2. Selected mouse models suitable for studying tumors belonging to the particular CMS group. Since CMS4 tumors are mainly characterized by activation of the transforming growth factor β (TGFβ) pathway in stromal cells, we did not include any mouse model to this category. It should be noted that mouse strains allowing downregulation of TGFβ signaling are available. However, tumors developed in these mice fit well into the CMS2 group. N/A, not available.

	Generated Allele or Strain Name	Advantages	Disadvantages	Reference
CMS1	$Braf^{V600E}$	crypt hyperproliferation, high incidence of tumors, mucinous phenotype	not all the animals develop tumors	[29]
	$Mlh1^{-/-}$	100% tumor development within 4 months	tumors develop in many other tissues, short lifespan	[30]
	$Msh2^{loxP/loxP}$ Villin-Cre	90 % of mice developed adenomas and adenocarcinomas, tumor formation is restricted to the intestine	mosaic recombination in the tissue	[31]
CMS2	Apc^{Min}	multiple intestinal tumors, early tumor development, recapitulates human FAP syndrome	relatively rare tumorigenesis in the colon	[32]
	$Apc^{cKO/cKO}$ Lgr5-EGFP-IRES-CreERT2	inducible tumor initiation, all tumors develop during the same (and defined) time period	tamoxifen dose-dependent variability of the phenotype	[33]
	$Catnb^{+/lox(ex3)}$ Krt1-19-Cre	early tumor development, large amount of tumors, microadenomas in the colon	short lifespan due to extensive tumorigenesis	[34]
	Apc^{Min} $p53^{-/-}$	increased number and invasivity of intestinal tumors	tumors develop in many other tissues, short lifespan	[35]
CMS3	$Apc^{2lox14/+}$ LSL-$Kras^{G12D}$ Rapbp1-Cre	combination of Apc and Kras mutations, adenomas in the colon	crossbreeding	[36]
	Apc^{Min} K-ras^{Asp12} Ah-Cre	increased number of intestinal tumors with higher effect in the colon	crossbreeding	[37]
CMS4	N/A			

2. Mouse Models of Chemically Induced Colorectal Tumorigenesis

Since different chemical compounds cause different mutations, utilization of chemical mutagens results in generation of a variety of tumors that fall into all CMS groups. Consequently, chemically induced tumors mimic the wide range of genetic alterations found in sporadic CRC and CAC. Additionally, chemical induction of intestinal tumors can be used to study the tumorigenic properties of chemical substances commonly found in the human diet or environment. One group of such chemical substances are heterocyclic aromatic amines that are present in grilled or roasted meat. For example, 2-amino-1-methyl-6-phenylimidazol[4,5-b] pyridine (PhIP) was used several times to induce tumors in the mouse or rat colons; however, the tumor incidence was relatively low [38,39], although the tumor incidence was increased when PhIP treatment was combined with a high-fat diet [40]. Other tumorigenic substances are alkylnitrosamide compounds such as methylnitrosourea. This topical carcinogen does not require metabolic activation and, thus, may be administered directly into the colon lumen. Tumors induced by methylnitrosourea are formed mainly in the distal colon and rectum [41]. The lesions are well differentiated and frequently invade the submucosa. However, tumor induction by intrarectal administration of the mutagen is not high, and reproducibility of such experiments depends on the skill of the experimenter (reviewed in Reference [42]). The most frequently used chemicals for CRC induction are 1,2-dimethylhydrazine (DMH) [43] or its metabolite azoxymethane (AOM). AOM is a potent carcinogen that causes a wide spectrum of mutations in key genes encoding components of multiple intracellular signal transduction cascades [44–47]. Upon administration, AOM is metabolized to methylazoxymethanol, and subsequently to formaldehyde and a methyldiazonium ion. The latter is highly reactive and causes alkylation of DNA bases. Repetitive administration of AOM leads to development of epithelial neoplasia initiated by abnormal colonic crypts, so-called aberrant crypt foci (ACF); ACF further progress to adenoma and malignant adenocarcinoma [48]. AOM-treated mice generate tumors predominantly in the distal colon; the tumors reach the advanced carcinoma stage within a few months after the mutagen administration. This can be considered an advantage, since the majority of genetic mouse models—in contrast to humans—produce tumors mainly in the small intestine. Moreover, as described in the following chapters, genetic manipulations of tumor suppressors or oncogenes predominantly induce multiple tumors that severely disturb the absorptive function of the epithelium. The tumor burden leads to preconscious animal death before individual tumors reach advanced stages [49]. Interestingly, it was reported that various laboratory mouse strains displayed different sensitivity to AOM (the sensitivity is manifested by the number of induced lesions) [50].

To create a model of colorectal tumors associated with chronic inflammation, a protocol combining AOM with an inflammatory agent, dextran sulfate sodium (DSS) salt, was introduced. Chronic inflammation leads to the formation of a microenvironment enriched with immune cells that produce pro-inflammatory cytokines and growth factors and, simultaneously, increase the local levels of reactive oxygen species. Subsequently, cell proliferation and the risk of DNA damage are increased. In the case of a long-lasting inflammatory response, cell transformation and tumorigenesis occur with high frequency. The inflammatory response and cell survival are promoted by the NF-κB signaling pathway. As shown in mice with conditional deletion of IκB kinase β (*IKKβ*), impairment of NF-κB signaling in colonic epithelial cells led to decreased tumor incidence without affecting the level of inflammation in AOM/DSS-treated mice [51]. Another advantage of the AOM and DSS combination is further reduction in the time needed for tumor formation. A single dose of AOM followed by five days of DSS treatment resulted in development of multiple colon tumors within 10 weeks [52,53]. This procedure proved to be very reliable and reproducible and was used to induce CAC in mice. Given the different mutation site in genes such as *Ctnnb1* (the *Ctnnb1* gene encodes β-catenin), it is evident that the combination of AOM and an inflammatory agent induces a different spectrum of tumors in comparison to induction by the carcinogen alone (reviewed in Reference [54]; all indicated models of chemically induced colorectal tumorigenesis are summarized in Table S1, Supplementary Materials).

3. Mouse Models of Aberrant Wnt Signaling

The canonical (i.e., β-catenin-dependent) Wnt signaling pathway maintains the balance between proliferation and differentiation of intestinal epithelial cells. Consequently, mutations resulting in aberrant activation of Wnt signaling initiate and promote tumorigenesis. Tumor suppressor gene *APC* encodes a key negative regulator of the pathway and it represents the most frequently mutated gene in CRC (reviewed in Reference [55]). Mutations in *APC* occur in all CMS tumor groups, with the highest representation in CMS2 (83%) and the lowest in CMS1 (40%). Concordantly, hyperactivation of the canonical Wnt signaling pathway was observed predominantly in CMS2 group tumors [24]. This chapter presents mouse models carrying (inducible) mutations in the *Apc* and *Ctnnb1* genes, as well as models enabling hyperactivation of the Wnt pathway by Wnt agonists R-spondins (RSPOs; corresponding models are summarized in Table S2, Supplementary Materials).

Wnt signaling is initiated upon Wnt ligand binding to the cell surface receptor Frizzled and co-receptor low-density lipoprotein receptor-related protein 5/6 (LRP5/6). The binding initiates a cascade of events leading to disintegration of the so-called β-catenin destruction complex, a cytosolic protein complex that regulates β-catenin stability (reviewed in Reference [56]). The APC protein interacts with β-catenin and establishes a protein core for the destruction complex, which further contains glycogen synthase kinase 3β (GSK3β), casein kinase 1 (CK1), and scaffold proteins axis inhibition 1 and 2 (AXIN1 and AXIN2) (reviewed in References [57–59]). Mutations in the *APC* or *CTNNB1* genes prevent formation of the destruction complex. This results in β-catenin stabilization and β-catenin entry into the nucleus. Nuclear β-catenin, together with transcription factors from the T-cell factor/lymphoid enhancer-binding factor (TCF/LEF) family, activates transcription of genes important for cell proliferation and cell survival [60–62] (Figure 1). Approximately 90% of sporadic colorectal tumors carry a mutation in *APC* and up to 5% in the *CTNNB1* gene (reviewed in References [63,64]). Relatively rare are mutations in Wnt negative regulators *AXIN1/2* and in transcription factor *TCF4* (reviewed in References [65,66]).

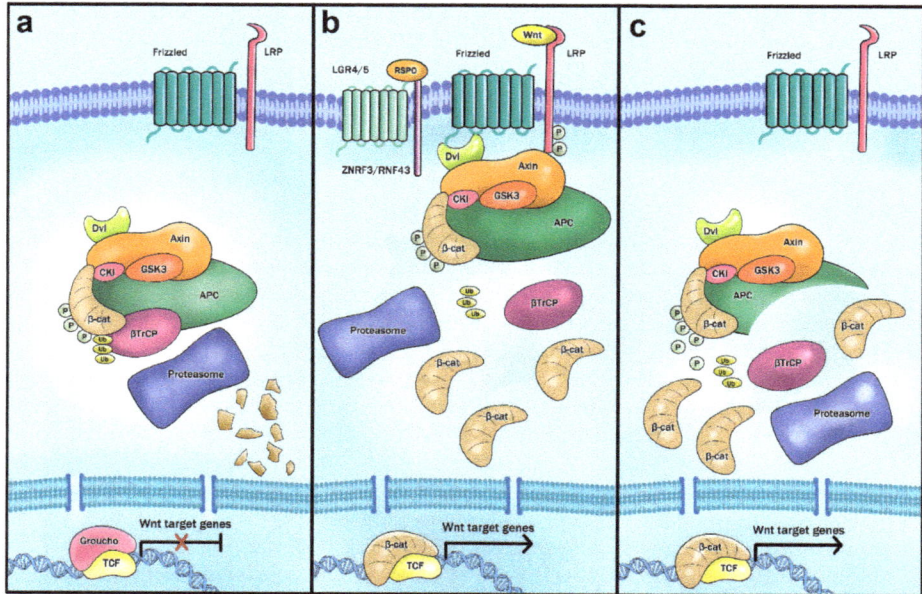

Figure 1. The canonical Wnt signaling pathway. (**a**) In the absence of Wnt ligand, a cytosolic protein complex composed of adenomatous polyposis coli (APC), axis inhibition (Axin), casein kinase 1 α (CK1α), glycogen synthase kinase 3 β (GSK3β), and β-transducin repeat-containing E3 ubiquitin protein ligase (βTrCP) mediates phosphorylation and ubiquitination of β-catenin (β-cat). Phosphorylated β-catenin is subsequently degraded by the proteasome. In such a situation, transcription factors from the T-cell factor/lymphoid enhancer-binding factor (TCF/LEF) family are held in an inactive state by interaction with transcription repressor Groucho that blocks transcription of Wnt signaling target genes. (**b**) Binding of the Wnt ligand to receptor Frizzled and co-receptor low-density lipoprotein receptor-related protein (LRP) leads to LRP phosphorylation that induces Axin recruitment to the cell membrane. As a result, the destruction complex is disassembled and β-catenin translocates to the cell nucleus to activate, in cooperation with TCF/LEF factors, transcription of Wnt target genes. R-spondin (RSPO) ligand binds the leucine-rich repeat-containing G-protein coupled receptor (Lgr) 4/5, which results in internalization and subsequent proteasomal degradation of transmembrane E3 ubiquitin ligases zinc and ring finger 3 (ZNRF3) and ring finger 43 (RNF43). The ligases mediate turnover of the Wnt receptor Frizzled and their inhibition enhances Wnt signaling. (**c**) Truncated APC protein does not retain the ability to scaffold the destruction complex, resulting in β-catenin stabilization and aberrant expression of Wnt target genes, i.e., even without the presence of the Wnt ligand.

The *APC* locus was discovered by studying a rare hereditary syndrome, familial adenomatous polyposis (FAP) [67,68]. Inherited mutation in the *APC* gene leads to development of hundreds to thousands adenomatous polyps predominantly located in the colon and rectum; the occurrence of polyps in the small intestine is less common. Because of frequent random inactivation of the second *APC* allele and successive accumulation of additional tumor-promoting mutations, the polyps progress to carcinoma by the age of 35 (reviewed in Reference [69]). Since most colorectal tumors harbor a mutation in the *APC* gene, a large proportion of mouse genetic intestinal cancer models target (or involve) the *Apc* gene (Figure 2).

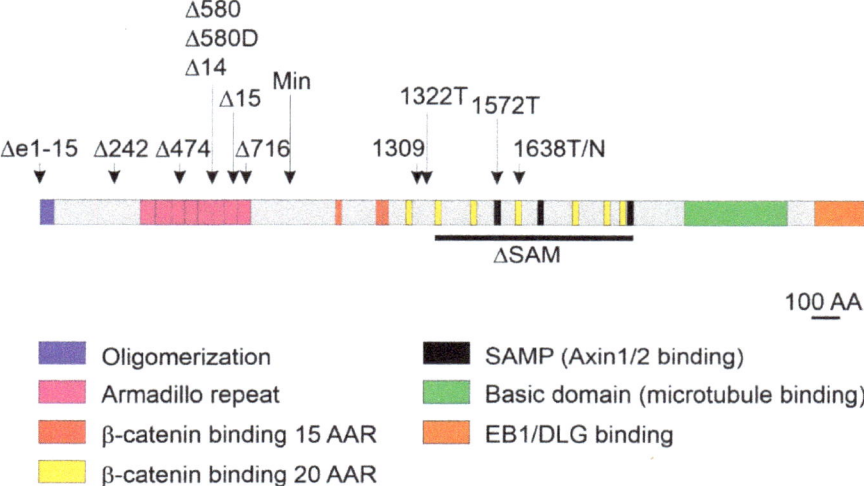

Figure 2. The domain structure and truncated variants of mouse adenomatous polyposis coli (Apc) protein. The scheme indicates positions of germline *Apc* mutations utilized in mouse models. The names of mutations correspond to the terms used in the studies describing a particular cancer model; the region which was deleted in the $Apc^{\Delta SAM}$ allele is underlined; Δ indicates deletion; AA, amino acid; AAR, amino-acid repeats; Axin, Axis inhibition; DLG, discs large; EB1, end-binding protein 1; SAMP, serine–alanine–methionine–proline.

The human APC protein consists of 2843 amino acids, and its interactions with other proteins of the β-catenin destruction complex are mediated by several domains (amino-acid repeats) located in the central part of the protein. There are three 15-amino-acid repeats (15AARs) that bind β-catenin constitutively and seven 20-amino-acid repeats (20AARs) that bind β-catenin inducibly (the interaction with 20AARs depends on the phosphorylation status of β-catenin) [70]. Three serine–alanine–methionine–proline (SAMP) amino-acid repeats are responsible for interactions with AXIN1/2 [71]. The N-terminal part of APC contains another protein interaction domain that includes eight so-called armadillo repeats. Finally, the C-terminus of the protein interacts with proteins involved in microtubule assembly, cell polarity, and chromosome segregation. More than 60% of *APC* mutations are located in a mutation cluster region (MCR) in exon 15, and, in most cases, the mutations result in loss of the C-terminal portion of APC protein [72,73]. The amino-acid sequence and domain composition of the Apc protein is evolutionarily conserved in metazoan species ranging from *Drosophila* to humans [74]. As the sequence identity of the human and mouse Apc proteins exceed 89%, the mouse represents a suitable mode to study the involvement of Apc truncations in intestinal cancer.

3.1. Multiple Intestinal Neoplasia (Min) Mice

The $Apc^{+/Min}$ mouse strain is a frequently used genetic mouse model to study CRC. Similarly to FAP patients, these mice (generated by random chemically induced mutagenesis) carry a nonsense germline mutation in one Apc allele that results in Apc truncation at codon 851 [32,75]. The Min mutation is autosomal dominant with 100% penetrance; while at homozygote state the mutation is embryonically lethal, the heterozygote animals are viable. After random inactivation of the second allele, adult $Apc^{+/Min}$ mice develop multiple intestinal polyps. The polyps predominantly develop in the small intestine, and to a much lesser extent in the colon. Occasionally, tumors might also appear in the mammary glands and stomach [76,77]. Importantly, the incidence of polyps is dependent on the genetic background and may be influenced by the diet. For example, intestinal polyps developed with 100% penetrance in $Apc^{+/Min}$ mice on the C57BL/6 background do not progress to carcinoma as the animals die at young age (16 to 18 weeks) due to anemia, inflammation, and other symptoms associated with digestive tract damage. In addition, the mice developed a large number of small intestinal tumors and a relatively low number of tumors in the colon [75]. In contrast, only 7% tumor incidence was observed in $Apc^{+/Min}$ mice of the FVB/Nj genetic background [78]. Recently, Sodrig and colleagues reported extensive colon carcinogenesis in $Apc^{+/Min}$ mice of the AKR/J background [79]. Strikingly, Cooper and co-workers documented that the presence of the Min allele in the animals (presumably) of the same genetic background but originating from separate colonies might be manifested by a remarkably differing phenotype. The authors of the study purchased $Apc^{+/Min}$ males of the C57BL/6 background from the Jackson Laboratory and crossed them with the wild-type (wt) C57BL/6 females originating from the Jackson Laboratory or from the domestic facility. The animals of the latter mouse "strain" designated $Apc^{+/Min-FCCC}$ developed more colorectal adenomas showing an increased rate of malignant progression and rectal prolapse [80]. Importantly, the animals were housed in the same animal facility and kept on the same diet, excluding exogenous sources of the observed phenotypic differences. Nevertheless, it was shown previously that the "Western type" of diet (increased fat and reduced fiber, calcium, and vitamin D content) significantly increased the incidence of Apc-deficient intestinal tumors [81–84]. Finally, different gene variants were examined to either enhance or attenuate the $Apc^{+/Min}$ phenotype. More than 10 genes called modifiers of Min (Mom) were discovered to date. The mechanism of action of Mom genes was described elsewhere [85].

3.2. Models Producing Mutant Apc Variants Longer Than Apc Protein Expressed from the Apc^{Min} Allele

Although the $Apc^{+/Min}$ strain is a commonly used model for intestinal neoplasia, most human mutations present in sporadic or hereditary intestinal neoplasms generate a longer form of APC protein than the one expressed from the Apc^{Min} allele. In human tumors, at least one APC allele produces a truncated protein retaining a functional β-catenin binding 20AAR motif [86,87]. Therefore, two mouse alleles—designated Apc^{1322T} and Apc^{1309} (original allele names are used throughout the review)—were generated; the alleles express the truncated Apc protein retaining one 20AAR. $Apc^{+/1322T}$ mice produced over 200 small intestinal polyps by the age of 10 to 12 weeks, which represented a more severe phenotype than the one observed in $Apc^{+/Min}$ animals. Surprisingly, although expression profiling showed that the messenger RNA (mRNA) levels of stem-cell marker leucine-rich repeat-containing G-protein coupled receptor 5 ($Lgr5$) were increased, nuclear β-catenin levels were lower than in $Apc^{+/Min}$ mice [88,89]. Since both strains, i.e., $Apc^{+/1322T}$ and $Apc^{+/Min}$ mice, were backcrossed with C57BL/6 animals, the discrepancy between the smaller amount of nuclear β-catenin and the more severe phenotype observed in $Apc^{+/1322T}$ mice cannot be explained by different genetic backgrounds. Nevertheless, the above observation can be explained by the finding that, when a certain level of nuclear β-catenin is exceeded, the production of intestinal tumors is (paradoxically) reduced [90]. In contrast, $Apc^{+/1309}$ mice have a milder intestinal phenotype than $Apc^{+/Min}$ mice, as they developed about 30 polyps by the age of 12 to 14 weeks. Moreover, the animals were affected by hyperlipidemia, a disorder characterized by abnormally elevated levels of lipids in the blood, at a younger age than

$Apc^{+/Min}$ mice [91,92]. The difference between the pathological manifestations documented in these mouse strains is striking, as the positions of the Apc protein truncation are only 13 amino acids apart. However, it might be explained by the differences in the gene targeting strategies used to generate the animals. Unfortunately, mice harboring the Apc^{1309} allele are not available in Europe or United States, and a detailed protocol describing the strain generation was not reported in English.

As mentioned, the C-terminus of APC is frequently lost in CRC, indicating that it is essential for the APC tumor suppressive role [93]. For functional studies of the C-terminal portion of the protein, a mouse model named $Apc^{\Delta SAMP}$ was created. In these mice, a central region of the Apc gene, which encodes six β-catenin binding 20AAR motives and all AXIN-binding SAMP repeats, was deleted, while the C-terminus was retained intact. $Apc^{+/\Delta SAMP}$ mice exhibited the same phenotype as mice harboring the Apc^{1322T} allele, which suggested that the presence of the C-terminal part of Apc is not sufficient to suppress tumorigenesis [94]. Moreover, three additional alleles were created; the alleles were designated Apc^{1638N}, Apc^{1638T}, and Apc^{1572T}. The Apc^{1638N} allele was generated by insertion of the phosphoglycerate kinase (PGK)–neomycin selectable marker cassette into exon 15 of Apc in reverse orientation. The insertion should have caused a truncating mutation at codon 1638. However, truncated Apc was not detectable by Western blotting, suggesting that Apc mRNA translation was possibly attenuated by the anti-sense transcript generated from the neomycin expression cassette; thus, the Apc^{1638N} allele is, in fact, a null allele [95]. While $Apc^{1638N/1638N}$ homozygotes died prenatally, heterozygous $Apc^{+/1638N}$ mice were viable and developed several (five to six) adenomas and adenocarcinomas located close to the periampullary area of the small intestine. Moreover, all $Apc^{+/1638N}$ mice developed cutaneous follicular cysts and desmoid tumors [96]. Therefore, $Apc^{+/1638N}$ mice phenocopied some of the symptoms observed in humans with the attenuated adenomatous polyposis coli (AAPC) syndrome. Hereditary AAPC is manifested by fewer than intestinal 100 polyps, delayed age of the polyp onset, and presence of severe desmoid tumors, osteosarcomas, and epidermoid cysts [97–99]. The Apc^{1638T} allele was generated by insertion of the PGK–hygromycin resistance cassette into exon 15 of the Apc gene in the sense orientation. In this arrangement, a truncated 1638-amino-acid-long polypeptide was indeed produced from the Apc locus. Surprisingly, $Apc^{1638T/1638T}$ mice were viable and tumor-free, thus displaying a remarkably different phenotype than that observed in $Apc^{1638N/1638N}$ and $Apc^{+/1638N}$ strains. Nevertheless, when compared to wild-type (wt) mice, the small intestine of $Apc^{1638T/1638T}$ animals was significantly shorter, migration and proliferation of intestinal epithelial cells was faster, and the numbers of Paneth and goblet cells were increased [100]. Moreover, $Apc^{1638T/1638N}$ and $Apc^{1638T/Min}$ heterozygotes died prenatally, indicating haploinsufficiency of the Apc^{1638T} allele [101]. Heterozygous $Apc^{+/1572T}$ animals producing the Apc protein truncated at codon 1572 were viable, but developed multifocal mammary adenocarcinomas with pulmonary metastases; homozygous $Apc^{1572T/1572T}$ died during embryonic development. Interestingly, in the tumor cells derived from this particular strain, a β-catenin/TCF luciferase reporter assay (TOP-FLASH) [102] and co-immunoprecipitation of β-catenin and APC indicated intermediate activation of the Wnt/β-catenin pathway. Such a level of Wnt signaling is possibly insufficient for development of intestinal neoplasia, but it might initiate breast cancer [103].

3.3. Models Producing Mutant Apc Variants Shorter Than Apc Protein Expressed from the Apc^{Min} Allele and a Strain with Complete Apc Deletion

This chapter discusses seven mouse models that carry a short form of Apc, i.e., shorter than the protein expressed from the Apc^{Min} allele. Additionally, we discuss the phenotype observed in animals after complete loss of the Apc protein, i.e., after removal of all Apc exons. The $Apc^{\Delta 242}$ allele was generated by inserting a β-geo gene trap cassette between exons 7 and 8. The targeting results in production of a fusion protein containing a truncated 242-amino-acid-long polypeptide lacking the armadillo repeat domain. $Apc^{+/\Delta 242}$ mice developed adenomas in the small intestine and colon with higher frequency than $Apc^{+/Min}$ mice, suggesting that the loss of the armadillo repeats increased tumorigenesis [104]. The $Apc^{\Delta 474}$ allele was created by duplication of exons 7–10 that cause a frameshift and immature stop in the Apc coding sequence. $Apc^{+/\Delta 474}$ heterozygotes exhibited a phenotype similar to $Apc^{+/Min}$ mice (polyps mainly in the small intestine and occasional mammary tumors) [33]. The $Apc^{\Delta 716}$ allele was constructed by insertion of the PGK–diphtheria toxin receptor selectable marker cassette into the Apc locus. The insertion leads to expression of a truncated transcript encoding a 716-amino-acid-long Apc polypeptide. Interestingly, although the protein produced in $Apc^{+/\Delta 716}$ mice is longer than in $Apc^{+/\Delta 242}$ and $Apc^{+/\Delta 474}$ animals, the number of polyps (>400) in $Apc^{+/\Delta 716}$ mice was remarkably higher than in the first two mouse strains [105].

Three independent research groups generated mouse strains harboring conditional knock-out (cKO) alleles of the Apc gene with exon 14 flanked, i.e., "floxed", by $loxP$ sequences [106–108]. Non-recombined homozygotes of all three strains (the non-recombined alleles were termed Apc^{580S}, Apc^{cKO}, and Apc^{3lox14}, respectively) were viable without any phenotype. Cre-mediated excision of exon 14 results in formation of the stop codon and production of a truncated Apc protein; Cre-recombined alleles were indicated as Apc^{580D}, $Apc^{\Delta 580}$, and $Apc^{\Delta 14}$, respectively. Shibata and colleagues injected a Cre-expressing adenovirus into the lumen of the colorectal region of $Apc^{580S/580S}$ mice, which resulted in formation of colorectal adenomas in 80% of experimental animals [106]. To generate heterozygous animals harboring a germline knock-out Apc allele, Apc^{cKO} and $Apc^{3lox14/+}$ mice were crossed with *EIIA-Cre-* and *MeuCre40*-expressing animals, respectively. In *EIIA-Cre* transgenic mice, Cre is expressed in the preimplantation embryo from early adenoviral (*EIIA*) promoter active in all tissues; in MeuCre40 mice, the Cre recombinase is expressed in all tissues. Animals from both strains developed numerous intestinal tumors, and subsequent analysis indicated that the wt Apc allele was inactivated by allelic loss [34,107]. Moreover, tamoxifen-induced recombination of the Apc^{cKO} alleles in $Apc^{cKO/cKO}$ *Lgr5-EGFP-IRES-CreERT2* and $Apc^{cKO/cKO}$ *Villin-CreERT2* animals allowed tissue-specific Apc inactivation in intestinal stem cells or in all intestinal epithelium cells, respectively [109,110]. In the latter strains, massive crypt hyperproliferation followed by intestinal microadenoma formation was observed already several days after tamoxifen administration (Figure 3) [111].

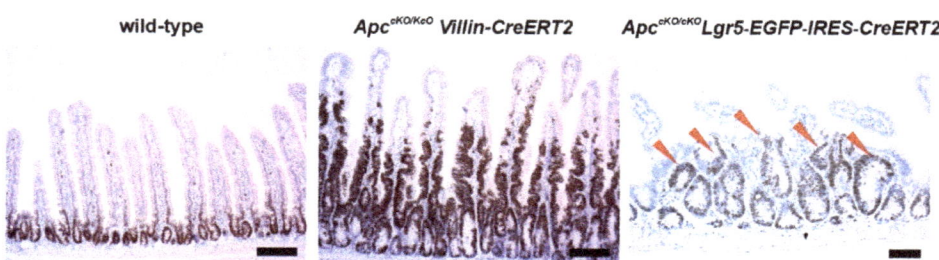

Figure 3. Crypt hyperplasia and microadenomas arising in the Apc-deficient small intestine. Immunohistochemical localization of proliferating cell nuclear antigen (PCNA; brown cell nuclei) in mice of the indicated genetic background. The middle microphotograph shows the hyperplastic crypt compartment developed in $Apc^{cKO/cKO}$ *Villin-CreERT2* mice seven days after tamoxifen administration; the right image shows microadenomas (red arrowheads) formed in the $Apc^{cKO/cKO}$ *Lgr5-EGFP-IRES-CreERT2* small intestine 21 days after tamoxifen administration. Sections were counterstained with hematoxylin (blue nuclear signal); scale bar: 0.3 mm (adopted from Reference [111]).

In addition to the mouse strains harboring floxed exon 14, Robanus-Maandag and colleagues generated a strain with floxed exon 15 (Apc^{15lox}). Deletion of this particular exon in germ cells generated $Apc^{+/\Delta 15}$ mice that displayed a phenotype reminding of $Apc^{+/Min}$ mice. Additionally, the $Apc^{+/15lox}$ mice were crossed to transgenic mice expressing Cre recombinase from the fatty acid-binding protein (*Fabpl*) gene promoter; the promoter is active in epithelial cells of the distal small intestine and colon. These mice survived longer (than $Apc^{+/\Delta 15}$) and developed about 40 tumors in the ileum, colon, and rectum [112].

Whereas the majority of human colorectal tumors harbor truncated *APC*, the null variant of the *APC* gene is relatively uncommon. In order to study the effect of complete loss of APC, Cheung and colleagues produced a mouse strain harboring cKO alleles allowing deletion of all 15 *Apc* exons (the recombined allele was designated $Apc^{\Delta e1-15}$). $Apc^{+/\Delta e1-15}$ heterozygotes had a more severe intestinal phenotype than $Apc^{+/Min}$ mice. Importantly, as the wt *Apc* allele was inactivated in $Apc^{+/\Delta e1-15}$ animals by *Apc* promoter hypermethylation or loss of heterozygosity, it was evident that, in the mouse model, the presence of a truncated Apc protein is not required for intestinal tumor development. Interestingly, although the amount of β-catenin protein was similar in tumors of $Apc^{+/\Delta e1-15}$ and $Apc^{+/Min}$ mice, the levels of β-catenin-dependent transcription seemed to be lower in $Apc^{+/\Delta e1-15}$ animals [113]. This confirmed that the "just optimal" β-catenin level is necessary for tumor initiation and growth [90].

3.4. Models Expressing Stabilized β-Catenin

Although *APC* mutations initiate the majority of human CRCs, a subset of human colorectal tumors with intact *APC* carries protein-stabilizing mutations in *CTNNB1*. For β-catenin ubiquitination and subsequent proteasomal degradation, the conserved N-terminal serine and threonine residues (S33, S37, T41, and S45) have to be phosphorylated. These amino acids are encoded by exon 3 of the *CTNNB1* gene; the same exon is considered to be a mutation hotspot in human CRC. Missense mutations or short deletion affecting the critical amino-acid residues (the mutational changes preserve the open reading frame) prevent β-catenin phosphorylation and, thus, lead to production of a stable protein (reviewed in References [114,115]). In order to model tumors that are initiated by alterations in the *CTNNB1* gene, Harada and colleagues generated mice harboring a conditional *Ctnnb1* allele where exon 3 was flanked by loxP sites ($Ctnnb1^{lox(ex3)/lox(ex3)}$). These mice were crossed with knock-in mice expressing Cre recombinase under the control of the cytokeratin 19 promoter ($Krt1-19^{Cre}$); the promoter drives Cre expression in the intestinal epithelium starting at early embryonic stages. Heterozygous $Ctnnb1^{+/lox(ex3)}$ $Krt1-19^{+/Cre}$ animals developed over 3000 polyps in the duodenum and proximal jejunum and only microadenomas in the colon by the third week after birth. Alternatively, $Ctnnb1^{lox(ex3)/lox(ex3)}$ mice were crossed with the $Fabpl^{Cre}$ strain; heterozygous $Ctnnb1^{+/lox(ex3)}$ $Fabpl^{Cre}$ animals developed 200 to 700 polyps in the small intestine by the age of 4–5 weeks [116]. In summary, the models of β-catenin oncogenic activation recapitulated a severe phenotype observed in some Apc-deficient mice.

3.5. Alleles Allowing Aberrant (Over) Expression of Wnt Agonists R-Spondins

Secreted RSPOs bind the Lgr 4/5/6 receptor to potentiate the Wnt signaling pathway output. The signaling function of the RSPO/LGR complex has multiple effects and, inter alia, leads to inhibition of transmembrane E3 ubiquitin ligases zinc and ring finger 3 (ZNRF3) and ring finger 43 (RNF43). These ligases act on Wnt receptor Frizzled, mediating its turnover. However, binding of the RSPO ligand to the LGR receptor results in ZNRF3 and RNF3 internalization and subsequent degradation in lysosomes. The mechanism leads to increased availability of the Frizzled receptors on the cell surface and, thus, enhanced Wnt signaling (Figure 1b) (reviewed in Reference [117]).

Approximately 10% of CRC specimens harbor chromosomal rearrangements that involve loci encoding *RSPO* genes. These chromosomal rearrangements are mainly based on gene fusions of *RSPO2* or *RSPO3* with another highly expressed gene, such as protein tyrosine phosphatase receptor type K (*PTPRK*), eukaryotic translation initiation factors 3e (*EIF3E*), and piezo-type mechanosensitive ion channel component 1 (*PIEZO1*) [118,119]. All these gene fusions result in aberrant *RSPO2/3* overexpression. To investigate this type of CRC, Hilkens and colleagues developed a conditional *Rspo3* transgenic mouse ($Rspo3^{inv}$) where *Rspo3* was expressed in cells producing Cre recombinase. The mice were crossed to *Lgr5-EGFP-IRES-CreERT2* [110] mice, and Cre-mediated *Rspo* expression was induced by tamoxifen. The animals developed hyperplasia in the small intestine, cecum, and proximal colon. The incidence of neoplasia (mainly adenoma and adenocarcinoma) was 2.5 tumors per mouse on average, and moderate upregulation of Wnt target genes was observed [120]. Additional mouse models were generated by Cas9-mediated fusion of *Rspo2* or *Rspo3* with *EIF3E* and *Ptprk*, respectively, using the tetracycline-inducible clustered regularly interspaced short palindromic repeats (CRISPR)/Cas9 system. Since the chromosomal rearrangements occurred randomly after the Cas9-mediated DNA cleavage, this model adequately reproduced the condition that is commonly found in human CRC. Two weeks after doxycycline administration, i.e., after Cas9 induction, adenomas were observed in the mouse small intestine. Nevertheless, in both models, tumor growth was rather attenuated, and hyperplastic or dysplastic lesions were formed only. Surprisingly, contrary to the model of Hilkens and co-workers, no significant increase in Wnt target gene expression in the *EIF3E-Rspo2* or *Ptprk-Rspo3* intestines was noted [121].

4. Mouse Models of Inactive Hippo Signaling

The Hippo signaling pathway was originally discovered in *Drosophila* as a signaling mechanism controlling the organ size. However, later studies identified involvement of the Hippo signaling in other important processes such as cell division, differentiation, and maintenance of cell pluripotency [122]. The core complex of the mammalian Hippo signaling pathway includes serine/threonine STE20-like protein kinase 1 (MST1; alternative name STK4) and related MST2 (STK3), large tumor suppressor kinase 1/2 (LATS1/2), scaffold proteins salvador family WW domain-containing protein 1 (SAV1), and mono-polar spindle-1 one binder kinase activator 1A/1B (MOB1A/1B). When the Hippo pathway is not active, the effectors yes-associated protein 1 (YAP1) and tafazzin (TAZ) can freely enter the cell nucleus, where they associate with transcription co-factors from the transcriptional enhancer factor 1 and abacus A family (TEAD). The YAP1 (TAZ)–TEAD complex activates transcription of pro-proliferative and anti-apoptotic genes. Conversely, when Hippo signaling is activated (by growth inhibiting signals), YAP and TAZ are phosphorylated by LATS1/2. The modification prevents their transport to the nucleus and drives their ubiquitination and degradation (reviewed in Reference [123]). The pathway is further controlled by ubiquitination-independent proteasome activator subunit 3 (PSME3, alternative name regenerating islet-derived protein 3 (REGγ)), which can degrade LATS1 and, thus, activate YAP1.

Neither deregulation of the Hippo pathway nor mutations in genes encoding the pathway components were reported in relation to a particular CMS group. Nevertheless, some CRCs show a positive correlation between poorer prognosis and overexpression of *YAP1*, *TAZ*, *TEAD4*, and *REGγ* [124–128]. In addition, YAP1 and TAZ proteins interact with β-catenin. The interaction leads to inhibition of β-catenin nuclear localization and results in downregulation of Wnt signaling. Moreover, since active Hippo signaling inhibits cells growth and proliferation, the signaling in fact opposes pro-proliferative Wnt pathway-mediated cellular processes. Consequently, models altering the Hippo pathway status might complement studies involving aberrant Wnt signaling.

The first model simulating the inactive Hippo pathway was represented by a transgenic mouse strain allowing doxycycline-inducible *Yap1* production/activation. Upon doxycycline administration, the mice ubiquitously expressed a mutated form of Yap1 (Yap1^{S127A}), which is not phosphorylated on critical serine 127 and, thus, escapes degradation. The mice (examined five days after activation of Yap1 expression) displayed massive cell proliferation in multiple organs. The most pronounced phenotype was observed in the intestine, where the entire epithelium appeared dysplastic. Interestingly, the proliferation was not restricted to the intestinal crypts, but dividing cells were also detected in the villus region. In addition, mature goblet or Paneth cells were absent throughout the intestine [129]. Additionally, the same research group generated a mouse strain with Yap1^{S127A} expression regulated by intestinal epithelium-specific expression of reverse tetracycline transactivator (rtTA). Interestingly, the phenotype of these mice was fundamentally different from the animals expressing Yap1^{S127A} ubiquitously. Strikingly, seven days after induction of Yap1^{S127A}, the intestinal epithelium exhibited progressive degeneration associated with loss of dividing cells in the crypts [130]. It was suggested that, in the whole-body Yap1 activation model, paracrine Yap1-dependent signals originated from stromal cells might support adjacent epithelial cells, and this type of support is absent in animals with tissue-specific Yap1^{S127A} expression [123]. Nevertheless, the discrepancy between the phenotypes observed in the above-described models remains unclear. Another model of the inactive Hippo pathway was based on null alleles of the *Mst1* gene (*Mst1^{null}*) and conditional *Mst2* alleles (*Mst2^{ff}*); to achieve epithelial inactivation of Mst2, the latter strain was intercrossed with transgenic *Villin-Cre* mice [109]. The *Mst1^{null}* or *Mst2^{ff} Villin-Cre* mice were born in Mendelian ratios, but their average lifespan was 13 weeks only. The mice displayed a significantly expanded stem-cell compartment and reduced numbers of differentiated cells in both small intestine and colon; moreover, adenomas were present in the distal part of the colon. Interestingly, whereas the total amount of β-catenin was not—in comparison to control wt mice—changed, the level of nuclear β-catenin was increased. Additionally, the phenotype of *Mst1^{null} Mst2^{ff} Villin-Cre* mice was suppressed after inactivation of one or both *Yap1* alleles [131]. Rather surprisingly, inactivation of *Yap1* per se in the intestine had no obvious phenotype. However, when subjected to DSS treatment, the regenerative capacity of the Yap1-deficient intestinal epithelium animals was abolished [132]. Enhanced Hippo signaling was also investigated in *REGγ$^{-/-}$* mice. REGγ deficiency increased expression of Lats1, and, as a consequence, the cellular level of phosphorylated Yap1 was upregulated. Nevertheless, after DSS-induced colitis, *REGγ$^{-/-}$* mice developed lower amounts of smaller and less proliferating colorectal tumors when compared to wt mice [128]. In summary, the described models (the corresponding strains are listed in Table S3, Supplementary Materials) indicated that impaired Hippo signaling via Yap1 is involved in intestinal tumorigenesis.

5. Mouse Models of p53 Pathway Deficiency

Activation of tumor suppressor p53 represents a fundamental mechanism blocking cancer cell proliferation and/or survival. Consequently, p53 loss is associated with initiation, progression, and invasiveness of various malignancies (reviewed in Reference [133]). In a healthy cell, the p53 level is kept low by action of E3 ubiquitin ligase mouse double minute 2 homolog (MDM2) [134]. Nevertheless, when the cell is exposed to adverse conditions such as oxidative stress, DNA damage, or replication stress, p53 is stabilized and induces apoptotic pathways (reviewed in Reference [135]). Moreover, to block cell-cycle progression, p53 activates transcription of many target genes involved in cell-cycle regulation. A prototypic p53-induced gene is represented by cyclin-dependent kinase inhibitor 1A (*CDKN1A*), which encodes cyclin-dependent kinase (CDK) inhibitor p21 (alternative name CIP1/WAF1); p21 prevents cells from entering the synthesis (S) phase (reviewed in Reference [136]). Loss of the p53 function was detected in 50–70% of all colorectal tumors [16,137]; nevertheless, p53 mutations were mostly detected in advanced tumors. Thus, p53 inactivation represents one of the crucial events in adenoma-carcinoma transition. Moreover, *TP53*-mutant tumors appear to be more resistant to chemotherapy, resulting in poorer prognosis of the treated patient (reviewed in Reference [24]). Mutations in the *TP53* gene were found in tumors of all CMS types, ranging from 27% to 62% in the CMS1 or CMS2 group, respectively [24]. The most frequently mutated region of the *TP53* gene consisted of exons 5–8 that encode a sequence-specific DNA-binding domain. Intriguingly, mutations in codons 175, 245, 248, 273, and 282 were repeatedly identified in several studies [35,138,139]. These predominantly missense mutations affect the p53 ability to bind target DNA, and consequently they inhibit the transcriptional regulatory role of p53. Interestingly, different *TP53* mutations might impact CRC properties, especially lymphatic or vascular invasion and metastasis (reviewed in Reference [140]). Inactivation of the p53 target gene *CDKN1A* was detected in 79% of colorectal tumors, and it showed a clear correlation with *TP53* deficiency [141]. Strikingly, p21 loss inversely correlated with high CIMP and MSI. Moreover, in CIMP- and MSI-high CRCs, the deficiency was independent of the *TP53* status [142]. Therefore, colorectal tumors with mutated p21 were assigned to the CMS2 or CMS4 groups that display low CIMP and MSI and contain a high proportion of p53-mutated tumors [24].

A whole-body knockout of the *Trp53* gene in the mouse was described more than 25 years ago. The study confirmed the tumor suppressive role of p53; p53-deficient mice were predisposed to formation of many different types of tumors, predominantly lymphomas, osteosarcomas, and adenocarcinomas [143,144]. Combinations of p53 deficiency with other mouse tumor models modulated the rate, localization, and number of gastrointestinal tumors. For example, $Apc^{+/Min}$ $Trp53^{-/-}$ mice developed increased amounts of more invasive intestinal adenomas than $Apc^{+/Min}$ mice harboring wt p53 [145]. In addition, $Trp53^{-/-}$ $Tcr\beta^{-/-}$ mice suffered from more severe colitis than $Tcr\beta^{-/-}$ mice and developed inflammation-associated adenocarcinomas in the cecum and colon [146]. Interestingly, AOM/DSS treatment in p53-deficient mice resulted in nuclear accumulation of β-catenin accompanied by robust activation of Wnt-responsive genes. However, increased Wnt/β-catenin-dependent transcription was not seen when animals were treated with DSS only [147].

Interestingly, in the case of CAC, p53 deficiency influenced not only the incidence, but also the morphology of the tumors. Comparison of tumors isolated from DSS-treated $Trp53^{-/-}$, $Trp53^{+/-}$, and $Trp53^{+/+}$ mice showed that $Trp53^{-/-}$ tumors are rather flat (84.6%), while $Trp53^{+/-}$ and $Trp53^{+/+}$ lesions are mostly polypoid (83.3% and 100%, respectively; polypoid tumors represent neoplastic lesions whose height is greater than one-half of their diameter). Moreover, polypoid neoplasia often carried (in 75% of cases) mutations in the *Ctnnb1* gene, and tumor cells displayed nuclear localization of β-catenin. The results suggest that different tumorigenic mechanisms affect not only the formation, but also the morphology of CAC [148].

In addition to the FAP syndrome, there are several other hereditary polyposis syndromes including the Peutz–Jeghers syndrome (PJS). Individuals with PJS develop gastrointestinal hamartomatous polyps due to an inactivating germline mutation in the liver kinase B1 (*LKB1*) gene (alternative name serine/threonine kinase 11 (*STK11*)). In contrast to the polyps developed in FAP patients, malignant transformation of PJS hamartomas is very rare (reviewed in Reference [149]). LKB1 physically associates with p53 and promotes p53-dependent apoptosis [150]. Importantly, restoration of LKB1 activity in (originally) LKB1-defective cancer cells induced p21 expression followed by cell-cycle arrest [151,152]. In order to investigate the LKB1 function in PJS, mice harboring mutation in the *Lkb1* gene were generated. Homozygous germline deletion of *Lkb1* was embryonic lethal; however, heterozygous mice developed hamartomatous gastric and small intestinal polyps [153]. In addition, $Lkb1^{+/-}$ $Trp53^{-/-}$ mice displayed increased incidence and earlier formation of tumors that retained a hamartomatous character [154], indicating that combined deficiency in both genes might accelerate tumor formation.

As already indicated, CDK inhibitor p21 (*Cdkn1a*) is important regulatory protein involved in cell proliferation. Surprisingly, although $p53^{-/-}$ mice develop multiple tumors, spontaneous tumor development was not observed in young $Cdkn1a^{-/-}$ mice [155,156]. However, when the mice were reared for one year or longer, formation of hematopoietic, endothelial, and epithelial tumors was noted [157]. Importantly, *Cdkn1a*-deficient mice developed increased numbers of ACFs along the entire length of the colon after treatment with AOM [158]. Moreover, tumor incidence and metastatic potential was further potentiated by whole-body irradiation [159]. Similarly to $Trp53^{-/-}$ $Apc^{+/Min}$ mice, the increased tumor burden was observed in $Cdkn1a^{-/-}$ $Apc^{+/1638}$ animals [160]. The results suggested that the p53–p21 pathway plays an important role in the inhibition of growth of Apc-deficient tumors. Indeed, in human tumors, p21 loss indicates poor prognosis [161]. In conclusion, mutations inactivating p53 were manifested by increased incidence of neoplasia in other organs than the intestine. Therefore, to model CRC, p53 pathway-deficient mice were mainly employed in combination with other genetic modifications (or with irradiation and mutagen exposure) to provoke (or accelerate) intestinal tumor development and progression. Models described in this chapter are listed in Table S4 (Supplementary Materials).

6. Mouse Models of Aberrant Activation of the Epidermal Growth Factor Signaling Pathway

The signaling pathway initiated by interaction of the epidermal growth factor (EGF) ligand and the EGF receptor [(EGFR; alternative names avian erythroblastic leukemia viral (v-erb-b) oncogene homolog (ERBB1) or human epidermal growth factor receptor 2 (HER1)] represents a signaling cascade inducing pleiotropic effects in the target cell. The effects include proliferation and inhibition of apoptosis; therefore, the pathway activity is tightly regulated (reviewed in Reference [162]). Ligand binding to EGFR triggers sequential activation of mitogen-activated protein kinases (MAPKs), which transduces the signal to the cell nucleus. In more detail, EGFR functions as a transmembrane receptor tyrosine kinase that undergoes autophosphorylation upon interaction with EGF. A phosphorylated intracellular portion of the receptor interacts with the Src homology 2 (SH2) domain of the cytoplasmic proteins growth factor receptor-bound protein 2 (GRB2) and son of sevenless (SOS). Receptor complex-bound SOS promotes the exchange of guanosine diphosphate (GDP) to guanosine triphosphate (GTP) associated with small G-proteins from the RAS family. GTP-loaded Ras proteins in turn activate Raf protein kinases, the initial kinases in the MAPK cascade (reviewed in Reference [162]).

In human sporadic CRC, several principal components of the MAPK pathway, i.e., *EGFR*, *KRAS*, *NRAS*, and *BRAF*, are recurrently mutated. Generally, activating mutations in proto-oncogenes *KRAS* and *BRAF* were present in human tumors corresponding to the CMS3 (68%) and CMS1 (42%) groups, respectively. Whereas *BRAF* mutations were almost exclusively present in these CMS groups, *KRAS* mutations were also detected, although to a lesser extent, in the CMS2 and CMS4 groups. Interestingly, in tumor-derived intestinal organoid cultures, *KRAS* mutations were found in all CMS groups except for CMS3 [26]. Mutations in *NRAS* were mostly detected in the CMS3 group (9%) [24].

To analyze the impact of genetic alterations in the EGFR pathway on CRC initiation or progression, a number of mouse models were used. According to mouse studies, mutations in the EGFR pathway alone are not sufficient to initiate colon tissue transformation [163,164]. Nevertheless, oncogenic mutations in genes involved in EGFR-mediated signaling are considered to be driver mutations as they emerge in early (pre-neoplastic) lesions. In fact, activating mutations in *KRAS* and *BRAF* were already detected in tumor-initiating cells [165,166]. Additionally, when these genetic alterations are combined with mutations in genes encoding *Trp53* or Wnt pathway components, they facilitate colorectal tumor progression.

6.1. Mouse Strains Expressing Mutant Epidermal Growth Factor Receptor

Activating mutations in the *EGFR* gene were found in 10% of the analyzed human tumor specimens. Moreover, 7% of CRCs harbored activating mutations in EGFR paralog ERBB2/HER2 [167]. The EGFR function in CRC was assessed using mice carrying the $Egfr^{wa2}$ [168] and $Egfr^{wa5}$ [169] loss-of-function alleles, and $Egfr^{tm1Mag}$ [170] null allele using various genetic backgrounds. Whereas *EGFR* gene amplification and activating mutations in the receptor kinase domain are frequent in human CRC samples [171,172], experiments in mice showed that the EGFR activity is indispensable for tumors developed in $Apc^{+/Min}$ mice [170] or in AOM/DSS-induced neoplasia [168]. To assess the Egfr function in immune-mediated colitis, $Egfr^{wa5/wa5}$ mice were treated with AOM/DSS and crossed with interleukin 10 (Il10)-deficient ($Il10^{-/-}$) mice, a strain that represents a model of spontaneous colitis with many characteristics of human inflammatory bowel disease (IBD). Although the incidence of tumors in AOM/DSS-treated $Egfr^{wa5/wa5}$ mice was comparable to wt controls, tumor progression was significantly increased. In 40% of AOM/DSS-treated $Egfr^{wa5/wa5}$ mice, invasive adenocarcinomas were formed; tumors in wt mice remained non-invasive. In contrast, $Il10^{-/-}$ $Egfr^{wa5/wa5}$ mice exhibited elevated tumor formation and progression in comparison to $Il10^{-/-}$ $Egfr^{+/+}$ mice. Since the tumors in $Il10^{-/-}$ $Egfr^{wa5/wa5}$ animals developed without administration of (any) mutagen, this model might be more applicable to studying tumorigenesis in IBD patients. Nevertheless, the results of these experiments paradoxically indicated an unexpected tumor-suppressive function of EGFR signaling in chronic colitis [169].

6.2. Mouse Models Producing Mutant Kras *and* Nras

KRAS mutations that "lock" the protein in the active GTP-bound state were detected in approximately 40% of human CRCs [173]. Mutations in the homologous *NRAS* gene were identified in less than 5% of sporadic CRCs. As *KRAS* is the most frequently mutated oncogene participating in EGFR signaling in human CRC, great effort was made to characterize the *KRAS* function using animal models. In human tumors, activating *KRAS* mutations are localized to the region that encodes the GTP-binding domain, specifically to codons 12 and 13. Accordingly, mouse alleles harboring substitutions in amino-acid glycine at position 12 or 13 (G12 and G13) were used to model colorectal carcinogenesis. In general, phenotypical and histological analyses of the *Kras*-mutant colonic epithelium converged on the fact that the *Kras* oncogene enhanced proliferation but was insufficient for cell transformation. However, in combination with other driver mutations, such as in *Apc* or *Trp53*, mutant *Kras* indeed promoted tumor progression [164,174]. Additionally, several research groups generated mouse strains carrying *Kras* alleles with inducible substitution of the glycine 12 residue to aspartate (G12D) or valine (D12V). Johnson and colleagues prepared two "latent" alleles ($Kras^{LA1}$ and $Kras^{LA2}$), which were activated by spontaneous (mutual) recombination of wt and oncogenic $Kras^{G12D}$ variant of exon 1. The $Kras^{LA1}$ allele contains only one copy of the mutated exon 1, while the $Kras^{LA2}$ allele contains two copies. Thus, in vivo recombination of the $Kras^{LA1}$ allele produces both wt and $Kras^{G12D}$ allele (in a 1:1 ratio), whereas the $Kras^{LA2}$ allele generates the oncogenic $Kras^{G12D}$ allele only. The frequency of recombination ranged from 10^{-3} to 10^{-7} per cell generation, which (surpassingly) ensured sufficient cell numbers expressing mutant Kras. Mice harboring the latent allele developed colonic aberrant crypt foci (ACF), which represent pre-neoplastic epithelial lesions with enhanced proliferation and potential for malignant growth [165]. However, ACF found in $Kras^{LA1}$ and $Kras^{LA2}$ mice did not progress to form more advanced tumors. This suggested that *Kras* was not sufficient for malignant transformation of epithelial cells [164]. Interestingly, the presence of $Kras^{LA1}$ and $Kras^{LA2}$ alleles on the $Apc^{+/Min}$ and $Trp53^{-/-}$ genetic background had—presumably due to the low incidence of oncogenic *Kras* allele activation—no or little effect on ACF progression, The only detectable effect was occurrence of several adenocarcinomas in the duodenum [164].

In order to maximize the effect of oncogenic *Kras*, additional alleles were designed. Guerra and colleagues generated mice harboring the conditional $Kras^{G12V}$-IRES-β-geo allele and crossed the animals with mice that expressed tamoxifen-inducible Cre-ERT2 recombinase from the promoter of the large subunit of RNA polymerase II (*RERTn*); the allele produced upon Cre-mediated recombination was named $Kras^{V12}$. Since the homozygous $Kras^{V12/V12}$ animals died during embryonic development, heterozygous $Kras^{+/V12}$ $RERTn^{+/ERT}$ mice were utilized in further experiments. However, these mice did not reveal any pathologic changes in the intestinal epithelium [175]. In contrast, the similar inducible $Kras^{G12D}$ allele, which was specifically activated in the intestinal epithelium, caused hyperproliferation of cells in the colon crypts of $Kras^{G12D}$ $Fabpl^{cre}$ mice [163,174]. Moreover, the oncogenic form of *Kras* in the colon of Apc-deficient mice ($Apc^{2lox14/+}$ $Kras^{G12D/+}$ *Fapbl-Cre* strain) markedly increased the number of tumors, and, by blocking cell differentiation, $Kras^{V12}$ induced tumor progression [174]. Interestingly, the $Nras^{G12D}$ allele in the analogous genetic background neither enhanced proliferation of the healthy colonic epithelia nor promoted progression of Apc-deficient adenomas. However, the mutant $Nras^{G12D}$ allele had the capacity to suppress DSS-mediated apoptosis in the colonic epithelium [174]. Finally, mice harboring the $Kras^{G12D}$-IRES-EGFP allele (the allele was designated $Kras^{Asp12}$) were crossed with *Ah-Cre* mice that produce Cre in various tissues after induction with β-naphthoflavone [176]. The $Kras^{Asp12}$ *Ah-Cre* mice developed several adenomas in the small intestine and colon within two years after Cre induction. However, after crossing with $Apc^{+/Min}$ mice and Cre induction with β-naphthoflavone, the compound mutants ($Kras^{Asp12}$ *Ah-Cre* $Apc^{+/Min}$) displayed a much severer phenotype than $Apc^{+/Min}$ mice, i.e., decreased lifespan and elevated amounts of small intestinal and colonic tumors [177]. As an alternative approach to Cre-expressing mouse strains, Hung and colleagues accelerated colon adenocarcinoma progression by injection of adenoviral Cre into the colon of $Apc^{cKO/cKO}$ $Kras^{+/G12D}$ mice [178]. Most recently, a novel $Kras^{A146T}$ allele that mimics less frequent mutation in the Kras guanine nucleotide-binding domain found in human CRC was established and expressed after $Fabp1^{cre}$-mediated recombination in the colon of wt and $Apc^{2lox14/+}$ mice. However, the effect of the mutated protein on the intestinal epithelium was milder when compared to the phenotype observed in animals expressing the $Kras^{G12D}$ allele [179].

6.3. Mouse Models Harboring Mutant Braf Alleles

Another recurrently mutated gene in the EGFR pathway that was genetically manipulated in mice is *BRAF* [180]. The *BRAF* gene was mutated in approximately 10% of colorectal adenocarcinomas [37].

The majority of *BRAF* mutations in human cancers are localized to the region encoding a kinase domain; the gene alterations mainly result in amino-acid substitution from valine (V) to glutamic acid (G) in codon 600 (V600E missense mutation; the mutation was formerly known as V599E) [180,181]. To study the function of aberrantly activated *BRAF* in tumorigenesis, Mercer and colleagues generated the mouse allele *Braf*^{V600E} that allows Cre-inducible expression of the oncogenic *Braf* variant [36]. Shortly after the study was published, Dankort and colleagues produced a similar Cre-inducible *Braf*^{V600E} allele and used the allele to analyze the *Braf* function in lung adenocarcinomas [182]. Unfortunately, none of these mouse models were employed to study colon tumorigenesis. Finally, in 2013, intestine-specific recombination of the third version of the *Braf*^{V600E} allele was carried out by cross-breeding of *Braf*$^{+/V600}$ mice with the *Villin-Cre* strain. Expression of the *Braf*^{V600E} oncogene in the mouse intestinal epithelium resulted in crypt hyperplasia with a high rate of tumor progression. Although the presence of the *Braf*^{V600} allele was sufficient to transform cells, gene expression and immunohistochemical analysis of advanced tumors showed that additional mutations in genes encoding the Wnt and p53 pathways components were required for tumor progression [183]. Additionally, organoids derived from the *Braf*^{V600E} mouse were employed in experiments (the allele activation was achieved by infection of organoid cells with Cre-expressing lentivirus) showing that age-related epigenetic changes are an important oncogenic driver in intestinal cells expressing mutant *Braf* [184].

Interestingly, CIMP- and MSI-high tumors, which fall to the CMS1 group of CRC with mutations in *BRAF*, often exhibit significant mucinous cell differentiation [29,185]. Moreover, a correlation between enhanced expression of mucins and the presence of somatic *BRAF*^{V600E} mutation was reported recently [186]. Major glycoprotein secreted by intestinal goblet cells Mucin-2 functions as an important homeostasis-preserving protein involved in formation of the mucinous layer protecting the intestinal epithelium [187]. The protective role of Mucin-2 against tissue damage was documented in *Muc2*$^{-/-}$ mice that developed adenomas in the small intestine, colon, and rectum [188]. Since mucinous tumors frequently display poorer prognosis, we might speculate that elevated mucin expression results in increased tumor resistance towards treatment.

In addition to MAPK signaling, the EGFR pathway activates the phosphoinositide 3-kinase (PI3K)/protein kinase B (PKB/AKT)/mammalian target of rapamycin (mTOR) signaling cascade (reviewed in Reference [162]). Mutations of critical components involved in PI3K-mediated signaling, i.e., in *PIK3*, phosphatase and tensin homolog (*PTEN*; the gene encodes a dual-specificity phosphatase that antagonizes PI3K signaling [189]), and *AKT* occurred in 13–32%, 14%, and 1–6% of human CRC samples, respectively [190,191]. Recently, Mitchell and Phillips reviewed the mouse models of mutant PI3K in disease, covering CRC in detail [192]. In addition, mouse models mimicking mutations in the *Pten* and *Akt* genes were described elsewhere [193–196]. Thus, for the sake of brevity, we do not discuss the mouse models of aberrant EGF signaling that include alterations in the *Pik3*, *PTEN*, and *AKT* genes; the mouse strains that are mentioned in this chapter are listed in Table S5 (Supplementary Materials).

7. Mouse Models of Impaired TGFβ Signaling

The TGFβ signaling pathway is indispensable for intestinal homeostasis as it inhibits proliferation and supports differentiation of intestinal epithelial cells. Hence, the pathway represents an important tumor-suppressive mechanism. Therefore, TGFβ signaling is often altered in sporadic CRC (reviewed in Reference [197]). In brief, TGFβ ligands exist in three isoforms (TGFβ1/2/3) and form active homo- or heterodimers. The ligand dimers bind to TGFβ receptors type II (TGFβ-RII) that subsequently recruit and phosphorylate the TGFβ-RI receptors. In the cytoplasm, phosphorylated TGFβ-RI further bind receptor-regulated SMAD signal transducers (R-SMADs), which upon phosphorylation bind the common partner SMAD4. The R-SMAD/SMAD4 complexes then shuttle into the nucleus, where they interact with a variety of transcriptional factors and regulate gene expression (reviewed in Reference [198]).

The most common mutations of the TGFβ pathway in CRC are in the *TGFBR2* gene encoding the type II receptor (nearly 30% of CRCs). Since the *TGFBR2* gene contains a microsatellite sequence in its coding region, mutated *TGFBR2* was found in more than 80% of MSI-high tumors (reviewed in Reference [199]). Mutations in individual *SMAD* genes are present in approximately 10% of CRC and predict—due to their association with disease progression and lymph node metastasis—poor prognosis [200]. Mutations in *SMAD4* are the most frequent and are associated with mucinous tumor histology [201]. Increasing incidence of *SMAD4* mutations in advanced malignancies also suggests that this transcription co-factor is involved in tumor progression [202,203]. In addition, hereditary germline *SMAD4* mutations are associated with the juvenile polyposis syndrome characterized by increased incidence of hamartomatous intestinal polyps that gradually progress to carcinomas [204]. Mutations in *SMAD2* and *SMAD3* are less frequent than in *SMAD4*, although they are very similar with respect to the mutation type and distribution in the gene region [201].

Intriguingly, the CMS4 group tumors indicated the gene expression signature of active TGFβ signaling [24]. Similarly, gene set enrichment analysis of CRC cell lines and tumor-derived organoids revealed increased activation of the TGFβ pathway in the CMS4 group cell lines and organoids. Recent studies identified cancer-associated fibroblasts (CAFs) present in the tumor stroma as a "source" of the gene expression signature, indicating elevated TGFβ signaling [205,206]. Importantly, active TGFβ signaling in the tumor microenvironment increases the count of tumor-initiating cells in the tumor [205]. Moreover, tumors enriched in TGFβ-specific transcription tend to form metastases, resulting in poor prognosis [207]. Interestingly, mutations in the TGFβ pathway are less frequent in commercially available cell lines and tumor organoids than expected from the analysis of human tumor specimens [26]. This is consistent with the fact that the tumor stroma is primarily responsible for the TGFβ signaling gene signature.

In accordance with the fact that the TGFβ pathway is involved in the immune response regulation, $Tgfb1^{-/-}$ mice displayed extensive inflammation and died within one month after birth [208,209]. However, cross-breeding of $Tgfb1^{-/-}$ mice with immunodeficient $Rag2^{-/-}$ mice generated viable animals that developed tumors in the cecum and colon [210]. Homozygous knock-out of the *Smad2* and *Smad4* genes was embryonic lethal; however, deletion of one *Smad4* allele only yielded gastrointestinal hamartomas in the stomach and duodenum with histopathological features reminding of JPS [211]. In contrast, *Smad3* homozygous deletion did not affect embryogenesis; however, Smad3-deficient mice developed invasive colorectal tumors that metastasized to the lymph nodes [212].

Colorectal tumors arising as a result of impaired TGFβ signaling did not display elevated Wnt signaling [213]. This mirrored the fact that upregulation of the TGFβ and Wnt signaling pathways was observed in different CMS groups (CMS4 vs. CMS2 group, respectively) [24]. Nevertheless, deficiency in *Tgfbr1/2* or *Smad3/4* further accelerated intestinal tumor development and increased malignancy of lesions formed in the Apc-deficient intestine [214–218]. Analogously, compound heterozygous disruption of the *Apc* and *Smad2* genes enhanced tumor progression and invasiveness [219]. Interestingly, mice with conditional *Tgfbr2* knock-out in the intestinal epithelium ($Tgfbr2^{E2flox/E2flox}$ *Villin-CreERT2*) displayed impaired mucosal regeneration after irradiation and, moreover, developed invasive carcinomas in the colon upon colitis-inducing DSS treatment. Thus, the genetic alteration of the TGFβ pathway appears to be sufficient to generate CAC in the inflammatory microenvironment without any need for Apc inactivation [30]. Mouse strains described in this chapter are listed in Table S6 (Supplementary Materials).

8. Mouse Models of DNA Mismatch Repair Deficiency

The mismatch repair (MMR) mechanism provides corrections of base–base mismatches and loops in DNA strands that originate from incorrect base insertions (or deletions) during DNA replication. Nucleotide selectivity and polymerase proofreading result in the error rate of approximately 10^{-5} to 10^{-6} mismatches during DNA replication. Importantly, the functional MMR system further decreases the error rates to as low as 10^{-10} [220]. The canonical MMR pathway in humans consists of two major functional components having names derived from homologous bacterial genes, mutator S (*MutS*) and mutator L (*MutL*). MutS contains the MutS homolog 2 (MSH2) protein, which forms a heterodimer with the MSH6 protein, in the case of base substitutions and small loop repairs, or with MSH3, in the case of larger DNA loops. Heterodimer MutL, formed with MutL homolog 1 (MLH1) in combination with postmeiotic segregation increased 1/2 (PMS1/2) or MLH3, is involved in the recognition and repair of non-Watson–Crick base pairs. MMR deficiency leads to a higher mutation rate and occurs in cancers with MSI. Thus, intestinal tumors with mutations in the MMR pathway genes were assigned to the CMS1 group. As might be expected, the increased presence of neoantigens generated as a result of non-functional MMR also leads to significant infiltration of the CMS1 group tumors by immune cells. Impaired MMR is also associated with hereditary nonpolyposis colorectal cancer, so-called Lynch syndrome. Moreover, increased MSI was found in patients with ulcerative colitis [221].

Loss of the MMR function is mainly caused by inactivating mutations in the *MLH1*, *MSH2*, *MSH3*, *MSH6*, and *PMS1/2* genes. Additionally, epigenetic changes, e.g., hypermethylation of the *MLH1* promoter, may also be involved in silencing of gene expression of some MMR pathway components (reviewed in Reference [222]). Colorectal tumors associated with MMR deficiency exhibit several characteristic features such as proximal colon localization, mucinous or undifferentiated phenotype, and lymphocytic infiltrations [223]. In mice, homozygous deletion of the MMR genes is mostly compatible with the animal life; however, inactivation of the genes might result in lymphomas and other tumor types including adenomas formed in all segments of the gastrointestinal tract (the corresponding models of the deficient MMR pathway are listed in Table S7, Supplementary Materials). For example, *Mlh1*$^{-/-}$ and *Msh2*$^{-/-}$ mice developed tumors predominantly in the small intestine and survived no longer than one year [31,224]. *Msh3*$^{-/-}$ mice did not exhibit any cancer predispositions; nevertheless, *Msh6*$^{-/-}$ mice developed lymphomas of the skin and uterine carcinomas. Interestingly, combination of *Msh6* and *Msh3* null alleles promoted intestinal tumorigenesis [225]. In addition, no neoplastic lesions were observed in *Pms1*$^{-/-}$ mice; in contrast, *Pms2*$^{-/-}$ animals developed lymphomas and sarcomas and died (without any occurrence of intestinal neoplasia) at the age of 17 months [226]. The absence of the *Mlh3* gene product caused MSI accompanied by impaired DNA damage response and tumor development throughout the lower gastrointestinal tract. In these animals, tumor incidence was further increased by a simultaneous germline deletion of the *Pms2* gene; the resulting phenotype then mirrored the situation observed in *Mlh1*$^{-/-}$ mice [227]. Mice harboring *Msh2* cKO alleles and *EIIa-Cre* transgene (the transgene allows constitutive gene recombination of floxed sequences in the zygote [228]) recapitulated the phenotype observed in *Msh2*$^{-/-}$ mice, i.e., they displayed MMR deficiency and developed intestinal tumors. In contrast, intestinal inactivation of *Msh2* in *Msh2*$^{cKO/cKO}$ *Villin-Cre* mice was compatible with near-standard life expectancy. Strikingly, these mice developed intestinal tumors with truncating somatic *Apc* mutations [229]. Intriguingly, somatic mutations truncating Apc were also detected in tumors developed in *Msh2*$^{-/-}$ mice [230].

It is evident that MMR deficiency leads to increased predisposition of intestinal cells to mutations that further potentiate tumor growth. For example, *Msh2*$^{-/-}$ mice harboring the inducible oncogenic *Kras*^{V12} allele developed a higher number of colon adenomas when compared to *Msh2*$^{-/-}$ animals producing wt *Kras* [231]. Similarly, germline deletion of *Mlh1* or *Msh2* increased colon tumor incidence in *Apc*$^{+/1638N}$ and *Apc*$^{+/Min}$ mice, respectively [224,230]. Moreover, mutations in the particular "MMR gene" might also influence the way in which the second (wt) *Apc* allele is inactivated. For example, similarly as in the case of Msh2-deficient mice, *Mlh3*$^{-/-}$ *Apc*$^{+/1638N}$ mice showed increased frequency of frameshift mutations in the wt *Apc* allele; however, these frameshift mutations were, in contrast to mutations induced by MSI, in the non-repetitive sequences. Furthermore, combined homozygous deletion of *Mlh3* and *Pms2* caused increased incidence of base substitutions in *Apc*. Moreover, the position of the genetic changes in the wt *Apc* allele was also dependent on which MMR gene was mutated. For example, *Apc* mutations in *Mlh3*$^{-/-}$ *Pms2*$^{-/-}$ or *Mlh1*$^{-/-}$ mice occurred preferentially in the mutation hotspot in codons 854, 929, 1211, and 1464 [227,232,233]. In conclusion, although all of the "MMR genes" belong to one signaling pathway, the phenotype caused by their (combined) mutations varies with respect to the genetic change, tumor type, and tumor incidence.

9. Future Perspectives

In this review, we summarized some currently available mouse models of intestinal tumorigenesis. We also attempted to assign the models to the recently introduced CMS system used for classification of human CRCs. Although many mouse strains develop different types of neoplasia as a result of a single mutational event, multiple genetic alterations are necessary to obtain a progressed solid tumor in a "reasonable" time period. Since the initial mutation in the majority of human sporadic colorectal carcinomas occur in the *APC* gene, the effect of mutations in other possibly driver genes is often studied on the Apc-deficient genetic background. Alternatively, to mimic human CAC, the gene of interest can be modified in animals with DSS-induced colitis.

In relation to assignment of individual CRCs to one of the CMS groups, the question arises whether such an assignment, which indicates the gene expression profile of the resected tumor, is retained during tumor progression. Numerous experiments showed that combination of multiple genetic changes and the inflammatory response have a profound influence on the gene expression profile and cell composition of the primary lesion. This fact indicates that CMS group "switching" is common. Consequently, the necessity for sequential (multiple) genetic changes (or epigenetic alterations) limits the usage of the mouse cancer models. Nevertheless, there are recent examples showing that these limitations can be overcome. For example, mouse models using sleeping beauty (*SB*) transposon-based insertional mutagenesis allowed simultaneous inactivation of multiple genes. Moreover, usage of the *SB* system in mice that already carried a driver mutation were employed to either study the importance of the order of certain genetic changes, or to detect low-frequency mutations in the genes that cooperate with the particular driver mutation [234,235]. In addition, intestinal organoid cultures were used to introduce multiple genetic alterations into the genome of intestinal epithelium cells. The indisputable advantage of using organoids is the possibility to work with primary human cells obtained directly from the tumor (or healthy) tissue. Moreover, organoid preparation and genetic manipulations are much faster than generation of a new genetically modified mouse strain. For example, in 2015, two laboratories used the CRISPR/Cas9 system to sequentially introduce four mutations in *APC*, *TP53*, *KRAS*, and *SMAD4* genes into human cells growing as colon organoids [236,237]. We anticipate that organoids, although a very suitable in vitro model, do not contain all cell types present in a tumor growing in a particular organ. Thus, conclusions drawn from the results obtained in organoids do not necessarily correspond to the situation in vivo. Nevertheless, to obtain a more comprehensive and detailed picture, the existing mouse cancer models should be more thoroughly characterized. A high-throughput gene expression and proteomic analysis of mouse tumors induced by different genetic alterations would undoubtedly yield more accurate information on the tumor characteristics developed in a given mouse model.

Supplementary Materials: The following supplementary tables are available online at http://www.mdpi.com/2073-4425/10/10/788/s1: Table S1: Chemically induced colitis and intestinal tumors; Table S2: Mouse models of hyperactivated Wnt signaling; Table S3: Mouse models of the deregulated Hippo pathway; Table S4: Mouse models of the impaired p53 pathway; Table S5: Mouse strains modeling aberrant EGF signaling; Table S6: Mouse models of impaired TGFβ signaling; Table S7: Mouse models of DNA mismatch repair deficiency.

Author Contributions: D.H., L.J., M.S., and V.K. wrote the draft; M.S. and V.K. wrote the final version.

Funding: This research was funded by the Czech Science Foundation (grant number 18-26324S), by the Ministry of Education, Youth, and Sports (MEYS; project LO1419), and by the Academy of Sciences of the Czech Republic (RVO 68378050).

Acknowledgments: We thank Sarka Takacova for critically reading the manuscript.

Conflicts of Interest: The authors declare no conflicts of interest.

References

1. Siegel, R.L.; Miller, K.D.; Jemal, A. Cancer statistics, 2019. *CA Cancer J. Clin.* **2019**, *69*, 7–34. [CrossRef] [PubMed]
2. Kinzler, K.W.; Vogelstein, B. Lessons from hereditary colorectal cancer. *Cell* **1996**, *87*, 159–170. [CrossRef]

3. Jen, J.; Powell, S.M.; Papadopoulos, N.; Smith, K.J.; Hamilton, S.R.; Vogelstein, B.; Kinzler, K.W. Molecular determinants of dysplasia in colorectal lesions. *Cancer Res.* **1994**, *54*, 5523–5526. [PubMed]
4. Janssen, K.P.; Alberici, P.; Fsihi, H.; Gaspar, C.; Breukel, C.; Franken, P.; Rosty, C.; Abal, M.; El Marjou, F.; Smits, R.; et al. APC and oncogenic KRAS are synergistic in enhancing Wnt signaling in intestinal tumor formation and progression. *Gastroenterology* **2006**, *131*, 1096–1109. [CrossRef] [PubMed]
5. Smith, A.J.; Stern, H.S.; Penner, M.; Hay, K.; Mitri, A.; Bapat, B.V.; Gallinger, S. Somatic APC and K-ras codon 12 mutations in aberrant crypt foci from human colons. *Cancer Res.* **1994**, *54*, 5527–5530.
6. Rodrigues, N.R.; Rowan, A.; Smith, M.E.; Kerr, I.B.; Bodmer, W.F.; Gannon, J.V.; Lane, D.P. p53 mutations in colorectal cancer. *Proc. Natl. Acad. Sci. USA* **1990**, *87*, 7555–7559. [CrossRef] [PubMed]
7. Vogelstein, B.; Fearon, E.R.; Hamilton, S.R.; Kern, S.E.; Preisinger, A.C.; Leppert, M.; Nakamura, Y.; White, R.; Smits, A.M.; Bos, J.L. Genetic alterations during colorectal-tumor development. *N. Engl. J. Med.* **1988**, *319*, 525–532. [CrossRef]
8. Weinberg, R.A. Oncogenes, antioncogenes, and the molecular bases of multistep carcinogenesis. *Cancer Res.* **1989**, *49*, 3713–3721.
9. Mattar, M.C.; Lough, D.; Pishvaian, M.J.; Charabaty, A. Current management of inflammatory bowel disease and colorectal cancer. *Gastrointest. Cancer Res.* **2011**, *4*, 53–61.
10. Van Der Kraak, L.; Gros, P.; Beauchemin, N. Colitis-associated colon cancer: Is it in your genes? *World J. Gastroenterol.* **2015**, *21*, 11688–11699. [CrossRef]
11. Brentnall, T.A.; Crispin, D.A.; Rabinovitch, P.S.; Haggitt, R.C.; Rubin, C.E.; Stevens, A.C.; Burmer, G.C. Mutations in the p53 gene: An early marker of neoplastic progression in ulcerative colitis. *Gastroenterology* **1994**, *107*, 369–378. [CrossRef]
12. Shenoy, A.K.; Fisher, R.C.; Butterworth, E.A.; Pi, L.; Chang, L.J.; Appelman, H.D.; Chang, M.; Scott, E.W.; Huang, E.H. Transition from colitis to cancer: High Wnt activity sustains the tumor-initiating potential of colon cancer stem cell precursors. *Cancer Res.* **2012**, *72*, 5091–5100. [CrossRef] [PubMed]
13. Yaeger, R.; Shah, M.A.; Miller, V.A.; Kelsen, J.R.; Wang, K.; Heins, Z.J.; Ross, J.S.; He, Y.; Sanford, E.; Yantiss, R.K.; et al. Genomic Alterations Observed in Colitis-Associated Cancers Are Distinct From Those Found in Sporadic Colorectal Cancers and Vary by Type of Inflammatory Bowel Disease. *Gastroenterology* **2016**, *151*, 278–287. [CrossRef] [PubMed]
14. Ullman, T.A.; Itzkowitz, S.H. Intestinal inflammation and cancer. *Gastroenterology* **2011**, *140*, 1807–1816. [CrossRef] [PubMed]
15. Andreyev, H.J.; Norman, A.R.; Cunningham, D.; Oates, J.R.; Clarke, P.A. Kirsten ras mutations in patients with colorectal cancer: The multicenter "RASCAL" study. *J. Natl. Cancer Inst.* **1998**, *90*, 675–684. [CrossRef] [PubMed]
16. Smith, G.; Carey, F.A.; Beattie, J.; Wilkie, M.J.; Lightfoot, T.J.; Coxhead, J.; Garner, R.C.; Steele, R.J.; Wolf, C.R. Mutations in APC, Kirsten-ras, and p53—Alternative genetic pathways to colorectal cancer. *Proc. Natl. Acad. Sci. USA* **2002**, *99*, 9433–9438. [CrossRef] [PubMed]
17. Robles, A.I.; Traverso, G.; Zhang, M.; Roberts, N.J.; Khan, M.A.; Joseph, C.; Lauwers, G.Y.; Selaru, F.M.; Popoli, M.; Pittman, M.E.; et al. Whole-Exome Sequencing Analyses of Inflammatory Bowel Disease-Associated Colorectal Cancers. *Gastroenterology* **2016**, *150*, 931–943. [CrossRef] [PubMed]
18. Budinska, E.; Popovici, V.; Tejpar, S.; D'Ario, G.; Lapique, N.; Sikora, K.O.; Di Narzo, A.F.; Yan, P.; Hodgson, J.G.; Weinrich, S.; et al. Gene expression patterns unveil a new level of molecular heterogeneity in colorectal cancer. *J. Pathol.* **2013**, *231*, 63–76. [CrossRef]
19. Marisa, L.; de Reynies, A.; Duval, A.; Selves, J.; Gaub, M.P.; Vescovo, L.; Etienne-Grimaldi, M.C.; Schiappa, R.; Guenot, D.; Ayadi, M.; et al. Gene expression classification of colon cancer into molecular subtypes: Characterization, validation, and prognostic value. *PLoS Med.* **2013**, *10*, e1001453. [CrossRef]
20. Roepman, P.; Schlicker, A.; Tabernero, J.; Majewski, I.; Tian, S.; Moreno, V.; Snel, M.H.; Chresta, C.M.; Rosenberg, R.; Nitsche, U.; et al. Colorectal cancer intrinsic subtypes predict chemotherapy benefit, deficient mismatch repair and epithelial-to-mesenchymal transition. *Int. J. Cancer* **2014**, *134*, 552–562. [CrossRef]
21. De Sousa, E.M.F.; Wang, X.; Jansen, M.; Fessler, E.; Trinh, A.; de Rooij, L.P.; de Jong, J.H.; de Boer, O.J.; van Leersum, R.; Bijlsma, M.F.; et al. Poor-prognosis colon cancer is defined by a molecularly distinct subtype and develops from serrated precursor lesions. *Nat. Med.* **2013**, *19*, 614–618. [CrossRef] [PubMed]

22. Sadanandam, A.; Lyssiotis, C.A.; Homicsko, K.; Collisson, E.A.; Gibb, W.J.; Wullschleger, S.; Ostos, L.C.; Lannon, W.A.; Grotzinger, C.; Del Rio, M.; et al. A colorectal cancer classification system that associates cellular phenotype and responses to therapy. *Nat. Med.* **2013**, *19*, 619–625. [CrossRef] [PubMed]
23. Schlicker, A.; Beran, G.; Chresta, C.M.; McWalter, G.; Pritchard, A.; Weston, S.; Runswick, S.; Davenport, S.; Heathcote, K.; Castro, D.A.; et al. Subtypes of primary colorectal tumors correlate with response to targeted treatment in colorectal cell lines. *BMC Med. Genom.* **2012**, *5*, 66. [CrossRef] [PubMed]
24. Guinney, J.; Dienstmann, R.; Wang, X.; de Reynies, A.; Schlicker, A.; Soneson, C.; Marisa, L.; Roepman, P.; Nyamundanda, G.; Angelino, P.; et al. The consensus molecular subtypes of colorectal cancer. *Nat. Med.* **2015**, *21*, 1350–1356. [CrossRef] [PubMed]
25. Ning, C.; Li, Y.Y.; Wang, Y.; Han, G.C.; Wang, R.X.; Xiao, H.; Li, X.Y.; Hou, C.M.; Ma, Y.F.; Sheng, D.S.; et al. Complement activation promotes colitis-associated carcinogenesis through activating intestinal IL-1β/IL-17A axis. *Mucosal Immunol.* **2015**, *8*, 1275–1284. [CrossRef] [PubMed]
26. Linnekamp, J.F.; Hooff, S.R.V.; Prasetyanti, P.R.; Kandimalla, R.; Buikhuisen, J.Y.; Fessler, E.; Ramesh, P.; Lee, K.; Bochove, G.G.W.; de Jong, J.H.; et al. Consensus molecular subtypes of colorectal cancer are recapitulated in in vitro and in vivo models. *Cell Death Differ.* **2018**, *25*, 616–633. [CrossRef] [PubMed]
27. Phesse, T.J.; Durban, V.M.; Sansom, O.J. Defining key concepts of intestinal and epithelial cancer biology through the use of mouse models. *Carcinogenesis* **2017**, *38*, 953–965. [CrossRef] [PubMed]
28. Taketo, M.M.; Edelmann, W. Mouse models of colon cancer. *Gastroenterology* **2009**, *136*, 780–798. [CrossRef] [PubMed]
29. Park, S.Y.; Lee, H.S.; Choe, G.; Chung, J.H.; Kim, W.H. Clinicopathological characteristics, microsatellite instability, and expression of mucin core proteins and p53 in colorectal mucinous adenocarcinomas in relation to location. *Virchows Arch.* **2006**, *449*, 40–47. [CrossRef] [PubMed]
30. Oshima, H.; Nakayama, M.; Han, T.S.; Naoi, K.; Ju, X.; Maeda, Y.; Robine, S.; Tsuchiya, K.; Sato, T.; Sato, H.; et al. Suppressing TGFβ signaling in regenerating epithelia in an inflammatory microenvironment is sufficient to cause invasive intestinal cancer. *Cancer Res.* **2015**, *75*, 766–776. [CrossRef]
31. Reitmair, A.H.; Redston, M.; Cai, J.C.; Chuang, T.C.; Bjerknes, M.; Cheng, H.; Hay, K.; Gallinger, S.; Bapat, B.; Mak, T.W. Spontaneous intestinal carcinomas and skin neoplasms in *Msh2*-deficient mice. *Cancer Res.* **1996**, *56*, 3842–3849. [PubMed]
32. Su, L.K.; Kinzler, K.W.; Vogelstein, B.; Preisinger, A.C.; Moser, A.R.; Luongo, C.; Gould, K.A.; Dove, W.F. Multiple intestinal neoplasia caused by a mutation in the murine homolog of the APC gene. *Science* **1992**, *256*, 668–670. [CrossRef] [PubMed]
33. Sasai, H.; Masaki, M.; Wakitani, K. Suppression of polypogenesis in a new mouse strain with a truncated $Apc^{\Delta 474}$ by a novel COX-2 inhibitor, JTE-522. *Carcinogenesis* **2000**, *21*, 953–958. [CrossRef] [PubMed]
34. Colnot, S.; Niwa-Kawakita, M.; Hamard, G.; Godard, C.; Le Plenier, S.; Houbron, C.; Romagnolo, B.; Berrebi, D.; Giovannini, M.; Perret, C. Colorectal cancers in a new mouse model of familial adenomatous polyposis: Influence of genetic and environmental modifiers. *Lab. Investig. J. Tech. Methods Pathol.* **2004**, *84*, 1619–1630. [CrossRef] [PubMed]
35. Russo, A.; Bazan, V.; Iacopetta, B.; Kerr, D.; Soussi, T.; Gebbia, N. The TP53 colorectal cancer international collaborative study on the prognostic and predictive significance of *p53* mutation: Influence of tumor site, type of mutation, and adjuvant treatment. *J. Clin. Oncol.* **2005**, *23*, 7518–7528. [CrossRef] [PubMed]
36. Mercer, K.; Giblett, S.; Green, S.; Lloyd, D.; DaRocha Dias, S.; Plumb, M.; Marais, R.; Pritchard, C. Expression of endogenous oncogenic V600EB-raf induces proliferation and developmental defects in mice and transformation of primary fibroblasts. *Cancer Res.* **2005**, *65*, 11493–11500. [CrossRef] [PubMed]
37. Samowitz, W.S.; Sweeney, C.; Herrick, J.; Albertsen, H.; Levin, T.R.; Murtaugh, M.A.; Wolff, R.K.; Slattery, M.L. Poor survival associated with the *BRAF* V600E mutation in microsatellite-stable colon cancers. *Cancer Res.* **2005**, *65*, 6063–6069. [CrossRef] [PubMed]
38. Ito, N.; Hasegawa, R.; Sano, M.; Tamano, S.; Esumi, H.; Takayama, S.; Sugimura, T. A new colon and mammary carcinogen in cooked food, 2-amino-1-methyl-6-phenylimidazo[4,5-b]pyridine (PhIP). *Carcinogenesis* **1991**, *12*, 1503–1506. [CrossRef] [PubMed]
39. Ochiai, M.; Imai, H.; Sugimura, T.; Nagao, M.; Nakagama, H. Induction of intestinal tumors and lymphomas in C57BL/6N mice by a food-borne carcinogen, 2-amino-1-methyl-6-phenylimidazo[4,5-b]pyridine. *Jpn. J. Cancer Res.* **2002**, *93*, 478–483. [CrossRef] [PubMed]

40. Nakagama, H.; Nakanishi, M.; Ochiai, M. Modeling human colon cancer in rodents using a food-borne carcinogen, PhIP. *Cancer Sci.* **2005**, *96*, 627–636. [CrossRef] [PubMed]
41. Yang, J.; Shikata, N.; Mizuoka, H.; Tsubura, A. Colon carcinogenesis in shrews by intrarectal infusion of N-methyl-N-nitrosourea. *Cancer Lett.* **1996**, *110*, 105–112. [CrossRef]
42. Rosenberg, D.W.; Giardina, C.; Tanaka, T. Mouse models for the study of colon carcinogenesis. *Carcinogenesis* **2009**, *30*, 183–196. [CrossRef] [PubMed]
43. Deschner, E.E.; Long, F.C. Colonic neoplasms in mice produced with six injections of 1,2-dimethylhydrazine. *Oncology* **1977**, *34*, 255–257. [CrossRef] [PubMed]
44. Maltzman, T.; Whittington, J.; Driggers, L.; Stephens, J.; Ahnen, D. AOM-induced mouse colon tumors do not express full-length APC protein. *Carcinogenesis* **1997**, *18*, 2435–2439. [CrossRef] [PubMed]
45. Takahashi, M.; Nakatsugi, S.; Sugimura, T.; Wakabayashi, K. Frequent mutations of the β-catenin gene in mouse colon tumors induced by azoxymethane. *Carcinogenesis* **2000**, *21*, 1117–1120. [PubMed]
46. Vivona, A.A.; Shpitz, B.; Medline, A.; Bruce, W.R.; Hay, K.; Ward, M.A.; Stern, H.S.; Gallinger, S. K-ras mutations in aberrant crypt foci, adenomas and adenocarcinomas during azoxymethane-induced colon carcinogenesis. *Carcinogenesis* **1993**, *14*, 1777–1781. [CrossRef] [PubMed]
47. Wang, Q.S.; Papanikolaou, A.; Sabourin, C.L.; Rosenberg, D.W. Altered expression of cyclin D1 and cyclin-dependent kinase 4 in azoxymethane-induced mouse colon tumorigenesis. *Carcinogenesis* **1998**, *19*, 2001–2006. [CrossRef] [PubMed]
48. Chen, J.; Huang, X.F. The signal pathways in azoxymethane-induced colon cancer and preventive implications. *Cancer Biol. Ther.* **2009**, *8*, 1313–1317. [CrossRef] [PubMed]
49. Waaler, J.; Machon, O.; Tumova, L.; Dinh, H.; Korinek, V.; Wilson, S.R.; Paulsen, J.E.; Pedersen, N.M.; Eide, T.J.; Machonova, O.; et al. A novel tankyrase inhibitor decreases canonical Wnt signaling in colon carcinoma cells and reduces tumor growth in conditional APC mutant mice. *Cancer Res.* **2012**, *72*, 2822–2832. [CrossRef] [PubMed]
50. Bissahoyo, A.; Pearsall, R.S.; Hanlon, K.; Amann, V.; Hicks, D.; Godfrey, V.L.; Threadgill, D.W. Azoxymethane is a genetic background-dependent colorectal tumor initiator and promoter in mice: Effects of dose, route, and diet. *Toxicol. Sci.* **2005**, *88*, 340–345. [CrossRef] [PubMed]
51. Greten, F.R.; Eckmann, L.; Greten, T.F.; Park, J.M.; Li, Z.W.; Egan, L.J.; Kagnoff, M.F.; Karin, M. IKKβ links inflammation and tumorigenesis in a mouse model of colitis-associated cancer. *Cell* **2004**, *118*, 285–296. [CrossRef] [PubMed]
52. Neufert, C.; Becker, C.; Neurath, M.F. An inducible mouse model of colon carcinogenesis for the analysis of sporadic and inflammation-driven tumor progression. *Nat. Protoc.* **2007**, *2*, 1998–2004. [CrossRef] [PubMed]
53. Tanaka, T.; Kohno, H.; Suzuki, R.; Yamada, Y.; Sugie, S.; Mori, H. A novel inflammation-related mouse colon carcinogenesis model induced by azoxymethane and dextran sodium sulfate. *Cancer Sci.* **2003**, *94*, 965–973. [CrossRef] [PubMed]
54. De Robertis, M.; Massi, E.; Poeta, M.L.; Carotti, S.; Morini, S.; Cecchetelli, L.; Signori, E.; Fazio, V.M. The AOM/DSS murine model for the study of colon carcinogenesis: From pathways to diagnosis and therapy studies. *J. Carcinog.* **2011**, *10*, 9. [CrossRef] [PubMed]
55. Aoki, K.; Taketo, M.M. Adenomatous polyposis coli (APC): A multi-functional tumor suppressor gene. *J. Cell Sci.* **2007**, *120*, 3327–3335. [CrossRef] [PubMed]
56. Valenta, T.; Hausmann, G.; Basler, K. The many faces and functions of β-catenin. *EMBO J.* **2012**, *31*, 2714–2736. [CrossRef] [PubMed]
57. Kimelman, D.; Xu, W. β-catenin destruction complex: Insights and questions from a structural perspective. *Oncogene* **2006**, *25*, 7482–7491. [CrossRef]
58. Stamos, J.L.; Weis, W.I. The β-catenin destruction complex. *Cold Spring Harb. Perspect. Biol.* **2013**, *5*, a007898. [CrossRef]
59. Saito-Diaz, K.; Chen, T.W.; Wang, X.; Thorne, C.A.; Wallace, H.A.; Page-McCaw, A.; Lee, E. The way Wnt works: Components and mechanism. *Growth Factors* **2013**, *31*, 1–31. [CrossRef]
60. He, T.C.; Sparks, A.B.; Rago, C.; Hermeking, H.; Zawel, L.; da Costa, L.T.; Morin, P.J.; Vogelstein, B.; Kinzler, K.W. Identification of c-MYC as a target of the APC pathway. *Science* **1998**, *281*, 1509–1512. [CrossRef]
61. Shtutman, M.; Zhurinsky, J.; Simcha, I.; Albanese, C.; D'Amico, M.; Pestell, R.; Ben-Ze'ev, A. The cyclin D1 gene is a target of the β-catenin/LEF-1 pathway. *Proc. Natl. Acad. Sci. USA* **1999**, *96*, 5522–5527. [CrossRef] [PubMed]

62. Wielenga, V.J.; Smits, R.; Korinek, V.; Smit, L.; Kielman, M.; Fodde, R.; Clevers, H.; Pals, S.T. Expression of CD44 in Apc and Tcf mutant mice implies regulation by the WNT pathway. *Am. J. Pathol.* **1999**, *154*, 515–523. [CrossRef]
63. Coppede, F.; Lopomo, A.; Spisni, R.; Migliore, L. Genetic and epigenetic biomarkers for diagnosis, prognosis and treatment of colorectal cancer. *World J. Gastroenterol.* **2014**, *20*, 943–956. [CrossRef] [PubMed]
64. Segditsas, S.; Tomlinson, I. Colorectal cancer and genetic alterations in the Wnt pathway. *Oncogene* **2006**, *25*, 7531–7537. [CrossRef] [PubMed]
65. Shimizu, Y.; Ikeda, S.; Fujimori, M.; Kodama, S.; Nakahara, M.; Okajima, M.; Asahara, T. Frequent alterations in the Wnt signaling pathway in colorectal cancer with microsatellite instability. *Genes Chromosomes Cancer* **2002**, *33*, 73–81. [CrossRef] [PubMed]
66. Mazzoni, S.M.; Fearon, E.R. AXIN1 and AXIN2 variants in gastrointestinal cancers. *Cancer Lett.* **2014**, *355*, 1–8. [CrossRef] [PubMed]
67. Nishisho, I.; Nakamura, Y.; Miyoshi, Y.; Miki, Y.; Ando, H.; Horii, A.; Koyama, K.; Utsunomiya, J.; Baba, S.; Hedge, P. Mutations of chromosome 5q21 genes in FAP and colorectal cancer patients. *Science* **1991**, *253*, 665–669. [CrossRef] [PubMed]
68. Groden, J.; Thliveris, A.; Samowitz, W.; Carlson, M.; Gelbert, L.; Albertsen, H.; Joslyn, G.; Stevens, J.; Spirio, L.; Robertson, M.; et al. Identification and characterization of the familial adenomatous polyposis coli gene. *Cell* **1991**, *66*, 589–600. [CrossRef]
69. Galiatsatos, P.; Foulkes, W.D. Familial adenomatous polyposis. *Am. J. Gastroenterol.* **2006**, *101*, 385–398. [CrossRef] [PubMed]
70. Rubinfeld, B.; Albert, I.; Porfiri, E.; Fiol, C.; Munemitsu, S.; Polakis, P. Binding of GSK3β to the APC-β-catenin complex and regulation of complex assembly. *Science* **1996**, *272*, 1023–1026. [CrossRef] [PubMed]
71. Behrens, J.; Jerchow, B.A.; Wurtele, M.; Grimm, J.; Asbrand, C.; Wirtz, R.; Kuhl, M.; Wedlich, D.; Birchmeier, W. Functional interaction of an axin homolog, conductin, with β-catenin, APC, and GSK3β. *Science* **1998**, *280*, 596–599. [CrossRef] [PubMed]
72. Miyoshi, Y.; Nagase, H.; Ando, H.; Horii, A.; Ichii, S.; Nakatsuru, S.; Aoki, T.; Miki, Y.; Mori, T.; Nakamura, Y. Somatic mutations of the APC gene in colorectal tumors: Mutation cluster region in the APC gene. *Hum. Mol. Genet.* **1992**, *1*, 229–233. [PubMed]
73. Miyaki, M.; Konishi, M.; Kikuchi-Yanoshita, R.; Enomoto, M.; Igari, T.; Tanaka, K.; Muraoka, M.; Takahashi, H.; Amada, Y.; Fukayama, M.; et al. Characteristics of somatic mutation of the adenomatous polyposis coli gene in colorectal tumors. *Cancer Res.* **1994**, *54*, 3011–3020. [PubMed]
74. Hayashi, S.; Rubinfeld, B.; Souza, B.; Polakis, P.; Wieschaus, E.; Levine, A.J. A *Drosophila* homolog of the tumor suppressor gene adenomatous polyposis coli down-regulates β-catenin but its zygotic expression is not essential for the regulation of Armadillo. *Proc. Natl. Acad. Sci. USA* **1997**, *94*, 242–247. [CrossRef] [PubMed]
75. Moser, A.R.; Pitot, H.C.; Dove, W.F. A dominant mutation that predisposes to multiple intestinal neoplasia in the mouse. *Science* **1990**, *247*, 322–324. [CrossRef]
76. Moser, A.R.; Mattes, E.M.; Dove, W.F.; Lindstrom, M.J.; Haag, J.D.; Gould, M.N. ApcMin, a mutation in the murine Apc gene, predisposes to mammary carcinomas and focal alveolar hyperplasias. *Proc. Natl. Acad. Sci. USA* **1993**, *90*, 8977–8981. [CrossRef]
77. Tomita, H.; Yamada, Y.; Oyama, T.; Hata, K.; Hirose, Y.; Hara, A.; Kunisada, T.; Sugiyama, Y.; Adachi, Y.; Linhart, H.; et al. Development of gastric tumors in $Apc^{Min/+}$ mice by the activation of the β-catenin/Tcf signaling pathway. *Cancer Res.* **2007**, *67*, 4079–4087. [CrossRef]
78. Svendsen, C.; Alexander, J.; Knutsen, H.K.; Husoy, T. The min mouse on FVB background: Susceptibility to spontaneous and carcinogen-induced intestinal tumourigenesis. *Anticancer Res.* **2011**, *31*, 785–788.
79. Sodring, M.; Gunnes, G.; Paulsen, J.E. Spontaneous initiation, promotion and progression of colorectal cancer in the novel A/J Min/+ mouse. *Int. J. Cancer* **2016**, *138*, 1936–1946. [CrossRef]
80. Cooper, H.S.; Chang, W.C.; Coudry, R.; Gary, M.A.; Everley, L.; Spittle, C.S.; Wang, H.; Litwin, S.; Clapper, M.L. Generation of a unique strain of multiple intestinal neoplasia ($Apc^{+/Min-FCCC}$) mice with significantly increased numbers of colorectal adenomas. *Mol. Carcinog.* **2005**, *44*, 31–41. [CrossRef]
81. Bashir, O.; FitzGerald, A.J.; Goodlad, R.A. Both suboptimal and elevated vitamin intake increase intestinal neoplasia and alter crypt fission in the $Apc^{Min/+}$ mouse. *Carcinogenesis* **2004**, *25*, 1507–1515. [CrossRef] [PubMed]

82. Lawrance, A.K.; Deng, L.; Brody, L.C.; Finnell, R.H.; Shane, B.; Rozen, R. Genetic and nutritional deficiencies in folate metabolism influence tumorigenicity in $Apc^{min/+}$ mice. *J. Nutr. Biochem.* **2007**, *18*, 305–312. [CrossRef] [PubMed]
83. Mutanen, M.; Pajari, A.M.; Oikarinen, S.I. Beef induces and rye bran prevents the formation of intestinal polyps in Apc^{Min} mice: Relation to β-catenin and PKC isozymes. *Carcinogenesis* **2000**, *21*, 1167–1173. [CrossRef] [PubMed]
84. Yang, K.; Lamprecht, S.A.; Shinozaki, H.; Fan, K.; Yang, W.; Newmark, H.L.; Kopelovich, L.; Edelmann, W.; Jin, B.; Gravaghi, C.; et al. Dietary calcium and cholecalciferol modulate cyclin D1 expression, apoptosis, and tumorigenesis in intestine of *adenomatous polyposis coli*$^{1638N/+}$ mice. *J. Nutr.* **2008**, *138*, 1658–1663. [CrossRef] [PubMed]
85. Kwong, L.N.; Dove, W.F. APC and its modifiers in colon cancer. *Adv. Exp. Med. Biol.* **2009**, *656*, 85–106. [PubMed]
86. Lamlum, H.; Ilyas, M.; Rowan, A.; Clark, S.; Johnson, V.; Bell, J.; Frayling, I.; Efstathiou, J.; Pack, K.; Payne, S.; et al. The type of somatic mutation at APC in familial adenomatous polyposis is determined by the site of the germline mutation: A new facet to Knudson's 'two-hit' hypothesis. *Nat. Med.* **1999**, *5*, 1071–1075. [CrossRef] [PubMed]
87. Sieber, O.M.; Heinimann, K.; Gorman, P.; Lamlum, H.; Crabtree, M.; Simpson, C.A.; Davies, D.; Neale, K.; Hodgson, S.V.; Roylance, R.R.; et al. Analysis of chromosomal instability in human colorectal adenomas with two mutational hits at APC. *Proc. Natl. Acad. Sci. USA* **2002**, *99*, 16910–16915. [CrossRef]
88. Lewis, A.; Segditsas, S.; Deheragoda, M.; Pollard, P.; Jeffery, R.; Nye, E.; Lockstone, H.; Davis, H.; Clark, S.; Stamp, G.; et al. Severe polyposis in Apc^{1322T} mice is associated with submaximal Wnt signalling and increased expression of the stem cell marker *Lgr5*. *Gut* **2010**, *59*, 1680–1686. [CrossRef]
89. Pollard, P.; Deheragoda, M.; Segditsas, S.; Lewis, A.; Rowan, A.; Howarth, K.; Willis, L.; Nye, E.; McCart, A.; Mandir, N.; et al. The Apc^{1322T} mouse develops severe polyposis associated with submaximal nuclear β-catenin expression. *Gastroenterology* **2009**, *136*, 2204–2213. [CrossRef]
90. Bakker, E.R.; Hoekstra, E.; Franken, P.F.; Helvensteijn, W.; van Deurzen, C.H.; van Veelen, W.; Kuipers, E.J.; Smits, R. β-Catenin signaling dosage dictates tissue-specific tumor predisposition in Apc-driven cancer. *Oncogene* **2013**, *32*, 4579–4585. [CrossRef]
91. Quesada, C.F.; Kimata, H.; Mori, M.; Nishimura, M.; Tsuneyoshi, T.; Baba, S. Piroxicam and acarbose as chemopreventive agents for spontaneous intestinal adenomas in APC gene 1309 knockout mice. *Jpn. J. Cancer Res.* **1998**, *89*, 392–396. [CrossRef] [PubMed]
92. Niho, N.; Takahashi, M.; Kitamura, T.; Shoji, Y.; Itoh, M.; Noda, T.; Sugimura, T.; Wakabayashi, K. Concomitant suppression of hyperlipidemia and intestinal polyp formation in Apc-deficient mice by peroxisome proliferator-activated receptor ligands. *Cancer Res.* **2003**, *63*, 6090–6095. [PubMed]
93. Deka, J.; Kuhlmann, J.; Muller, O. A domain within the tumor suppressor protein APC shows very similar biochemical properties as the microtubule-associated protein tau. *Eur. J. Biochem.* **1998**, *253*, 591–597. [CrossRef] [PubMed]
94. Lewis, A.; Davis, H.; Deheragoda, M.; Pollard, P.; Nye, E.; Jeffery, R.; Segditsas, S.; East, P.; Poulsom, R.; Stamp, G.; et al. The C-terminus of Apc does not influence intestinal adenoma development or progression. *J. Pathol.* **2012**, *226*, 73–83. [CrossRef] [PubMed]
95. Fodde, R.; Edelmann, W.; Yang, K.; van Leeuwen, C.; Carlson, C.; Renault, B.; Breukel, C.; Alt, E.; Lipkin, M.; Khan, P.M.; et al. A targeted chain-termination mutation in the mouse Apc gene results in multiple intestinal tumors. *Proc. Natl. Acad. Sci. USA* **1994**, *91*, 8969–8973. [CrossRef] [PubMed]
96. Smits, R.; van der Houven van Oordt, W.; Luz, A.; Zurcher, C.; Jagmohan-Changur, S.; Breukel, C.; Khan, P.M.; Fodde, R. Apc^{1638N}: A mouse model for familial adenomatous polyposis-associated desmoid tumors and cutaneous cysts. *Gastroenterology* **1998**, *114*, 275–283. [CrossRef]
97. Caspari, R.; Olschwang, S.; Friedl, W.; Mandl, M.; Boisson, C.; Boker, T.; Augustin, A.; Kadmon, M.; Moslein, G.; Thomas, G.; et al. Familial adenomatous polyposis: Desmoid tumours and lack of ophthalmic lesions (CHRPE) associated with APC mutations beyond codon 1444. *Hum. Mol. Genet.* **1995**, *4*, 337–340. [CrossRef]
98. Davies, D.R.; Armstrong, J.G.; Thakker, N.; Horner, K.; Guy, S.P.; Clancy, T.; Sloan, P.; Blair, V.; Dodd, C.; Warnes, T.W.; et al. Severe Gardner syndrome in families with mutations restricted to a specific region of the APC gene. *Am. J. Hum. Genet.* **1995**, *57*, 1151–1158.

99. Ikenoue, T.; Yamaguchi, K.; Komura, M.; Imoto, S.; Yamaguchi, R.; Shimizu, E.; Kasuya, S.; Shibuya, T.; Hatakeyama, S.; Miyano, S.; et al. Attenuated familial adenomatous polyposis with desmoids caused by an APC mutation. *Hum. Genome Var.* **2015**, *2*, 15011. [CrossRef]
100. Wang, T.; Onouchi, T.; Yamada, N.O.; Matsuda, S.; Senda, T. A disturbance of intestinal epithelial cell population and kinetics in APC1638T mice. *Med. Mol. Morphol.* **2017**, *50*, 94–102. [CrossRef]
101. Smits, R.; Kielman, M.F.; Breukel, C.; Zurcher, C.; Neufeld, K.; Jagmohan-Changur, S.; Hofland, N.; van Dijk, J.; White, R.; Edelmann, W.; et al. *Apc*1638T: A mouse model delineating critical domains of the adenomatous polyposis coli protein involved in tumorigenesis and development. *Genes Dev.* **1999**, *13*, 1309–1321. [CrossRef] [PubMed]
102. Xu, Q.; Wang, Y.S.; Dabdoub, A.; Smallwood, P.M.; Williams, J.; Woods, C.; Kelley, M.W.; Jiang, L.; Tasman, W.; Zhang, K.; et al. Vascular development in the retina and inner ear: Control by Norrin and Frizzled-4, a high-affinity ligand-receptor pair. *Cell* **2004**, *116*, 883–895. [CrossRef]
103. Gaspar, C.; Franken, P.; Molenaar, L.; Breukel, C.; van der Valk, M.; Smits, R.; Fodde, R. A targeted constitutive mutation in the APC tumor suppressor gene underlies mammary but not intestinal tumorigenesis. *PLoS Genet.* **2009**, *5*, e1000547. [CrossRef] [PubMed]
104. Crist, R.C.; Roth, J.J.; Baran, A.A.; McEntee, B.J.; Siracusa, L.D.; Buchberg, A.M. The armadillo repeat domain of Apc suppresses intestinal tumorigenesis. *Mamm. Genome Off. J. Int. Mamm. Genome Soc.* **2010**, *21*, 450–457. [CrossRef] [PubMed]
105. Oshima, M.; Oshima, H.; Kitagawa, K.; Kobayashi, M.; Itakura, C.; Taketo, M. Loss of Apc heterozygosity and abnormal tissue building in nascent intestinal polyps in mice carrying a truncated Apc gene. *Proc. Natl. Acad. Sci. USA* **1995**, *92*, 4482–4486. [CrossRef] [PubMed]
106. Shibata, H.; Toyama, K.; Shioya, H.; Ito, M.; Hirota, M.; Hasegawa, S.; Matsumoto, H.; Takano, H.; Akiyama, T.; Toyoshima, K.; et al. Rapid colorectal adenoma formation initiated by conditional targeting of the Apc gene. *Science* **1997**, *278*, 120–123. [CrossRef] [PubMed]
107. Kuraguchi, M.; Wang, X.P.; Bronson, R.T.; Rothenberg, R.; Ohene-Baah, N.Y.; Lund, J.J.; Kucherlapati, M.; Maas, R.L.; Kucherlapati, R. Adenomatous polyposis coli (APC) is required for normal development of skin and thymus. *PLoS Genet.* **2006**, *2*, e146. [CrossRef]
108. Colnot, S.; Decaens, T.; Niwa-Kawakita, M.; Godard, C.; Hamard, G.; Kahn, A.; Giovannini, M.; Perret, C. Liver-targeted disruption of Apc in mice activates β-catenin signaling and leads to hepatocellular carcinomas. *Proc. Natl. Acad. Sci. USA* **2004**, *101*, 17216–17221. [CrossRef]
109. El Marjou, F.; Janssen, K.P.; Chang, B.H.; Li, M.; Hindie, V.; Chan, L.; Louvard, D.; Chambon, P.; Metzger, D.; Robine, S. Tissue-specific and inducible Cre-mediated recombination in the gut epithelium. *Genesis* **2004**, *39*, 186–193. [CrossRef]
110. Barker, N.; van Es, J.H.; Kuipers, J.; Kujala, P.; van den Born, M.; Cozijnsen, M.; Haegebarth, A.; Korving, J.; Begthel, H.; Peters, P.J.; et al. Identification of stem cells in small intestine and colon by marker gene *Lgr5*. *Nature* **2007**, *449*, 1003–1007. [CrossRef]
111. Horazna, M.; Janeckova, L.; Svec, J.; Babosova, O.; Hrckulak, D.; Vojtechova, M.; Galuskova, K.; Sloncova, E.; Kolar, M.; Strnad, H.; et al. Msx1 loss suppresses formation of the ectopic crypts developed in the Apc-deficient small intestinal epithelium. *Sci. Rep.* **2019**, *9*, 1629. [CrossRef] [PubMed]
112. Robanus-Maandag, E.C.; Koelink, P.J.; Breukel, C.; Salvatori, D.C.; Jagmohan-Changur, S.C.; Bosch, C.A.; Verspaget, H.W.; Devilee, P.; Fodde, R.; Smits, R. A new conditional Apc-mutant mouse model for colorectal cancer. *Carcinogenesis* **2010**, *31*, 946–952. [CrossRef] [PubMed]
113. Cheung, A.F.; Carter, A.M.; Kostova, K.K.; Woodruff, J.F.; Crowley, D.; Bronson, R.T.; Haigis, K.M.; Jacks, T. Complete deletion of Apc results in severe polyposis in mice. *Oncogene* **2010**, *29*, 1857–1864. [CrossRef] [PubMed]
114. Gao, C.; Wang, Y.M.; Broaddus, R.; Sun, L.H.; Xue, F.X.; Zhang, W. Exon 3 mutations of CTNNB1 drive tumorigenesis: A review. *Oncotarget* **2018**, *9*, 5492–5508. [CrossRef] [PubMed]
115. Kim, S.; Jeong, S. Mutation Hotspots in the β-Catenin Gene: Lessons from the Human Cancer Genome Databases. *Mol. Cells* **2019**, *42*, 8–16. [CrossRef] [PubMed]
116. Harada, N.; Tamai, Y.; Ishikawa, T.; Sauer, B.; Takaku, K.; Oshima, M.; Taketo, M.M. Intestinal polyposis in mice with a dominant stable mutation of the β-catenin gene. *EMBO J.* **1999**, *18*, 5931–5942. [CrossRef] [PubMed]

117. Kriz, V.; Korinek, V. Wnt, RSPO and Hippo Signalling in the Intestine and Intestinal Stem Cells. *Genes* **2018**, *9*, 20. [CrossRef] [PubMed]
118. Seshagiri, S.; Stawiski, E.W.; Durinck, S.; Modrusan, Z.; Storm, E.E.; Conboy, C.B.; Chaudhuri, S.; Guan, Y.; Janakiraman, V.; Jaiswal, B.S.; et al. Recurrent R-spondin fusions in colon cancer. *Nature* **2012**, *488*, 660–664. [CrossRef] [PubMed]
119. Hashimoto, T.; Ogawa, R.; Yoshida, H.; Taniguchi, H.; Kojima, M.; Saito, Y.; Sekine, S. EIF3E-RSPO2 and PIEZO1-RSPO2 fusions in colorectal traditional serrated adenoma. *Histopathology* **2019**. [CrossRef]
120. Hilkens, J.; Timmer, N.C.; Boer, M.; Ikink, G.J.; Schewe, M.; Sacchetti, A.; Koppens, M.A.J.; Song, J.Y.; Bakker, E.R.M. RSPO3 expands intestinal stem cell and niche compartments and drives tumorigenesis. *Gut* **2017**, *66*, 1095–1105. [CrossRef]
121. Han, T.; Schatoff, E.M.; Murphy, C.; Zafra, M.P.; Wilkinson, J.E.; Elemento, O.; Dow, L.E. R-Spondin chromosome rearrangements drive Wnt-dependent tumour initiation and maintenance in the intestine. *Nat. Commun.* **2017**, *8*, 15945. [CrossRef] [PubMed]
122. Zhao, B.; Tumaneng, K.; Guan, K.L. The Hippo pathway in organ size control, tissue regeneration and stem cell self-renewal. *Nat. Cell Boil.* **2011**, *13*, 877–883. [CrossRef] [PubMed]
123. Yu, F.X.; Meng, Z.; Plouffe, S.W.; Guan, K.L. Hippo pathway regulation of gastrointestinal tissues. *Annu. Rev. Physiol.* **2015**, *77*, 201–227. [CrossRef] [PubMed]
124. Wang, L.; Shi, S.; Guo, Z.; Zhang, X.; Han, S.; Yang, A.; Wen, W.; Zhu, Q. Overexpression of YAP and TAZ is an independent predictor of prognosis in colorectal cancer and related to the proliferation and metastasis of colon cancer cells. *PLoS ONE* **2013**, *8*, e65539. [CrossRef]
125. Yuen, H.F.; McCrudden, C.M.; Huang, Y.H.; Tham, J.M.; Zhang, X.; Zeng, Q.; Zhang, S.D.; Hong, W. TAZ expression as a prognostic indicator in colorectal cancer. *PLoS ONE* **2013**, *8*, e54211. [CrossRef] [PubMed]
126. Avruch, J.; Zhou, D.; Bardeesy, N. YAP oncogene overexpression supercharges colon cancer proliferation. *Cell Cycle* **2012**, *11*, 1090–1096. [CrossRef] [PubMed]
127. Cho, S.Y.; Gwak, J.W.; Shin, Y.C.; Moon, D.; Ahn, J.; Sol, H.W.; Kim, S.; Kim, G.; Shin, H.M.; Lee, K.H.; et al. Expression of Hippo pathway genes and their clinical significance in colon adenocarcinoma. *Oncol. Lett.* **2018**, *15*, 4926–4936. [CrossRef] [PubMed]
128. Wang, Q.; Gao, X.; Yu, T.; Yuan, L.; Dai, J.; Wang, W.; Chen, G.; Jiao, C.; Zhou, W.; Huang, Q.; et al. REGγ Controls Hippo Signaling and Reciprocal NF-κB-YAP Regulation to Promote Colon Cancer. *Clin. Cancer Res.* **2018**, *24*, 2015–2025. [CrossRef]
129. Camargo, F.D.; Gokhale, S.; Johnnidis, J.B.; Fu, D.; Bell, G.W.; Jaenisch, R.; Brummelkamp, T.R. YAP1 increases organ size and expands undifferentiated progenitor cells. *Curr. Boil. CB* **2007**, *17*, 2054–2060. [CrossRef]
130. Barry, E.R.; Morikawa, T.; Butler, B.L.; Shrestha, K.; de la Rosa, R.; Yan, K.S.; Fuchs, C.S.; Magness, S.T.; Smits, R.; Ogino, S.; et al. Restriction of intestinal stem cell expansion and the regenerative response by YAP. *Nature* **2013**, *493*, 106–110. [CrossRef]
131. Zhou, D.; Zhang, Y.; Wu, H.; Barry, E.; Yin, Y.; Lawrence, E.; Dawson, D.; Willis, J.E.; Markowitz, S.D.; Camargo, F.D.; et al. Mst1 and Mst2 protein kinases restrain intestinal stem cell proliferation and colonic tumorigenesis by inhibition of Yes-associated protein (Yap) overabundance. *Proc. Natl. Acad. Sci. USA* **2011**, *108*, E1312–E1320. [CrossRef] [PubMed]
132. Cai, J.; Zhang, N.; Zheng, Y.; de Wilde, R.F.; Maitra, A.; Pan, D. The Hippo signaling pathway restricts the oncogenic potential of an intestinal regeneration program. *Genes Dev.* **2010**, *24*, 2383–2388. [CrossRef] [PubMed]
133. Muller, P.A.; Vousden, K.H. Mutant p53 in cancer: New functions and therapeutic opportunities. *Cancer Cell* **2014**, *25*, 304–317. [CrossRef] [PubMed]
134. Oliner, J.D.; Pietenpol, J.A.; Thiagalingam, S.; Gyuris, J.; Kinzler, K.W.; Vogelstein, B. Oncoprotein MDM2 conceals the activation domain of tumour suppressor p53. *Nature* **1993**, *362*, 857–860. [CrossRef] [PubMed]
135. Amaral, J.D.; Xavier, J.M.; Steer, C.J.; Rodrigues, C.M. The role of p53 in apoptosis. *Discov. Med.* **2010**, *9*, 145–152. [PubMed]
136. Abukhdeir, A.M.; Park, B.H. P21 and p27: Roles in carcinogenesis and drug resistance. *Expert Rev. Mol. Med.* **2008**, *10*, e19. [CrossRef] [PubMed]
137. Baker, S.J.; Preisinger, A.C.; Jessup, J.M.; Paraskeva, C.; Markowitz, S.; Willson, J.K.; Hamilton, S.; Vogelstein, B. p53 gene mutations occur in combination with 17p allelic deletions as late events in colorectal tumorigenesis. *Cancer Res.* **1990**, *50*, 7717–7722. [PubMed]

138. Hainaut, P.; Hollstein, M. p53 and human cancer: The first ten thousand mutations. *Adv. Cancer Res.* **2000**, *77*, 81–137.
139. Lopez, I.; Oliveira, L.P.; Tucci, P.; Alvarez-Valin, F.; Coudry, R.A.; Marin, M. Different mutation profiles associated to P53 accumulation in colorectal cancer. *Gene* **2012**, *499*, 81–87. [CrossRef]
140. Li, X.L.; Zhou, J.; Chen, Z.R.; Chng, W.J. P53 mutations in colorectal cancer—Molecular pathogenesis and pharmacological reactivation. *World J. Gastroenterol.* **2015**, *21*, 84–93. [CrossRef]
141. Ogino, S.; Nosho, K.; Shima, K.; Baba, Y.; Irahara, N.; Kirkner, G.J.; Hazra, A.; De Vivo, I.; Giovannucci, E.L.; Meyerhardt, J.A.; et al. p21 expression in colon cancer and modifying effects of patient age and body mass index on prognosis. *Cancer Epidemiol. Biomark. Prev.* **2009**, *18*, 2513–2521. [CrossRef]
142. Ogino, S.; Kawasaki, T.; Kirkner, G.J.; Ogawa, A.; Dorfman, I.; Loda, M.; Fuchs, C.S. Down-regulation of p21 (CDKN1A/CIP1) is inversely associated with microsatellite instability and CpG island methylator phenotype (CIMP) in colorectal cancer. *J. Pathol.* **2006**, *210*, 147–154. [CrossRef]
143. Jacks, T.; Remington, L.; Williams, B.O.; Schmitt, E.M.; Halachmi, S.; Bronson, R.T.; Weinberg, R.A. Tumor spectrum analysis in *p53*-mutant mice. *Curr. Boil. CB* **1994**, *4*, 1–7. [CrossRef]
144. Lang, G.A.; Iwakuma, T.; Suh, Y.A.; Liu, G.; Rao, V.A.; Parant, J.M.; Valentin-Vega, Y.A.; Terzian, T.; Caldwell, L.C.; Strong, L.C.; et al. Gain of function of a p53 hot spot mutation in a mouse model of Li-Fraumeni syndrome. *Cell* **2004**, *119*, 861–872. [CrossRef] [PubMed]
145. Halberg, R.B.; Katzung, D.S.; Hoff, P.D.; Moser, A.R.; Cole, C.E.; Lubet, R.A.; Donehower, L.A.; Jacoby, R.F.; Dove, W.F. Tumorigenesis in the multiple intestinal neoplasia mouse: Redundancy of negative regulators and specificity of modifiers. *Proc. Natl. Acad. Sci. USA* **2000**, *97*, 3461–3466. [CrossRef] [PubMed]
146. Funabashi, H.; Uchida, K.; Kado, S.; Matsuoka, Y.; Ohwaki, M. Establishment of a *Tcrb* and *Trp53* genes deficient mouse strain as an animal model for spontaneous colorectal cancer. *Exp. Anim.* **2001**, *50*, 41–47. [CrossRef]
147. Cooks, T.; Pateras, I.S.; Tarcic, O.; Solomon, H.; Schetter, A.J.; Wilder, S.; Lozano, G.; Pikarsky, E.; Forshew, T.; Rosenfeld, N.; et al. Mutant p53 prolongs NF-κB activation and promotes chronic inflammation and inflammation-associated colorectal cancer. *Cancer Cell* **2013**, *23*, 634–646. [CrossRef]
148. Chang, W.C.; Coudry, R.A.; Clapper, M.L.; Zhang, X.; Williams, K.L.; Spittle, C.S.; Li, T.; Cooper, H.S. Loss of p53 enhances the induction of colitis-associated neoplasia by dextran sulfate sodium. *Carcinogenesis* **2007**, *28*, 2375–2381. [CrossRef]
149. Vyas, M.; Yang, X.; Zhang, X. Gastric Hamartomatous Polyps-Review and Update. *Clin. Med. Insights Gastroenterol.* **2016**, *9*, 3–10. [CrossRef]
150. Karuman, P.; Gozani, O.; Odze, R.D.; Zhou, X.C.; Zhu, H.; Shaw, R.; Brien, T.P.; Bozzuto, C.D.; Ooi, D.; Cantley, L.C.; et al. The Peutz-Jegher gene product LKB1 is a mediator of p53-dependent cell death. *Mol. Cell* **2001**, *7*, 1307–1319. [CrossRef]
151. Tiainen, M.; Vaahtomeri, K.; Ylikorkala, A.; Makela, T.P. Growth arrest by the LKB1 tumor suppressor: Induction of p21(WAF1/CIP1). *Hum. Mol. Genet.* **2002**, *11*, 1497–1504. [CrossRef] [PubMed]
152. Tiainen, M.; Ylikorkala, A.; Makela, T.P. Growth suppression by Lkb1 is mediated by a G_1 cell cycle arrest. *Proc. Natl. Acad. Sci. USA* **1999**, *96*, 9248–9251. [CrossRef] [PubMed]
153. Miyoshi, H.; Nakau, M.; Ishikawa, T.O.; Seldin, M.F.; Oshima, M.; Taketo, M.M. Gastrointestinal hamartomatous polyposis in Lkb1 heterozygous knockout mice. *Cancer Res.* **2002**, *62*, 2261–2266. [PubMed]
154. Wei, C.J.; Amos, C.I.; Stephens, L.C.; Campos, I.; Deng, J.M.; Behringer, R.R.; Rashid, A.; Frazier, M.L. Mutation of *Lkb1* and *p53* genes exert a cooperative effect on tumorigenesis. *Cancer Res.* **2005**, *65*, 11297–11303. [CrossRef] [PubMed]
155. Deng, C.; Zhang, P.; Harper, J.W.; Elledge, S.J.; Leder, P. Mice lacking p21$^{CIP1/WAF1}$ undergo normal development, but are defective in G1 checkpoint control. *Cell* **1995**, *82*, 675–684. [CrossRef]
156. Brugarolas, J.; Chandrasekaran, C.; Gordon, J.I.; Beach, D.; Jacks, T.; Hannon, G.J. Radiation-induced cell cycle arrest compromised by p21 deficiency. *Nature* **1995**, *377*, 552–557. [CrossRef]
157. Martin-Caballero, J.; Flores, J.M.; Garcia-Palencia, P.; Serrano, M. Tumor susceptibility of *p21*$^{Waf1/Cip1}$-deficient mice. *Cancer Res.* **2001**, *61*, 6234–6238. [PubMed]
158. Poole, A.J.; Heap, D.; Carroll, R.E.; Tyner, A.L. Tumor suppressor functions for the Cdk inhibitor p21 in the mouse colon. *Oncogene* **2004**, *23*, 8128–8134. [CrossRef]
159. Jackson, R.J.; Engelman, R.W.; Coppola, D.; Cantor, A.B.; Wharton, W.; Pledger, W.J. p21^{Cip1} nullizygosity increases tumor metastasis in irradiated mice. *Cancer Res.* **2003**, *63*, 3021–3025.

160. Yang, W.C.; Mathew, J.; Velcich, A.; Edelmann, W.; Kucherlapati, R.; Lipkin, M.; Yang, K.; Augenlicht, L.H. Targeted inactivation of the $p21^{WAF1/cip1}$ gene enhances Apc-initiated tumor formation and the tumor-promoting activity of a Western-style high-risk diet by altering cell maturation in the intestinal mucosal. *Cancer Res.* **2001**, *61*, 565–569.
161. Zirbes, T.K.; Baldus, S.E.; Moenig, S.P.; Nolden, S.; Kunze, D.; Shafizadeh, S.T.; Schneider, P.M.; Thiele, J.; Hoelscher, A.H.; Dienes, H.P. Prognostic impact of p21/waf1/cip1 in colorectal cancer. *Int. J. Cancer* **2000**, *89*, 14–18. [CrossRef]
162. Wee, P.; Wang, Z. Epidermal Growth Factor Receptor Cell Proliferation Signaling Pathways. *Cancers* **2017**, *9*, 52. [CrossRef]
163. Tuveson, D.A.; Shaw, A.T.; Willis, N.A.; Silver, D.P.; Jackson, E.L.; Chang, S.; Mercer, K.L.; Grochow, R.; Hock, H.; Crowley, D.; et al. Endogenous oncogenic K-ras^{G12D} stimulates proliferation and widespread neoplastic and developmental defects. *Cancer Cell* **2004**, *5*, 375–387. [CrossRef]
164. Johnson, L.; Mercer, K.; Greenbaum, D.; Bronson, R.T.; Crowley, D.; Tuveson, D.A.; Jacks, T. Somatic activation of the *K-ras* oncogene causes early onset lung cancer in mice. *Nature* **2001**, *410*, 1111–1116. [CrossRef] [PubMed]
165. Yamashita, N.; Minamoto, T.; Ochiai, A.; Onda, M.; Esumi, H. Frequent and characteristic K-*ras* activation and absence of p53 protein accumulation in aberrant crypt foci of the colon. *Gastroenterology* **1995**, *108*, 434–440. [CrossRef]
166. Roerink, S.F.; Sasaki, N.; Lee-Six, H.; Young, M.D.; Alexandrov, L.B.; Behjati, S.; Mitchell, T.J.; Grossmann, S.; Lightfoot, H.; Egan, D.A.; et al. Intra-tumour diversification in colorectal cancer at the single-cell level. *Nature* **2018**, *556*, 457–462. [CrossRef] [PubMed]
167. Kavuri, S.M.; Jain, N.; Galimi, F.; Cottino, F.; Leto, S.M.; Migliardi, G.; Searleman, A.C.; Shen, W.; Monsey, J.; Trusolino, L.; et al. HER2 activating mutations are targets for colorectal cancer treatment. *Cancer Discov.* **2015**, *5*, 832–841. [CrossRef]
168. Dougherty, U.; Cerasi, D.; Taylor, I.; Kocherginsky, M.; Tekin, U.; Badal, S.; Aluri, L.; Sehdev, A.; Cerda, S.; Mustafi, R.; et al. Epidermal growth factor receptor is required for colonic tumor promotion by dietary fat in the azoxymethane/dextran sulfate sodium model: Roles of transforming growth factor-α and PTGS2. *Clin. Cancer Res.* **2009**, *15*, 6780–6789. [CrossRef] [PubMed]
169. Dube, P.E.; Yan, F.; Punit, S.; Girish, N.; McElroy, S.J.; Washington, M.K.; Polk, D.B. Epidermal growth factor receptor inhibits colitis-associated cancer in mice. *J. Clin. Investig.* **2012**, *122*, 2780–2792. [CrossRef]
170. Roberts, R.B.; Min, L.; Washington, M.K.; Olsen, S.J.; Settle, S.H.; Coffey, R.J.; Threadgill, D.W. Importance of epidermal growth factor receptor signaling in establishment of adenomas and maintenance of carcinomas during intestinal tumorigenesis. *Proc. Natl. Acad. Sci. USA* **2002**, *99*, 1521–1526. [CrossRef]
171. Nagahara, H.; Mimori, K.; Ohta, M.; Utsunomiya, T.; Inoue, H.; Barnard, G.F.; Ohira, M.; Hirakawa, K.; Mori, M. Somatic mutations of epidermal growth factor receptor in colorectal carcinoma. *Clin. Cancer Res.* **2005**, *11*, 1368–1371. [CrossRef] [PubMed]
172. Moroni, M.; Veronese, S.; Benvenuti, S.; Marrapese, G.; Sartore-Bianchi, A.; Di Nicolantonio, F.; Gambacorta, M.; Siena, S.; Bardelli, A. Gene copy number for epidermal growth factor receptor (EGFR) and clinical response to antiEGFR treatment in colorectal cancer: A cohort study. *Lancet Oncol.* **2005**, *6*, 279–286. [CrossRef]
173. Brink, M.; de Goeij, A.F.; Weijenberg, M.P.; Roemen, G.M.; Lentjes, M.H.; Pachen, M.M.; Smits, K.M.; de Bruine, A.P.; Goldbohm, R.A.; van den Brandt, P.A. *K-ras* oncogene mutations in sporadic colorectal cancer in The Netherlands Cohort Study. *Carcinogenesis* **2003**, *24*, 703–710. [CrossRef] [PubMed]
174. Haigis, K.M.; Kendall, K.R.; Wang, Y.; Cheung, A.; Haigis, M.C.; Glickman, J.N.; Niwa-Kawakita, M.; Sweet-Cordero, A.; Sebolt-Leopold, J.; Shannon, K.M.; et al. Differential effects of oncogenic K-Ras and N-Ras on proliferation, differentiation and tumor progression in the colon. *Nat. Genet.* **2008**, *40*, 600–608. [CrossRef]
175. Guerra, C.; Mijimolle, N.; Dhawahir, A.; Dubus, P.; Barradas, M.; Serrano, M.; Campuzano, V.; Barbacid, M. Tumor induction by an endogenous *K-ras* oncogene is highly dependent on cellular context. *Cancer Cell* **2003**, *4*, 111–120. [CrossRef]
176. Ireland, H.; Kemp, R.; Houghton, C.; Howard, L.; Clarke, A.R.; Sansom, O.J.; Winton, D.J. Inducible Cre-mediated control of gene expression in the murine gastrointestinal tract: Effect of loss of β-catenin. *Gastroenterology* **2004**, *126*, 1236–1246. [CrossRef]

177. Luo, F.; Brooks, D.G.; Ye, H.; Hamoudi, R.; Poulogiannis, G.; Patek, C.E.; Winton, D.J.; Arends, M.J. Mutated K-ras^{Asp12} promotes tumourigenesis in Apc^{Min} mice more in the large than the small intestines, with synergistic effects between K-ras and Wnt pathways. *Int. J. Exp. Pathol.* **2009**, *90*, 558–574. [CrossRef]
178. Hung, K.E.; Maricevich, M.A.; Richard, L.G.; Chen, W.Y.; Richardson, M.P.; Kunin, A.; Bronson, R.T.; Mahmood, U.; Kucherlapati, R. Development of a mouse model for sporadic and metastatic colon tumors and its use in assessing drug treatment. *Proc. Natl. Acad. Sci. USA* **2010**, *107*, 1565–1570. [CrossRef]
179. Poulin, E.J.; Bera, A.K.; Lu, J.; Lin, Y.J.; Strasser, S.D.; Paulo, J.A.; Huang, T.Q.; Morales, C.; Yan, W.; Cook, J.; et al. Tissue-Specific Oncogenic Activity of KRAS^{A146T}. *Cancer Discov.* **2019**. [CrossRef]
180. Davies, H.; Bignell, G.R.; Cox, C.; Stephens, P.; Edkins, S.; Clegg, S.; Teague, J.; Woffendin, H.; Garnett, M.J.; Bottomley, W.; et al. Mutations of the *BRAF* gene in human cancer. *Nature* **2002**, *417*, 949–954. [CrossRef]
181. Rajagopalan, H.; Bardelli, A.; Lengauer, C.; Kinzler, K.W.; Vogelstein, B.; Velculescu, V.E. Tumorigenesis—*RAF/RAS* oncogenes and mismatch-repair status. *Nature* **2002**, *418*, 934. [CrossRef] [PubMed]
182. Dankort, D.; Filenova, E.; Collado, M.; Serrano, M.; Jones, K.; McMahon, M. A new mouse model to explore the initiation, progression, and therapy of *BRAF*^{V600E}-induced lung tumors. *Genes Dev.* **2007**, *21*, 379–384. [CrossRef] [PubMed]
183. Rad, R.; Cadinanos, J.; Rad, L.; Varela, I.; Strong, A.; Kriegl, L.; Constantino-Casas, F.; Eser, S.; Hieber, M.; Seidler, B.; et al. A Genetic Progression Model of Braf^{V600E}-Induced Intestinal Tumorigenesis Reveals Targets for Therapeutic Intervention. *Cancer Cell* **2013**, *24*, 15–29. [CrossRef] [PubMed]
184. Tao, Y.; Kang, B.; Petkovich, D.A.; Bhandari, Y.R.; In, J.; Stein-O'Brien, G.; Kong, X.; Xie, W.; Zachos, N.; Maegawa, S.; et al. Aging-like Spontaneous Epigenetic Silencing Facilitates Wnt Activation, Stemness, and Braf^{V600})-Induced Tumorigenesis. *Cancer Cell* **2019**, *35*, 315–328.e6. [CrossRef] [PubMed]
185. Biemer-Huttmann, A.E.; Walsh, M.D.; McGuckin, M.A.; Simms, L.A.; Young, J.; Leggett, B.A.; Jass, J.R. Mucin core protein expression in colorectal cancers with high levels of microsatellite instability indicates a novel pathway of morphogenesis. *Clin. Cancer Res.* **2000**, *6*, 1909–1916.
186. Walsh, M.D.; Clendenning, M.; Williamson, E.; Pearson, S.A.; Walters, R.J.; Nagler, B.; Packenas, D.; Win, A.K.; Hopper, J.L.; Jenkins, M.A.; et al. Expression of MUC2, MUC5AC, MUC5B, and MUC6 mucins in colorectal cancers and their association with the CpG island methylator phenotype. *Mod. Pathol.* **2013**, *26*, 1642–1656. [CrossRef]
187. Winterford, C.M.; Walsh, M.D.; Leggett, B.A.; Jass, J.R. Ultrastructural localization of epithelial mucin core proteins in colorectal tissues. *J. Histochem. Cytochem.* **1999**, *47*, 1063–1074. [CrossRef] [PubMed]
188. Velcich, A.; Yang, W.; Heyer, J.; Fragale, A.; Nicholas, C.; Viani, S.; Kucherlapati, R.; Lipkin, M.; Yang, K.; Augenlicht, L. Colorectal cancer in mice genetically deficient in the mucin Muc2. *Science* **2002**, *295*, 1726–1729. [CrossRef] [PubMed]
189. Stambolic, V.; Suzuki, A.; de la Pompa, J.L.; Brothers, G.M.; Mirtsos, C.; Sasaki, T.; Ruland, J.; Penninger, J.M.; Siderovski, D.P.; Mak, T.W. Negative regulation of PKB/Akt-dependent cell survival by the tumor suppressor PTEN. *Cell* **1998**, *95*, 29–39. [CrossRef]
190. Velho, S.; Oliveira, C.; Ferreira, A.; Ferreira, A.C.; Suriano, G.; Schwartz, S., Jr.; Duval, A.; Carneiro, F.; Machado, J.C.; Hamelin, R.; et al. The prevalence of PIK3CA mutations in gastric and colon cancer. *Eur. J. Cancer* **2005**, *41*, 1649–1654. [CrossRef] [PubMed]
191. Samuels, Y.; Waldman, T. Oncogenic mutations of PIK3CA in human cancers. *Curr. Top. Microbiol. Immunol.* **2010**, *347*, 21–41. [CrossRef] [PubMed]
192. Mitchell, C.B.; Phillips, W.A. Mouse Models for Exploring the Biological Consequences and Clinical Significance of PIK3CA Mutations. *Biomolecules* **2019**, *9*, 158. [CrossRef] [PubMed]
193. Goel, A.; Arnold, C.N.; Niedzwiecki, D.; Carethers, J.M.; Dowell, J.M.; Wasserman, L.; Compton, C.; Mayer, R.J.; Bertagnolli, M.M.; Boland, C.R. Frequent inactivation of PTEN by promoter hypermethylation in microsatellite instability-high sporadic colorectal cancers. *Cancer Res.* **2004**, *64*, 3014–3021. [CrossRef] [PubMed]
194. Berg, M.; Danielsen, S.A.; Ahlquist, T.; Merok, M.A.; Agesen, T.H.; Vatn, M.H.; Mala, T.; Sjo, O.H.; Bakka, A.; Moberg, I.; et al. DNA sequence profiles of the colorectal cancer critical gene set KRAS-BRAF-PIK3CA-PTEN-TP53 related to age at disease onset. *PLoS ONE* **2010**, *5*, e13978. [CrossRef] [PubMed]

195. Carpten, J.D.; Faber, A.L.; Horn, C.; Donoho, G.P.; Briggs, S.L.; Robbins, C.M.; Hostetter, G.; Boguslawski, S.; Moses, T.Y.; Savage, S.; et al. A transforming mutation in the pleckstrin homology domain of AKT1 in cancer. *Nature* **2007**, *448*, 439–444. [CrossRef] [PubMed]
196. Bleeker, F.E.; Felicioni, L.; Buttitta, F.; Lamba, S.; Cardone, L.; Rodolfo, M.; Scarpa, A.; Leenstra, S.; Frattini, M.; Barbareschi, M.; et al. $AKT1^{E17K}$ in human solid tumours. *Oncogene* **2008**, *27*, 5648–5650. [CrossRef] [PubMed]
197. Xu, Y.; Pasche, B. TGF-β signaling alterations and susceptibility to colorectal cancer. *Hum. Mol. Genet.* **2007**, *16*, R14–R20. [CrossRef]
198. Meulmeester, E.; Ten Dijke, P. The dynamic roles of TGF-β in cancer. *J. Pathol.* **2011**, *223*, 205–218. [CrossRef] [PubMed]
199. Lampropoulos, P.; Zizi-Sermpetzoglou, A.; Rizos, S.; Kostakis, A.; Nikiteas, N.; Papavassiliou, A.G. TGF-β signalling in colon carcinogenesis. *Cancer Lett.* **2012**, *314*, 1–7. [CrossRef]
200. Xie, W.; Rimm, D.L.; Lin, Y.; Shih, W.J.; Reiss, M. Loss of Smad signaling in human colorectal cancer is associated with advanced disease and poor prognosis. *Cancer J.* **2003**, *9*, 302–312. [CrossRef]
201. Fleming, N.I.; Jorissen, R.N.; Mouradov, D.; Christie, M.; Sakthianandeswaren, A.; Palmieri, M.; Day, F.; Li, S.; Tsui, C.; Lipton, L.; et al. SMAD2, SMAD3 and SMAD4 mutations in colorectal cancer. *Cancer Res.* **2013**, *73*, 725–735. [CrossRef]
202. Miyaki, M.; Iijima, T.; Konishi, M.; Sakai, K.; Ishii, A.; Yasuno, M.; Hishima, T.; Koike, M.; Shitara, N.; Iwama, T.; et al. Higher frequency of Smad4 gene mutation in human colorectal cancer with distant metastasis. *Oncogene* **1999**, *18*, 3098–3103. [CrossRef]
203. Takagi, Y.; Kohmura, H.; Futamura, M.; Kida, H.; Tanemura, H.; Shimokawa, K.; Saji, S. Somatic alterations of the DPC4 gene in human colorectal cancers in vivo. *Gastroenterology* **1996**, *111*, 1369–1372. [CrossRef]
204. Howe, J.R.; Roth, S.; Ringold, J.C.; Summers, R.W.; Jarvinen, H.J.; Sistonen, P.; Tomlinson, I.P.; Houlston, R.S.; Bevan, S.; Mitros, F.A.; et al. Mutations in the *SMAD4/DPC4* gene in juvenile polyposis. *Science* **1998**, *280*, 1086–1088. [CrossRef]
205. Calon, A.; Lonardo, E.; Berenguer-Llergo, A.; Espinet, E.; Hernando-Momblona, X.; Iglesias, M.; Sevillano, M.; Palomo-Ponce, S.; Tauriello, D.V.; Byrom, D.; et al. Stromal gene expression defines poor-prognosis subtypes in colorectal cancer. *Nat. Genet.* **2015**, *47*, 320–329. [CrossRef]
206. Nakagawa, H.; Liyanarachchi, S.; Davuluri, R.V.; Auer, H.; Martin, E.W., Jr.; de la Chapelle, A.; Frankel, W.L. Role of cancer-associated stromal fibroblasts in metastatic colon cancer to the liver and their expression profiles. *Oncogene* **2004**, *23*, 7366–7377. [CrossRef]
207. Calon, A.; Espinet, E.; Palomo-Ponce, S.; Tauriello, D.V.; Iglesias, M.; Cespedes, M.V.; Sevillano, M.; Nadal, C.; Jung, P.; Zhang, X.H.; et al. Dependency of colorectal cancer on a TGF-β-driven program in stromal cells for metastasis initiation. *Cancer Cell* **2012**, *22*, 571–584. [CrossRef]
208. Kulkarni, A.B.; Huh, C.G.; Becker, D.; Geiser, A.; Lyght, M.; Flanders, K.C.; Roberts, A.B.; Sporn, M.B.; Ward, J.M.; Karlsson, S. Transforming Growth Factor-β-1 Null Mutation in Mice Causes Excessive Inflammatory Response and Early Death. *Proc. Natl. Acad. Sci. USA* **1993**, *90*, 770–774. [CrossRef]
209. Shull, M.M.; Ormsby, I.; Kier, A.B.; Pawlowski, S.; Diebold, R.J.; Yin, M.Y.; Allen, R.; Sidman, C.; Proetzel, G.; Calvin, D.; et al. Targeted Disruption of the Mouse Transforming Growth Factor-β-1 Gene Results in Multifocal Inflammatory Disease. *Nature* **1992**, *359*, 693–699. [CrossRef]
210. Engle, S.J.; Hoying, J.B.; Boivin, G.P.; Ormsby, I.; Gartside, P.S.; Doetschman, T. Transforming growth factor β1 suppresses nonmetastatic colon cancer at an early stage of tumorigenesis. *Cancer Res.* **1999**, *59*, 3379–3386.
211. Takaku, K.; Miyoshi, H.; Matsunaga, A.; Oshima, M.; Sasaki, N.; Taketo, M.M. Gastric and duodenal polyps in *Smad4* (*Dpc4*) knockout mice. *Cancer Res.* **1999**, *59*, 6113–6117.
212. Zhu, Y.; Richardson, J.A.; Parada, L.F.; Graff, J.M. *Smad3* mutant mice develop metastatic colorectal cancer. *Cell* **1998**, *94*, 703–714. [CrossRef]
213. Kaiser, S.; Park, Y.K.; Franklin, J.L.; Halberg, R.B.; Yu, M.; Jessen, W.J.; Freudenberg, J.; Chen, X.; Haigis, K.; Jegga, A.G.; et al. Transcriptional recapitulation and subversion of embryonic colon development by mouse colon tumor models and human colon cancer. *Genome Biol.* **2007**, *8*, R131. [CrossRef]
214. Zeng, Q.; Phukan, S.; Xu, Y.; Sadim, M.; Rosman, D.S.; Pennison, M.; Liao, J.; Yang, G.Y.; Huang, C.C.; Valle, L.; et al. *Tgfbr1* haploinsufficiency is a potent modifier of colorectal cancer development. *Cancer Res.* **2009**, *69*, 678–686. [CrossRef]
215. Alberici, P.; Jagmohan-Changur, S.; De Pater, E.; Van Der Valk, M.; Smits, R.; Hohenstein, P.; Fodde, R. *Smad4* haploinsufficiency in mouse models for intestinal cancer. *Oncogene* **2006**, *25*, 1841–1851. [CrossRef]

216. Sodir, N.M.; Chen, X.; Park, R.; Nickel, A.E.; Conti, P.S.; Moats, R.; Bading, J.R.; Shibata, D.; Laird, P.W. Smad3 deficiency promotes tumorigenesis in the distal colon of $Apc^{Min/+}$ mice. *Cancer Res.* **2006**, *66*, 8430–8438. [CrossRef]
217. Aguilera, O.; Fraga, M.F.; Ballestar, E.; Paz, M.F.; Herranz, M.; Espada, J.; Garcia, J.M.; Munoz, A.; Esteller, M.; Gonzalez-Sancho, J.M. Epigenetic inactivation of the Wnt antagonist *DICKKOPF-1* (*DKK-1*) gene in human colorectal cancer. *Oncogene* **2006**, *25*, 4116–4121. [CrossRef]
218. Takaku, K.; Oshima, M.; Miyoshi, H.; Matsui, M.; Seldin, M.F.; Taketo, M.M. Intestinal tumorigenesis in compound mutant mice of both *Dpc4* (*Smad4*) and *Apc* genes. *Cell* **1998**, *92*, 645–656. [CrossRef]
219. Hamamoto, T.; Beppu, H.; Okada, H.; Kawabata, M.; Kitamura, T.; Miyazono, K.; Kato, M. Compound disruption of *Smad2* accelerates malignant progression of intestinal tumors in *Apc* knockout mice. *Cancer Res.* **2002**, *62*, 5955–5961.
220. Kunkel, T.A. Evolving views of DNA replication (in)fidelity. *Cold Spring Harb. Symp. Quant. Biol.* **2009**, *74*, 91–101. [CrossRef]
221. O'Sullivan, J.N.; Bronner, M.P.; Brentnall, T.A.; Finley, J.C.; Shen, W.T.; Emerson, S.; Emond, M.J.; Gollahon, K.A.; Moskovitz, A.H.; Crispin, D.A.; et al. Chromosomal instability in ulcerative colitis is related to telomere shortening. *Nat. Genet.* **2002**, *32*, 280–284. [CrossRef]
222. Poulogiannis, G.; Frayling, I.M.; Arends, M.J. DNA mismatch repair deficiency in sporadic colorectal cancer and Lynch syndrome. *Histopathology* **2010**, *56*, 167–179. [CrossRef]
223. Boland, C.R.; Goel, A. Microsatellite instability in colorectal cancer. *Gastroenterology* **2010**, *138*, 2073–2087. [CrossRef]
224. Edelmann, W.; Yang, K.; Kuraguchi, M.; Heyer, J.; Lia, M.; Kneitz, B.; Fan, K.; Brown, A.M.; Lipkin, M.; Kucherlapati, R. Tumorigenesis in *Mlh1* and *Mlh1/Apc1638N* mutant mice. *Cancer Res.* **1999**, *59*, 1301–1307.
225. de Wind, N.; Dekker, M.; Claij, N.; Jansen, L.; van Klink, Y.; Radman, M.; Riggins, G.; van der Valk, M.; van't Wout, K.; te Riele, H. HNPCC-like cancer predisposition in mice through simultaneous loss of Msh3 and Msh6 mismatch-repair protein functions. *Nat. Genet.* **1999**, *23*, 359–362. [CrossRef]
226. Prolla, T.A.; Baker, S.M.; Harris, A.C.; Tsao, J.L.; Yao, X.; Bronner, C.E.; Zheng, B.; Gordon, M.; Reneker, J.; Arnheim, N.; et al. Tumour susceptibility and spontaneous mutation in mice deficient in Mlh1, Pms1 and Pms2 DNA mismatch repair. *Nat. Genet.* **1998**, *18*, 276–279. [CrossRef]
227. Chen, P.C.; Dudley, S.; Hagen, W.; Dizon, D.; Paxton, L.; Reichow, D.; Yoon, S.R.; Yang, K.; Arnheim, N.; Liskay, R.M.; et al. Contributions by MutL homologues *Mlh3* and *Pms2* to DNA mismatch repair and tumor suppression in the mouse. *Cancer Res.* **2005**, *65*, 8662–8670. [CrossRef]
228. Lakso, M.; Pichel, J.G.; Gorman, J.R.; Sauer, B.; Okamoto, Y.; Lee, E.; Alt, F.W.; Westphal, H. Efficient in vivo manipulation of mouse genomic sequences at the zygote stage. *Proc. Natl. Acad. Sci. USA* **1996**, *93*, 5860–5865. [CrossRef]
229. Kucherlapati, M.H.; Lee, K.; Nguyen, A.A.; Clark, A.B.; Hou, H., Jr.; Rosulek, A.; Li, H.; Yang, K.; Fan, K.; Lipkin, M.; et al. An *Msh2* conditional knockout mouse for studying intestinal cancer and testing anticancer agents. *Gastroenterology* **2010**, *138*, 993–1002. [CrossRef]
230. Reitmair, A.H.; Cai, J.C.; Bjerknes, M.; Redston, M.; Cheng, H.; Pind, M.T.; Hay, K.; Mitri, A.; Bapat, B.V.; Mak, T.W.; et al. MSH2 deficiency contributes to accelerated APC-mediated intestinal tumorigenesis. *Cancer Res.* **1996**, *56*, 2922–2926.
231. Luo, F.; Brooks, D.G.; Ye, H.; Hamoudi, R.; Poulogiannis, G.; Patek, C.E.; Winton, D.J.; Arends, M.J. Conditional expression of mutated K-*ras* accelerates intestinal tumorigenesis in *Msh2*-deficient mice. *Oncogene* **2007**, *26*, 4415–4427. [CrossRef]
232. Kuraguchi, M.; Edelmann, W.; Yang, K.; Lipkin, M.; Kucherlapati, R.; Brown, A.M. Tumor-associated *Apc* mutations in $Mlh1^{-/-} Apc^{1638N}$ mice reveal a mutational signature of Mlh1 deficiency. *Oncogene* **2000**, *19*, 5755–5763. [CrossRef]
233. Kuraguchi, M.; Yang, K.; Wong, E.; Avdievich, E.; Fan, K.; Kolodner, R.D.; Lipkin, M.; Brown, A.M.; Kucherlapati, R.; Edelmann, W. The distinct spectra of tumor-associated *Apc* mutations in mismatch repair-deficient Apc^{1638N} mice define the roles of MSH3 and MSH6 in DNA repair and intestinal tumorigenesis. *Cancer Res.* **2001**, *61*, 7934–7942.
234. Takeda, H.; Rust, A.G.; Ward, J.M.; Yew, C.C.; Jenkins, N.A.; Copeland, N.G. Sleeping Beauty transposon mutagenesis identifies genes that cooperate with mutant *Smad4* in gastric cancer development. *Proc. Natl. Acad. Sci. USA* **2016**, *113*, E2057–E2065. [CrossRef]

235. Starr, T.K.; Allaei, R.; Silverstein, K.A.; Staggs, R.A.; Sarver, A.L.; Bergemann, T.L.; Gupta, M.; O'Sullivan, M.G.; Matise, I.; Dupuy, A.J.; et al. A transposon-based genetic screen in mice identifies genes altered in colorectal cancer. *Science* **2009**, *323*, 1747–1750. [CrossRef]
236. Drost, J.; van Jaarsveld, R.H.; Ponsioen, B.; Zimberlin, C.; van Boxtel, R.; Buijs, A.; Sachs, N.; Overmeer, R.M.; Offerhaus, G.J.; Begthel, H.; et al. Sequential cancer mutations in cultured human intestinal stem cells. *Nature* **2015**, *521*, 43–47. [CrossRef]
237. Matano, M.; Date, S.; Shimokawa, M.; Takano, A.; Fujii, M.; Ohta, Y.; Watanabe, T.; Kanai, T.; Sato, T. Modeling colorectal cancer using CRISPR-Cas9-mediated engineering of human intestinal organoids. *Nat. Med.* **2015**, *21*, 256–262. [CrossRef]

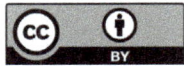

© 2019 by the authors. Licensee MDPI, Basel, Switzerland. This article is an open access article distributed under the terms and conditions of the Creative Commons Attribution (CC BY) license (http://creativecommons.org/licenses/by/4.0/).

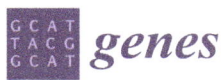

Review

Experimental Modeling of Myeloproliferative Neoplasms

Lucie Lanikova [1,*], **Olga Babosova** [1] **and Josef T. Prchal** [1,2,*]

[1] Laboratory of Cell and Developmental Biology, Institute of Molecular Genetics of the Czech Academy of Sciences, Videnska 1083, 142 20 Prague 4, Czech Republic; ola.babosova@gmail.com

[2] Division of Hematology & Hematologic Malignancies, Department of Internal Medicine, University of Utah, School of Medicine and VAH, Salt Lake City, UT 84132, USA

* Correspondence: lucie.lanikova@img.cas.cz (L.L.); josef.prchal@hsc.utah.edu (J.T.P.); Tel.: +420-241-063-107 (L.L.); Tel.: +1-801-585-2626 (J.T.P.)

Received: 28 August 2019; Accepted: 12 October 2019; Published: 15 October 2019

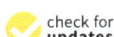

Abstract: Myeloproliferative neoplasms (MPN) are genetically very complex and heterogeneous diseases in which the acquisition of a somatic driver mutation triggers three main myeloid cytokine receptors, and phenotypically expresses as polycythemia vera (PV), essential thrombocytosis (ET), and primary myelofibrosis (PMF). The course of the diseases may be influenced by germline predispositions, modifying mutations, their order of acquisition and environmental factors such as aging and inflammation. Deciphering these contributory elements, their mutual interrelationships, and their contribution to MPN pathogenesis brings important insights into the diseases. Animal models (mainly mouse and zebrafish) have already significantly contributed to understanding the role of several acquired and germline mutations in MPN oncogenic signaling. Novel technologies such as induced pluripotent stem cells (iPSCs) and precise genome editing (using CRISPR/*Cas9*) contribute to the emerging understanding of MPN pathogenesis and clonal architecture, and form a convenient platform for evaluating drug efficacy. In this overview, the genetic landscape of MPN is briefly described, with an attempt to cover the main discoveries of the last 15 years. Mouse and zebrafish models of the driver mutations are discussed and followed by a review of recent progress in modeling MPN with patient-derived iPSCs and CRISPR/*Cas9* gene editing.

Keywords: MPN (myeloproliferative neoplasms); zebrafish; mice; iPSCs; *JAK2*; *MPL*; *CALR*; thrombosis

1. Introduction

Philadelphia chromosome-negative classical myeloproliferative disorders (more recently coined as neoplasms, MPN) are represented by polycythemia vera (PV), essential thrombocytosis (ET), and primary myelofibrosis (PMF). They are characterized by hyperplasia of at least one myeloid lineage in the bone marrow and an increased number of mature and entirely functional erythrocytes, platelets, or leukocytes, as popularized by Dameshek in the early 50s [1]. MPNs arise from a single somatically mutated hematopoietic stem cell (HSC), and the expansion of the mutated clone is accompanied by hyperplasia of a single phenotype-defining lineage. A high hemoglobin (Hb%) constitutes PV, and normal Hb% and high platelets constitute ET; however, PV patients often have elevated platelet counts, and both PV and ET may also have an elevated leukocyte count. In PMF, typical findings are anemia, neutrophilia, and thrombocytosis, or in a minority, thrombocytopenia and leukopenia, splenomegaly, immature granulocytes, increased clusters of differentiation 34+ cells (CD^{34+}), nucleated red cells, teardrop-shaped red cells (dacrocytes) in the blood, marrow fibrosis, and often osteosclerosis. The high rate of proliferation is driven by the so-called 'driver mutation' in genes that are important for normal myeloproliferation, Janus kinase 2 (*JAK2*), and thrombopoietin receptor (*C-MPL, MPL*), or in ET and PMF, mutated calreticulin gene (*CALR*), which has acquired a novel *MPL*-activating function [2,3]. The fact that the clonal architecture, microenvironment, and mutational profile change in a given patient over time results in different phenotypes, supports the idea that MPNs are not distinct biological entities but rather a continuum in which ET transforms to PV, or chronic phase PV and ET transform to PMF, and all three transform to acute leukemia [4].

In addition to the driver mutations, loss-of-function or neomorph mutations in genes that code for epigenetic regulators, and that are shared with myelodysplastic syndromes (MDS) and acute myeloid leukemia (AML), can act as disease modifiers in MPN [5]. Besides somatic mutations, other factors such as germline variants can modulate the risk of MPN development, favor the acquisition of somatic mutations, and influence the clinical course of the disease. Furthermore, several germline mutations have been described in hereditary erythrocytosis and hereditary thrombocytosis, benign conditions represented by polyclonal hematopoiesis that, clinically, can mimic MPN and pose a difficulty in diagnosis and therapeutic management [6].

2. Mutational Landscape of MPN

Precise diagnosis of MPN is often challenging and has been shown to occur years after the initiation of the disease (5–10–15 years) [7]. It has been proposed that about 95–98% of PV patients carry a mutation in the *JAK2* gene, with an occurrence in ET patients of about 60% and in PMF patients of about 55% [8]. Somatic mutation *MPL* W515 occurs in 3–8% of patients with ET and PMF. Mutations in *CALR* occur in 20–35% patients with ET and PMF [3]. Noticeably, the activation of thrombopoietin (TPO) receptor (TPOR) leads to a phenotype of ET and PMF, not the PV phenotype. There are also MPN patients who do not carry any of the aforementioned mutations, so-called 'triple-negative' MPN patients. Triple-negative patients either carry a mutation that is as yet unknown or remains to be elucidated, or are influenced by another factor affecting their HSCs and progenitors. In fact, it has been shown that acquiring a somatic driver mutation is rather a late event in the disease process, and that other factors, such as chronic inflammation, can predispose patients' cells to MPN transmission [9–11]. Additionally, polymorphisms in genes involved in DNA damage response and in the JAK/STAT pathway may increase the risk of MPN development. This includes the polymorphisms in the *JAK2* gene known as the *JAK2* 46/1 haplotype. The 46/1 haplotype was discovered by a genome-wide association study, and is a 280 Kb-long region of chromosome 9p that includes three genes in their entirety: the *JAK2* gene, insulin like 4 (*INSL4*), and insulin like 6 (*INSL6*). Surprisingly, *INSL4* and *INSL6* genes are not expressed in hematopoietic cells. There seems to be a strong association between the 46/1 haplotype and the occurrence of the *JAK2* V617F mutation; however, the precise mechanism remains to be elucidated [2,12–14]. A subset of patients carrying the *JAK2* 46/1 haplotype may also be predisposed to homologous recombinations of *JAK2*, followed or not by a mutation in the *JAK2* gene on the recombined allele [15].

The most frequently occurring gain-of-function *JAK2* V617F mutation gives rise to a constitutively active JAK2 kinase, which drives the JAK/STAT signaling that leads to excessive proliferation and survival of myeloid progenitor cells and accounts for >95% of driver mutations in PV and >55% in ET and PMF. Exon 12 of the *JAK2* gene is a less-frequent PV driver mutation (about 1%). Other *JAK2* mutations contributing to the MPN phenotype are under investigation [16,17]. These mutations lead to the PV phenotype and include non-synonymous substitutions, deletions and duplications, all affecting a region adjacent to the pseudokinase domain located between F533 and F547 [4,18]. The germline *JAK2* mutations were identified both in the pseudokinase (V617I, R564Q S755R) and in the kinase (R867Q, R938Q) domain [19–21], giving rise to the thrombocytosis phenotype. In some cases, the germline *JAK2* mutations were found to co-exist with *JAK2* V617F, further enhancing its signaling and likely predisposing the progenitor cells to the acquisition of *JAK2* V617F [22,23]. Further, two germline *JAK2* mutations, E846D and R1063H, were described in a case of hereditary erythrocytosis accompanied by megakaryocytic atypia [24], with R1063H being initially described in three out of 93 PV patients that were positive for *JAK2* V617F [17].

Mutations in the *JAK2* gene have been found to occur in all the cells of the hematopoietic tree starting from the HSC population, including not only a myeloid but also a lymphoid lineage [25]. Several studies point to the fact that *JAK2* V617F does not provide the HSC population with a proliferation advantage [26–29]. Patient *JAK2*-mutant xenografts in immunodeficient animal models suggest that *JAK2* mutations do not result in a self-renewal advantage. Instead, rather than enhanced self-renewal, *JAK2* V617F-positive cells expand at the progenitor level. These observations suggest that the *JAK2* V617F mutation alone is not sufficient to initiate MPN diseases, and that additional factors are required [30,31]. This is consistent with the fact that *JAK2* V617F mutation occurs in the normal population [32,33], accounting for the so-called entity of clonal hematopoiesis of indeterminate potential (CHIP) [34,35]. Intriguingly, these individuals bearing *JAK2* V617F and other CHIP somatic mutations, typically at a very low allelic burden, have increased risk of cardiovascular disease and some (but not an inevitable) risk of MPN progression. An alternative plausible explanation would be that the expansion of the progenitor pool, rather than the stem cell pool, is sufficient to induce the pathogenesis of MPN when driven by the *JAK2* mutation. This theory is supported by studies of native clonal hematopoiesis showing that a pool of long-term multipotent progenitors are the main drivers of adult hematopoiesis [36].

Activating mutations in the myeloproliferative leukemia virus (*MPL*) gene, encoding TPOR, can be either germline, such as in rare cases of familial essential thrombocytosis (*MPL* S505N) [37], or somatic. Surprisingly, the *MPL* S505N mutation has also been reported to be acquired in some rare cases of ET [38]. The most frequent somatic mutation in *MPL* is a mutation of the tryptophan residue at the 515 position (*MPL* W515) [39,40]. The mechanism by which these mutations alter TPOR signaling lies in modifying the geometry of the TPOR dimers, thus leading to transphosphorylation of the pre-bound JAK2 proteins. This results in constitutively active JAK2/STAT signaling initiated through TPOR [41,42].

Calreticulin is a multifunctional protein. It plays a role in calcium homeostasis as it binds calcium ions, rendering them inactive. Calreticulin also serves as a chaperone in the endoplasmic reticulum. However, the ET and PMF *CALR* mutations (more than 50 have been described) are all insertions or deletions that lead to frameshift mutations, resulting in their different 3'protein tails (an entirely different peptide downstream from *CALR* mutations) that acquire unique properties. This new C-terminal sequence is rich in positively charged amino acids and, unlike unmutated *CALR* (which is located in the cytoplasm), these unique *CALR*-mutated peptides are transported to the cellular membrane and activate thrombopoietin receptor. They are even secreted and activate non-mutated cells, thus acting as the *roque* cytokines [43,44].

There are other acquired mutations often reported in MPN patients. These are not restricted to MPN and frequently also occur in other hematological malignancies. They do not directly drive the clonal proliferation; nevertheless, they influence the course and progression of the disease and thus contribute to the heterogeneity of MPN. Among the most frequently reported are mutations in epigenetic regulators, splicing factors, and transcription factors, such as the tumor protein 53 (*TP53*). Out of these, the most frequently mutated are epigenetic regulators TET methylcytosine dioxygenase 2 (*TET2*) and DNA (cytosine-5)-methyltransferase 3A (*DNMT3A*). Mutations in epigenetic regulators such as enhancer of zeste homolog 2 (*EZH2*), additional sex combs like 1 (*ASXL1*), and a splicing factor, arginine/serine-rich 2 (*SRSF2*), are associated with poor prognosis and risk of AML transformation [2].

As the *JAK2* V617F mutation can drive the pathogenesis of all three classical MPNs, the question arises of how the progression of the disease differs in persons with the same mutation. A correlation between the level of expression and the phenotype has been found, with low expression being associated with an ET-like phenotype, and higher expression with a PV-like phenotype [2]. This is supported by the fact that *JAK2* exon 12 mutations exclusively lead to the PV phenotype and have been shown to activate STAT5 signaling to a greater extent [45]. Secondly, uniparental disomy (UPD) of chromosome 9 giving rise to *JAK2* V617F homozygosity is more likely associated with PV and PMF, and only rarely with ET [46,47]. This theory is also supported by knock-in mouse models, in which the ratio of mutant to wild-type Jak2 correlates with the degree of erythrocytosis [30,48]. This is also replicated in vivo in ET, when the patients that show greater *JAK2* V617F allele burden have a higher degree of erythrocytosis and leukocytosis [49].

JAK2 V617F binds to, and stimulates, all three receptors involved in the pathogenesis of MPN erythropoietin receptor (EPOR), TPOR and granulocyte-colony stimulating factor receptor (G-CSFR). In cases of familial MPN exhibiting hereditary thrombocytosis and triple-negative MPN, it is proposed that the inherited *JAK2* mutations signal through TPOR rather than EPOR [20,21]. Differential signaling of STATs might induce differential clinical phenotypes, such as thrombocytosis being induced by TPOR/STAT1 signaling and erythrocytosis by EPOR/STAT5 [2,21,50,51]. The acquisition of somatic mutations in disease modifiers also influences the course of the disease. Further, the order of the mutation acquisition matters. It was shown that prior mutation of *TET2* altered the transcriptional program activated by *JAK2* V617F in a cell-intrinsic manner and induced the ET phenotype. In contrast, patients in whom the *JAK2* V617F was acquired first more likely present PV [52].

3. Experimental Models of MPN

In addition to the clinical data, mutational landscape exploration in patients' samples, and in vitro experiments with cell lines simulating the impact of known alterations on hematopoietic signaling pathways, several experimental models were also created to unravel the myeloproliferative diseases' mechanisms and dynamics. In brief, among all animal models, zebrafish have offered unsurpassed tools for in vivo functional testing of genetic variants at the cell and organism level. Zebrafish (*Danio rerio*) have been used as a model organism to study vertebrate hematopoiesis during the past two decades. They display many appealing features—easy manipulation with transparent embryos and the capacity to carry out large-scale genetic and chemical screens, allowing convenient genetic manipulation and in vivo imaging of normal and aberrant hematopoiesis [53]. The majority of hematological malignancies modeled by zebrafish represent lymphoblastic and myeloid leukemias where the transgenic lines express oncogenic fusion genes and mutations commonly found in patients [54]. MPN modeling in zebrafish introduced *jak2a* V581F (an ortholog of human *JAK2* V617F), which shared features with human PV [55]. Meanwhile, zebrafish expressing *calr* mutants have developed mpl-dependent thrombocytosis [56], and a subset of zebrafish with disrupted *asxl* genes increased their numbers of myelomonocytes [57]. These models illustrate that the signaling machinery related to the MPN phenotype is conserved between human and zebrafish and has a great potential to uncover the unique mechanisms underlying MPN.

Several mouse models have been created to characterize the role of aberrant *Jak2* signaling within the hematopoietic compartment. Retroviral transduction models, transgenic and knock-in mice bearing *Jak2* V617F concomitantly with epigenetic modifier mutations were used to study MPN maintenance and progression (reviewed elsewhere in detail [58]). The early retroviral transduction models [59–62] confirmed the role of mutated Jak2 protein in MPN pathology, in which all mice developed a PV-like disease with noticeable erythrocytosis, leukocytosis, and splenomegaly, demonstrating that the *Jak2* V617F mutation is sufficient to induce an MPN-like condition in mice. The more advanced transgenic mouse models allowing quantitative expression of *Jak2* V617F [48,63,64] indicated a correlation between the mutant Jak2 protein expression levels and MPN phenotypes progressing from ET to PV and PMF with increasing *Jak2* V617F allelic burden, thus emulating the continuous progression in MPN sub-types. In 2010, four independent groups recreated *Jak2* V617F expression in the bone marrow compartment through knock-in models with Cre-mediated recombination under the control of a specific hematopoietic promoter [58]. These mice allowed the impact of *Jak2* mutation to be studied in its endogenous environment with the native expression ratio. Once again, all studies confirmed the pivotal role of the *Jak2* V617F mutation in the onset of MPN disease and recapitulated earlier observation that the *Jak2* allele burden might affect the disease phenotype. Interestingly, all models developed a severe

PV-like disorder that later progressed to myelofibrosis. Only the model by Li et al. using a human *JAK2* V617F cDNA construct under the control of endogenous murine *Jak2* promoter showed a modest ET-like phenotype, as in human ET, with only 10% of mice developing a PV-like disease, and only after 26 weeks, with marked erythrocytosis or bone marrow fibrosis [65]. Considering the crucial role of erythropoietin signaling in development of the disease [66,67], it is possible that the extensive polycythemia phenotype in these models (more severe than expected from patient studies) might reflect stronger signaling triggered by the murine EpoR when compared to human EPOR [68,69]. Double-mutant mouse models of *Jak2* V617F and epigenetic regulator *Tet2* loss-of-function, xenotransplantation-based models [70], and models using fetal liver cells expressing one or both alleles transplanted into lethally irradiated recipients [71], developed an aggressive MPN-like phenotype with rapid progression to myelofibrosis, and exhibited decreased overall survival. Detailed analysis of double-mutant early stem cells (so-called LSK, Lin$^-$Sca1$^+$cKit$^+$) showed a strong competitive advantage over wild-type cells, suggesting that mutated *Tet2* cooperates with *Jak2* V617F in vivo to promote stem cell self-renewal and proliferation while enhancing production of late-stage stem/progenitors and resulting in disease progression through combinatorial effects [70,71]. Similar to *Tet2*, mouse models combining the loss-of-function mutation of *Ezh2* with *Jak2* V617F developed an aggressive MPN-like phenotype with an overall expansion of the LSK stem/progenitor compartment [58].

Thrombotic events are very frequent and significantly contribute to morbidity and mortality in patients with MPN, mainly PV and ET [72]. However, the pathological processes associated with thromboembolic complications in these patients are not completely understood. Several experimental evidences suggest that *JAK2* V617F-associated abnormalities in erythrocytes, leukocytes, and platelets, as well as dysfunctions of endothelial cells, might play a role [72,73]. It was shown that *Jak2* V617F mice had increased atherosclerosis caused by cellular defects in erythrocytes and macrophages, leading to increased erythrophagocytosis but defective efferocytosis [74]. Zhao et al. identified the important role of pleckstrin-2 (*Plek2*) in erythroid cell survival and enucleation during terminal erythroid differentiation [75]. By crossing *Plek2*-knock-out mice with *Jak2* V617F-knock-in mice, they were able to ameliorate the myeloproliferative phenotype and additionally rescue *Jak2* V617F-induced widespread vascular occlusion and lethality in mice [76]. *Jak2* V617F-driven MPN mouse models have also increased neutrophil extracellular trap formation, which promotes the pro-thrombotic phenotype [77]. The pathologic thrombus formation in a thrombosis model using *Jak2* V617F mice was also suppressed by blocking β1 and β2 integrin activity [78]. Remarkably, *JAK2* V617F mutation can be present not only in blood cells, but also in endothelial cells of *JAK2* V617F-positive MPN patients [79,80]. Mouse models that allow the expression of *Jak2* V617F only in endothelial cells have shown that vascular endothelial cell expression of *Jak2* V617F is sufficient to promote a pro-thrombotic state. Furthermore, treatment with hydroxyurea has reduced thrombosis and decreased the pathological interaction between leukocytes and *Jak2* V617F-expressing endothelial cells through direct reduction of endothelial P-selectin expression [81]. Overall, these findings have identified new key players in blood clotting activation in MPNs, and suggest new therapeutic targets (e.g., *Plek2*, β1/β2 integrins) and applications (e.g., achieving lower levels of hematocrit in patients due to the direct role of *JAK2* V617F-positive erythrocytes in promoting advanced atherosclerosis [74]).

The pathogenic role of increased ectopic expression of murine *Tpo* receptor [82] or high thrombopoietin production by hematopoietic cells [83] were known long before *MPL* mutations were discovered in MPN patients [38,39]. In 2006, the retroviral transduction mouse model generated by Pikman et al. [39] expressing the most common *Mpl* mutation, W515L, resulted in a fully penetrant myeloproliferative disorder characterized by marked thrombocytosis, which increased reticulin fibrosis and induced splenomegaly due to extramedullary hematopoiesis. Importantly, the effect of *Mpl* W515L was lost when *Jak2* was deleted from recipient cells (Mx-Cre-Jak2$^{flox/flox}$ knock-out cells) [84], and *Jak2* V617F/Mpl$^{-/-}$ transgenic mice [85] exhibited reduced thrombocythemia, neutrophilia, splenomegaly, and neoplastic stem cell pools. This suggests that *Mpl* expression, but not TPO, has a fundamental effect on MPN development and severity. In addition, these results have demonstrated that the *Mpl*

W515L clone relies on the presence of wild-type Jak2 kinase to maintain the MPN phenotype and vice versa, that wild-type *Mpl* is indispensable in the development of *Jak2* V617F MPN-like diseases in mice. The mouse models with mutated *Calr* cover the two most commonly seen mutations in humans, *CALR*del52 and *CALR*ins5 [86], and are consistent with the ET phenotype in humans—all the models displayed isolated thrombocytosis with no significant effect on erythrocyte or leukocyte counts [58].

In conclusion, mouse models are a useful tool for studying the impact of the most prominent mutations on progression of MPN diseases. Since there are only limited data available describing the biochemical compatibility of human and mouse cytokines and their interaction with appropriate receptors (EPOR, MPL, or G-CSFR), it is important, particularly in murine models and derived cell lines, to co-express same-species receptors and use same-species cytokines, or to appropriately describe and discuss the experimental set-up. In addition, advances in understanding the critical role of JAK2/STAT signaling have allowed the design of potential MPN therapies, such as JAK2 inhibitors and murine models, which have been proven to be suitable candidates for screening and testing new promising compounds, although these do not fully allow the MPN heterogeneity seen in human patients to be addressed.

The derivation of human-induced pluripotent stem cells (iPSCs) in 2007 [87] began a new era in the modeling of human diseases, and introduced the generation of disease- and clone-specific iPSC lines that preserve the genetic identity of hematopoietic stem/progenitor clones. The first MPN-specific iPSCs were derived from $CD34^+$ cells isolated from the peripheral blood of both PV and PMF patients with heterozygous *JAK2* V617F mutations and an allele burden of approximately 50% [88]. The reprogramming protocol was based on Yamanaka retroviral factors (*Oct4, Sox2, Klf4* and *c-Myc*), which were transduced to pre-activated $CD34^+$ cells, and in total 11 clones were expanded and characterized. The expanded *JAK2* V617F iPSC clones displayed characteristics of pluripotent human embryonic stem cells with normal karyotypes and allowed direct differentiation into hematopoietic cells ($CD34^+/CD45^+$). Further evaluation of erythroid potential identified a two-fold proliferation advantage in the *JAK2* V617F clones over the normal controls. In addition, PV-iPSC-generated hematopoietic progenitor cells showed a PV-unique gene expression pattern corresponding to the primary $CD34^+$ cells. This pivotal experiment showed that, similar to human iPSCs derived from fibroblasts and normal $CD34^+$ cells, MPN cells can be directly reprogrammed with efficiencies comparable to those of normal cells. In contrast, MDS and AML cells are significantly more refractory to the reprogramming [89]. While bone marrow genetic heterogeneity hampers the isolation of individual oncogenic subclones, generation of MPN-iPSCs allows reconstruction of the clonal hierarchy and investigation of the effects of the mutations in their endogenous loci. In addition, advanced genome editing techniques (e.g., CRISPR/*Cas9* technology) offer allele-specific gene targeting based on homologous donors and the generation of isogenic corrected lines. It has already been shown that the efficacy of the CRISPR/*Cas9* system in targeting the *JAK2* V617F allele in PV-iPSCs is more than 80% [90]. Whereas high-frequency off-target mutagenesis induced by CRISPR/*Cas9* nucleases have been reported in some human cells [91], the targeted deep sequencing of edited PV-iPSCs clones has revealed high specificity with only minimal off-target effects [90,92].

The attempt to decipher the pre-*JAK2* V617F predisposing genetic lesions by PV-iPSCs has identified several candidate genes that, however, await further functional characterization [93]. Isogenic human erythroblasts and hematopoietic progenitors generated from PV patient-specific iPSCs have been used to examine responses to clinically used kinase inhibitors, especially JAK2 inhibitors. Saliba et al. used inhibitors targeting different signaling pathways (INCB018424 (Ruxolitinib)—JAK2 and JAK1; TG101348 (SAR302503)—JAK2 and FLT3; Ly294002—PI3K; RAD001—mTOR and AUY922—HSP90) and showed inhibition of erythroid growth in a dose- dependent manner in all the generated cell lines, regardless of their *JAK2* status [94]. The main disadvantage of retrovirally generated iPSCs is the methylation-induced silencing of transgenes and the random integration of retroviruses, which may affect the differentiation potential of the derived iPSC lines. Non-integrational, virus-free iPSC derivation by episomal vectors can overcome these problems, and was used by Ye et al. to generate iPSCs with distinct *JAK2* V617F allele compositions from one female PV patient [95]. The authors investigated the capacity of INCB018424 (Ruxolitinib), TG101348 (SAR302503), and CYT387 to suppress mutated *JAK2* V617F in PV-iPSC-derived myeloid and erythroid cells. Similar to the previous study and to the clinical findings [96,97], all three drugs non-selectively inhibited erythropoiesis in normal and PV-iPSC lines; however, the JAK inhibitors had a lower inhibitory effect on the self-renewal of iPSC-derived CD^{34+} hematopoietic progenitors, explaining the failure to eradicate the *JAK2* V617F clones after the treatment. Generation of human iPSCs from ET and PMF patients carrying *MPL* V501L and *CALR*ins5 has been reported, but detailed analysis of their erythroid and megakaryocytic differentiation potential is still ongoing [98,99]. Transcriptomic and proteomic analyses of megakaryocyte progenitors derived from *CALR* mutants and CRISPR/*Cas9*-corrected isogenic iPSC lines are ongoing as well [100]. Overall, MPN-iPSCs recapitulate the disease phenotype in vitro, and have been proven suitable for studying MPN pathogenesis, clonal architecture, and drug efficacy.

4. Conclusions

MPN molecular pathogenesis has been extensively elucidated by discoveries of MPN driver and modifier mutations during the last 15 years. Thanks to the combination of in vitro studies and animal modeling, it is now clear that aberrant hematopoietic cytokine receptors/JAK2 cooperation and, consequently, abnormal signaling of their downstream partners, can replicate most of the MPN phenotypes. Nevertheless, the molecular mechanisms of the disease's initiation are still not completely understood, and the exact role of the contribution of important disease-modifying factors such as aging, inflammation, and germline genetic predisposition await further study. Undoubtedly, *JAK2* V617F mutation is frequently present, but has insufficient penetrance to give rise to the MPN disease or three different MPN phenotypes. Therefore, it will be important in the future to model the oncogenic cooperation between MPN driver and other acquired or germline mutations with extrinsic factors and genetic abnormalities (e.g., by using a combination of CRISPR/*Cas9* and iPSCs techniques). Initial studies have already produced interesting new insights by modelling the DNA-damaging inflammatory microenvironment using induced pluripotent stem cell-derived CD^{34+} progenitor-enriched cultures from a *JAK2* V617F PV patient. It was shown that *JAK2* V617F PV progenitors utilize dual-specificity phosphatase 1 (DUSP1) activity as a protection mechanism against DNA damage accumulation, promoting their proliferation and survival in the inflammatory microenvironment [101].

Author Contributions: All authors listed have made a substantial, direct, and intellectual contribution to the work and approved it for publication.

Funding: This research was funded by the Ministry of Education, Youth and Sports, Czech Republic, grant number LO1419, Program NPU I, and by the Czech Science Foundation, grant number GACR 17-05988S.

Acknowledgments: We thank Sarka Takacova for critically reading the manuscript.

Conflicts of Interest: The authors declare no conflict of interest.

References

1. Dameshek, W. Some speculations on the myeloproliferative syndromes. *Blood* **1951**, *6*, 372–375. [CrossRef] [PubMed]
2. Vainchenker, W.; Kralovics, R. Genetic basis and molecular pathophysiology of classical myeloproliferative neoplasms. *Blood* **2017**, *129*, 667–679. [CrossRef] [PubMed]
3. Skoda, R.; Duek, A.; Grisouard, J. Pathogenesis of myeloproliferative neoplasms. *Exp. Hematol.* **2015**, *43*, 599–608. [CrossRef] [PubMed]
4. Grinfeld, J.; Nangalia, J.; Green, A. Molecular determinants of pathogenesis and clinical phenotype in myeloproliferative neoplasms. *Haematologica* **2017**, *102*, 7–17. [CrossRef]
5. Rumi, E.; Cazzola, M. Diagnosis, risk stratification, and response evaluation in classical myeloproliferative neoplasms. *Blood* **2017**, *129*, 680–692. [CrossRef]

6. Harutyunyan, A.; Kralovics, R. Role of germline genetic factors in MPN pathogenesis. *Hematol. Oncol. Clin. N. Am.* **2012**, *26*, 1037–1051. [CrossRef]
7. Hasselbalch, H.; Bjørn, M. MPNs as Inflammatory Diseases: The Evidence, Consequences, and Perspectives. *Mediat. Inflamm.* **2015**, *2015*, 102476. [CrossRef]
8. Tefferi, A. Myeloproliferative neoplasms: A decade of discoveries and treatment advances. *Am. J. Hematol.* **2016**, *91*, 50–58. [CrossRef]
9. Kralovics, R.; Teo, S.S.; Li, S.; Theocharides, A.; Buser, A.; Tichelli, A.; Skoda, R. Acquisition of the V617F mutation of JAK2 is a late genetic event in a subset of patients with myeloproliferative disorders. *Blood* **2006**, *108*, 1377–1380. [CrossRef]
10. Hermouet, S.; Bigot-Corbel, E.; Gardie, B. Pathogenesis of Myeloproliferative Neoplasms: Role and Mechanisms of Chronic Inflammation. *Mediat. Inflamm.* **2015**, *2015*, 145293. [CrossRef]
11. Maxson, J.; Gotlib, J.; Pollyea, D.; Fleischman, A.; Agarwal, A.; Eide, C.; Bottomly, D.; Wilmot, B.; McWeeney, S.; Tognon, C.; et al. Oncogenic CSF3R Mutations in Chronic Neutrophilic Leukemia and Atypical CML. *N. Engl. J. Med.* **2013**, *368*, 1781–1790. [CrossRef] [PubMed]
12. Olcaydu, D.; Harutyunyan, A.; Jäger, R.; Berg, T.; Gisslinger, B.; Pabinger, I.; Gisslinger, H.; Kralovics, R. A common JAK2 haplotype confers susceptibility to myeloproliferative neoplasms. *Nat. Genet.* **2009**, *41*, 450–454. [CrossRef] [PubMed]
13. Jones, A.; Chase, A.; Silver, R.; Oscier, D.; Zoi, K.; Wang, L.; Cario, H.; Pahl, H.; Collins, A.; Reiter, A.; et al. JAK2 haplotype is a major risk factor for the development of myeloproliferative neoplasms. *Nat. Genet.* **2009**, *41*, 446–449. [CrossRef] [PubMed]
14. Kilpivaara, O.; Mukherjee, S.; Schram, A.; Wadleigh, M.; Mullally, A.; Ebert, B.; Bass, A.; Marubayashi, S.; Heguy, A.; Garcia-Manero, G.; et al. A germline JAK2 SNP is associated with predisposition to the development of JAK2(V617F)-positive myeloproliferative neoplasms. *Nat. Genet.* **2009**, *41*, 455–459. [CrossRef]
15. Vilaine, M.; Olcaydu, D.; Harutyunyan, A.; Bergeman, J.; Tiab, M.; Ramée, J.-F.; Jian-Min, C.; Kralovics, R.; Hermouet, S. Homologous recombination of wild-type JAK2, a novel early step in the development of myeloproliferative neoplasm. *Blood* **2011**, *118*, 6468–6470. [CrossRef]
16. James, C.; Ugo, V.; Le Couédic, J.-P.; Staerk, J.; Delhommeau, F.; Lacout, C.; Garçon, L.; Raslova, H.; Berger, R.; Bennaceur-Griscelli, A.; et al. A unique clonal JAK2 mutation leading to constitutive signalling causes polycythaemia vera. *Nature* **2005**, *434*, 1144–1148. [CrossRef]
17. Levine, R.; Wadleigh, M.; Cools, J.; Ebert, B.; Wernig, G.; Huntly, B.; Boggon, T.; Wlodarska, I.; Clark, J.; Moore, S.; et al. Activating mutation in the tyrosine kinase JAK2 in polycythemia vera, essential thrombocythemia, and myeloid metaplasia with myelofibrosis. *Cancer Cell* **2005**, *7*, 387–397. [CrossRef]
18. Scott, L. The JAK2 exon 12 mutations: A comprehensive review. *Am. J. Hematol.* **2011**, *86*, 668–676. [CrossRef]
19. Mead, A.; Rugless, M.; Jacobsen, S.; Schuh, A. Germline JAK2 mutation in a family with hereditary thrombocytosis. *N. Engl. J. Med.* **2012**, *366*, 967–969. [CrossRef]
20. Etheridge, S.L.; Cosgrove, M.; Sangkhae, V.; Corbo, L.; Roh, M.; Seeliger, M.; Chan, E.; Hitchcock, I. A novel activating, germline JAK2 mutation, JAK2R564Q, causes familial essential thrombocytosis. *Blood* **2013**, *123*, 1059–1068. [CrossRef]
21. Marty, C.; Saint Martin, C.; Pecquet, C.; Grosjean, S.; Saliba, J.; Mouton, C.; Leroy, E.; Harutyunyan, A.; Abgrall, J.-F.; Favier, R.; et al. Germ-line JAK2 mutations in the kinase domain are responsible for hereditary thrombocytosis and are resistant to JAK2 and HSP90 inhibitors. *Blood* **2014**, *123*, 1372–1383. [CrossRef] [PubMed]
22. Lanikova, L.; Babosova, O.; Swierczek, S.; Wang, L.; Wheeler, D.; Divoky, V.; Korinek, V.; Prchal, J. Coexistence of gain-of-function JAK2 germline mutations with JAK2V617F in polycythemia vera. *Blood* **2016**, *128*, 2266–2270. [CrossRef] [PubMed]
23. Mambet, C.; Babosova, O.; Defour, J.-P.; Leroy, E.; Necula, L.; Stanca, O.; Tatic, A.; Berbec, N.; Coriu, D.; Belickova, M.; et al. Co-occurring JAK2 V617F and R1063H mutations increase JAK2 signaling and neutrophilia in MPN patients. *Blood* **2018**, *132*, 2695–2699. [CrossRef] [PubMed]
24. Kapralova, K.; Horvathova, M.; Pecquet, C.; Fialova Kucerova, J.; Pospíšilová, D.; Leroy, E.; Kralova, B.; Milosevic Feenstra, J.; Schischlik, F.; Kralovics, R.; et al. Cooperation of germline JAK2 mutations E846D and R1063H in hereditary erythrocytosis with megakaryocytic atypia. *Blood* **2016**, *128*, 1418–1423. [CrossRef]

25. Lundberg, P.; Takizawa, H.; Kubovcakova, L.; Guo, G.; Hao-Shen, H.; Dirnhofer, S.; Orkin, S.; Manz, M.; Skoda, R. Myeloproliferative neoplasms can be initiated from a single hematopoietic stem cell expressing JAK2-V617F. *J. Exp. Med.* **2014**, *211*, 2213–2230. [CrossRef]
26. Anand, S.; Stedham, F.; Beer, P.; Gudgin, E.; Ortmann, C.; Bench, A.; Erber, W.; Green, A.; Huntly, B. Effects of the JAK2 mutation on the hematopoietic stem and progenitor compartment in human myeloproliferative neoplasms. *Blood* **2011**, *118*, 177–181. [CrossRef]
27. James, C.; Mazurier, F.; Dupont, S.; Chaligne, R.; Lamrissi-Garcia, I.; Tulliez, M.; Lippert, E.; Mahon, F.-X.; Pasquet, J.; Etienne, G.; et al. The hematopoietic stem cell compartment of JAK2V617F-positive myeloproliferative disorders is a reflection of disease heterogeneity. *Blood* **2008**, *112*, 2429–2438. [CrossRef]
28. Larsen, T.; Christensen, J.; Hasselbalch, H.; Pallisgaard, N. The JAK2 V617F mutation involves B- and T-lymphocyte lineages in a subgroup of patients with Philadelphia-chromosome negative chronic myeloproliferative disorders. *Br. J. Haematol.* **2007**, *136*, 745–751. [CrossRef]
29. Mullally, A.; Lane, S.; Ball, B.; Megerdichian, C.; Okabe, R.; Al-Shahrour, F.; Paktinat, M.; Haydu, E.; Housman, E.; Lord, A.; et al. Physiological Jak2V617F Expression Causes a Lethal Myeloproliferative Neoplasm with Differential Effects on Hematopoietic Stem and Progenitor Cells. *Cancer Cell* **2010**, *17*, 584–596. [CrossRef]
30. Li, J.; Kent, D.; Godfrey, A.; Manning, H.; Nangalia, J.; Aziz, A.; Chen, E.; Saeb-Parsy, K.; Fink, J.; Sneade, R.; et al. JAK2V617F homozygosity drives a phenotypic switch in myeloproliferative neoplasms, but is insufficient to sustain disease. *Blood* **2014**, *123*, 3139–3151. [CrossRef]
31. Kent, D.; Li, J.; Tanna, H.; Fink, J.; Kirschner, K.; Pask, D.; Silber, Y.; Hamilton, T.; Sneade, R.; Simons, B.; et al. Self-Renewal of Single Mouse Hematopoietic Stem Cells Is Reduced by JAK2V617F Without Compromising Progenitor Cell Expansion. *PLoS Biol.* **2013**, *11*, e1001576. [CrossRef] [PubMed]
32. McKerrell, T.; Park, N.; Moreno, T.; Grove, C.; Ponstingl, H.; Stephens, J.; Crawley, C.; Craig, J.; Scott, M.; Hodkinson, C.; et al. Leukemia-Associated Somatic Mutations Drive Distinct Patterns of Age-Related Clonal Hemopoiesis. *Cell Rep.* **2015**, *10*, 1239–1245. [CrossRef] [PubMed]
33. Genovese, G.; Kähler, A.; Handsaker, R.; Lindberg, J.; Rose, S.; Bakhoum, S.; Chambert, K.; Mick, E.; Neale, B.; Fromer, M.; et al. Clonal Hematopoiesis and Blood-Cancer Risk Inferred from Blood DNA Sequence. *N. Engl. J. Med.* **2014**, *371*, 2477–2487. [CrossRef] [PubMed]
34. Jaiswal, S.; Libby, P. Clonal haematopoiesis: Connecting ageing and inflammation in cardiovascular disease. *Nat. Rev. Cardiol.* **2019**. [CrossRef]
35. Prchal, J. The Significance of JAK2-Positive Test Results in a Healthy Patient. In ASH Clinical News, American Society of Hematology. 2019. Available online: https://www.ashclinicalnews.org (accessed on 1 August 2019).
36. Sun, J.; Ramos, A.; Chapman, B.; Johnnidis, J.; Le, L.; Ho, Y.-J.; Klein, A.; Hofmann, O.; Camargo, F. Clonal dynamics of native haematopoiesis. *Nature* **2014**, *514*, 322–327. [CrossRef]
37. Ding, J.; Komatsu, H.; Wakita, A.; Kato-Uranishi, M.; Ito, M.; Satoh, A.; Tsuboi, K.; Nitta, M.; Miyazaki, H.; Iida, S.; et al. Familial essential thrombocythemia associated with a dominant-positive activating mutation of the c-MPL gene, which encodes for the receptor for thrombopoietin. *Blood* **2004**, *103*, 4198–4200. [CrossRef]
38. Beer, P.; Campbell, P.; Scott, L.; Bench, A.; Erber, W.; Bareford, D.; Wilkins, B.; Reilly, J.; Hasselbalch, H.; Bowman, R.; et al. MPL mutations in myeloproliferative disorders: Analysis of the PT-1 cohort. *Blood* **2008**, *112*, 141–149. [CrossRef]
39. Pikman, Y.; Lee, B.; Mercher, T.; McDowell, E.; Ebert, B.; Gozo, M.; Cuker, A.; Wernig, G.; Moore, S.; Galinsky, I.; et al. MPLW515L Is a Novel Somatic Activating Mutation in Myelofibrosis with Myeloid Metaplasia. *PLoS Med.* **2006**, *3*, e270. [CrossRef]
40. Pardanani, A.; Lasho, T.; McClure, R.; Lacy, M.; Tefferi, A. Discordant distribution of JAK2V617F mutation in siblings with familial myeloproliferative disorders. *Blood* **2006**, *107*, 4572–4573. [CrossRef]
41. Staerk, J.; Defour, J.-P.; Pecquet, C.; Leroy, E.; Poirel, H.; Brett, I.; Itaya, M.; Smith, S.; Vainchenker, W.; Constantinescu, S. Orientation-specific signalling by thrombopoietin receptor dimers. *EMBO J.* **2011**, *30*, 4398–4413. [CrossRef]
42. Constantinescu, S.; Keren, T.; Socolovsky, M.; Nam, H.; Henis, Y.; Lodish, H.; Constantinescu, S.N.; Keren, T.; Socolovsky, M.; Nam, H.; et al. Ligand-independent oligomerization of cell-surface erythropoietin receptor is mediated by the transmembrane domain. *Proc. Natl. Acad. Sci. USA* **2001**, *98*, 4379–4384. [CrossRef] [PubMed]

43. Pecquet, C.; Chachoua, I.; Roy, A.; Balligand, T.; Vertenoeil, G.; Leroy, E.; Albu, R.-I.; Defour, J.-P.; Nivarthi, H.; Hug, E.; et al. Calreticulin mutants as oncogenic rogue chaperones for TpoR and traffic-defective pathogenic TpoR mutants. *Blood* **2019**, *133*, 2669–2681. [CrossRef] [PubMed]
44. Pecquet, C.; Balligand, T.; Chachoua, I.; Roy, A.; Vertenoeil, G.; Colau, D.; Fertig, E.; Marty, C.; Nivarthi, H.; Defour, J.-P.; et al. Secreted Mutant Calreticulins As Rogue Cytokines Trigger Thrombopoietin Receptor Activation Specifically in CALR Mutated Cells: Perspectives for MPN Therapy. *Blood* **2018**, *132*, 4. [CrossRef]
45. Scott, L.; Tong, W.; Levine, R.; Scott, M.; Beer, P.; Stratton, M.; Andrew Futreal, P.; Erber, W.; McMullin, M.; Harrison, C.; et al. JAK2 Exon 12 Mutations in Polycythemia Vera and Idiopathic Erythrocytosis. *N. Engl. J. Med.* **2007**, *356*, 459–468. [CrossRef] [PubMed]
46. Kralovics, R.; Guan, Y.; Prchal, J. Acquired uniparental disomy of chromosome 9p is a frequent stem cell defect in polycythemia vera. *Exp. Hematol.* **2002**, *30*, 229–236. [CrossRef]
47. Scott, L.; Scott, M.; Campbell, P.; Green, A. Progenitors homozygous for the V617F mutation occur in most patients with polycythemia vera, but not essential thrombocythemia. *Blood* **2006**, *108*, 2435–2437. [CrossRef]
48. Tiedt, R.; Hao-Shen, H.; Sobas, M.; Looser, R.; Dirnhofer, S.; Schwaller, J.; Skoda, R. Ratio of mutant JAK2-V617F to wild-type Jak2 determines the MPD phenotypes in transgenic mice. *Blood* **2008**, *111*, 3931–3940. [CrossRef]
49. Vannucchi, A.; Antonioli, E.; Guglielmelli, P.; Rambaldi, A.; Barosi, G.; Marchioli, R.; Marfisi, R.; Finazzi, G.; Guerini, V.; Fabris, F.; et al. Clinical profile of homozygous JAK2 617V>F mutation in patients with polycythemia vera or essential thrombocythemia. *Blood* **2007**, *110*, 840–846. [CrossRef]
50. Yao, H.; Ma, Y.; Hong, Z.; Zhao, L.; Monaghan, A.S.; Hu, M.; Huang, L.-S. Activating JAK2 mutants reveal cytokine receptor coupling differences that impact outcomes in myeloproliferative neoplasm. *Leukemia* **2017**, *31*, 2122–2131. [CrossRef]
51. Chen, E.; Beer, P.; Godfrey, A.; Ortmann, C.; Li, J.; Costa-Pereira, A.; Ingle, C.; Dermitzakis, E.; Campbell, P.; Green, A. Distinct Clinical Phenotypes Associated with JAK2V617F Reflect Differential STAT1 Signaling. *Cancer Cell* **2010**, *18*, 524–535. [CrossRef]
52. Ortmann, C.; Kent, D.; Nangalia, J.; Silber, Y.; Wedge, D.; Grinfeld, J.; Baxter, E.; Massie, C.; Papaemmanuil, E.; Menon, S.; et al. Effect of Mutation Order on Myeloproliferative Neoplasms. *N. Engl. J. Med.* **2015**, *372*, 601–612. [CrossRef] [PubMed]
53. Lieschke, G.; Currie, P. Animal models of human disease: Zebrafish swim into view. *Nat. Rev. Genet.* **2007**, *8*, 353–367. [CrossRef] [PubMed]
54. Baeten, J.; de Jong, J. Genetic Models of Leukemia in Zebrafish. *Front. Cell Dev. Biol.* **2017**, *6*, 115. [CrossRef] [PubMed]
55. Ma, A.; Fan, A.; Ward, A.; Liongue, C.; Lewis, R.; Cheng, S.; Chan, P.; Yip, S.-F.; Liang, R.; Leung, A. A novel zebrafish jak2aV581F model shared features of human JAK2V617F polycythemia vera. *Exp. Hematol.* **2009**, *37*, 1379–1386. [CrossRef]
56. Lim, K.-H.; Chang, Y.C.; Chiang, Y.H.; Lin, H.C.; Chang, C.-Y.; Lin, C.S.; Huang, L.; Wang, W.T.; Chen, G.-S.; Chou, W.C.; et al. Expression of CALR mutants causes mpl-dependent thrombocytosis in zebrafish. *Blood Cancer J.* **2016**, *6*, e481. [CrossRef]
57. Gjini, E.; Jing, C.-B.; Nguyen, A.; Reyon, D.; Gans, E.; Kesarsing, M.; Peterson, J.; Pozdnyakova, O.; Rodig, S.; Mansour, M.; et al. Disruption of asxl1 results in myeloproliferative neoplasms in zebrafish. *Dis. Models Mech.* **2019**, *12*, dmm035790. [CrossRef]
58. Dunbar, A.; Nazir, A.; Levine, R. Overview of Transgenic Mouse Models of Myeloproliferative Neoplasms (MPNs). *Curr. Protoc. Pharmacol.* **2017**, *77*, 11–19.
59. Bumm, T.; Elsea, C.; Corbin, A.; Loriaux, M.; Sherbenou, D.; Wood, L.; Deininger, J.; Silver, R.; Druker, B.; Deininger, M. Characterization of Murine JAK2V617F-Positive Myeloproliferative Disease. *Cancer Res.* **2007**, *66*, 11156–11165. [CrossRef]
60. Lacout, C.; Pisani, D.; Tulliez, M.; Moreau-Gachelin, F.; Vainchenker, W.; Villeval, J.-L.; Lacout, C.; Pisani, D.F.; Tulliez, M.; Gachelin, F.M.; et al. JAK2V617F expression in murine hematopoietic cells leads to MPD mimicking human PV with secondary myelofibrosis. *Blood* **2006**, *108*, 1652–1660. [CrossRef]
61. Wernig, G.; Mercher, T.; Okabe, R.; Levine, R.; Lee, B.; Gilliland, G. Expression of Jak2V617F causes a polycythemia vera-like disease with associated myelofibrosis in a murine bone marrow transplant model. *Blood* **2006**, *107*, 4274–4281. [CrossRef]
62. Zaleskas, V.; Krause, D.; Lazarides, K.; Patel, N.; Hu, Y.; Li, S.; Van Etten, R. Molecular Pathogenesis and Therapy of Polycythemia Induced in Mice by JAK2 V617F. *PLoS ONE* **2006**, *1*, e18. [CrossRef] [PubMed]

63. Shide, K.; Shimoda, H.; Kumano, T.; Karube, K.; Kameda, T.; Takenaka, K.; Oku, S.; Abe, H.; Katayose, K.; Kubuki, Y.; et al. Development of ET, primary myelofibrosis and PV in mice expressing JAK2 V617F. *Leukemia* **2008**, *22*, 87–95. [CrossRef] [PubMed]
64. Xing, S.; Wanting, T.; Zhao, W.; Ma, J.; Wang, S.; Xu, X.; Li, Q.; Fu, X.; Xu, M.; Zhao, Z. Transgenic expression of JAK2(V617F) causes myeloproliferative disorders in mice. *Blood* **2008**, *111*, 5109–5117. [CrossRef] [PubMed]
65. Li, J.; Spensberger, D.; Sook Ahn, J.; Anand, S.; Beer, P.; Ghevaert, C.; Chen, E.; Forrai, A.; Scott, L.; Ferreira, R.; et al. JAK2 V617F impairs hematopoietic stem cell function in a conditional knock-in mouse model of JAK2 V617F-positive essential thrombocythemia. *Blood* **2010**, *116*, 1528–1538. [CrossRef]
66. Lu, X.; Levine, R.; Tong, W.; Wernig, G.; Pikman, Y.; Zarnegar, S.; Gilliland, G.; Lodish, H. Expression of a homodimeric type I cytokine receptor is required for JAK2V617F-mediated transformation. *Proc. Natl. Acad. Sci. USA* **2006**, *102*, 18962–18967. [CrossRef]
67. Kota, J.; Caceres, N.; Constantinescu, S. Aberrant signal transduction pathways in myeloproliferative neoplasms. *Leukemia* **2008**, *22*, 1828–1840. [CrossRef]
68. Ebie, A.; Fleming, K. Dimerization of the Erythropoietin Receptor Transmembrane Domain in Micelles. *J. Mol. Biol.* **2007**, *366*, 517–524. [CrossRef]
69. Divoky, V.; Song, J.; Horvathova, M.; Kralova, B.; Bruchova Votavova, H.; Prchal, J.; Yoon, D. Delayed Hemoglobin Switching and Perinatal Neocytolysis in Mice with Gain-of-Function Erythropoietin Receptor. *J. Mol. Med.* **2015**, *94*, 597–608. [CrossRef]
70. Chen, E.; Schneider, R.; Breyfogle, L.; Rosen, E.; Poveromo, L.; Elf, S.; Ko, A.; Brumme, K.; Levine, R.; Ebert, B.; et al. Distinct effects of concomitant Jak2V617F expression and Tet2 loss in mice promote disease progression in myeloproliferative neoplasms. *Blood* **2014**, *125*, 327–335. [CrossRef]
71. Kameda, T.; Shide, K.; Yamaji, T.; Kamiunten, A.; Sekine, M.; Taniguchi, Y.; Hidaka, T.; Kubuki, Y.; Shimoda, H.; Marutsuka, K.; et al. Loss of TET2 has dual roles in murine myeloproliferative neoplasms: Disease sustainer and disease accelerator. *Blood* **2014**, *125*, 304–315. [CrossRef]
72. Falanga, A.; Marchetti, M. Thrombosis in Myeloproliferative Neoplasms. *Semin. Thromb. Hemost.* **2014**, *40*, 348–358. [PubMed]
73. Vannucchi, A.; Guglielmelli, P. JAK2 Mutation-Related Disease and Thrombosis. *Semin. Thromb. Hemost.* **2013**, *39*, 496–506. [PubMed]
74. Wang, W.; Liu, W.; Fidler, T.; Wang, Y.; Tang, Y.; Woods, B.; Welch, C.; Cai, B.; Silvestre-Roig, C.; Ai, D.; et al. Macrophage Inflammation, Erythrophagocytosis, and Accelerated Atherosclerosis in Jak2V617F Mice. *Circ. Res.* **2018**, *123*, e35–e47. [CrossRef] [PubMed]
75. Zhao, B.; Keerthivasan, G.; Mei, Y.; Yang, J.; McElherne, J.; Wong, P.; Doench, J.; Feng, G.; Root, D.; Ji, P. Targeted shRNA screening identified critical roles of pleckstrin-2 in erythropoiesis. *Haematologica* **2014**, *99*, 1157–1167. [CrossRef] [PubMed]
76. Zhao, B.; Mei, Y.; Cao, L.; Zhang, J.; Sumagin, R.; Yang, J.; Gao, J.; Schipma, M.; Wang, Y.; Thorsheim, C.; et al. Loss of pleckstrin-2 reverts lethality and vascular occlusions in JAK2V617F-positive myeloproliferative neoplasms. *J. Clin. Investig.* **2017**, *128*, 125–140. [CrossRef] [PubMed]
77. Wolach, O.; Sellar, R.; Martinod, K.; Cherpokova, D.; McConkey, M.; Chappell, R.; Silver, A.; Adams, D.; Castellano, C.; Schneider, R.; et al. Increased neutrophil extracellular trap formation promotes thrombosis in myeloproliferative neoplasms. *Sci. Transl. Med.* **2018**, *10*, eaan8292. [CrossRef]
78. Edelmann, B.; Gupta, N.; Schnoeder, T.; Oelschlegel, A.; Shahzad, K.; Goldschmidt, J.; Philipsen, L.; Weinert, S.; Ghosh, A.; Saalfeld, F.; et al. JAK2-V617F promotes venous thrombosis through β1/β2 integrin activation. *J. Clin. Investig.* **2018**, *128*, 4359–4371. [CrossRef]
79. Teofili, L.; Martini, M.; Iachininoto, M.; Capodimonti, S.; Nuzzolo, E.; Torti, L.; Cenci, T.; Larocca, L.; Leone, G. Endothelial progenitor cells are clonal and exhibit the JAK2(V617F) mutation in a subset of thrombotic patients with Ph-negative myeloproliferative neoplasms. *Blood* **2011**, *117*, 2700–2707. [CrossRef]
80. Rosti, V.; Villani, L.; Riboni, R.; Poletto, V.; Bonetti, E.; Tozzi, L.; Bergamaschi, G.; Catarsi, P.; Dallera, E.; Novara, F.; et al. Spleen endothelial cells from patients with myelofibrosis harbor the JAK2V617F mutation. *Blood* **2012**, *121*, 360–368. [CrossRef]
81. Guy, A.; Gourdou-Latyszenok, V.; Lay, N.; Peghaire, C.; Kilani, B.; Dias, J.; Duplaa, C.; Renault, M.-A.; Denis, C.; Villeval, J.; et al. Vascular endothelial cell expression of JAK2V617F is sufficient to promote a pro-thrombotic state due to increased P-selectin expression. *Haematologica* **2018**, *104*, 70–81. [CrossRef]

82. Cocault, L.; Bouscary, D.; Le Bousse Kerdiles, C.; Clay, D.; Picard, F.; Gisselbrecht, S.; Souyri, M. Ectopic expression of murine TPO receptor (c-Mpl) in mice is pathogenic and induces erythroblastic proliferation. *Blood* **1996**, *88*, 1656–1665. [CrossRef] [PubMed]
83. Villeval, J.-L.; Cohen-Solal, K.; Tulliez, M.; Giraudier, S.; Guichard, J.; Burstein, S.A.; Cramer, E.; Vainchenker, W.; Wendling, F. High thrombopoietin production by hematopoietic cells induces a fatal myeloproliferative syndrome in mice. *Blood* **1998**, *90*, 4369–4383. [CrossRef]
84. Bhagwat, N.; Koppikar, P.; Keller, M.; Marubayashi, S.; Shank, K.; Rampal, R.; Qi, J.; Kleppe, M.; Patel, H.; Shah, S.; et al. Improved targeting of JAK2 leads to increased therapeutic efficacy in myeloproliferative neoplasms. *Blood* **2014**, *123*, 2075–2083. [CrossRef] [PubMed]
85. Sangkhae, V.; Etheridge, S.; Kaushansky, K.; Hitchcock, I. The thrombopoietin receptor, MPL, is critical for development of a JAK2V(617)F-induced myeloproliferative neoplasm. *Blood* **2014**, *124*, 3956–3963. [CrossRef]
86. Klampfl, T.; Gisslinger, H.; Harutyunyan, A.; Nivarthi, H.; Rumi, E.; Milosevic Feenstra, J.; Them, N.; Berg, T.; Gisslinger, B.; Pietra, D.; et al. Somatic Mutations of Calreticulin in Myeloproliferative Neoplasms. *N. Engl. J. Med.* **2013**, *369*, 2379–2390. [CrossRef] [PubMed]
87. Takahashi, K.; Tanabe, K.; Ohnuki, M.; Narita, M.; Ichisaka, T.; Tomoda, K.; Yamanaka, S. Induction of Pluripotent Stem Cells from Adult Human Fibroblasts by Defined Factors. *Cell* **2007**, *131*, 861–872. [CrossRef]
88. Ye, Z.; Zhan, H.; Mali, P.; Dowey, S.; Williams, D.; Jang, Y.; Dang, C.; Spivak, J.; Moliterno, A.; Cheng, L. Human-induced pluripotent stem cells from blood cells of healthy donors and patients with acquired blood disorders. *Blood* **2009**, *114*, 5473–5480. [CrossRef]
89. Papapetrou, E. Modeling myeloid malignancies with patient-derived iPSCs. *Exp. Hematol.* **2018**, *71*, 77–84. [CrossRef]
90. Smith, C.; Abalde-Atristain, L.; He, C.; Brodsky, R.; Braunstein, E.; Chaudhari, P.; Jang, Y.; Cheng, L.; Ye, Z. Efficient and Allele-Specific Genome Editing of Disease Loci in Human iPSCs. *Mol. Ther.* **2014**, *23*, 570–577. [CrossRef]
91. Fu, Y.; Foden, J.; Khayter, C.; Maeder, M.; Reyon, D.; Joung, J.; Sander, J. High-frequency off-target mutagenesis induced by CRISPR-Cas nucleases in human cells. *Nat. Biotechnol.* **2013**, *31*, 822–826. [CrossRef]
92. Smith, C.; Gore, A.; Yan, W.; Abalde-Atristain, L.; Li, Z.; He, C.; Wang, Y.; Brodsky, R.; Zhang, K.; Cheng, L.; et al. Whole-genome sequencing analysis reveals high specificity of CRISPR/Cas9 and TALEN-based genome editing in human iPSCs. *Cell Stem Cell* **2014**, *15*, 12–13. [CrossRef] [PubMed]
93. Tian, L.; Piterkova, L.; Wang, L.; Ye, Z.; Cheng, L.; Wheeler, D.A.; Hakonarson, H.; Prchal, J. Whole Genome Sequencing of Four CD34+-Derived iPSC Polycythemia Vera Clones from a Single Female. *Blood* **2012**, *120*, 1755. [CrossRef]
94. Saliba, J.; Hamidi, S.; Lenglet, G.; Langlois, T.; Yin, J.; Cabagnols, X.; Secardin, L.; Legrand, C.; Galy, A.; Opolon, P.; et al. Heterozygous and Homozygous JAK2V617F States Modeled by Induced Pluripotent Stem Cells from Myeloproliferative Neoplasm Patients. *PLoS ONE* **2013**, *8*, e74257. [CrossRef] [PubMed]
95. Ye, Z.; Liu, C.; Lanikova, L.; Dowey, S.; He, C.; Huang, X.; Brodsky, R.; Spivak, J.; Prchal, J.; Cheng, L. Differential Sensitivity to JAK Inhibitory Drugs by Isogenic Human Erythroblasts and Hematopoietic Progenitors Generated from Patient-Specific Induced Pluripotent Stem Cells. *Stem Cells* **2014**, *32*, 269–278. [CrossRef] [PubMed]
96. Verstovsek, S.; Kantarjian, H.; Mesa, R.; Pardanani, A.; Cortes-Franco, J.; Thomas, D.A.; Estrov, Z.; Fridman, J.; Bradley, E.; Erickson-Viitanen, S.; et al. Safety and efficacy of INCB018424, a JAK1 and JAK2 inhibitor, in myelofibrosis. *N. Engl. J. Med.* **2010**, *363*, 1117–1127. [CrossRef] [PubMed]
97. Verstovsek, S.; Kantarjian, H.; Estrov, Z.; Cortes, J.; Thomas, D.; Kadia, T.; Pierce, S.; Jabbour, E.; Borthakur, G.; Rumi, E.; et al. Long-term outcomes of 107 patients with myelofibrosis receiving JAK1/JAK2 inhibitor ruxolitinib: Survival advantage in comparison to matched historical controls. *Blood* **2012**, *120*, 1202–1209. [CrossRef]
98. Senquan, L.; Williams, D.; Moliterno, A.; Spivak, J.; Huang, H.; Gao, Y.; Ye, Z.; Cheng, L. Generation, Characterization and Genetic Modification of Human iPSCs Containing Calr, MPL and JAK2 Mutations Found in MPN Patients. *Blood* **2016**, *128*, 3139. [CrossRef]
99. Liu, S.; Ye, Z.; Gao, Y.; He, C.; Rowley, D.; Moliterno, A.; Spivak, J.; Huang, H.; Cheng, L. Generation of human iPSCs from an essential thrombocythemia patient carrying a V501L mutation in the MPL gene. *Stem Cell Res.* **2017**, *18*, 57–59. [CrossRef]

100. Wang, W.; Wang, T.; Kotini, A.; Iancu-Rubin, C.; Hoffman, R.; Papapetrou, E. Modeling Calreticulin-Mutant Myeloproliferative Neoplasms with Isogenic Induced Pluripotent Stem Cells. *Blood* **2018**, *132*, 4319. [CrossRef]
101. Štetka, J.; Vyhlidalova, P.; Lanikova, L.; Koralkova, P.; Gursky, J.; Hlusi, A.; Flodr, P.; Hubackova, S.; Bartek, J.; Hodny, Z.; et al. Addiction to DUSP1 protects JAK2V617F-driven polycythemia vera progenitors against inflammatory stress and DNA damage, allowing chronic proliferation. *Oncogene* **2019**, *38*, 1. [CrossRef]

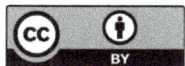

© 2019 by the authors. Licensee MDPI, Basel, Switzerland. This article is an open access article distributed under the terms and conditions of the Creative Commons Attribution (CC BY) license (http://creativecommons.org/licenses/by/4.0/).

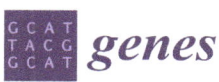 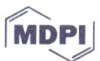

Review

Ubiquitin Ligases Involved in the Regulation of Wnt, TGF-β, and Notch Signaling Pathways and Their Roles in Mouse Development and Homeostasis

Nikol Baloghova, Tomas Lidak and Lukas Cermak *

Laboratory of Cancer Biology, Division BIOCEV, Institute of Molecular Genetics of the Czech Academy of Sciences, 252 42 Vestec, Czech Republic; nikol.baloghova@img.cas.cz (N.B.); tomas.lidak@img.cas.cz (T.L.)
* Correspondence: lukas.cermak@img.cas.cz

Received: 8 September 2019; Accepted: 13 October 2019; Published: 16 October 2019

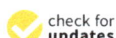

Abstract: The Wnt, TGF-β, and Notch signaling pathways are essential for the regulation of cellular polarity, differentiation, proliferation, and migration. Differential activation and mutual crosstalk of these pathways during animal development are crucial instructive forces in the initiation of the body axis and the development of organs and tissues. Due to the ability to initiate cell proliferation, these pathways are vulnerable to somatic mutations selectively producing cells, which ultimately slip through cellular and organismal checkpoints and develop into cancer. The architecture of the Wnt, TGF-β, and Notch signaling pathways is simple. The transmembrane receptor, activated by the extracellular stimulus, induces nuclear translocation of the transcription factor, which subsequently changes the expression of target genes. Nevertheless, these pathways are regulated by a myriad of factors involved in various feedback mechanisms or crosstalk. The most prominent group of regulators is the ubiquitin–proteasome system (UPS). To open the door to UPS-based therapeutic manipulations, a thorough understanding of these regulations at a molecular level and rigorous confirmation in vivo are required. In this quest, mouse models are exceptional and, thanks to the progress in genetic engineering, also an accessible tool. Here, we reviewed the current understanding of how the UPS regulates the Wnt, TGF-β, and Notch pathways and we summarized the knowledge gained from related mouse models.

Keywords: ubiquitin–proteasome system; cancer; mouse model; gene inactivation

---

1. Introduction

As revealed by the analysis of The Cancer Genome Atlas (TCGA), the Wnt, transforming growth factor-β (TGF-β), and Notch signaling pathways belong among the ten evaluated and curated canonical signaling pathways that are altered in most cancers [1]. It is the central role in governing and controlling cell proliferation which makes these pathways as well as their regulators vulnerable to cancer-associated somatic mutations [2–4]. The ubiquitin–proteasome system (UPS)-dependent regulation of Wnt, TGF-β, and Notch signaling is well known and established. Importantly, it represents a gateway for therapeutic modification and micromanagement of these signaling pathways, especially in the context of cancer [5,6]. To understand and exploit these possibilities it is necessary to evaluate the knowledge in vivo. Thus, the ambition of this review was to summarize the current understanding of how the UPS regulates Wnt, TGF-β, and Notch signaling. Additionally, we wanted to highlight the physiological roles of the ubiquitin ligases responsible for these regulations as they have been reported from currently available mouse models. Of note, the role of deubiquitinases (DUBs) was out of the scope of this text and is reviewed elsewhere [7].

2. The Ubiquitin–Proteasome System

The ubiquitin–proteasome system regulates many cellular processes, including cell cycle, differentiation, DNA repair, and the immune response (for a review, see Reference [8]). Its main function is to achieve the precise temporal and spatial expression of a diverse repertoire of proteins. Essentially, the UPS delivers unneeded or damaged proteins to the proteasome where they are unfolded and ultimately chopped into small peptides. At a molecular level, the proteasome is a multisubunit protein complex with a central hollow part involved in the proteolysis and two proximal parts involved in the recognition of the substrate and its ATP-dependent unfolding. The selectivity of the UPS is accomplished by specific recognition of the target protein (i.e., substrate) which has to be covalently modified by a chain of small protein ubiquitin—polyubiquitinated (Figure 1a).

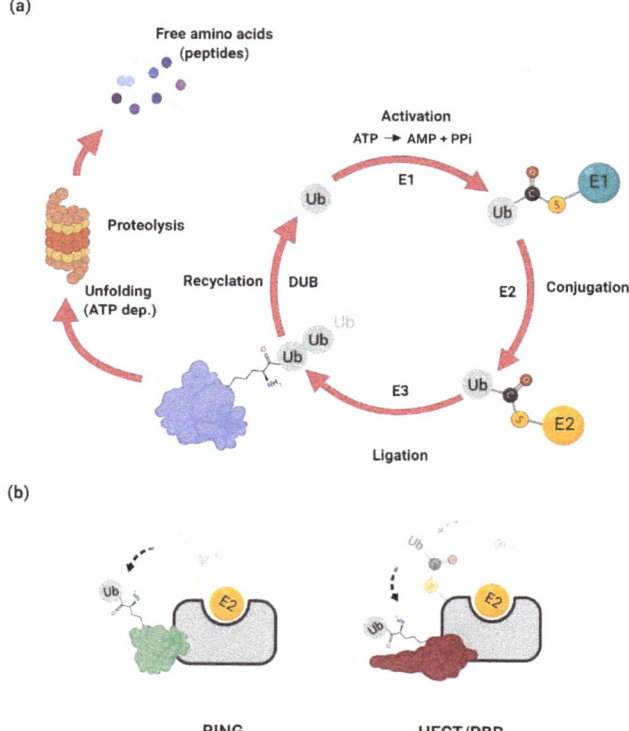

Figure 1. The ubiquitin–proteasome system. (**a**) The mature free ubiquitin monomer protein is either recycled from the ubiquitinated substrate or cleaved from the polyubiquitin precursor. Both of these reactions are catalyzed by deubiquitinases (DUBs). Ubiquitin is then activated (E1), conjugated (E2), and finally ligated to the cognate substrate via ubiquitin ligases (E3). The polyubiquitinated substrate is later transferred to the proteasome, unfolded, and proteolytically degraded to small peptides or free amino acids. For more details see the text. (**b**) RING E3s catalyze the direct transfer of ubiquitin from E2~ubiquitin to the substrate. HECT (homologous to E6AP C-terminus), and RBR (RING-between-RING) E3s accept ubiquitin from E2 to form an E3~ubiquitin thioester intermediate via transthiolation reaction. For more details see the text.

2.1. Ubiquitination

The ubiquitination is achieved via an enzymatic cascade in which ubiquitin is activated by covalent linkage to the E1 ubiquitin-activating enzyme. This activation is dependent on ATP-driven adenylation of ubiquitin followed by the covalent association of ubiquitin with the E1 enzyme via a thioester bond and subsequent transfer of the activated ubiquitin to the E2 ubiquitin-conjugating enzyme through trans-thioesterification [9]. In the final step, the E3 ubiquitin ligase mediates the transfer of ubiquitin to the lysine residue in the substrate [10]. The covalently linked ubiquitin then serves as an acceptor for another ubiquitin molecule, ultimately producing long polyubiquitin chains. The polyubiquitin chains can be linked via different lysine residues in the ubiquitin. At least for certain E3 ubiquitin ligases the type of polyubiquitin chain seems to be dependent on the different usage of the specific E2 enzyme [11]. Currently, there are more than thirty genes in human genome encoding proteins harboring E2 activity [12]. Some of them specifically modify proteins with linear ubiquitin chains (e.g., lysine 63–K63) that are not recognized by the proteasome but are involved in cellular signaling [13]. Others (e.g., K48, K11) are involved in proteasome-dependent degradation or their role is currently not clear (e.g., K27) [14]. Notably, a key regulatory step of the ubiquitination reaction is dictated by the E3 ubiquitin ligase, which determines substrate selection and a choice of polyubiquitin chain.

2.2. Ubiquitin Ligases

The human genome encodes between 600–1000 E3 ubiquitin ligases. They are responsible for substrate selection and coordination towards the E2 enzyme (for a review, see References [15,16]). Currently, there are four main classes of ubiquitin ligases classified on the basis of the functional and structural features: RING (really interesting new gene), U-box, HECT (homologous to E6AP C-terminus), and RBR (RING-between-RING) [9]. The RING E3s catalyze the direct transfer of ubiquitin from E2~ubiquitin to the substrate. The HECT and RBR E3s harbor a catalytic cysteine residue in their structure that accepts ubiquitin from E2 to form an E3~ubiquitin thioester intermediate via transthiolation reaction (Figures 1b and 2). This step is followed by the transfer of ubiquitin to the substrate lysine via aminolysis reaction.

The E3 ligases recognize the cognate substrates using different mechanisms. The specificity of ubiquitination is achieved via protein–protein interaction between a ubiquitin ligase and a substrate. This interaction can be direct or indirectly mediated by a protein or a small molecule adapter. The direct interaction is usually regulated by post-translational modification of the substrate or the ubiquitin ligase. In certain cellular processes, ubiquitin ligases have to be locally enriched to effectively bind and mediate substrate ubiquitination. A typical example is the RING finger 8 (RNF8) ubiquitin ligase, which is sequestrated at DNA damage sites where it targets a diverse spectrum of proteins (including histones) [17,18].

2.2.1. RING-Type Ubiquitin Ligases

The RING ubiquitin ligases constitute two main classes based on the number of subunits (for a review, see References [6,19]). Monosubunit RING ligases form homo- and heterodimers or act as monomers. A typical example of these ubiquitin ligases is the mouse double minute 2 homolog (MDM2) protein. In the absence of DNA damage, MDM2 binds the p53 tumor suppressor and mediates its ubiquitination, with consequent proteasomal degradation [20]. The DNA damage-activated Ataxia-telangiectasia mutated (ATM) kinase inhibits MDM2–p53 interaction leading to p53 stabilization and activation of p53-dependent DNA damage response [21,22].

Multisubunit E3 ubiquitin ligase complexes, such as Cullin-RING ligases (CRLs), mediate ubiquitination of numerous substrates via variable substrate recognition modules [19]. They represent a dominant group of ubiquitin ligases. In mammals, there are eight different cullins which associate with large numbers of adaptor proteins, forming more than 200 CRLs. Many of these ubiquitin ligases are deregulated in a wide range of disorders including cancer and autoimmune syndromes [6,23,24].

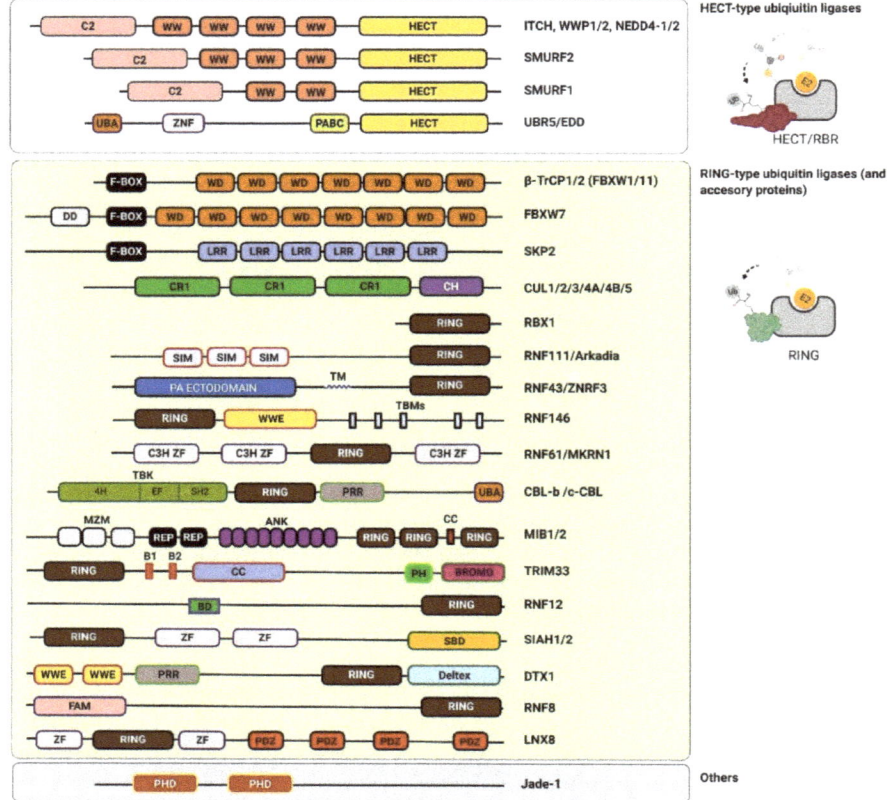

Figure 2. The modular structure of ubiquitin ligases involved in the Wnt, TGF-β, and Notch pathways.

2.2.2. U-box-Type Ubiquitin Ligases

A specific group of RING-type ubiquitin ligases is U-box, containing ubiquitin ligases (for a review, see Reference [25]). A U-box is a 70 amino acid long domain with a similar fold as the RING domain. In contrast to RING, the U-box domain lacks conserved cysteine residues and it is not coordinated with zinc atoms. Nevertheless, the molecular mechanism underlying ubiquitination is similar for both U-box and RING-type ubiquitin ligases.

A typical example of U-box-type ubiquitin ligase is the C terminus of the Hsc70-interacting protein (CHIP) [26]. Upon heat stress, CHIP recognizes its substrates in the context of activated heat shock proteins, controlling the stability and fate of misfolded proteins.

2.2.3. HECT-Type Ubiquitin Ligases

The human genome encodes 28 HECT ubiquitin ligases (for a review, see Reference [27]). They are characterized by a modular structure which comprises the N-terminal substrate-binding domain and the C-terminal HECT domain [27]. The HECT domain contains two lobes connected by a flexible hinge loop. The N-terminal lobe binds E2~ubiquitin and the C-terminal lobe harbors the catalytic cysteine involved in the transfer of ubiquitin to substrates lysines. There are three different HECT-type ligase families: the NEDD (neural precursor cell expressed, developmentally downregulated) family, characterized by the tryptophan-rich WW domain involved in recognition of the PY motif; the HERC

(HECT and RCC domain) family, which contains the regulator of chromosome condensation (RCC) 1-like domains; and the HECT family, with a spectrum of different protein–protein interaction domains.

A typical example of the HECT-type ubiquitin ligase is Smad ubiquitination regulatory factor 2 (SMURF2) protein [28]. The SMURF2 protein is a HECT-type E3 ubiquitin ligase from the NEDD4 subfamily. The WW domain, located in the N-terminal part of SMURF2 ubiquitin ligase, recognizes PPxY (PY) motifs in SMURF–targeted substrates [29]. One of the SMURF2 substrates is a TGF-β receptor I (TGF-βRI) [30]. The SMURF2 protein binds this receptor indirectly via Small mothers against decapentaplegic 7 (Smad7), an inhibitor of TGF-β signaling. The SMURF2 interacts with Smad7 in the nucleus. The complex of SMURF2 and Smad7 is then translocated to the cytosol where it recognizes and ubiquitinates TGF-βRI. This represents the strong negative feedback necessary to control TGF-β signaling and its dynamics.

2.2.4. RBR-Type Ubiquitin Ligases

There are 14 RBR E3s identified in the human genome (for a review, see Reference [31]). They all contain a RING1–IBR–RING2 motif. The RING1 domain interacts with E2~ubiquitin and mediates the transfer of ubiquitin to the catalytic cysteine of the RING2 domain. It was shown that RING2 forms a thioester intermediate with the C terminus of ubiquitin in a HECT E3-like manner and, consequently, transfers ubiquitin on the lysines of the selected substrates. An example of an RBR ubiquitin ligase is Parkin [32]. Parkin is involved in the recognition of proteins on the outer mitochondrial membrane [33]. Upon stress exposure, Parkin mediates mitochondria ubiquitination and its clearance via mitophagy [34].

3. Wnt Signaling Pathway and Its Regulation by Ubiquitin Ligases

Wnt ligands are extracellular soluble proteins. They are secreted by a diverse spectrum of cells and they are instrumental in the regulation of cell identity, migration, and proliferation [35,36]. Genes encoding the components of the Wnt signaling pathway are often misregulated or mutated in human cancers, especially in tissues with fast cellular renewal (e.g., breast, intestine, skin, prostate or lung). This is due to the central role of the Wnt signaling pathway in stem cell recovery and progenitor cell pool formation.

The Wnt signaling pathway is initiated upon Wnt binding to its cognate receptor. This is followed by the sequence of activation steps which lead to translocation of the β-catenin transcription co-activator to the nucleus (Figure 3). Nuclear β-catenin associates with DNA-binding transcriptional factors from the T-cell factor/lymphoid enhancer-binding factor (TCF/LEF) family and activates the Wnt-dependent transcriptional program.

In more detail, the intracellular signaling is triggered by Wnt binding to the complex of its receptor Frizzled (Fzd) and co-receptor from the lipoprotein receptor-related protein family (LRP5/6) [37]. When inactive, the Fzd protein level and its membrane localization are regulated negatively by two closely related ubiquitin ligases, RNF43 and Zinc–RING finger 3 (ZNRF3) [38,39]. These transmembrane ligases from the RING family interact with Fzd in the extracellular part and mediate ubiquitination of its cytosolic loops via the intracellular RING domain. This interaction is dependent on the intracellular protein Dishevelled, which (in the absence of Wnt stimulation) promotes Fzd degradation [40]. Upon the Wnt ligand engagement to Fzd, RNF43/ZNRF3 is inhibited by sequestration to the complex of leucine-rich repeat-containing G-protein coupled receptor (LGR4/5) transmembrane proteins. This interaction is mediated by a Wnt agonist from the R-spondin family [38].

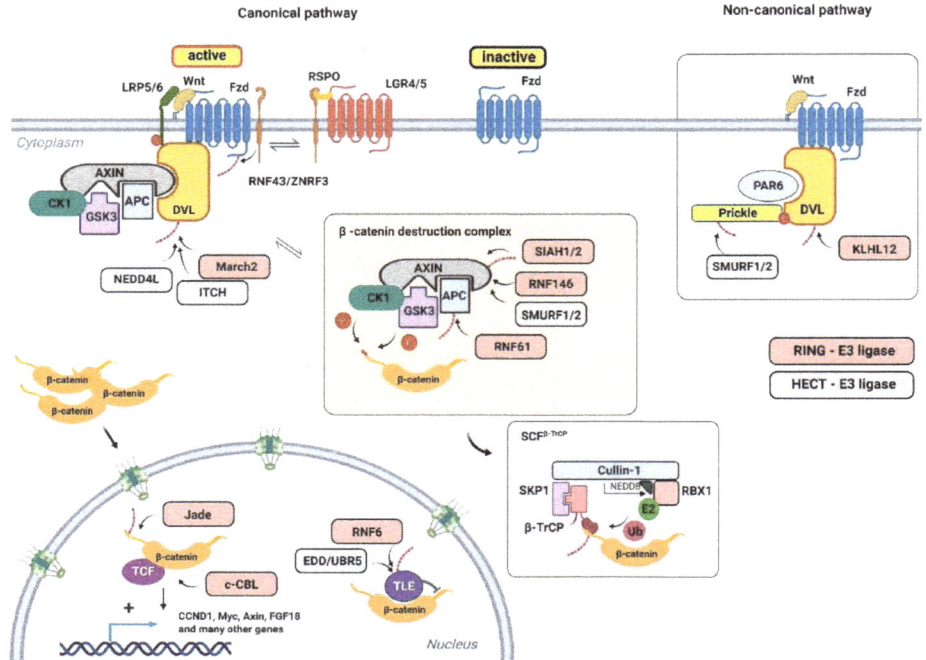

Figure 3. The Wnt signaling pathway and its regulation by ubiquitination The canonical Wnt signaling pathway is triggered by Wnt ligand binding to the complex of its receptor, Frizzled, and co-receptors LRP5/6. The activated receptor associates with the Dishevelled (DVL) protein and inhibits the β-catenin destruction complex. The stabilized β-catenin translocates and accumulates in the nucleus, where it activates the Wnt-dependent transcriptional program. For details see the text.

The essential part of signal transduction initiated from the Fzd receptor relies on β-catenin destruction complex inhibition. This multisubunit complex consists of several regulatory and accessory proteins. Its major role is to mediate β-catenin phosphorylation by coordination of priming casein kinase 1 (CK1) and functionally redundant processing kinases glycogen synthase kinase 3α and 3β (GSK3α and GSK3β, respectively) [41–43]. Adapter proteins adenomatous polyposis coli (APC) and AXIN are responsible for this dynamic and precise phosphorylation machinery [44,45]. In detail, AXIN allows β-catenin Ser45 to be phosphorylated by CK1. This phosphorylation creates a docking site for GSK-3α/β, which subsequently phosphorylates β-catenin at Thr41, Ser37, and Ser33. The phosphorylated N-terminal part of β-catenin serves as a binding site (degron) for a β-transducin repeat-containing protein (β-TrCP) [46,47]. The β-TrCP is a canonical Cullin 1 (CUL1)-dependent F-box-containing substrate adapter. It associates via the S-phase kinase-associated protein 1 (SKP1) adapter and CUL1 scaffold proteins with the RING protein Ring-box 1 (RBX1). The RBX1 mediates β-catenin ubiquitination and degradation.

The Fzd activation by Wnt ligands results in Dishevelled-dependent oligomerization of LRP6 co-receptor and its CK1γ/GSK3-mediated phosphorylation [48,49]. In the AXIN-dependent manner, the cytosolic destruction complex is sequestered to the membrane. This process inhibits the interaction of the destruction complex with β-catenin. Importantly, it was suggested that upon the activation of the Wnt signaling, the destruction complex is not inhibited per se. Rather, it leads to the inhibition of β-TrCP-dependent ubiquitination. Phosphorylated non-ubiquitinated β-catenin stays in the complex and blocks the association of newly translated molecules [50]. Stabilized (non-phosphorylated) β-catenin then translocates and accumulates in the nucleus, where it interacts with DNA-binding transcriptional factors from the TCF/LEF family [45]. The sustained Wnt signaling leads to the strong association of the β-catenin/TCF complex with target gene promoters, engagement of transcriptional co-activators, and, ultimately, to the activation of the Wnt-dependent transcriptional program.

The β-catenin destruction complex itself is a target for several ubiquitin ligases. The main substrate of the UPS-dependent regulation is the AXIN protein. The seven in absentia homolog 1 (SIAH1) ubiquitin ligase mediates ubiquitination of the AXIN protein [51]. The SIAH1 recognizes the AXIN VxP (Val-x-Pro) motif involved in AXIN–GSK3 interaction. The GSK3 counteracts SIAH-dependent AXIN ubiquitination, and, correspondingly, SIAH inactivation leads to the Wnt signaling attenuation. This regulatory process is important for sustained Wnt/β-catenin signaling. In a similar manner, poly ADP-ribosylated (PARylated) AXIN is a target of the ubiquitin ligase RNF146. PARylation of AXIN is dependent on the Tankyrase enzyme [52]. It was shown that RNF146 interacts directly with poly-ADP-ribose through its WWE domain and promotes degradation of many PARylated proteins [53,54]. The AXIN RNF146-dependent degradation seems to be dependent on a physiological context [55]. Both *Xenopus* and *Drosophila* models have shown the role of Tankyrase in AXIN degradation, but based on the findings from *Drosophila* studies, there seems to be redundancy on the RNF146 side [56,57]. HECT-type ubiquitin ligase, SMURF1, was shown to ubiquitinate the AXIN protein in a cell-cycle-dependent manner. Its interaction with AXIN is inhibited during G2/M which correlates with increased Wnt signaling [58]. The SMURF1-mediated AXIN ubiquitination does not lead to its degradation. Instead, Lys29-linked polyubiquitination of AXIN disrupts its interaction with the Wnt coreceptors LRP5/6, consequentially inhibiting Wnt signaling activation [59]. Close homolog of SMURF1, SMURF2, interacts with AXIN in a canonical WW-dependent manner. Ectopic expression of SMURF2 leads to AXIN protein level downregulation, and SMURF2 mediates AXIN ubiquitination in vitro [60]. The other subunit of the β-catenin destruction complex, APC, is also a target for the UPS. The RNF61 ubiquitin ligase, otherwise known as Makorin 1 (Mkrn1), binds to the armadillo repeats region of APC and targets it for proteasomal degradation. Inactivation of RNF61 leads to Wnt signaling inhibition, and this inhibition is rescued by concurrent APC knockdown [61].

The Dishevelled (Dishevelled 1–3) protein level is regulated by three other HECT-like ubiquitin ligases NEDD4L, NEDD4, and ITCH [62–64]. They were all shown to promote Dishevelled ubiquitination. Ubiquitin ligase NEDD4 positively regulates the maturation of cell–cell junctions in cooperation with the small GTPase Ras-related C3 botulinum toxin substrate 1 (Rac1). Activated Rac1 promotes Nedd4-mediated ubiquitination and degradation of Dishevelled 1 [64]. A close homolog of NEDD4, NEDD4L, attenuates Wnt/β-catenin signaling by regulation of Dishevelled 2 stability. The Wnt5a-induced c-Jun N-terminal kinase (JNK)-dependent phosphorylation of NEDD4L is critical for its activity towards Dishevelled 2 [62]. The inhibition of Wnt signaling via the ubiquitin ligase NEDD4L was observed in both *Xenopus* and human models [62,65]. The mammalian ortholog of *Drosophila* Suppressor of Deltex (Su(Dx)), ITCH, inhibits Wnt signaling upstream of β-catenin, by targeting activated Dishevelled 2 to proteasomal degradation [63]. The role of Dishevelled protein is not limited to the β-catenin destruction complex inhibition and its sequestration to the activated receptor. It is also involved in activation of the non-canonical pathway controlling planar polarity and proper tissue architecture. This pathway is β-catenin-independent and it is actively inhibited by ubiquitin ligase RNF43 and its interaction with Dishevelled protein. Transmembrane RING-type ubiquitin ligase RNF43 inhibits the non-canonical pathway in a ubiquitination-independent manner, and cancer-associated mutations of RNF43 do not have any effect on this activity [66]. Another E3 ubiquitin ligase promoting Dishevelled ubiquitination and degradation in the non-canonical pathway is the Cullin3-dependent substrate-binding adapter Kelch-like protein 12 (KLHL12). The KLHL12 binds Dishevelled in a Wnt-dependent manner, and KLHL12-dependent degradation of Dishevelled antagonizes the convergent extension movements of cells during gastrulation in zebrafish [67]. The study in the *Xenopus* model shows that another RING-type ubiquitin ligase membrane-associated ring-CH-type finger (MARCH2) is targeting Dishevelled during head development. The MARCH2 interaction with Dishevelled is dependent on the Dishevelled interaction partner Dapper1, and ubiquitinated Dishevelled is degraded in the lysosomal compartment [68].

Nuclear bound β-catenin is a target of several ubiquitin ligases. They mostly serve as crosstalk hubs from different pathways and signaling checkpoints involved in the control of the proper shutdown of the activated pathway. In hypoxic conditions, the Von Hippel–Lindau (VHL) tumor suppressor inhibits the Wnt pathway via promoting degradation of activated β-catenin. It is dependent on VHL-induced stabilization of the ubiquitin ligase Jade1 [69]. This is relevant for clear cell renal cell carcinomas (CCRCCs) with mutated VHL. The active VHL stabilizes Jade1 by interaction with its α- and β-domain. The stabilized Jade1 interacts with the β-catenin N-terminus and mediates its ubiquitination and degradation [70,71]. Of note, Jade1 does not belong to either HECT- or RING-type ligases. It contains two pleckstrin homology domain (PHD) fingers, and its intrinsic ubiquitin ligase activity has not yet been supported by independent observations. Casitas B-lineage lymphoma (c-CBL) is another ligase that binds preferentially to active β-catenin [72,73]. Wnt-dependent nuclear c-CBL seems to selectively inhibit pro-angiogenic Wnt effects [72].

One of the paradigms in Wnt signaling is that in the absence of Wnt stimulation, TCF/LEF factors are acting as transcription repressors and that this repression is abrogated by β-catenin binding. Mechanistically, TCF factors associate with repressors from the TLE (transducin-like enhancer) family in the absence of Wnt signaling, and this interaction is blocked by competitive binding between TLE repressors and activated β-catenin. The TLE factors are subsequently targeted by the E3 isolated by differential display/ubiquitin protein ligase E3 component n-recognin 5 (EDD/UBR5) ubiquitin ligase from the HECT family for ubiquitination and degradation [74]. Besides TLE factors, EDD ubiquitinates phosphorylated β-catenin, as well. Instead of degradation, it was observed that in the context of β-catenin, EDD promotes the growth of Lys29- and Lys11-linked ubiquitin chains, supposedly to potentiate β-catenin stability and signaling [75]. This pathway is probably redundant or cell context-dependent, as it was shown that in colorectal cancer it is rather the ubiquitin ligase RNF6 which promotes Wnt signaling via controlling the stability of the TLE3 factor [76].

The UPS-based quality control is another regulatory mechanism in the Wnt signaling pathway. This is important for endoplasmatic reticulum (ER)-associated protein production and restricted to secreted and transmembrane proteins. It was shown that in the absence of Wnt ligands, the cargo protein EVI is degraded via ER-associated degradation (ERAD) [77]. Additionally, the Wnt co-receptor LRP6 is targeted to the ERAD pathway as well [78,79]. Upon ubiquitination of its intracellular part, LRP6 presumably interacts with a ubiquitin-binding protein which acts as a chaperone for its correct folding. The successfully folded LRP6 is palmitoylated and transported to the cell surface [80]. If folding is impaired, another round of polyubiquitination targets LRP6 to the ERAD pathway.

The Wnt signaling pathway is also sensitive to common stress-inducers such as heat stress. Activation of heat shock proteins leads to activation of the U-box ubiquitin ligase CHIP, which is involved in ubiquitin-dependent clearance of misfolded proteins [81]. One of the substrates of CHIP ubiquitin ligase is β-catenin [82]. The recognition of β-catenin via CHIP rather represents a general mechanism involved in unfolded protein and heat shock response than specific regulation of the Wnt signaling pathway.

3.1. Mouse Models of Ubiquitin Ligases Involved in the Wnt Signaling Pathway

As mentioned above, Wnt signaling plays a crucial role in an array of developmental and homeostatic processes. Mouse models defective in the Wnt signaling pathway reflect this fact and display various defects. The phenotypes span from higher cancer incidence, stem cell depletion to defects in tissue polarity and anteroposterior patterning [45,83–85]. The role of several ubiquitin ligases that have been shown to regulate the Wnt signaling pathway in vitro was confirmed in the cognate mouse models. This was true for ZNRF3/RNF43, RNF146, RNF61, SMURF1/2, and partially for β-TrCP1/2 and Nedd4 ubiquitin ligases [39,55,86–89]. However, the mouse models of other ubiquitin ligases did not confirm the function in Wnt signaling and show either different or more general physiological functions. These observations probably arise from the fact that these ubiquitin ligases have other physiological substrates and control different processes. The other possible explanation is that the involvement of these ligases in physiological Wnt signaling is subtle. Therefore, these mouse models require more detailed analysis or challenges such as aging or stress response to show and confirm in vitro observations.

3.1.1. β-Transducin Repeat-Containing Protein (β-TrCP)

Both β-TrCP1 and β-TrCP2 (also known as F-box and WD repeat domain, containing 1/11) are highly evolutionarily conserved F-box proteins [23]. They serve as substrate adapters for the CRL ubiquitin ligase. They both recognize a phosphodegron through seven WD-repeats assembled to a typical propeller structure. They are currently assigned to many different substrates including NFκB Inhibitor α (IκBα), β-catenin, and a canonical regulator of circadian rhythm Period2 [23,90]. Both β-TrCP1 and β-TrCP2 are biochemically indistinguishable in vitro and it is not clear if they recognize a unique set of substrates in vivo.

Mice deficient in β-TrCP1-are viable, with normal circadian rhythm and only minor defects in fertility. Animals do not exhibit any apparent defects up to 16 months of age [86,91–93]. Isolated mouse embryonic fibroblasts (MEFs) have a reduced growth rate, increased size, and abnormal ploidy. Upon Wnt3a stimulation, they show more stable nuclear β-catenin accumulation.

The β-TrCP-deficient male germ cells do not enter meiosis but instead undergo apoptosis. The early mitotic inhibitor 1 (Emi1) accumulation appears to contribute to the slight impairment in spermatogenesis and male fertility [23,92]. Another study shows that simultaneous inactivation of β-TrCP2 expression via inducible shRNA (which reduced β-TrCP2 to ~10% of the original level) leads to more severe testicular defects in otherwise viable and healthy animals. Authors of the study were able to rescue the defect by β-TrCP2 restoration and attributed the observed defect to ineffective degradation of the Snail1 transcription factor [94]. This transcription factor is important for epithelial–mesenchymal transition and its degradation is necessary for the proper development of cell adhesion within the seminiferous tubules. Depletion of Snail1 completely rescues spermatogenesis in β-TrCP1-deficient mice. Another research group used testis-specific inactivation of β-TrCP2 in the context of β-TrCP1-deficient mice. The authors also observed spermatogenesis impairment but attributed this defect to inappropriate degradation of the Doublesex- and mab-3-related transcription factor 1 (Dmrt1) involved in the mitosis–meiosis transition in mouse male germ cells [91].

Ubiquitin ligase β-TrCP1 is also an important factor in other tissues' homeostasis. Contrary to the epidermal or intestinal epithelium, mammary glands of β-TrCP1-deficient female mice display a hypoplastic phenotype [95]. A β-TrCP1-deficient retina shows a complete absence of cholinergic amacrine cells (CACs), decrease in tyrosine hydroxylase-expressing amacrine cells, and reduction in the number of retinal ganglion cells. The population of precursors of CACs is reduced, whereas the population of precursors of retinal ganglion cells increases [96]. The intestine-specific tamoxifen-inducible ablation of both β-TrCP1 and β-TrCP2 results in β-catenin and IκBα stabilization and leads to mucositis, a deleterious gut mucosal inflammation resulting in mucosal barrier defects. The increased NF-κB-independent production of interleukin 1β (IL-1β) is responsible for mucosal barrier defects, and inhibition of IL-1β partially rescues the inflammatory phenotype [97].

Contrary to the mild phenotype of β-TrCP1 deficiency, inactivation of β-TrCP2 results in the developmental arrest and the embryonic death before E10.5 [98]. Embryos lacking β-TrCP2 manifest accumulation of the cyclin-dependent kinase (CDK) inhibitor p19Arf in the yolk sac, but the concomitant inactivation of p19Arf does not rescue the lethal phenotype.

3.1.2. Zinc and RING Finger 3/ RING Finger 43 (ZNRF3/RNF43)

Both ZNRF3/RNF43 are RING-type transmembrane ubiquitin ligases containing the protease-associated ectodomain in the extracellular part. As mentioned, they target the Fzd receptor and mediate its ubiquitination and degradation which leads to attenuation of Wnt signaling. Both RNF43 and ZNRF3 are mutated in pancreatic carcinomas and colorectal and endometrial cancer [99,100].

Mice deficient in Znrf3 die shortly after birth. They have impaired lens development and about 20% of embryos show neural tube closure defects [38]. Simultaneous deletion of both genes (Znrf3 and RNF43) in the intestine leads to the epithelial hyperproliferation phenotype similar to one observed in Apc^{min} mice with constitutively active β-catenin [39]. This phenotype is dependent on paracrine delivery of Wnt3, and the simultaneous inactivation of the Wnt-secretion co-factor Porcupine abrogates the enhanced epithelial proliferation [101]. Expectedly, the adrenocortical deletion of ZNRF3, but not RNF43 (which is not expressed at a significant level in the adrenal cortex), leads to a hyperproliferative phenotype as well. The ZNFR3-dependent expansion is restricted only to the inner zone of the adrenal cortex and does not phenocopy β-catenin hyperactivation [102]. A ZNRF3 deficiency also leads to a disrupted testis determination. This is in agreement with the observation that testis development depends on Wnt signaling inhibition [103]. Mice without Znrf3 have a gonadal reversal in E12.5 and it depends on ectopic Wnt signaling during sex determination [104].

3.1.3. RING Finger 146 (RNF146)

Ubiquitin ligase RNF146 contains the N-terminal RING domain and the WWE domain. It mediates the ubiquitination of proteins PARylated by Tankyrase and its expression level was significantly elevated in a subset of non-small cell lung cancer and colorectal cancer [105].

Mice deficient in RNF146 die during embryogenesis. They are smaller with a delayed bone formation in the calvarium [55]. Mice with the osteoblast-specific RNF146 deletion die perinatally due to the fact of respiratory failure. Embryos have a short stature, fail to close fontanelles, exhibit hypomineralization of the calvarium, have small clavicles, and are osteopenic, with low serum levels of osteocalcin. The phenotype mimics some features observed in patients with cleidocranial dysplasia. Loss of RNF146 results in AXIN stabilization in osteoblasts and inhibition of the Wnt signaling pathway. Defective expression of the Wnt target fibroblasts growth factor 18 (FGF18) leads to inhibition of mitogen-activated protein kinase (MAPK) activity and, subsequently, to decreased osteoblast proliferation. As a consequence of reduced osteocalcin production, the osteoblasts-specific Rnf146-deficient mice exhibit an increase in bone marrow fat stores and glucose intolerance [55].

Contrary to its role in osteoblasts, Wnt signaling inhibits osteoclastogenesis [106]. A major osteoclast factor Rankl restricts Wnt activation via suppression of Rnf146 expression and Axin stabilization. Accordingly, macrophage-specific deletion of Rnf146 triggers accelerated osteoclastogenesis [107]. Besides Axin, RNF146 is responsible for the degradation of the SH3 domain-binding protein 2 (SH3BP2). Stabilized SH3BP2 potentiates RANKL signaling and osteoclastogenesis, mimicking its "gain-of-function" mutations found in patients with hereditary cherubism [108,109].

3.1.4. RING Finger 61 (RNF61)

Ubiquitin ligase RNF61 is a member of the putative RNA-binding protein family characterized by unusual C3H-Zinc finger domains and the RING domain. Telomerase reverse transcriptase (TERT), phosphatase and tensin homolog (PTEN), adenomatous polyposis coli (APC) or AMP-activated protein kinase (AMPK) are among its potential substrates.

Mice deficient in Rnf61 show chronic AMPK activation in both liver and adipose tissue, resulting in significant suppression of the diet-induced metabolic syndrome [88]. Although no clear connection exists between this phenotype and deregulated Wnt signaling, there is well-described crosstalk between AMPK and β-catenin activity [110–112]. Moreover, AMPK activation by metformin was recently shown to inhibit β-catenin stabilization [113]. Thus, Rnf61-dependent ubiquitination and degradation of AMPK and APC could represent an interesting feedback mechanism between Wnt signaling and metabolism activity.

3.1.5. Seven in Absentia Homolog (SIAH)

Seven in Absentia Homolog 1/2 ubiquitin ligases are homologous proteins consisting of the N-terminal RING domain, two zinc-finger domains, and the substrate-binding domain. There is a number of substrates subjected to degradation mediated by SIAH1/2 ubiquitin ligases. Under hypoxic conditions, SIAH1/2 mediate ubiquitination and degradation of prolyl hydroxylase 1 (PHD1) and PHD3. As a consequence, the hypoxia-inducible factor 1-α (HIF1α) is stabilized and the hypoxia response transcription program is initiated [114].

Seven in Absentia Homolog 1a-deficient mice exhibit growth retardation or early lethality (about 70% of SIAH1a-deficient pups die during the nursing period). They are sterile with defective spermatogenesis due to the impairment of meiotic progression [115]. Mice deficient in Siah1a suffer from osteopenia [116]. Interestingly, Siah2-deficient mice are normal, healthy, and fertile. They have a significant expansion of myeloid progenitor cells and osteoclasts in the bone marrow [117]. Embryos lacking both *SIAH* genes die within several hours of birth. They do not have any obvious defects, and the cause of death remains to be determined. Notably, both Siah1 and Siah2 have been shown to play a role in hypoxia and unfolded protein response (UPR) and their absence can result in a complex phenotype caused by oxidative and proteotoxic cellular stress [117–120].

3.1.6. E3 Isolated by Differential Display (EDD)

The EDD/UBR5 ubiquitin ligase belongs to the HECT ligase family. It has the UBA (ubiquitin-associated) domain in its N-terminus, a centrally located UBR-type zinc finger involved in the recognition of N-terminal degrons and the C-terminal HECT domain. E3 isolated by differential display is predominantly localized in the nucleus. The EDD was shown to target RNF168 ubiquitin ligase and TLE/Groucho repressors for proteasomal degradation [121]. It is deregulated in many types of cancer, e.g., breast and ovarian cancer or mantle cell carcinoma [122].

E3 isolated by differential display-deficient mice have significant developmental arrest characterized by defective vascular development in the yolk sac and allantois, along with defective chorioallantoic fusion [123]. The authors discussed that these extraembryonic defects presumably compromise fetal–maternal circulation, leading to a general failure of embryonic cell proliferation and widespread apoptosis. It is of note that mice deficient in Wnt receptor Fzd5 have similar defects in the yolk sac and placental vasculogenesis [124]. Nevertheless, there is no study of Wnt signaling deregulation in Edd-deficient mice. To investigate the EDD physiologic role in this pathway and generally in mouse development, it is necessary to prepare conditional mouse models. So far only limb bud-specific *Edd* deletion has been reported with no obvious morphological or developmental defects [125].

3.1.7. Neural Precursor Cell Expressed, Developmentally Downregulated 4 (Nedd4)

The Nedd4 ubiquitin ligase belongs to the NEDD-type HECT ligase family. It has a characteristic structure common for all NEDD4 family members: the N-terminal C2 domain, four WW domains, and the C-terminal HECT domain. The NEDD4 was proposed to interact with the tumor suppressor PTEN and to mediate its ubiquitination. It has been also shown to play a role in the regulation of Epithelial Na^+ channel (ENaC) and RNA polymerase 2. The NEDD4 is often overexpressed in many types of human malignancies, e.g., prostate, bladder, colorectal, gastric or breast carcinoma [126].

Mice heterozygous for Nedd4 are moderately insulin-resistant but protected against high-fat diet (HFD)-induced obesity. They show less body weight gain, less fat mass, and smaller adipocytes [127]. Knockout mice die perinatally [128–130]. They are growth-retarded around E11.5 with signs of subcutaneous bleeding in more than half of embryos. At E18.5, embryos do not display any spontaneous movement. The neural circuits are still active as the embryos react to mild pinches. Diaphragm muscles are significantly thinner and fragile with wavy and disorganized muscle fibers. Mice have an impaired innervation pattern in diaphragm muscles, leaving a gap at its ventral region. The Schwann cells differentiation is intact but they have a lower number of axons and motoneurons, impaired formation of neuromuscular synapses, and abnormal neuromuscular synaptic activity [128]. In another study, Nedd4-deficient neurons had more immature dendrites and showed significantly reduced apical dendrite branching, synaptic transmission, and synapse numbers. The authors revealed that the major substrate of Nedd4 involved in neuronal branching regulation is the Ras-related protein 2a (Rap2a) and that the expression of dominant-negative Rap2A rescues correct dendritogenesis [129]. Another research group presents that Nedd4-deficient mice show prominent heart defects (double-outlet right ventricle and atrioventricular cushion defects) and vasculature abnormalities [131]. Follow-up research pinpointed that the inhibitor of insulin signaling the growth factor receptor-bound protein 10 (Grb10) is a major substrate of the Nedd4 ubiquitin ligase. Its stabilization is responsible for delayed embryonic development, reduced growth, body weight, and neonatal lethality. Mechanistically, the stabilized Grb10 inhibits the insulin-like growth factor 1 receptor (Igf1R) cell surface localization. The Grb10 heterozygosity rescues the Nedd4 deficiency lethal phenotype [130]. Vascular-specific deletion of *Nedd4* displays deformed aortas with disarranged elastin fibers. It also results in increased vascular calcification and bone-related marker expression in aortas [132]. The bone-specific Nedd4-mutant mice show enhanced bone mass accrual and upregulated gene expression of osteogenic markers in the bone. Bone formation is decreased, and the proliferation of primary osteoblasts isolated from calvaria is higher. The number and surface area of tibial osteoblasts are higher as well [133]. The neural crest cell-specific Nedd4 deficiency results in significant craniofacial defects with reduction of a cranial bone and decrease in osteoblasts numbers. The Nedd4 seems to be essential for neural crest stem cell self-renewal and survival [134,135]. T cells from Nedd4-deficient fetal liver chimeras display a naïve T cell phenotype. T cells develop normally but proliferate less and their ability to activate B cells is diminished. Biochemically, upon CD28 co-stimulation, Nedd4 controls the stability of another ubiquitin ligase Cbl-b. Inappropriately stabilized Cbl-b ligase targets the T cell receptor (TCR) and its components and ultimately blocks T cell activation and function [136]. Interestingly, Nedd4 deficiency abrogates T cell hyperactivity in Cbl-b-deficient mice [137]. Animals with intestine-specific deletion of *Nedd4* when crossed with APC$^{+/min}$ mice have enhanced tumor growth and Wnt signaling [89].

3.1.8. Neural Precursor Cell Expressed, Developmentally Downregulated 4-Like (NEDD4L)

The NEDD4L ubiquitin ligase is a close homolog to NEDD4 and they share a common structure. The NEDD4L regulates numerous ion channels, especially ENaC [29]. As mentioned in Section 4.1., NEDD4L also mediates degradation of phosphorylated Smad2 and Smad3, and associates with TGF-βRI via the Smad7 adaptor leading to destabilization of the receptor. The polymorphism causing premature truncation of the NEDD4L protein is associated with essential hypertension [138].

Neural precursor cell expressed, developmentally downregulated 4-like heterozygous mice are viable but hyperactive [139]. The mouse model of NEDD4L with complete deficiency suggests that the Nedd4L major ubiquitination target is ENaC [140,141]. This sodium channel is involved in the reabsorption of sodium ions in the kidney, colon, and lungs [142]. It is also necessary for the saltiness perception associated with taste buds [143]. Neural precursor cell expressed, developmentally downregulated 4-like binds to the PY motifs of ENaC subunits via its WW domains. This interaction is responsible for ENaC ubiquitination and subsequent downregulation on the apical membrane. There are two independent mouse models of Nedd4L deficiency. The possibly hypomorphic Nedd4L knockout model has a relatively mild phenotype with higher blood pressure in both normal and high-salt diets. Concurrent administration of the ENaC inhibitor amiloride rescues the hypertension phenotype. Moreover, a chronic high-salt diet leads to cardiac hypertrophy [144]. In the second model of Nedd4L deficiency, the embryos have collapsed alveolar spaces and die perinatally [145]. The kidney-specific knockout mice suffer from a progressive kidney injury phenotype associated with increased sodium ion reabsorption, hypertension, and reduced levels of aldosterone. The phenotype is manifested by fibrosis, higher apoptosis, and cystic tubules [146]. In the mast cell-specific knockout, NEDD4L limits the intensity and duration of immunoglobulin E (IgE)-Fc$_\varepsilon$RI-induced positive signal transduction. It appears that in mast cells, the tyrosine kinase Syk is the main substrate for the NEDD4L ligase [147].

3.1.9. ITCH

The ITCH ubiquitin ligase belongs to the NEDD-type HECT ligase family. It contains the N-terminal C2 domain, four WW domains, and the HECT domain. Ubiquitin ligase ITCH regulates the stability of transmembrane receptors through monoubiquitination and intracellular proteins through polyubiquitination. It drives the monoubiquitinated and polyubiquitinated substrates to lysosomal and proteasomal degradation, respectively [148]. Reportedly, for proliferation- and survival-associated proteins c-Jun, JunB, p63, Notch, and glioma-associated oncogene homolog 1 (GLI1), TGF-β activated kinase 1 binding protein 1 (TAB1) belong to their substrates [149,150]. Mutations in ITCH cause inflammation, including inflammatory bowel disease or nephritis, and the ITCH deficiency is associated with multisystem autoimmune disease [151].

The non-agouti-lethal *Itchy* mice suffer from severe immune and inflammatory defects which result in persistent scratching of the skin [152,153]. On the C57BL/10 background, Itch deficiency is associated with the spontaneous development of a late-onset and progressively lethal systemic autoimmune-like disease, characterized by lymphoproliferation in the spleen, lymph nodes, and medulla of the thymus and by chronic pulmonary interstitial inflammation. The usual cause of death of these animals is hypoxia. On the JU/Ct background, *Itchy* mice develop an inflammatory disease of the large intestine [153].

For *Itchy* mice, T cells proliferate and adopt an activated phenotype. Production of the Th2 (T helper cell type 2) cytokines IL-4 and IL-5 is augmented upon stimulation, and the Th2-dependent serum concentrations of IgG1 and IgE are increased [154]. The phenotype is partially caused by the dysregulation of regulatory T (Treg) cells in the absence of the ITCH ligase. Treg cell-specific ablation of the Itch E3 ubiquitin ligase causes massive multiorgan lymphocyte infiltration and skin lesions, chronic Th2 cell activation, and the development of severe antigen-induced airway inflammation. The Itch-deficient Treg cells express a higher amount of Th2 cytokines and they are able to instruct naïve T cells to differentiate into Th2 effector cells [155]. The follow-up research has shown that Itch is essential for the differentiation of follicular B helper T cells (T$_{FH}$), germinal center response, and IgG production following acute viral infection. The development of T$_{FH}$ cells is halted in early stages, and Itch acts intrinsically in CD4+ T cells. At the molecular level, during T$_{FH}$ cell development, the Itch ubiquitin ligase controls the stability of the transcription factor Foxo1 [156]. Mice deficient in the E3 ubiquitin ligases CBL-b and Itch show an increase in T cell activation and display spontaneous autoimmunity. The double-mutant T cells show increased phosphorylation of the TCR-ζ chain, but TCR complex stability and membrane location are intact [157].

Keratinocyte-specific knockout of ITCH revealed its contribution to skin development and wound healing which is independent of the immunological phenotype observed in *Itchy* mice [158]. Moreover, *Itchy* females have reduced implantation sites, decreased corpora lutea, and increased estrous cycle length [159]. Mice deficient in Itch fed a HFD do not gain weight and do not show insulin resistance. It seems that Itch deficiency protects mice from obesity-related non-alcoholic fatty liver disease. Deficient animals have an accelerated metabolism and higher expression of genes involved in fatty acid oxidation. As a result of aberrant T helper cells activation, mutant mice exhibit a lower amount of M2 (obese adipose tissue)-type macrophages [160]. Moreover, Itch deficiency renders mice resistant to tumor necrosis factor-α (TNF-α)-induced acute liver failure in three distinct models [161].

The E3 ubiquitin ligase Itch negatively regulates the development and function of hematopoietic stem cells (HSCs). Specifically, HSCs deficient in Itch are more competent, have longer repopulating activity, accelerated proliferation rates, and sustained progenitor properties. They also display an accumulation of the activated Notch1 receptor. Consistently, knockdown of Notch1 in Itch-deficient HSCs results in reversion of the phenotype [162].

3.1.10. Casitas B-Lineage Lymphoma (CBL)

Both c-CBL and CBL-b are close homologs from the CBL family and share the N-terminal tyrosine-kinase-binding domain, a linker, and the RING domain [163,164]. Expression of c-CBL is broad with the highest level in the thymus and testes. In activated T cells, it is a prominent target of tyrosine kinases [165].

Mice deficient for either c-CBL or CBL-b show T cell hyperactivation, which is driven by lowering the TCR affinity/avidity threshold and loss of the co-receptor signal requirement [166–169]. While c-Cbl-deficient mice have hyperactive thymocytes, CBL-b-deficient mice have activated mature T cells. Double-positive (CD4+CD8+) thymocytes lacking c-CBL display a higher amount of the membrane-bound TCR/CD3 complex—CD4 and CD8 receptors and tyrosine kinases Lck and Fyn [166]. An elevated level of the TCR complex can be a result of TCR ζ-chain stabilization [170,171]. Mice deficient in Cbl-b have a normal thymus and thymocyte development, but they display hyperproliferation of peripheral T cells. Similarly to CBL-b deficiency, there is no requirement for the second signal, and sole CD3 stimulation leads to T cell activation and proliferation. As a result of inadequate control of T cell activation, the CBL-b mouse model is susceptible to experimentally induced or spontaneous autoimmune diseases such as arthritis and diabetes [172]. Effector T cells in these animals are also insensitive to Treg on the cellular level mediated suppression of its mediator TGF-β [173].

As mentioned above, the c-CBL-deficient mice phenotype is mainly associated with thymocytes hyperactivation and proliferation. On the biochemical level, they display increased protein activation of the tyrosine kinase Lck and Zap-70 and the downstream effectors linker for activation of T cells (Lat) and SH2 domain containing leukocyte protein of 76 kDa (Slp-76). Protein kinase Zap-70 is able to mediate c-CBL interaction with TCRζ but it is probably not the direct target of its ubiquitin ligase activity [170]. Based on the results from c-CBL-deficient thymocytes, it seems that c-CBL can regulate different stages of T cell development, maturation, and selection processes.

The mammary fat pads of c-CBL–mutant female mice show increased ductal density and branching [167]. The decrease in motility of c-CBL-deficient osteoclasts results in a decreased ability of osteoclasts to invade and resorb bone and mineralized cartilage in vivo [174]. Mice deficient in c-Cbl exhibit an increase in whole-body energy expenditure, decrease in adiposity, and an increase in food intake, reduced circulating insulin, leptin, and triglyceride levels and improved glucose tolerance [175]. These changes are accompanied by a significant increase in mouse activity (2 to 3 fold).

Both c-CBL and CBL-b double knockout (DKO) mice are embryonically lethal before E10.5, which suggests that these ligases have important overlapping functions in embryonic development. T cell-specific DKO leads to an exaggeration of the immune phenotype as T cells become hyperresponsive upon CD3 stimulation [168]. The DKO T cells do not downregulate surface TCR after antibody engagement, which results in continuous TCR signaling [168]. The germinal center B cells deficient in both ligases display an early exit of high-affinity antigen-specific B cells from the germinal center reaction and, therefore, impaired clonal expansion [176]. The mouse model of mast cell-specific deficiency of both ligases shows that CBL-b, but not c-CBL, functions as a negative regulator of FcεRI-induced degranulation [177]. The mouse DKO model in HSCs develops a myeloproliferative disorder. The HSCs of c-CBL-deficient mice exhibit only an augmented pool size, hyperproliferation, greater competence, and enhanced long-term repopulating capacity [178]. The mammary gland-specific DKO shows CBL-b and c-CBL redundant function in mammary stem cell renewal [179].

4. TGF-β Signaling Pathway

Transforming growth factor-β belongs to a distinct family of extracellular soluble protein ligands involved in diverse developmental and homeostatic processes of higher eukaryotes [180]. During maturation, TGF-β homodimer forms a complex with a LAP (latency-associated peptide) originally derived from the region of the TGF-β protein between the signaling peptide and the C-terminally located active TGF-β ligand. This small latent complex (SLC) associates with latent TGF-β-binding protein 1 (LTBP1) and it is sequestrated to the fibronectin-based extracellular matrix [181]. Following proteolytic activation, the released TGF-β binds to the TGF-β receptor II (TGF-βRII) and initiates transphosphorylation of the associated TGF-β receptor I (TGF-βRI) (Figure 4) [182]. These events lead to full activation of the serine/threonine kinase located in the intracellular part of TGF-βRI. The activated receptor transduces the signal to downstream factors belonging to the family of regulatory-Smad (r-Smad) transcription factors—Smad2 and Smad3. Phosphorylation of these factors depends on the FYVE (Fab1p, YOTB, Vac1p and EEA1) domain containing protein Smad anchor for receptor activation (SARA) or hepatocyte growth-factor-regulated tyrosine kinase substrate (HGS) [183,184]. These membrane-associated proteins are responsible for delivering Smad factors to the vicinity of the activated receptor complex. Once phosphorylated, Smad2/3 form a trimer complex with Smad4 (co-Smad4) and translocate to the nucleus. The Smads mad homology 1 (MH1) domain is responsible for the specific association with target gene promoters, whereas the mad homology 2 (MH2) domain is responsible for interactions with transcriptional co-factors, transactivators, and other regulators [185,186]. The fully assembled complex initiates expression of TGF-β target genes and, ultimately, activates transcriptional programs which govern and execute tasks like cell cycle inhibition or transdifferentiation [187,188].

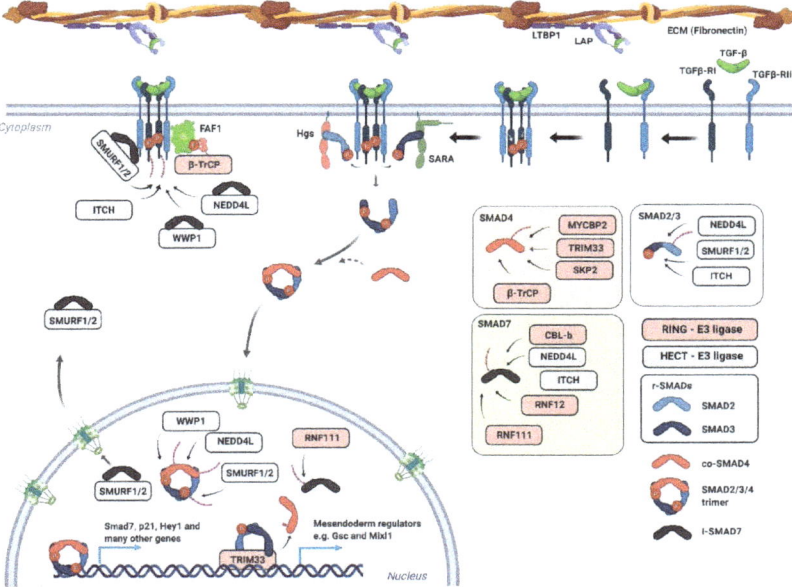

Figure 4. The TGF-β signaling pathway and its regulation by ubiquitination TGF-β released from the LTBP1 complex binds to TGF-β receptor II (TGF-βRII) and initiates transphosphorylation and activation of the associated TGF-β receptor I (TGF-βRI). The fully activated receptor transduces the signal to downstream factors belonging to the family of r-Smad (regulatory-Small mothers against decapentaplegic) transcription factors—Smad2 and Smad3. Smad2/3 form a trimer complex with Smad4 (co-Smad), translocate to the nucleus, and initiate transcription of TGF-β target genes. For details see the text.

4.1. TGF-β Signaling Pathway and its Regulation by Ubiquitin Ligases

The Smad homolog *Smad7* is one of the early target genes of TGF-β signaling [189]. It lacks the N-terminally located MH1 domain but still contains the receptor-binding MH2 domain. In the linker region between N- and C-terminal parts, Smad7 contains the PPxY motif which is responsible for E3 ubiquitin ligase SMURF2 (Smad ubiquitination regulatory factor 2) association [190,191].

Ubiquitin ligase SMURF2 associates with Smad7 in the nucleus and their complex subsequently translocates to the cytosol. The complex then interacts with the activated receptor and causes its proteasome-dependent degradation, which ultimately leads to the inhibition or attenuation of TGF-β signaling. During the TGF-β stimulated epithelial–mesenchymal transition (EMT), SMURF-dependent ubiquitination and degradation of TGF-βRI is blocked by concurrent action of another ubiquitin ligase TNF receptor-associated factor 4 (TRAF4), a member of the RING domain containing E3 ubiquitin ligase family [192–194]. Transforming growth factor β receptor-associated TRAF4 potentiates TGF-β signaling by mediating ubiquitination and proteasome degradation of SMURF. At the same time, it was shown that TRAF4 is also responsible for signaling-type Lys63-linked ubiquitination of TGF-βR, leading to its association with TGF-β activated kinase 1 (TAK1). Ubiquitin ligase SMURF2 also interacts with Smad2/3. It mediates Smad2 ubiquitination and targets it for degradation [195]. Its activity towards Smad3 is much weaker and leads to multiple monoubiquitinations of Smad3. This seems to have no effect on Smad3 stability, but rather on its ability to form a complex with Smad4 [196]. Interestingly, SMURF2 also targets Smad inhibitors Sloan–Kettering Institute (SKI) proteins. It binds them indirectly using Smad2 as an adapter [197].

Another E3 ubiquitin ligase that has been shown to effectively regulate the canonical TGF-β pathway is NEDD4L (NEDD4-like). The activated Smad complex is phosphorylated in the nucleus in a series of events initiated by CDK8/9 [198]. These transcription-associated kinases prime the Smad complex to another round of phosphorylation via GSK3β. The GSK3β-phosphorylated motif is recognized by the WW domain of the HECT-type ubiquitin ligase NEDD4L [199]. NEDD4L-dependent ubiquitination leads to the proteasome-dependent degradation of Smad2/3 and attenuation of TGF-β signaling. Interestingly, the WW domain is flanked by two serines targeted by serum/glucocorticoid regulated kinase 1 (SGK1). This phosphorylation inhibits NEDD4L interaction with Smads and promotes their stability. The ubiquitin ligase NEDD4L and another HECT-type ligase WW domain containing E3 ubiquitin protein ligase 1 (WWP1) were also shown to recognize TGF-βRI in a similar manner as SMURF (Smad7–dependent). The receptor ubiquitination decreases its stability on the membrane and leads to its internalization and subsequent degradation.

Additionally, the HECT-type ITCH ligase positively regulates TGF-β signaling as well. It binds Smad2 but does not have any effect on its stability. It rather promotes, in a HECT-dependent manner, its association with TGF-βR [200]. A possible explanation can be drawn from other studies which have shown that ITCH promotes TGF-β signaling by mediating TGF-βR-dependent degradation of Smad-signaling inhibitors, Smad7 and Ras association domain family 1 isoform A (RASSF1A) [201,202].

The Smad7 protein is also a substrate for ubiquitin ligases RNF111 (Arkadia) and RNF12 (RLIM), which both localize to the nucleus and most probably target Smad7 in this compartment [203–206]. Importantly, RNF111 has a chain of Small ubiquitin-like modifier (SUMO)-interacting motifs in its N-terminal part, and it is possible that it recognizes its substrates once they are sumoylated. Moreover, it has displayed activity towards Smad transcriptional co-repressors SKIL and SKI [207–209]. The protein involved in β-catenin degradation, AXIN, was shown to be a scaffold protein linking the RNF111 ubiquitin ligase and Smad7 [205]. It seems that Rnf12 can recognize Smad7 in the context of its interaction with SMURF [210]. In T cells, CBL-b is another RING ligase targeting Smad7. CBL-b and Smad7 interact physically and genetically, as it was shown that Smad7 inactivation restores the TGF-β signaling defect in CBL-b-deficient T cells [211].

Cullin1-dependent ubiquitin ligase β-TrCP was shown to mediate degradation of TGF-βR. The β-TrCP protein does not bind to the receptor directly but via the linker protein FAS-associated factor 1 (FAF1) [212]. Upon phosphorylation by the AKT kinase, FAF1 relocates to the plasma membrane where it interacts with TGF-βR and mediates its ubiquitination via the β-TrCP-ubiquitin ligase. This represents interesting crosstalk between PI3-K and TGF-β signaling.

Additionally, the E3 ubiquitin ligase TRIM33 (TIF-1γ or ectodermin) was also shown to interact with the Smad2/3 complex [213,214]. There are conflicting studies regarding its role in TGF-β signaling. It was proposed that TRIM33 and Smad4 associate with the r-Smads in a mutually exclusive manner [215]. Another study suggests that TRIM33 is a bona fide ubiquitin ligase for Smad4 which mediates chromatin-associated Smad4 monoubiquitination [216].

Last two ubiquitin ligases involved in TGF-β signaling are MYC binding protein 2 (MYCBP2) and S-phase kinase associated protein 2 (SKP2) [217–219]. Putative RING finger E3 ubiquitin ligase MYCBP2 could regulate Smad stability in neurons. *Drosophila* MYCBP2 homolog Highwire (Hiw) interacts with the *Drosophila* Smad homolog Medea. Highwire-mutant flies have also unrestrained synaptic growth [218]. Biochemically, Hiw controls the level of *Drosophila* TGF-βR (Tkv) and this could be involved in restricting Medea signalization in *Drosophila* neurons and intestinal stem cells [217]. The cullin1 ubiquitin ligase-dependent substrate adapter SKP2 mediates degradation of Smad4. It preferentially binds cancer-associated forms of Smad4 [219].

4.2. Mouse Models of Ubiquitin Ligases Involved in the TGF-β Signaling Pathway

Since the TGF-β signalling pathway has a crucial role in diverse developmental processes, mouse models deficient in its core components exhibit a wide range of developmental defects [220,221]. As mentioned above, several ubiquitin ligases have been suggested to regulate the TGF-β signalling pathway. However, mouse models of their deficiency show that these ubiquitin ligases often have different functions. While phenotypes of RNF111 (Arkadia) and TRIM33-deficient mice supported a crucial role in the TGF-β signaling pathway, the mouse models examining the deficiencies of other ubiquitin ligases failed to bring evidence of involvement in TGF-β signaling [214,222]. They seem to have other physiological substrates instead and, thus, control different processes as discussed in more detail below.

4.2.1. Smad Ubiquitination Regulatory Factor (SMURF)

Ubiquitin ligases SMURF1/2 share a high protein sequence homology (>70%) and their domain architecture is similar. Structurally they belong to NEDD-type HECT ligases. The N-terminal protein kinase C (PKC)-related C2 domain is followed by two or three WW PPxY/substrate interacting domains, respectively, and the catalytical C-terminal HECT domain. As mentioned above, SMURF1–2 were implicated in activated Smad2/3 and TGF-βRI degradation. Intracellular localization of SMURF1/2 is ambiguous as they were found in both the cytosol and the nucleus. Overexpression of SMURF1/2 was found in many cancer tissues and is associated with worse patient survival.

Individual SMURF1- and SMURF2-deficient mice are viable and fertile without any noticeable defects in embryogenesis [223,224]. The SMURF1 absence leads to an age-dependent bone mass increase due to the enhanced osteoblast activity [223]. One line of evidence shows that SMURF1 inhibits mesenchymal stem cell (MSC) differentiation and their osteoblastic potential via controlling the stability of the transcriptional factor JunB. Simultaneous inactivation of JunB in vitro rescued the osteogenic potential of MSCs to the normal level [225]. Another group revealed that the osteoblast Smurf1 ubiquitin ligase activity was directed towards another factor, Map kinase kinase 2 (Mekk2), an upstream kinase in the Jnk signaling cascade. Hyperactive Jnk signalization was then responsible for the higher activity of osteoblasts [223]. It was also reported that bone loss observed in mice with artificially increased TNF-α signaling was dependent on SMURF1 activation [226]. Another age-dependent phenotype of SMURF1-deficient mice was the spontaneous development of hepatic steatosis. In hepatocytes, the SMURF1 deficiency leads to upregulation of the expression of peroxisome proliferator-activated receptor γ (PPARγ) and its target genes involved in lipid synthesis and fatty acid uptake. In this context, however, SMURF1 does not mediate protein degradation of PPARγ but rather inhibited its activity via the non-proteolytic K63-linked ubiquitin modification. Treatment of SMURF1-deficient mice with a PPARγ antagonist, GW9662, reversed the lipid accumulation in the mutant mice liver [227].

The SMURF2-deficient mice display an expanded HSC compartment in the bone marrow with a higher repopulating capacity especially in aged animals [224]. The Smurf2 deficiency renders mice susceptible to spontaneous tumorigenesis, most notably the B-cell lymphoma, which resembles human diffuse large B-cell (DLBC) lymphoma with molecular features of germinal or post-germinal center B cells [228]. Mechanistically, Smurf2 is responsible for the degradation of Yin Yang 1 (YY1), a key germinal center transcription factor. Stabilized YY1 is responsible for transactivation of the c-Myc oncogene and activation of B cell proliferation [229].

Transgenic mice deficient for both SMURF1 and SMURF2 display complex developmental defects. Approximately one-third of mutant embryos display gastrulation defects characterized by abnormal posterior structures. The rest of the embryos gastrulate normally but show gross developmental abnormalities including an open neural tube and lateral expansion of the neuroectoderm [87]. This is a feature characteristic for mice with defects in planar cell polarity (PCP) and convergent extension movements (CE). Indeed, mice with only one of the four *SMURFS* alleles (e.g., *SMURF1*$^{-/+}$; *SMURF2*$^{-/-}$) show stereocilia misalignment on the cochlear organ of Corti. Mechanistically, SMURF deficiency is responsible for inappropriate activation of the non-canonical Wnt signaling pathway. Wnt engagement to FZD receptor leads to Dishevelled 2 protein phosphorylation and its translocation to the membrane. The phosphorylated Dishevelled 2 binds the Prickle protein, a major regulator of PCP. This interaction is mediated by the Dishevelled 2 constitutive partner PAR6. The whole complex is later recognized by SMURF which is responsible for the ubiquitination and degradation of Prickle. Inappropriate Prickle degradation leads to PCP and CE defects in SMURF1/2 DKO mice [87].

4.2.2. RING Finger 111/Arkadia

As mentioned above, RNF111 contains several SUMO-binding motifs and it can possibly recognize sumoylated substrates [230]. Mutations affecting RNF111 function were documented in patients with ovarian and colorectal cancer [231].

In mice, the *Arkadia* recessive mutation was generated using gene-trap mutagenesis. Heterozygous *Arkadia* mice are normal and healthy, yet they have reduced expression of several TGF-β target genes [231]. Developmental abnormalities of homozygous animals appear early in mouse embryogenesis. An antero-visceral endoderm (AVE) is formed but the embryo lacks a node, has a reduced head, fails to undergo turning, and dies very early at midgestation [232]. Similarly to Trim33-deficient mice, *Arkadia* mice exhibit defects associated with deregulated Nodal signaling. Embryonic cells show an accumulation of phosphorylated Smad2/3 proteins, yet surprisingly most of Nodal/Smad target genes are downregulated. As a result, *Arkadia* mice have a very similar phenotype-like Smad2-deficient embryos [222].

4.2.3. S-Phase Kinase-Associated Protein 2 (SKP2)

S-phase kinase-associated protein 2 (SKP2) is the F-box protein which is characterized by five leucine-rich repeats in its N-terminus. S-phase kinase-associated protein 2 controls the stability of the CDK inhibitor p27 during the G1/S-phase transition [233]. The p27 protein is specifically recognized upon threonine phosphorylation and in the context of its complex with adapter proteins CDK regulatory subunit 1 (CKS1), CDK2, and cyclin E [234,235].

S-phase kinase-associated protein 2 knockout mice are small but viable [236]. Their cells have enlarged nuclei with polyploidy, aberrant centrosomes, and accumulated p27 protein. Simultaneous inactivation of the *CDKN1B/p27* gene reverts the phenotype [237]. When subjected to partial hepatectomy, SKP2-deficient mice exhibit proliferation-independent liver regeneration (via cellular enlargement) [238]. Similarly, scraping of the corneal epithelium in SKP2-deficient mice leads to defected wound healing [239]. Again, the phenotype was reversed by concurrent deletion of the *CDKN1B/p27* gene.

4.2.4. MYC Binding Protein 2 (MYCBP2)

The MYCBP2 is a putative atypical RING ligase. It is a large protein containing the RCC1-like GEF domain, two PHR-family-specific domains, the RAE1-binding domain, the F-box binding domain

1, the Myc binding domain, and the C-terminal RING domain. Expression of MYCBP2 was found to be reduced in patients with acute lymphoblastic leukemia [240].

In mice, the genetic screen and targeted inactivation revealed MYCBP2 function in motor neuron pathfinding. In *Magellan*-mutant embryos, with the mutation causing MYCBP2 protein truncation, motor axons display navigation defects [241]. Surprisingly, they respond to guidance cues with normal sensitivity in vitro. Motor and sensory neurons from *Magellan* mutants show abnormal axon and growth cone morphologies. The phenotype is probably caused due to the disruption of the polarized distribution of the dual leucine zipper kinase (DLK), which acts upstream from p38Mapk and regulates microtubule stability. In accordance, the *Magellan* phenotype could be reversed by stabilizing microtubules with taxol or inhibiting p38Mapk activity. In a parallel study, the targeted conditional mutant shows that, as in invertebrates, MYCBP2 function is essential for shaping motor neurons terminals and the formation of major CNS axon tracts including those of the internal capsule. Major CNS axon tract phenotypes are partially caused by cell-non-autonomous mechanisms in a Dlk-independent manner [242]. The discrepancies among these models could be a result of different genomic deletions in the *MYCBP2* gene locus. In comparison to the *Magellan* mutant with the C-terminally truncated protein, the motor neuron-specific knockout mice have only 70 amino acid region proximal to the RCC1 domain deleted [241,242]. A follow-up study took advantage of these two models and prepared their cross [243]. The study focused on the previous observation that the MYCBP2 regulates mTOR signaling [244]. In agreement with this observation, mTOR signaling is attenuated in both models but, surprisingly, there are no mTOR signaling alterations in the prepared cross. This suggests that Mycbp2 regulates mTOR signaling via two independent pathways. Moreover, defective mTOR signaling is responsible only for certain neurodevelopmental defects (corpus callosum) associated with MYCBP2 deficiency but does not rescue the whole phenotype (defects in axon fiber tracts of the internal capsule and anterior commissure). Additionally, another study revealed that loss of MYCBP2 results in prolonged survival of severed axons in both the peripheral and central nervous systems. Survival of these axons depends on stabilization of mononucleotide adenyltransferase 2 [245].

4.2.5. Tripartite Motif Containing 33 (TRIM33)

Tripartite motif containing 33 ubiquitin ligase is a member of the tripartite motif (TRIM) protein family. In its N-terminus, it has the RING finger, two B-box domains, and the coiled-coil domain. The C-terminal part of this protein is composed of the plant homeodomain (PHD) followed by the bromodomain. Tripartite motif containing 33 was found to be mutated or downregulated in several human cancers, like chronic myelomonocytic leukemia [246].

Mouse embryos deficient in Trim33 die at E9 [214,247]. They display a dramatic developmental delay. At E8.0–8.5 (3–6 somite pairs in controls), the TRIM33 mutant embryos are aligned at the base of the yolk sac, and, although they have formed the anterior-posterior body axis and recognizable head folds, it is difficult to identify any other embryonal structures. They are smaller and lack a clear distinction between epiblast and extra-embryonic ectoderm. Morphological and histological analyses demonstrated that TRIM33 mutants display remarkable defects in embryonic polarity and tissue patterning. The phenotype of mutant embryos was opposite to those observed in Nodal, Smad2, and Smad4 knockouts. Nodal induces and patterns the anterior visceral endoderm, and sustains trophoblast development. In TRIM33-deficient embryos, Nodal signaling becomes unrestricted leading to dramatic changes in the embryo body plan. In the epiblast, TRIM33 deficiency shifts mesoderm fates towards node/organizer fates. As a result of impaired primitive streak development embryos have defective mesoderm formation.

Mice with TRIM33 inactivation in monocytes, bone-marrow-derived macrophages, peritoneal macrophages, and neutrophils are normal and healthy. They show sustained expression of interferon-$\beta1$ at late stages of toll-like receptor-mediated activation in macrophages [248]. Hematopoietic stem cells' specific loss of TRIM33 resulted in significant changes in erythroid, B-lymphoid, and myeloid compartments and decreased HSC capacity in transplantation assays [249]. The following study shows that a block in erythroid maturation in bone marrow was compensated with enhanced spleen erythropoiesis [250]. Another study on TRIM33 deficiency in HSCs showed that four-month-old mutant mice develop an accelerated aging phenotype in HSCs. The authors suggested that TRIM33 inhibition of TGF-β signaling was important for the balance between lymphoid and myeloid lineage differentiation and that myeloid- and lymphoid-biased HSC populations respond differently to TGF-β signaling. As the TGF-β signaling pathway was involved in the inhibition of HSC reentry into the cell cycle, disturbance in this signaling in TRIM33-mutant HSCs could result in the aging phenotype [251]. Tripartite motif containing 33-null mammary gland development appeared to be normal with no obvious developmental defects during the lifespan of virgin mice. However, after giving birth, the mice developed a significant lactation defect. Therefore, TRIM33 is probably essential for the terminal differentiation of alveolar epithelial cells in the mammary gland at the end of pregnancy.

4.2.6. RING Finger 12 (RNF12)

Ubuquitin ligase RNF12 has the C-terminally located RING domain and the central basic domain (BD). It is involved in X-chromosome inactivation (XCI) and in mediating ubiquitination and degradation of pluripotency marker reduced expression protein 1 (REX1) [252,253]. Mutations in RNF12 were reported in X-linked intellectual disability.

Mice deficient in RNF12 mice display early embryonic lethality specific for female embryos due to the defectively imprinted XCI, precluding the development of embryonic trophoblast tissues. Males carrying a germline knockout of *RNF12* (Δ/Y) appear healthy and are fertile [254]. There is a study showing that only 50 percent of male neonates survive and those that die are significantly smaller, with altered lung branching and maturation [255]. Importantly, RNF12 is essential for triggering imprinted XCI but dispensable for random XCI [256]. Its crucial role is to maintain high Xist RNA levels, Xist clouds, and X-silencing in female embryos at blastocyst stages [257]. Mammary gland-specific knockout of RNF12 shows its requirement for alveolar morphogenesis and milk production. It acts as a survival factor for milk-producing alveolar cells. While mammary glands of virgin females contain many living RNF12-negative epithelial cells, lactating glands are only RNF12-positive. Moreover, decreased expression of RNF12 correlates with mammary gland involution [258].

4.2.7. WW Domain Containing E3 Ubiquitin Protein Ligase (WWP)

Ubiquitin ligases WWP1/2 belong to the NEDD-type HECT ligase family [259]. They contain the N-terminal C2 domain, four WW domains, and the C-terminal HECT domain. They are both cytosolic and nuclear. Potential WWP1 substrates include TGF-βRI, Smad2 or Erb-B2 receptor tyrosine kinase 4 (ERBB4). Moreover, WWP2 was shown to mediate degradation of PTEN or the transcription factor OCT4. Interestingly, WWP1 is overexpressed in many types of cancer, especially prostate, breast, and liver, whereas WWP2 is frequently overexpressed in oral cancer.

Mice deficient in Wwp1 are viable and fertile without any obvious abnormalities. Embryos are born at the normal Mendelian ratio and grow relatively healthily. They develop increased bone mass as they age. This phenotype is associated with increased bone formation rates and normal bone resorption parameters [260,261]. They develop malformations of the craniofacial region. At the molecular level, Wwp2 is associated with Goosecoid, a transcriptional activator of the key cartilage regulatory protein Sox6. Importantly, WWP2 facilitates Goosecoid monoubiquitination, a post-translational modification required for its optimal transcriptional activity [260]. Mice defiecent in WWP2 also have reduced body and organ size and they resemble PTEN transgenic mice (Super-PTEN). In support of this, they have elevated and stabilized PTEN protein levels and reduced phosphorylation of the AKT kinase [262]. The bone marrow-derived macrophages have a stronger response to poly(I:C) challenge (regarding secreted TNF-α and IL-6 cytokines) and are more susceptible to poly(I:C)-induced death. These findings suggest that WWP2 negatively regulates TLR3-mediated innate immune and inflammatory responses. Indeed, WWP2 was shown to target adapter protein in TLR3-mediated NF-κB and IRF3 activation pathways (TRIF) for ubiquitination and degradation [261].

Mice deficient in both WWP1 and WWP2 display defects in axon–dendrite polarity in pyramidal neurons and abnormal laminar cortical distribution [263]. Interestingly, knockout of *miR-140*, encoded in *WWP2* intron, displayed similar phenotypic changes as those upon *WWP1* and *WWP2* deletion. The authors of the study delineated a novel regulatory pathway that involves the Sox9 transcription factor as a major regulator of WWP1/WWP2/miR-140 locus expression, and consequentially, axon specification, acquisition of pyramidal morphology, and accurate laminar distribution of cortical neurons.

5. Notch Signaling Pathway

The highly conserved Notch signaling pathway is critical for cell fate determination during development and tissue homeostasis [264,265]. It translates extracellular stimuli to transcriptional programs involved in cell cycle regulation and cellular differentiation [266,267]. The core architecture of this pathway is simple with only a few important canonical proteins (Figure 5) [268]. The human genome encodes five Notch ligands (Jagged 1/2 and Delta-like 1/3/4) and four Notch receptors (Notch 1–4). Notch ligands are transmembrane proteins expressed by various types of cells and tissues. Notch receptors are single-pass type I transmembrane proteins. They have a different amount of EGF-like repeats in the extracellular part. During maturation, these repeats are fucosylated by *O*-fucosyltransferase, and fucosyl moieties are further modified by the Fringe family of 1,3 *N*-acetylglucosaminyltransferases [269]. Such glycosylations represent "the code" which is responsible for specific recognition of ligands by different receptors. After glycosylation, the extracellular part of the Notch receptor is cleaved by the furin-like convertase (S1 cleavage) [270]. The non-covalently linked heterodimer is subsequently transported from Golgi to the cell surface. There are two additional domains between the membrane and EGF-like repeats—Lin20-Notch repeats (LNR) and heterodimerization domain (HD). Both are involved in ligand-dependent receptor activation.

Upon the receptor binding, the endocytic system is activated in the ligand-bearing cell. This forcefully drags the ligand-receptor complex towards the interior of this cell and, consequently, relaxes the structure of the LNR/HD domains. Once relaxed, the membrane-proximal region of the Notch extracellular domain (NECD) becomes a substrate for a disintegrin and metalloprotease 10/17 (ADAM10/17) metalloproteinases (S2 cleavage) [271,272]. They subsequently cleave NECD, which is then engulfed by a ligand-presenting cell via a transendocytosis [273]. The residual extracellular part is cleaved in the last proteolytic step (S3 cleavage). This is accomplished by γ-secretase, a membrane-bound protein complex involved in intramembrane proteolytic cleavage [274]. After this step, the Notch intracellular domain (NICD) is released to the cytosol and transported to the nucleus. The NICD has several domains. The N-terminally located proline–glutamate–serine–threonine-rich (PEST) domain is followed by a nuclear localization signal, seven ankyrin repeats, transactivation domain (TAD), and C-terminal RBP-Jκ–associated molecule (RAM). Inside the nucleus, NICD interacts via the RAM domain and ankyrin repeats with the CSL/RBP-Jκ transcription factor and its co-factor Mastermind (MAML1) [275,276]. In the absence of Notch receptor activation, CSL interacts with the co-repressor complex (CoR) [277,278]. This complex is tethered to promoters of Notch target genes, actively repressing them. The interaction with NICD and MAML1 leads to the displacement of the CoR complex and the recruitment of transcription co-activators (e.g., p300). This is followed by activation of target genes' expression, including the Hairy enhancer of split 1 (HES1) family of transcriptional repressors, the CDK inhibitor p21, and others [266].

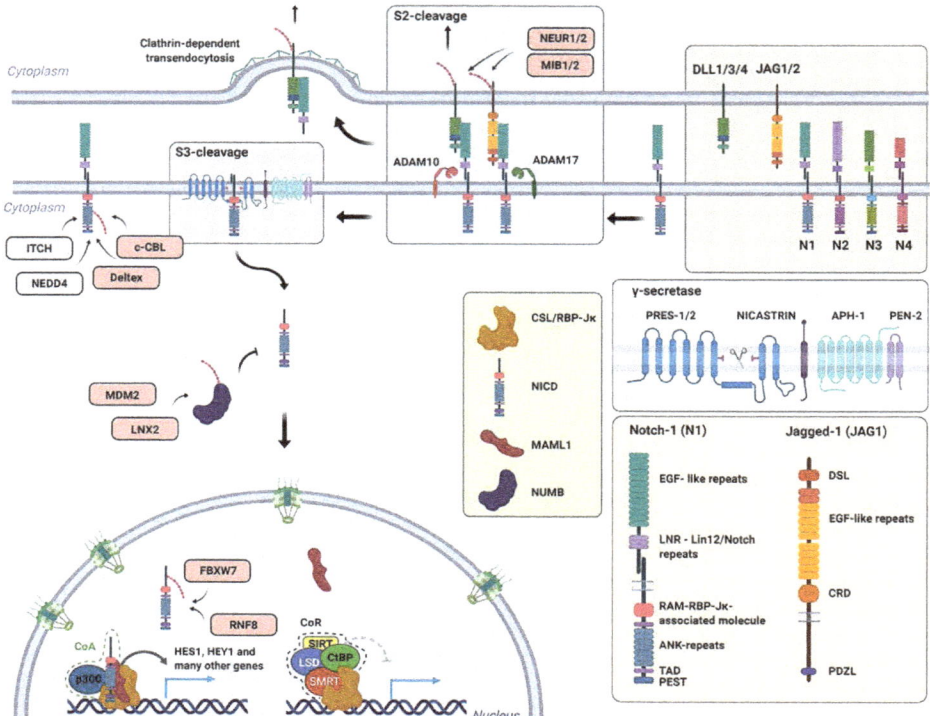

Figure 5. Notch signaling pathway by ubiquitination upon binding of Jagged/Delta (JAG/DLL) ligands to the Notch receptor (N1); the endocytic system is activated in the ligand-bearing cell. This leads to two sequential proteolytic events. The first is metalloproteinase-dependent (ADAM10/17) and it releases the extracellular domain of the Notch receptor which is afterward engulfed via transendocytosis. The second proteolytic cleavage is membrane bound and dependent on γ-secretase activity. After this step, NICD (the Notch intracellular part) is released to the cytosol and transported to the nucleus where it interacts with the CSL/RBP-Jκ transcription factor and its co-factor Mastermind (MAML1). The complex is tethered to promoters of Notch target genes. For details see the text.

5.1. Notch Signaling Pathway and its Regulation by Ubiquitin Ligases

The Notch receptor is a short-lived protein which is targeted by multiple ubiquitin ligases. Several HECT-type ubiquitin ligases regulate its membrane localization and endocytic recycling, promoting "non-activated Notch receptor degradation". Knockdown of the ITCH ubiquitin ligase leads to impaired Notch1 ubiquitination and lysosomal degradation [279]. Ubiquitin ligase ITCH interacts with the Notch receptor indirectly via the α-arrestin 1 (ARRDC1) and β-arrestins complex [280]. Interestingly, ITCH is also the main ubiquitin ligase involved in the NUMB-dependent Notch1 receptor inhibition [281]. Adapter protein NUMB, a major inhibitor of Notch signaling, is also a target of the RING-type ubiquitin ligase LNX2. This ubiquitin ligase, by mediating NUMB degradation, thus potentiates Notch signaling [282]. The WWP2 ubiquitin ligase was shown to mediate Notch1 polyubiquitination in a manner dependent on activated Dishevelled 2. Dishevelled 2 binds to the ubiquitin ligase WWP2 and unlocks its ligase activity from autoinhibition [283]. Of note, Dishevelled 2 involvement could point to possible signaling crosstalk between the Wnt and Notch1 pathways. Moreover, WWP2 also appeared in the screen for Notch3 interacting partners. It mediated ubiquitination of its active form and blocked Notch3 signaling in the context of ovarian cancer [284]. In general, ubiquitination of transmembrane receptors often regulates the receptor endocytosis and inappropriate activation. This was confirmed for Notch receptor. Its endocytosis is clathrin-dependent and requires epsin1 and the adaptor protein complex 2 (AP2) ubiquitin ligase Nedd4. Inactivation of Nedd4 leads to stabilization of membrane-bound Notch and signaling enhancement [285]. Another ubiquitin ligase involved in the regulation of the Notch cell surface stability is Deltex-1 (DTX1), which colocalizes with Notch1 on tubulovesicular recycling endosomes. Inactivation of DTX1 leads to Notch1 stabilization and cell surface relocation via the RAB4A-mediated transport route. Nevertheless, DTX1 does not mediate direct ubiquitination of the Notch receptor. The main DTX1 substrate in the endosomal compartment is PI5P4Kγ, a lipid kinase involved in PI(4,5)P2 production. It is PI5P4Kγ activity which is necessary for cell surface localization and stability of the Notch1 receptor [286]. The activated form of Notch (NICD) is also targeted by several other ubiquitin ligases, the most important being FBXW7. Phosphodegron-interacting protein FBXW7 belongs to the CRL family of RING-type ubiquitin ligases and recognizes the PEST region of NICD. This recognition is preceded by the sequence of priming and processing phosphorylations. The canonical priming kinase of the FBXW7 degron is CDK8, but integrin-linked kinase (ILK) is also able to phosphorylate it [287,288]. Like in other FBXW7 substrates, the processing kinase is GSK3β [289,290]. Moreover, the NUMB/ITCH complex and RNF8, a ubiquitin ligase involved in DNA damage response, are able to mediate NICD ubiquitination and degradation as well [281]. In support of RNF8 function as the Notch ubiquitin ligase, data from The Cancer Genome Atlas (TCGA) show an inverse correlation between RNF8 expression and Notch activity [291]. The ubiquitin ligase MDM2 targeting the p53 tumor suppressor plays an important role in potentiating the Notch signaling pathway via its interaction with Notch inhibitor NUMB. The mechanism remains to be elucidated [292,293].

Not only the receptors but also Notch ligands are regulated by ubiquitination. The ubiquitination is required for proper trafficking and presentation of the active ligands on the cell membrane and is provided by the E3 ubiquitin ligases Neuralized (NEUR) and Mindbomb (MIB) [273,294,295].

5.2. Mouse Models of Ubiquitin Ligases Involved in the Notch Signaling Pathway

Activation of the Notch receptor signaling pathway is important for embryonic development since it plays a critical role in cell fate determination. Expectedly, mice defective in this pathway often exhibit embryonic lethality and developmental abnormalities [296–298]. Several mouse models of ubiquitin ligases mentioned above confirm the role of these ligases in Notch signaling pathway in vivo. Mice deficient in Mib1 ubiquitin ligase clearly exhibit the Notch-defective phenotype, and mutant mice die early during embryogenesis with many developmental defects. On the other hand, mouse models of ubiquitin ligases which mediate degradation of many different proteins, for example FBW7, reflect this fact in their phenotypic complexity. Importantly, several mouse models do not support the importance of cognate ubiquitin ligases in the Notch signaling pathway, as discussed here [299–301].

5.2.1. F-box and WD Repeat Domain Containing 7 (Fbxw7)

Human FBXW7 is a well-characterized F-box protein that binds to its substrates in a similar manner like β-TrCP. It is also a haploinsufficient tumor suppressor with mutations found in many human cancers [302,303]. It regulates the stability of many substrates involved in the cell cycle and survival, including p100, c-Myc, c-Jun, cyclin E, NF1, and Notch [304,305].

F-box and WD repeat domain containing 7-deficient mouse embryos die around E10.5–11.5. The phenotype clearly reflects that endothelial tissues represent a major site of embryonic Fbxw7 expression. The embryos have significant abnormalities in brain and yolk sac vascular development [306,307]. They also exhibit defects in major trunk veins formation and heart chamber maturation. The animals have the upregulated endothelial cell-specific isoform of the Notch receptors family, Notch4, as well as Notch target genes *HEY1* and *HES1*. Although the phenotype suggests a potential involvement of the Notch signaling pathway hyperactivation, no genetic rescue experiment has been done yet [307]. The T cell-specific deletion of *FBXW7* leads to thymic hyperplasia and subsequent development of the thymic lymphoma. T cells from knockout mice are immature, accumulate the Myc protein—another canonical FBXW7 substrate—and fail to exit from the cell cycle [308]. The targeted deletion of *FBXW7* in HSCs revealed the essential role of Fbxw7 in maintaining the HSCs pool. In Fbxw7-deficient animals, HSCs are prematurely depleted due to the fact of active cell cycling and p53-dependent apoptosis. The HSC reconstitution capacity and quiescence are impaired [309]. Mice with conditionally inactivated intestinal *FBXW7* develop a hyperproliferative phenotype. They show impairment in goblet cell differentiation and the accumulation of highly proliferating progenitor cells [310]. The brain-specific deletion results in perinatal death of embryos. Animals lack suckling behavior and have morphological abnormalities in the brain structure. On the cellular level, they have a clear impairment of neural stem cells differentiation, resulting in a decrease of mature neurons. They also have disequilibrium in neural cell differentiation towards astrogenesis [311]. The hepatic inactivation results in hepatomegaly and steatohepatitis. Mutant hepatocytes accumulate SREBP and NOTCH1 proteins. The long-term Fbxw7 deficiency leads to the proliferation of the biliary system and appearance of hamartomas as well as the imbalanced ratio between cholangiocyte and hepatocyte lineages [312].

5.2.2. Mindbomb and Neuralized (Mib and Neur)

Mindbomb 1/2 proteins contain two substrate-recognizing domains—the ankyrin repeats domain and several RING domains. Neuralized 1/2 proteins consist of the neuralized homology repeats responsible for protein–protein interactions and the C-terminal RING domain. As described previously, Mib and Neur ubiquitin ligases target Notch ligands and influence Notch signaling.

Mindbomb 2-, NEUR1-, and NEUR2-deficient mice are viable with entirely normal appearance [299]. Mindbomb 1-deficient embryos are severely growth retarded at E9.5 and die at E10.5 from a lack of placental connection and defects in somitogenesis, vasculogenesis, and cardiogenesis [299–301]. The phenotype of these embryos clearly shows defective Notch signaling [296,313]. The yolk sacs have a blistered appearance with only small capillaries and complete lack of large vitelline-collecting vessels. Embryos lack heart looping and have an enlarged balloon-like pericardial sac and a smaller dorsal aorta. Other typical signs of Notch-related defects include irregular somitogenesis, absence of mesenchymal cells, and lack of second branchial arches. Knockout embryos show a strong neurogenic phenotype. The head of embryos appear normal but the neurons prematurely differentiate and undergo apoptosis. The reduction of progenitors leads to a loss of both astrocytes and oligodendrocytes. The embryos also lack intraembryonic hematopoietic progenitors [314]. Inducible inactivation of MIB1 (from E10 to E12), shows MIB1 continuous requirement in neuronal system development as it exhibits the suppression of glial differentiation [315].

The tissue-specific deletion of the *Mib1* gene shows its central role in Notch signaling and mouse development. Endoderm-specific inactivation causes a loss of endocrine progenitors and β-cells [316]. Its inactivation in the mouse myocardium mimics the phenotype of myocardial-specific deletion of *Jagged1*. Embryos have left ventricular non-compaction. They show reduced ventricular Notch1 activity, a dilated heart with a thin compact myocardium, and a large, non-compacted trabeculae protruding toward the ventricular lumen [317]. Mice with Mib1 inactivated in the bone marrow develop the myeloproliferative disease (MPD). They exhibit hepatosplenomegaly, accumulation of immature granulocytes, and anemia. Interestingly, the transplantation of wild-type bone marrow cells into the Mib1-null microenvironment results in a de novo MPD [318]. The absence of Mib1 during the development of the lymphatic system results in the developmental arrest of T cells and marginal zone B cells [319].

5.2.3. Deltex-1 (Dtx1)

Deltex-1 is a RING-finger ubiquitin ligase containing the proline-rich motif and the N-terminal Notch-binding WWE domains. Deltex-1 regulates Notch signaling by controlling PI5P4Kγ stability [286]. It is downregulated in a subset of gastric adenocarcinomas [320].

Deltex-1-deficient mice have diminished Treg-dependent T cell anergy resulting in autoantibody production, augmented T cell activation, and increased inflammatory response [321]. The mice are otherwise healthy and fertile and T and B cell development seems intact [322]. Biochemically, Treg-initiated T cell anergy is dependent on the Foxp3 transcriptional factor. Deltex-1, which is transcriptionally activated by the nuclear factor of activated T cells (Nfat), controls Foxp3 activity via degradation of the FOXP3 inhibitor Hif1α. In Deltex-1-deficient Treg cells, the stabilized Hif1α suppresses FOXP3 and, subsequently, Treg's ability to impose T cell anergy. Simultaneous knockout of Hif1α restores FOXP3 and rescues the defective suppressive activity in Deltex-1-deficient Treg cells in vivo [321,323]. It is not clear if Deltex-1 regulation of the Notch signaling pathway could be part of T cell anergy activation. As mentioned above, Deltex-1 is a positive regulator of Notch signaling [286]. Moreover, Notch was shown to act as the Foxp3 positive regulator [324,325]. Whether Deltex-1 activates Foxp3 also via potentiated Notch signaling or if Notch activation serves as positive feedback to sustain strong T cell anergy remains to be investigated.

5.2.4. RING finger 8 (RNF8)

Ubiquitin ligase RNF8 has the C-terminal RING domain and the N-terminal forkhead-associated (FHA)-domain [326]. The FHA-domain is necessary for DNA-damage association. It binds to the ATM-phosphorylated N-terminus of the mediator of DNA damage checkpoint protein 1 (MDC1) [327]. Specifically, RNF8 targets histones by K63-linked ubiquitination, which is recognized by another ubiquitin-ligase RNF168 and leads to the recruitment of DNA repair proteins.

Transgenic embryos lacking Rnf8 are growth retarded with reduced hematopoietic populations. They have impaired class switch recombination and accumulation of unresolved immunoglobulin heavy chain-associated DNA double-stranded breaks. They are more susceptible to ionizing radiation, exhibit increased genomic instability, and have elevated risk for tumorigenesis [328]. Mouse males deficient in Rnf8 are sterile with defective ubiquitination of the XY chromatin. They are proficient in meiotic sex chromosome inactivation but deficient in global nucleosome removal [329]. Mutant mice also exhibit neuronal degeneration and reactive astrocytosis. Importantly, Rnf8-deficient neurons appear more susceptible to X-ray-induced DNA damage and Rnf8-deficient mice display memory impairment and reduced exploratory behavior in the open-field test. This defect could correlate with higher neuronal loss in these animals [330]. Cerebellar granule cell-specific RNF8 knockout displays a higher number of parallel fiber presynaptic boutons and functional parallel fiber/Purkinje cell synapses. It also revealed that RNF8 is involved in suppression of granule neuron/Purkinje cell transmission [331].

5.2.5. Mouse double minute 2 (MDM2)

Mouse double minute 2 is a ubiquitin ligase with the C-terminal RING domain, the central acidic domain and the adjacent zinc finger region, and the N-terminal p53-binding domain that indicates its main function—to facilitate p53 ubiquitination and subsequent degradation. Despite some conflicting data, MDM2 was reported to be overexpressed in many different types of malignancies and it is usually related to a worse prognosis [332].

Mice with a hypomorphic allele of *MDM2* have defects in hematopoietic lineages. They develop mild anemia and the size of their lymphoid organs is significantly reduced due to the lower number of lymphocytes [333]. Mice with full inactivation of both *MDM2* alleles die early in development, and this phenotype is almost completely reversed with concurrent inactivation of murine *p53* [334]. Interestingly, mice with lowered levels of MDM2 were resistant to tumor formation, but otherwise were healthy and did not age prematurely [335].

6. Concluding Remarks

The importance of the ubiquitin–proteasome system has been emerging over the last three decades. Its discovery helped us to understand the biochemical nature of processes underlying major developmental and homeostatic events in the life domain. Each and every signaling pathway or cellular process depends on the UPS. The architecture of this system has both pleiotropic and specific facets. The pleiotropy is represented via proteasome while the specificity is ensured by a wide group of enzymes called ubiquitin ligases. Apparently, the UPS is essential for cellular and organismal homeostasis. This holds true especially for cancer cells which have to overcome the instability of the genetic information, and the control of the proteome is one way to do it. Therefore, they are fully dependent on proteasome function and this can be therapeutically exploited. The success of proteasome inhibitor bortezomib in multiple myeloma treatment fulfilled some of these expectations. Moreover, the re-discovery of thalidomide, a specific modulator of the ubiquitin ligase cereblon, for successful treatment of multiple myeloma initiated change of the focus towards the more specific approaches. It also proves that the right therapeutic options arise from fusion of the chemistry, the molecular biology, and the animal models. As presented in this review, there are numerous ubiquitin ligases which were found to be involved in the cancer-associated signaling pathways, but only few were confirmed to play the same role in vivo (Figure 6). Moreover, some of these ubiquitin ligases were shown to have a completely different function than expected. It is of the utmost importance to consider these observations and findings.

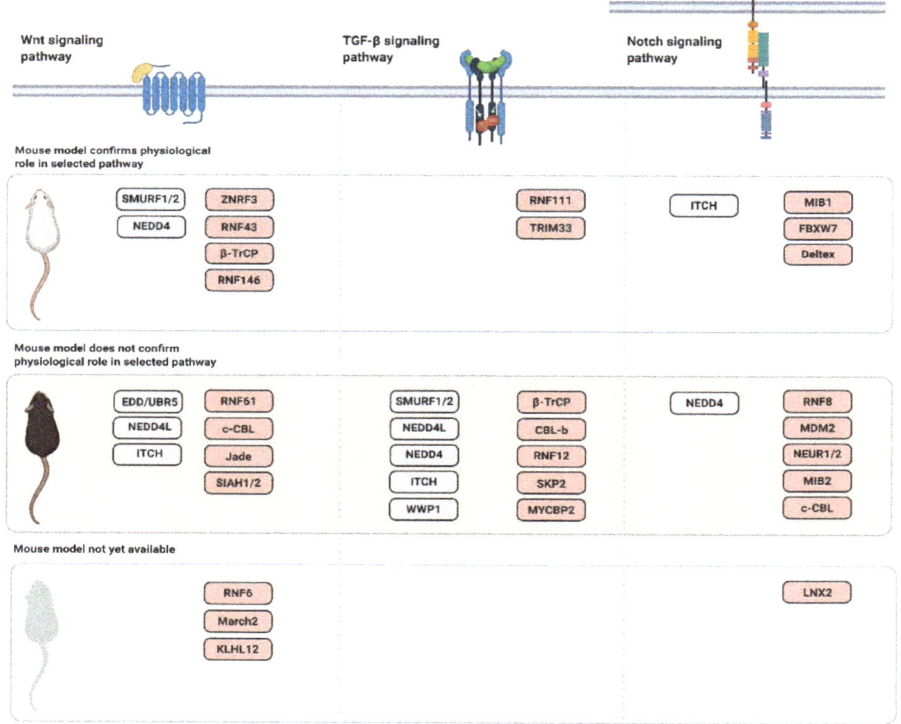

Figure 6. Schematic representation of mouse models of the selected ubiquitin ligases summarizing their physiological role in the Wnt, TGF-β, and Notch signaling pathways.

With the emerging technologies in genetic engineering, it should not be an option but a must to prove our results in mouse models. Because these models will not only confirm what we think we achieved in Petri dishes, they will be an important part of the next step—how to translate these results into better cancer therapy.

Author Contributions: L.C. prepared the manuscript and figures. N.B. and T.L. reviewed and edited the manuscript.

Funding: This work was supported by Grant Agency of Czech Republic (project: 18-27408S) and by the Ministry of Education, Youth and Sports (project LO1419); L.C. was supported by Marie Skłodowska-Curie Fellowship (LIGER).

Acknowledgments: We thank Marketa Vancurova, Emily Langore, Tadeas Cermak, and David Cermak for proofreading the manuscript. L.C. thanks Zuzana Stivinova for the support. L.C. acknowledges the databases OMIM (Online Mendelian Inheritance in Man) and MGI/MGD (Mouse Genome Database) [336,337]. The figures were created with BioRender.com.

Conflicts of Interest: The authors declare no conflict of interest.

References

1. Sanchez-Vega, F.; Mina, M.; Armenia, J.; Chatila, W.K.; Luna, A.; La, K.C.; Dimitriadoy, S.; Liu, D.L.; Kantheti, H.S.; Saghafinia, S.; et al. Oncogenic Signaling Pathways in The Cancer Genome Atlas. *Cell* **2018**, *173*, 321–337. [CrossRef]
2. Kinzler, K.W.; Nilbert, M.C.; Su, L.K.; Vogelstein, B.; Bryan, T.M.; Levy, D.B.; Smith, K.J.; Preisinger, A.C.; Hedge, P.; McKechnie, D.; et al. Identification of FAP locus genes from chromosome 5q21. *Science* **1991**, *253*, 661–665. [CrossRef]
3. Ellisen, L.W.; Bird, J.; West, D.C.; Soreng, A.L.; Reynolds, T.C.; Smith, S.D.; Sklar, J. TAN-1, the human homolog of the Drosophila notch gene, is broken by chromosomal translocations in T lymphoblastic neoplasms. *Cell* **1991**, *66*, 649–661. [CrossRef]
4. Yakicier, M.C.; Irmak, M.B.; Romano, A.; Kew, M.; Ozturk, M. Smad2 and Smad4 gene mutations in hepatocellular carcinoma. *Oncogene* **1999**, *18*, 4879–4883. [CrossRef]
5. Manasanch, E.E.; Orlowski, R.Z. Proteasome inhibitors in cancer therapy. *Nat. Rev. Clin. Oncol.* **2017**, *14*, 417–433. [CrossRef]
6. Skaar, J.R.; Pagan, J.K.; Pagano, M. SCF ubiquitin ligase-targeted therapies. *Nat. Rev. Drug Discov.* **2014**, *13*, 889–903. [CrossRef]
7. Kumari, N.; Jaynes, P.W.; Saei, A.; Iyengar, P.V.; Richard, J.L.C.; Eichhorn, P.J.A. The roles of ubiquitin modifying enzymes in neoplastic disease. *Biochim. Biophys. Acta Rev. Cancer* **2017**, *1868*, 456–483. [CrossRef]
8. Nalepa, G.; Rolfe, M.; Harper, J.W. Drug discovery in the ubiquitin-proteasome system. *Nat. Rev. Drug Discov.* **2006**, *5*, 596–613. [CrossRef]
9. Buetow, L.; Huang, D.T. Structural insights into the catalysis and regulation of E3 ubiquitin ligases. *Nat. Rev. Mol. Cell Biol.* **2016**, *17*, 626–642. [CrossRef]
10. Hershko, A.; Heller, H.; Elias, S.; Ciechanover, A. Components of ubiquitin-protein ligase system. Resolution, affinity purification, and role in protein breakdown. *J. Biol. Chem.* **1983**, *258*, 8206–8214.
11. Deol, K.K.; Lorenz, S.; Strieter, E.R. Enzymatic Logic of Ubiquitin Chain Assembly. *Front. Physiol.* **2019**, *10*, 835. [CrossRef]
12. Stewart, M.D.; Ritterhoff, T.; Klevit, R.E.; Brzovic, P.S. E2 enzymes: More than just middle men. *Cell Res.* **2016**, *26*, 423–440. [CrossRef]
13. Rittinger, K.; Ikeda, F. Linear ubiquitin chains: Enzymes, mechanisms and biology. *Open Biol.* **2017**, *7*. [CrossRef]
14. Akutsu, M.; Dikic, I.; Bremm, A. Ubiquitin chain diversity at a glance. *J. Cell Sci.* **2016**, *129*, 875–880. [CrossRef]
15. Nakayama, K.I.; Nakayama, K. Ubiquitin ligases: Cell-cycle control and cancer. *Nat. Rev. Cancer* **2006**, *6*, 369–381. [CrossRef]
16. Zheng, N.; Shabek, N. Ubiquitin Ligases: Structure, Function, and Regulation. *Annu. Rev. Biochem.* **2017**, *86*, 129–157. [CrossRef]
17. Lilley, C.E.; Chaurushiya, M.S.; Boutell, C.; Landry, S.; Suh, J.; Panier, S.; Everett, R.D.; Stewart, G.S.; Durocher, D.; Weitzman, M.D. A viral E3 ligase targets RNF8 and RNF168 to control histone ubiquitination and DNA damage responses. *EMBO J.* **2010**, *29*, 943–955. [CrossRef]
18. Huen, M.S.; Grant, R.; Manke, I.; Minn, K.; Yu, X.; Yaffe, M.B.; Chen, J. RNF8 transduces the DNA-damage signal via histone ubiquitylation and checkpoint protein assembly. *Cell* **2007**, *131*, 901–914. [CrossRef]

19. Skaar, J.R.; Pagan, J.K.; Pagano, M. Mechanisms and function of substrate recruitment by F-box proteins. *Nat. Rev. Mol. Cell Biol.* **2013**, *14*, 369–381. [CrossRef]
20. Honda, R.; Tanaka, H.; Yasuda, H. Oncoprotein MDM2 is a ubiquitin ligase E3 for tumor suppressor p53. *FEBS Lett.* **1997**, *420*, 25–27. [CrossRef]
21. de Toledo, S.M.; Azzam, E.I.; Dahlberg, W.K.; Gooding, T.B.; Little, J.B. ATM complexes with HDM2 and promotes its rapid phosphorylation in a p53-independent manner in normal and tumor human cells exposed to ionizing radiation. *Oncogene* **2000**, *19*, 6185–6193. [CrossRef] [PubMed]
22. Khosravi, R.; Maya, R.; Gottlieb, T.; Oren, M.; Shiloh, Y.; Shkedy, D. Rapid ATM-dependent phosphorylation of MDM2 precedes p53 accumulation in response to DNA damage. *Proc. Natl. Acad. Sci. USA* **1999**, *96*, 14973–14977. [CrossRef] [PubMed]
23. Frescas, D.; Pagano, M. Deregulated proteolysis by the F-box proteins SKP2 and beta-TrCP: Tipping the scales of cancer. *Nat. Rev. Cancer* **2008**, *8*, 438–449. [CrossRef] [PubMed]
24. Bulatov, E.; Ciulli, A. Targeting Cullin-RING E3 ubiquitin ligases for drug discovery: Structure, assembly and small-molecule modulation. *Biochem. J.* **2015**, *467*, 365–386. [CrossRef]
25. Aravind, L.; Koonin, E.V. The U box is a modified RING finger—A common domain in ubiquitination. *Curr. Biol.* **2000**, *10*, R132–R134. [CrossRef]
26. Wang, T.; Wang, W.; Wang, Q.; Xie, R.; Landay, A.; Chen, D. The E3 ubiquitin ligase CHIP in normal cell function and in disease conditions. *Ann. N. Y. Acad. Sci.* **2019**. [CrossRef]
27. Rotin, D.; Kumar, S. Physiological functions of the HECT family of ubiquitin ligases. *Nat. Rev. Mol. Cell Biol.* **2009**, *10*, 398–409. [CrossRef]
28. Podos, S.D.; Hanson, K.K.; Wang, Y.C.; Ferguson, E.L. The DSmurf ubiquitin-protein ligase restricts BMP signaling spatially and temporally during Drosophila embryogenesis. *Dev. Cell* **2001**, *1*, 567–578. [CrossRef]
29. Staub, O.; Dho, S.; Henry, P.; Correa, J.; Ishikawa, T.; McGlade, J.; Rotin, D. WW domains of Nedd4 bind to the proline-rich PY motifs in the epithelial Na+ channel deleted in Liddle's syndrome. *EMBO J.* **1996**, *15*, 2371–2380. [CrossRef]
30. Ebisawa, T.; Fukuchi, M.; Murakami, G.; Chiba, T.; Tanaka, K.; Imamura, T.; Miyazono, K. Smurf1 interacts with transforming growth factor-beta type I receptor through Smad7 and induces receptor degradation. *J. Biol. Chem.* **2001**, *276*, 12477–12480. [CrossRef]
31. Spratt, D.E.; Walden, H.; Shaw, G.S. RBR E3 ubiquitin ligases: New structures, new insights, new questions. *Biochem. J.* **2014**, *458*, 421–437. [CrossRef] [PubMed]
32. Marin, I.; Ferrus, A. Comparative genomics of the RBR family, including the Parkinson's disease-related gene parkin and the genes of the ariadne subfamily. *Mol. Biol. Evol.* **2002**, *19*, 2039–2050. [CrossRef] [PubMed]
33. Yoshii, S.R.; Kishi, C.; Ishihara, N.; Mizushima, N. Parkin mediates proteasome-dependent protein degradation and rupture of the outer mitochondrial membrane. *J. Biol. Chem.* **2011**, *286*, 19630–19640. [CrossRef] [PubMed]
34. Lee, J.Y.; Nagano, Y.; Taylor, J.P.; Lim, K.L.; Yao, T.P. Disease-causing mutations in parkin impair mitochondrial ubiquitination, aggregation, and HDAC6-dependent mitophagy. *J. Cell Biol.* **2010**, *189*, 671–679. [CrossRef]
35. Zhan, T.; Rindtorff, N.; Boutros, M. Wnt signaling in cancer. *Oncogene* **2017**, *36*, 1461–1473. [CrossRef]
36. Nusse, R.; Clevers, H. Wnt/beta-Catenin Signaling, Disease, and Emerging Therapeutic Modalities. *Cell* **2017**, *169*, 985–999. [CrossRef]
37. Tolwinski, N.S.; Wehrli, M.; Rives, A.; Erdeniz, N.; DiNardo, S.; Wieschaus, E. Wg/Wnt signal can be transmitted through arrow/LRP5,6 and Axin independently of Zw3/Gsk3beta activity. *Dev. Cell* **2003**, *4*, 407–418. [CrossRef]
38. Hao, H.X.; Xie, Y.; Zhang, Y.; Charlat, O.; Oster, E.; Avello, M.; Lei, H.; Mickanin, C.; Liu, D.; Ruffner, H.; et al. ZNRF3 promotes Wnt receptor turnover in an R-spondin-sensitive manner. *Nature* **2012**, *485*, 195–200. [CrossRef]
39. Koo, B.K.; Spit, M.; Jordens, I.; Low, T.Y.; Stange, D.E.; van de Wetering, M.; van Es, J.H.; Mohammed, S.; Heck, A.J.; Maurice, M.M.; et al. Tumour suppressor RNF43 is a stem-cell E3 ligase that induces endocytosis of Wnt receptors. *Nature* **2012**, *488*, 665–669. [CrossRef]
40. Jiang, X.; Charlat, O.; Zamponi, R.; Yang, Y.; Cong, F. Dishevelled promotes Wnt receptor degradation through recruitment of ZNRF3/RNF43 E3 ubiquitin ligases. *Mol. Cell* **2015**, *58*, 522–533. [CrossRef]
41. Peters, J.M.; McKay, R.M.; McKay, J.P.; Graff, J.M. Casein kinase I transduces Wnt signals. *Nature* **1999**, *401*, 345–350. [CrossRef] [PubMed]

42. Ikeda, S.; Kishida, S.; Yamamoto, H.; Murai, H.; Koyama, S.; Kikuchi, A. Axin, a negative regulator of the Wnt signaling pathway, forms a complex with GSK-3beta and beta-catenin and promotes GSK-3beta-dependent phosphorylation of beta-catenin. *EMBO J.* **1998**, *17*, 1371–1384. [CrossRef] [PubMed]
43. Doble, B.W.; Patel, S.; Wood, G.A.; Kockeritz, L.K.; Woodgett, J.R. Functional redundancy of GSK-3alpha and GSK-3beta in Wnt/beta-catenin signaling shown by using an allelic series of embryonic stem cell lines. *Dev. Cell* **2007**, *12*, 957–971. [CrossRef] [PubMed]
44. Morin, P.J.; Sparks, A.B.; Korinek, V.; Barker, N.; Clevers, H.; Vogelstein, B.; Kinzler, K.W. Activation of beta-catenin-Tcf signaling in colon cancer by mutations in beta-catenin or APC. *Science* **1997**, *275*, 1787–1790. [CrossRef]
45. Korinek, V.; Barker, N.; Morin, P.J.; van Wichen, D.; de Weger, R.; Kinzler, K.W.; Vogelstein, B.; Clevers, H. Constitutive transcriptional activation by a beta-catenin-Tcf complex in APC-/- colon carcinoma. *Science* **1997**, *275*, 1784–1787. [CrossRef]
46. Marikawa, Y.; Elinson, R.P. beta-TrCP is a negative regulator of Wnt/beta-catenin signaling pathway and dorsal axis formation in Xenopus embryos. *Mech. Dev.* **1998**, *77*, 75–80. [CrossRef]
47. Hart, M.; Concordet, J.P.; Lassot, I.; Albert, I.; del los Santos, R.; Durand, H.; Perret, C.; Rubinfeld, B.; Margottin, F.; Benarous, R.; et al. The F-box protein beta-TrCP associates with phosphorylated beta-catenin and regulates its activity in the cell. *Curr. Biol.* **1999**, *9*, 207–210. [CrossRef]
48. Zeng, X.; Huang, H.; Tamai, K.; Zhang, X.; Harada, Y.; Yokota, C.; Almeida, K.; Wang, J.; Doble, B.; Woodgett, J.; et al. Initiation of Wnt signaling: Control of Wnt coreceptor Lrp6 phosphorylation/activation via frizzled, dishevelled and axin functions. *Development* **2008**, *135*, 367–375. [CrossRef]
49. Pan, W.; Choi, S.C.; Wang, H.; Qin, Y.; Volpicelli-Daley, L.; Swan, L.; Lucast, L.; Khoo, C.; Zhang, X.; Li, L.; et al. Wnt3a-mediated formation of phosphatidylinositol 4,5-bisphosphate regulates LRP6 phosphorylation. *Science* **2008**, *321*, 1350–1353. [CrossRef]
50. Li, V.S.; Ng, S.S.; Boersema, P.J.; Low, T.Y.; Karthaus, W.R.; Gerlach, J.P.; Mohammed, S.; Heck, A.J.; Maurice, M.M.; Mahmoudi, T.; et al. Wnt signaling through inhibition of beta-catenin degradation in an intact Axin1 complex. *Cell* **2012**, *149*, 1245–1256. [CrossRef]
51. Ji, L.; Jiang, B.; Jiang, X.; Charlat, O.; Chen, A.; Mickanin, C.; Bauer, A.; Xu, W.; Yan, X.; Cong, F. The SIAH E3 ubiquitin ligases promote Wnt/beta-catenin signaling through mediating Wnt-induced Axin degradation. *Genes Dev.* **2017**, *31*, 904–915. [CrossRef] [PubMed]
52. Callow, M.G.; Tran, H.; Phu, L.; Lau, T.; Lee, J.; Sandoval, W.N.; Liu, P.S.; Bheddah, S.; Tao, J.; Lill, J.R.; et al. Ubiquitin ligase RNF146 regulates tankyrase and Axin to promote Wnt signaling. *PLoS ONE* **2011**, *6*, e22595. [CrossRef] [PubMed]
53. Zhang, Y.; Liu, S.; Mickanin, C.; Feng, Y.; Charlat, O.; Michaud, G.A.; Schirle, M.; Shi, X.; Hild, M.; Bauer, A.; et al. RNF146 is a poly(ADP-ribose)-directed E3 ligase that regulates axin degradation and Wnt signalling. *Nat. Cell Biol.* **2011**, *13*, 623–629. [CrossRef] [PubMed]
54. DaRosa, P.A.; Klevit, R.E.; Xu, W. Structural basis for tankyrase-RNF146 interaction reveals noncanonical tankyrase-binding motifs. *Protein Sci. A Publ. Protein Soc.* **2018**, *27*, 1057–1067. [CrossRef]
55. Matsumoto, Y.; La Rose, J.; Lim, M.; Adissu, H.A.; Law, N.; Mao, X.; Cong, F.; Mera, P.; Karsenty, G.; Goltzman, D.; et al. Ubiquitin ligase RNF146 coordinates bone dynamics and energy metabolism. *J. Clin. Investig.* **2017**, *127*, 2612–2625. [CrossRef]
56. Zhu, X.; Xing, R.; Tan, R.; Dai, R.; Tao, Q. The RNF146 E3 ubiquitin ligase is required for the control of Wnt signaling and body pattern formation in Xenopus. *Mech. Dev.* **2017**, *147*, 28–36. [CrossRef]
57. Wang, Z.; Tacchelly-Benites, O.; Noble, G.P.; Johnson, M.K.; Gagne, J.P.; Poirier, G.G.; Ahmed, Y. A Context-Dependent Role for the RNF146 Ubiquitin Ligase in Wingless/Wnt Signaling in Drosophila. *Genetics* **2019**, *211*, 913–923. [CrossRef]
58. Fei, C.; He, X.; Xie, S.; Miao, H.; Zhou, Z.; Li, L. Smurf1-mediated axin ubiquitination requires Smurf1 C2 domain and is cell cycle-dependent. *J. Biol. Chem.* **2014**, *289*, 14170–14177. [CrossRef]
59. Fei, C.; Li, Z.; Li, C.; Chen, Y.; Chen, Z.; He, X.; Mao, L.; Wang, X.; Zeng, R.; Li, L. Smurf1-mediated Lys29-linked nonproteolytic polyubiquitination of axin negatively regulates Wnt/beta-catenin signaling. *Mol. Cell. Biol.* **2013**, *33*, 4095–4105. [CrossRef]
60. Kim, S.; Jho, E.H. The protein stability of Axin, a negative regulator of Wnt signaling, is regulated by Smad ubiquitination regulatory factor 2 (Smurf2). *J. Biol. Chem.* **2010**, *285*, 36420–36426. [CrossRef]

61. Lee, H.K.; Lee, E.W.; Seo, J.; Jeong, M.; Lee, S.H.; Kim, S.Y.; Jho, E.H.; Choi, C.H.; Chung, J.Y.; Song, J. Ubiquitylation and degradation of adenomatous polyposis coli by MKRN1 enhances Wnt/beta-catenin signaling. *Oncogene* **2018**, *37*, 4273–4286. [CrossRef] [PubMed]
62. Ding, Y.; Zhang, Y.; Xu, C.; Tao, Q.H.; Chen, Y.G. HECT domain-containing E3 ubiquitin ligase NEDD4L negatively regulates Wnt signaling by targeting dishevelled for proteasomal degradation. *J. Biol. Chem.* **2013**, *288*, 8289–8298. [CrossRef] [PubMed]
63. Wei, W.; Li, M.; Wang, J.; Nie, F.; Li, L. The E3 ubiquitin ligase ITCH negatively regulates canonical Wnt signaling by targeting dishevelled protein. *Mol. Cell. Biol.* **2012**, *32*, 3903–3912. [CrossRef] [PubMed]
64. Nethe, M.; de Kreuk, B.J.; Tauriello, D.V.; Anthony, E.C.; Snoek, B.; Stumpel, T.; Salinas, P.C.; Maurice, M.M.; Geerts, D.; Deelder, A.M.; et al. Rac1 acts in conjunction with Nedd4 and dishevelled-1 to promote maturation of cell-cell contacts. *J. Cell Sci.* **2012**, *125*, 3430–3442. [CrossRef]
65. Zhang, Y.; Ding, Y.; Chen, Y.G.; Tao, Q. NEDD4L regulates convergent extension movements in Xenopus embryos via Disheveled-mediated non-canonical Wnt signaling. *Dev. Biol.* **2014**, *392*, 15–25. [CrossRef]
66. Tsukiyama, T.; Fukui, A.; Terai, S.; Fujioka, Y.; Shinada, K.; Takahashi, H.; Yamaguchi, T.P.; Ohba, Y.; Hatakeyama, S. Molecular Role of RNF43 in Canonical and Noncanonical Wnt Signaling. *Mol. Cell. Biol.* **2015**, *35*, 2007–2023. [CrossRef]
67. Angers, S.; Thorpe, C.J.; Biechele, T.L.; Goldenberg, S.J.; Zheng, N.; MacCoss, M.J.; Moon, R.T. The KLHL12-Cullin-3 ubiquitin ligase negatively regulates the Wnt-beta-catenin pathway by targeting Dishevelled for degradation. *Nat. Cell Biol.* **2006**, *8*, 348–357. [CrossRef]
68. Lee, H.; Cheong, S.M.; Han, W.; Koo, Y.; Jo, S.B.; Cho, G.S.; Yang, J.S.; Kim, S.; Han, J.K. Head formation requires Dishevelled degradation that is mediated by March2 in concert with Dapper1. *Development* **2018**, *145*. [CrossRef]
69. Zhou, M.I.; Wang, H.; Foy, R.L.; Ross, J.J.; Cohen, H.T. Tumor suppressor von Hippel-Lindau (VHL) stabilization of Jade-1 protein occurs through plant homeodomains and is VHL mutation dependent. *Cancer Res.* **2004**, *64*, 1278–1286. [CrossRef]
70. Shafique, S.; Rashid, S. Structural basis for renal cancer by the dynamics of pVHL-dependent JADE1 stabilization and beta-catenin regulation. *Prog. Biophys. Mol. Biol.* **2019**, *145*, 65–77. [CrossRef]
71. Chitalia, V.C.; Foy, R.L.; Bachschmid, M.M.; Zeng, L.; Panchenko, M.V.; Zhou, M.I.; Bharti, A.; Seldin, D.C.; Lecker, S.H.; Dominguez, I.; et al. Jade-1 inhibits Wnt signalling by ubiquitylating beta-catenin and mediates Wnt pathway inhibition by pVHL. *Nat. Cell Biol.* **2008**, *10*, 1208–1216. [CrossRef] [PubMed]
72. Shivanna, S.; Harrold, I.; Shashar, M.; Meyer, R.; Kiang, C.; Francis, J.; Zhao, Q.; Feng, H.; Edelman, E.R.; Rahimi, N.; et al. The c-Cbl ubiquitin ligase regulates nuclear beta-catenin and angiogenesis by its tyrosine phosphorylation mediated through the Wnt signaling pathway. *J. Biol. Chem.* **2015**, *290*, 12537–12546. [CrossRef] [PubMed]
73. Chitalia, V.; Shivanna, S.; Martorell, J.; Meyer, R.; Edelman, E.; Rahimi, N. c-Cbl, a ubiquitin E3 ligase that targets active beta-catenin: A novel layer of Wnt signaling regulation. *J. Biol. Chem.* **2013**, *288*, 23505–23517. [CrossRef] [PubMed]
74. Flack, J.E.; Mieszczanek, J.; Novcic, N.; Bienz, M. Wnt-Dependent Inactivation of the Groucho/TLE Co-repressor by the HECT E3 Ubiquitin Ligase Hyd/UBR5. *Mol. Cell* **2017**, *67*, 181–193. [CrossRef] [PubMed]
75. Hay-Koren, A.; Caspi, M.; Zilberberg, A.; Rosin-Arbesfeld, R. The EDD E3 ubiquitin ligase ubiquitinates and up-regulates beta-catenin. *Mol. Biol. Cell* **2011**, *22*, 399–411. [CrossRef] [PubMed]
76. Liu, L.; Zhang, Y.; Wong, C.C.; Zhang, J.; Dong, Y.; Li, X.; Kang, W.; Chan, F.K.L.; Sung, J.J.Y.; Yu, J. RNF6 Promotes Colorectal Cancer by Activating the Wnt/beta-Catenin Pathway via Ubiquitination of TLE3. *Cancer Res.* **2018**, *78*, 1958–1971. [CrossRef] [PubMed]
77. Glaeser, K.; Urban, M.; Fenech, E.; Voloshanenko, O.; Kranz, D.; Lari, F.; Christianson, J.C.; Boutros, M. ERAD-dependent control of the Wnt secretory factor Evi. *EMBO J.* **2018**, *37*. [CrossRef]
78. Perrody, E.; Abrami, L.; Feldman, M.; Kunz, B.; Urbe, S.; van der Goot, F.G. Ubiquitin-dependent folding of the Wnt signaling coreceptor LRP6. *Elife* **2016**, *5*. [CrossRef]
79. Feldman, M.; van der Goot, F.G. Novel ubiquitin-dependent quality control in the endoplasmic reticulum. *Trends Cell Biol.* **2009**, *19*, 357–363. [CrossRef]

80. Abrami, L.; Kunz, B.; Iacovache, I.; van der Goot, F.G. Palmitoylation and ubiquitination regulate exit of the Wnt signaling protein LRP6 from the endoplasmic reticulum. *Proc. Natl. Acad. Sci. USA* **2008**, *105*, 5384–5389. [CrossRef]
81. Joshi, V.; Amanullah, A.; Upadhyay, A.; Mishra, R.; Kumar, A.; Mishra, A. A Decade of Boon or Burden: What Has the CHIP Ever Done for Cellular Protein Quality Control Mechanism Implicated in Neurodegeneration and Aging? *Front. Mol. Neurosci.* **2016**, *9*, 93. [CrossRef] [PubMed]
82. Bhuripanyo, K.; Wang, Y.; Liu, X.; Zhou, L.; Liu, R.; Duong, D.; Zhao, B.; Bi, Y.; Zhou, H.; Chen, G.; et al. Identifying the substrate proteins of U-box E3s E4B and CHIP by orthogonal ubiquitin transfer. *Sci. Adv.* **2018**, *4*, e1701393. [CrossRef] [PubMed]
83. Rudloff, S.; Kemler, R. Differential requirements for beta-catenin during mouse development. *Development* **2012**, *139*, 3711–3721. [CrossRef] [PubMed]
84. Wang, Y.; Guo, N.; Nathans, J. The role of Frizzled3 and Frizzled6 in neural tube closure and in the planar polarity of inner-ear sensory hair cells. *J. Neurosci.* **2006**, *26*, 2147–2156. [CrossRef] [PubMed]
85. Korinek, V.; Barker, N.; Moerer, P.; van Donselaar, E.; Huls, G.; Peters, P.J.; Clevers, H. Depletion of epithelial stem-cell compartments in the small intestine of mice lacking Tcf-4. *Nat. Genet.* **1998**, *19*, 379–383. [CrossRef] [PubMed]
86. Nakayama, K.; Hatakeyama, S.; Maruyama, S.; Kikuchi, A.; Onoe, K.; Good, R.A.; Nakayama, K.I. Impaired degradation of inhibitory subunit of NF-kappa B (I kappa B) and beta-catenin as a result of targeted disruption of the beta-TrCP1 gene. *Proc. Natl. Acad. Sci. USA* **2003**, *100*, 8752–8757. [CrossRef] [PubMed]
87. Narimatsu, M.; Bose, R.; Pye, M.; Zhang, L.; Miller, B.; Ching, P.; Sakuma, R.; Luga, V.; Roncari, L.; Attisano, L.; et al. Regulation of planar cell polarity by Smurf ubiquitin ligases. *Cell* **2009**, *137*, 295–307. [CrossRef]
88. Lee, M.S.; Han, H.J.; Han, S.Y.; Kim, I.Y.; Chae, S.; Lee, C.S.; Kim, S.E.; Yoon, S.G.; Park, J.W.; Kim, J.H.; et al. Loss of the E3 ubiquitin ligase MKRN1 represses diet-induced metabolic syndrome through AMPK activation. *Nat. Commun.* **2018**, *9*, 3404. [CrossRef]
89. Lu, C.; Thoeni, C.; Connor, A.; Kawabe, H.; Gallinger, S.; Rotin, D. Intestinal knockout of Nedd4 enhances growth of Apc(min) tumors. *Oncogene* **2016**, *35*, 5839–5849. [CrossRef]
90. Grima, B.; Lamouroux, A.; Chelot, E.; Papin, C.; Limbourg-Bouchon, B.; Rouyer, F. The F-box protein slimb controls the levels of clock proteins period and timeless. *Nature* **2002**, *420*, 178–182. [CrossRef]
91. Nakagawa, T.; Zhang, T.; Kushi, R.; Nakano, S.; Endo, T.; Nakagawa, M.; Yanagihara, N.; Zarkower, D.; Nakayama, K. Regulation of mitosis-meiosis transition by the ubiquitin ligase beta-TrCP in male germ cells. *Development* **2017**, *144*, 4137–4147. [CrossRef] [PubMed]
92. Guardavaccaro, D.; Kudo, Y.; Boulaire, J.; Barchi, M.; Busino, L.; Donzelli, M.; Margottin-Goguet, F.; Jackson, P.K.; Yamasaki, L.; Pagano, M. Control of meiotic and mitotic progression by the F box protein beta-Trcp1 in vivo. *Dev. Cell* **2003**, *4*, 799–812. [CrossRef]
93. Ohsaki, K.; Oishi, K.; Kozono, Y.; Nakayama, K.; Nakayama, K.I.; Ishida, N. The role of {beta}-TrCP1 and {beta}-TrCP2 in circadian rhythm generation by mediating degradation of clock protein PER2. *J. Biochem.* **2008**, *144*, 609–618. [CrossRef] [PubMed]
94. Kanarek, N.; Horwitz, E.; Mayan, I.; Leshets, M.; Cojocaru, G.; Davis, M.; Tsuberi, B.Z.; Pikarsky, E.; Pagano, M.; Ben-Neriah, Y. Spermatogenesis rescue in a mouse deficient for the ubiquitin ligase SCF{beta}-TrCP by single substrate depletion. *Genes Dev.* **2010**, *24*, 470–477. [CrossRef] [PubMed]
95. Kudo, Y.; Guardavaccaro, D.; Santamaria, P.G.; Koyama-Nasu, R.; Latres, E.; Bronson, R.; Yamasaki, L.; Pagano, M. Role of F-box protein betaTrcp1 in mammary gland development and tumorigenesis. *Mol. Cell. Biol.* **2004**, *24*, 8184–8194. [CrossRef] [PubMed]
96. Baguma-Nibasheka, M.; Kablar, B. Abnormal retinal development in the Btrc null mouse. *Dev. Dyn.* **2009**, *238*, 2680–2687. [CrossRef]
97. Kanarek, N.; Grivennikov, S.I.; Leshets, M.; Lasry, A.; Alkalay, I.; Horwitz, E.; Shaul, Y.D.; Stachler, M.; Voronov, E.; Apte, R.N.; et al. Critical role for IL-1beta in DNA damage-induced mucositis. *Proc. Natl. Acad. Sci. USA* **2014**, *111*, E702–E711. [CrossRef]
98. Nakagawa, T.; Araki, T.; Nakagawa, M.; Hirao, A.; Unno, M.; Nakayama, K. S6 Kinase- and beta-TrCP2-Dependent Degradation of p19Arf Is Required for Cell Proliferation. *Mol. Cell. Biol.* **2015**, *35*, 3517–3527. [CrossRef]

99. Bond, C.E.; McKeone, D.M.; Kalimutho, M.; Bettington, M.L.; Pearson, S.A.; Dumenil, T.D.; Wockner, L.F.; Burge, M.; Leggett, B.A.; Whitehall, V.L. RNF43 and ZNRF3 are commonly altered in serrated pathway colorectal tumorigenesis. *Oncotarget* **2016**, *7*, 70589–70600. [CrossRef]
100. Giannakis, M.; Hodis, E.; Jasmine Mu, X.; Yamauchi, M.; Rosenbluh, J.; Cibulskis, K.; Saksena, G.; Lawrence, M.S.; Qian, Z.R.; Nishihara, R.; et al. RNF43 is frequently mutated in colorectal and endometrial cancers. *Nat. Genet.* **2014**, *46*, 1264–1266. [CrossRef]
101. Koo, B.K.; van Es, J.H.; van den Born, M.; Clevers, H. Porcupine inhibitor suppresses paracrine Wnt-driven growth of Rnf43;Znrf3-mutant neoplasia. *Proc. Natl. Acad. Sci. USA* **2015**, *112*, 7548–7550. [CrossRef] [PubMed]
102. Basham, K.J.; Rodriguez, S.; Turcu, A.F.; Lerario, A.M.; Logan, C.Y.; Rysztak, M.R.; Gomez-Sanchez, C.E.; Breault, D.T.; Koo, B.K.; Clevers, H.; et al. A ZNRF3-dependent Wnt/beta-catenin signaling gradient is required for adrenal homeostasis. *Genes Dev.* **2019**, *33*, 209–220. [CrossRef] [PubMed]
103. Jameson, S.A.; Lin, Y.T.; Capel, B. Testis development requires the repression of Wnt4 by Fgf signaling. *Dev. Biol.* **2012**, *370*, 24–32. [CrossRef] [PubMed]
104. Harris, A.; Siggers, P.; Corrochano, S.; Warr, N.; Sagar, D.; Grimes, D.T.; Suzuki, M.; Burdine, R.D.; Cong, F.; Koo, B.K.; et al. ZNRF3 functions in mammalian sex determination by inhibiting canonical WNT signaling. *Proc. Natl. Acad. Sci. USA* **2018**, *115*, 5474–5479. [CrossRef] [PubMed]
105. Shen, J.; Yu, Z.; Li, N. The E3 ubiquitin ligase RNF146 promotes colorectal cancer by activating the Wnt/beta-catenin pathway via ubiquitination of Axin1. *Biochem. Biophys. Res. Commun.* **2018**, *503*, 991–997. [CrossRef]
106. Wei, W.; Zeve, D.; Suh, J.M.; Wang, X.; Du, Y.; Zerwekh, J.E.; Dechow, P.C.; Graff, J.M.; Wan, Y. Biphasic and dosage-dependent regulation of osteoclastogenesis by beta-catenin. *Mol. Cell. Biol.* **2011**, *31*, 4706–4719. [CrossRef]
107. Matsumoto, Y.; Larose, J.; Kent, O.A.; Lim, M.; Changoor, A.; Zhang, L.; Storozhuk, Y.; Mao, X.; Grynpas, M.D.; Cong, F.; et al. RANKL coordinates multiple osteoclastogenic pathways by regulating expression of ubiquitin ligase RNF146. *J. Clin. Investig.* **2017**, *127*, 1303–1315. [CrossRef]
108. Ueki, Y.; Tiziani, V.; Santanna, C.; Fukai, N.; Maulik, C.; Garfinkle, J.; Ninomiya, C.; doAmaral, C.; Peters, H.; Habal, M.; et al. Mutations in the gene encoding c-Abl-binding protein SH3BP2 cause cherubism. *Nat. Genet.* **2001**, *28*, 125–126. [CrossRef]
109. Levaot, N.; Voytyuk, O.; Dimitriou, I.; Sircoulomb, F.; Chandrakumar, A.; Deckert, M.; Krzyzanowski, P.M.; Scotter, A.; Gu, S.; Janmohamed, S.; et al. Loss of Tankyrase-mediated destruction of 3BP2 is the underlying pathogenic mechanism of cherubism. *Cell* **2011**, *147*, 1324–1339. [CrossRef]
110. Zou, Y.F.; Xie, C.W.; Yang, S.X.; Xiong, J.P. AMPK activators suppress breast cancer cell growth by inhibiting DVL3-facilitated Wnt/beta-catenin signaling pathway activity. *Mol. Med. Rep.* **2017**, *15*, 899–907. [CrossRef]
111. Lee, H.; Kang, R.; Bae, S.; Yoon, Y. AICAR, an activator of AMPK, inhibits adipogenesis via the WNT/beta-catenin pathway in 3T3-L1 adipocytes. *Int. J. Mol. Med.* **2011**, *28*, 65–71. [CrossRef] [PubMed]
112. Inoki, K.; Ouyang, H.; Zhu, T.; Lindvall, C.; Wang, Y.; Zhang, X.; Yang, Q.; Bennett, C.; Harada, Y.; Stankunas, K.; et al. TSC2 integrates Wnt and energy signals via a coordinated phosphorylation by AMPK and GSK3 to regulate cell growth. *Cell* **2006**, *126*, 955–968. [CrossRef] [PubMed]
113. Park, S.Y.; Kim, D.; Kee, S.H. Metformin-activated AMPK regulates beta-catenin to reduce cell proliferation in colon carcinoma RKO cells. *Oncol. Lett.* **2019**, *17*, 2695–2702. [CrossRef] [PubMed]
114. Kondo, S.; Seo, S.Y.; Yoshizaki, T.; Wakisaka, N.; Furukawa, M.; Joab, I.; Jang, K.L.; Pagano, J.S. EBV latent membrane protein 1 up-regulates hypoxia-inducible factor 1alpha through Siah1-mediated down-regulation of prolyl hydroxylases 1 and 3 in nasopharyngeal epithelial cells. *Cancer Res.* **2006**, *66*, 9870–9877. [CrossRef]
115. Dickins, R.A.; Frew, I.J.; House, C.M.; O'Bryan, M.K.; Holloway, A.J.; Haviv, I.; Traficante, N.; de Kretser, D.M.; Bowtell, D.D. The ubiquitin ligase component Siah1a is required for completion of meiosis I in male mice. *Mol. Cell. Biol.* **2002**, *22*, 2294–2303. [CrossRef]
116. Frew, I.J.; Sims, N.A.; Quinn, J.M.; Walkley, C.R.; Purton, L.E.; Bowtell, D.D.; Gillespie, M.T. Osteopenia in Siah1a mutant mice. *J. Biol. Chem.* **2004**, *279*, 29583–29588. [CrossRef]
117. Frew, I.J.; Hammond, V.E.; Dickins, R.A.; Quinn, J.M.; Walkley, C.R.; Sims, N.A.; Schnall, R.; Della, N.G.; Holloway, A.J.; Digby, M.R.; et al. Generation and analysis of Siah2 mutant mice. *Mol. Cell. Biol.* **2003**, *23*, 9150–9161. [CrossRef]

118. Scortegagna, M.; Kim, H.; Li, J.L.; Yao, H.; Brill, L.M.; Han, J.; Lau, E.; Bowtell, D.; Haddad, G.; Kaufman, R.J.; et al. Fine tuning of the UPR by the ubiquitin ligases Siah1/2. *PLoS Genet.* **2014**, *10*, e1004348. [CrossRef]
119. Wang, D.; Wang, Y.; Kong, T.; Fan, F.; Jiang, Y. Hypoxia-induced beta-catenin downregulation involves p53-dependent activation of Siah-1. *Cancer Sci.* **2011**, *102*, 1322–1328. [CrossRef]
120. Simon, M.C. Siah proteins, HIF prolyl hydroxylases, and the physiological response to hypoxia. *Cell* **2004**, *117*, 851–853. [CrossRef]
121. Gudjonsson, T.; Altmeyer, M.; Savic, V.; Toledo, L.; Dinant, C.; Grofte, M.; Bartkova, J.; Poulsen, M.; Oka, Y.; Bekker-Jensen, S.; et al. TRIP12 and UBR5 suppress spreading of chromatin ubiquitylation at damaged chromosomes. *Cell* **2012**, *150*, 697–709. [CrossRef] [PubMed]
122. Shearer, R.F.; Iconomou, M.; Watts, C.K.; Saunders, D.N. Functional Roles of the E3 Ubiquitin Ligase UBR5 in Cancer. *Mol. Cancer Res.* **2015**, *13*, 1523–1532. [CrossRef] [PubMed]
123. Saunders, D.N.; Hird, S.L.; Withington, S.L.; Dunwoodie, S.L.; Henderson, M.J.; Biben, C.; Sutherland, R.L.; Ormandy, C.J.; Watts, C.K. Edd, the murine hyperplastic disc gene, is essential for yolk sac vascularization and chorioallantoic fusion. *Mol. Cell. Biol.* **2004**, *24*, 7225–7234. [CrossRef] [PubMed]
124. Ishikawa, T.; Tamai, Y.; Zorn, A.M.; Yoshida, H.; Seldin, M.F.; Nishikawa, S.; Taketo, M.M. Mouse Wnt receptor gene Fzd5 is essential for yolk sac and placental angiogenesis. *Development* **2001**, *128*, 25–33.
125. Kinsella, E.; Dora, N.; Mellis, D.; Lettice, L.; Deveney, P.; Hill, R.; Ditzel, M. Use of a Conditional Ubr5 Mutant Allele to Investigate the Role of an N-End Rule Ubiquitin-Protein Ligase in Hedgehog Signalling and Embryonic Limb Development. *PLoS ONE* **2016**, *11*, e0157079. [CrossRef]
126. Ye, X.; Wang, L.; Shang, B.; Wang, Z.; Wei, W. NEDD4: A promising target for cancer therapy. *Curr. Cancer Drug Targets* **2014**, *14*, 549–556. [CrossRef]
127. Li, J.J.; Ferry, R.J., Jr.; Diao, S.; Xue, B.; Bahouth, S.W.; Liao, F.F. Nedd4 haploinsufficient mice display moderate insulin resistance, enhanced lipolysis, and protection against high-fat diet-induced obesity. *Endocrinology* **2015**, *156*, 1283–1291. [CrossRef]
128. Liu, Y.; Oppenheim, R.W.; Sugiura, Y.; Lin, W. Abnormal development of the neuromuscular junction in Nedd4-deficient mice. *Dev. Biol.* **2009**, *330*, 153–166. [CrossRef]
129. Kawabe, H.; Neeb, A.; Dimova, K.; Young, S.M., Jr.; Takeda, M.; Katsurabayashi, S.; Mitkovski, M.; Malakhova, O.A.; Zhang, D.E.; Umikawa, M.; et al. Regulation of Rap2A by the ubiquitin ligase Nedd4-1 controls neurite development. *Neuron* **2010**, *65*, 358–372. [CrossRef]
130. Cao, X.R.; Lill, N.L.; Boase, N.; Shi, P.P.; Croucher, D.R.; Shan, H.; Qu, J.; Sweezer, E.M.; Place, T.; Kirby, P.A.; et al. Nedd4 controls animal growth by regulating IGF-1 signaling. *Sci. Signal.* **2008**, *1*. [CrossRef]
131. Fouladkou, F.; Lu, C.; Jiang, C.; Zhou, L.; She, Y.; Walls, J.R.; Kawabe, H.; Brose, N.; Henkelman, R.M.; Huang, A.; et al. The ubiquitin ligase Nedd4-1 is required for heart development and is a suppressor of thrombospondin-1. *J. Biol. Chem.* **2010**, *285*, 6770–6780. [CrossRef] [PubMed]
132. Lee, J.H.; Jeon, S.A.; Kim, B.G.; Takeda, M.; Cho, J.J.; Kim, D.I.; Kawabe, H.; Cho, J.Y. Nedd4 Deficiency in Vascular Smooth Muscle Promotes Vascular Calcification by Stabilizing pSmad1. *J. Bone Min. Res.* **2017**, *32*, 927–938. [CrossRef] [PubMed]
133. Jeon, S.A.; Lee, J.H.; Kim, D.W.; Cho, J.Y. E3-ubiquitin ligase NEDD4 enhances bone formation by removing TGFbeta1-induced pSMAD1 in immature osteoblast. *Bone* **2018**, *116*, 248–258. [CrossRef] [PubMed]
134. Wiszniak, S.; Harvey, N.; Schwarz, Q. Cell autonomous roles of Nedd4 in craniofacial bone formation. *Dev. Biol.* **2016**, *410*, 98–107. [CrossRef] [PubMed]
135. Wiszniak, S.; Kabbara, S.; Lumb, R.; Scherer, M.; Secker, G.; Harvey, N.; Kumar, S.; Schwarz, Q. The ubiquitin ligase Nedd4 regulates craniofacial development by promoting cranial neural crest cell survival and stem-cell like properties. *Dev. Biol.* **2013**, *383*, 186–200. [CrossRef] [PubMed]
136. Yang, B.; Gay, D.L.; MacLeod, M.K.; Cao, X.; Hala, T.; Sweezer, E.M.; Kappler, J.; Marrack, P.; Oliver, P.M. Nedd4 augments the adaptive immune response by promoting ubiquitin-mediated degradation of Cbl-b in activated T cells. *Nat. Immunol.* **2008**, *9*, 1356–1363. [CrossRef] [PubMed]
137. Guo, H.; Qiao, G.; Ying, H.; Li, Z.; Zhao, Y.; Liang, Y.; Yang, L.; Lipkowitz, S.; Penninger, J.M.; Langdon, W.Y.; et al. E3 ubiquitin ligase Cbl-b regulates Pten via Nedd4 in T cells independently of its ubiquitin ligase activity. *Cell Rep.* **2012**, *1*, 472–482. [CrossRef]
138. Russo, C.J.; Melista, E.; Cui, J.; DeStefano, A.L.; Bakris, G.L.; Manolis, A.J.; Gavras, H.; Baldwin, C.T. Association of NEDD4L ubiquitin ligase with essential hypertension. *Hypertension* **2005**, *46*, 488–491. [CrossRef]

139. Yanpallewar, S.; Wang, T.; Koh, D.C.; Quarta, E.; Fulgenzi, G.; Tessarollo, L. Nedd4-2 haploinsufficiency causes hyperactivity and increased sensitivity to inflammatory stimuli. *Sci. Rep.* **2016**, *6*, 32957. [CrossRef]
140. Harvey, K.F.; Dinudom, A.; Cook, D.I.; Kumar, S. The Nedd4-like protein KIAA0439 is a potential regulator of the epithelial sodium channel. *J. Biol. Chem.* **2001**, *276*, 8597–8601. [CrossRef]
141. Zhou, R.; Patel, S.V.; Snyder, P.M. Nedd4-2 catalyzes ubiquitination and degradation of cell surface ENaC. *J. Biol. Chem.* **2007**, *282*, 20207–20212. [CrossRef] [PubMed]
142. Hanukoglu, I.; Hanukoglu, A. Epithelial sodium channel (ENaC) family: Phylogeny, structure-function, tissue distribution, and associated inherited diseases. *Gene* **2016**, *579*, 95–132. [CrossRef] [PubMed]
143. Sun, C.; Hummler, E.; Hill, D.L. Selective Deletion of Sodium Salt Taste during Development Leads to Expanded Terminal Fields of Gustatory Nerves in the Adult Mouse Nucleus of the Solitary Tract. *J. Neurosci. Off. J. Soc. Neurosci.* **2017**, *37*, 660–672. [CrossRef] [PubMed]
144. Shi, P.P.; Cao, X.R.; Sweezer, E.M.; Kinney, T.S.; Williams, N.R.; Husted, R.F.; Nair, R.; Weiss, R.M.; Williamson, R.A.; Sigmund, C.D.; et al. Salt-sensitive hypertension and cardiac hypertrophy in mice deficient in the ubiquitin ligase Nedd4-2. *Am. J. Physiol. Ren. Physiol.* **2008**, *295*, F462–F470. [CrossRef] [PubMed]
145. Boase, N.A.; Rychkov, G.Y.; Townley, S.L.; Dinudom, A.; Candi, E.; Voss, A.K.; Tsoutsman, T.; Semsarian, C.; Melino, G.; Koentgen, F.; et al. Respiratory distress and perinatal lethality in Nedd4-2-deficient mice. *Nat. Commun.* **2011**, *2*, 287. [CrossRef] [PubMed]
146. Henshall, T.L.; Manning, J.A.; Alfassy, O.S.; Goel, P.; Boase, N.A.; Kawabe, H.; Kumar, S. Deletion of Nedd4-2 results in progressive kidney disease in mice. *Cell Death Differ.* **2017**, *24*, 2150–2160. [CrossRef] [PubMed]
147. Yip, K.H.; Kolesnikoff, N.; Hauschild, N.; Biggs, L.; Lopez, A.F.; Galli, S.J.; Kumar, S.; Grimbaldeston, M.A. The Nedd4-2/Ndfip1 axis is a negative regulator of IgE-mediated mast cell activation. *Nat. Commun.* **2016**, *7*, 13198. [CrossRef]
148. Infante, P.; Lospinoso Severini, L.; Bernardi, F.; Bufalieri, F.; Di Marcotullio, L. Targeting Hedgehog Signalling through the Ubiquitylation Process: The Multiple Roles of the HECT-E3 Ligase Itch. *Cells* **2019**, *8*. [CrossRef]
149. Liu, Y.C. The E3 ubiquitin ligase Itch in T cell activation, differentiation, and tolerance. *Semin. Immunol.* **2007**, *19*, 197–205. [CrossRef]
150. Gao, M.; Labuda, T.; Xia, Y.; Gallagher, E.; Fang, D.; Liu, Y.C.; Karin, M. Jun turnover is controlled through JNK-dependent phosphorylation of the E3 ligase Itch. *Science* **2004**, *306*, 271–275. [CrossRef]
151. Lohr, N.J.; Molleston, J.P.; Strauss, K.A.; Torres-Martinez, W.; Sherman, E.A.; Squires, R.H.; Rider, N.L.; Chikwava, K.R.; Cummings, O.W.; Morton, D.H.; et al. Human ITCH E3 ubiquitin ligase deficiency causes syndromic multisystem autoimmune disease. *Am. J. Hum. Genet.* **2010**, *86*, 447–453. [CrossRef]
152. Perry, W.L.; Hustad, C.M.; Swing, D.A.; O'Sullivan, T.N.; Jenkins, N.A.; Copeland, N.G. The itchy locus encodes a novel ubiquitin protein ligase that is disrupted in a18H mice. *Nat. Genet.* **1998**, *18*, 143–146. [CrossRef] [PubMed]
153. Hustad, C.M.; Perry, W.L.; Siracusa, L.D.; Rasberry, C.; Cobb, L.; Cattanach, B.M.; Kovatch, R.; Copeland, N.G.; Jenkins, N.A. Molecular genetic characterization of six recessive viable alleles of the mouse agouti locus. *Genetics* **1995**, *140*, 255–265. [PubMed]
154. Fang, D.; Elly, C.; Gao, B.; Fang, N.; Altman, Y.; Joazeiro, C.; Hunter, T.; Copeland, N.; Jenkins, N.; Liu, Y.C. Dysregulation of T lymphocyte function in itchy mice: A role for Itch in TH2 differentiation. *Nat. Immunol.* **2002**, *3*, 281–287. [CrossRef] [PubMed]
155. Jin, H.S.; Park, Y.; Elly, C.; Liu, Y.C. Itch expression by Treg cells controls Th2 inflammatory responses. *J. Clin. Investig.* **2013**, *123*, 4923–4934. [CrossRef] [PubMed]
156. Xiao, N.; Eto, D.; Elly, C.; Peng, G.; Crotty, S.; Liu, Y.C. The E3 ubiquitin ligase Itch is required for the differentiation of follicular helper T cells. *Nat. Immunol.* **2014**, *15*, 657–666. [CrossRef]
157. Huang, H.; Jeon, M.S.; Liao, L.; Yang, C.; Elly, C.; Yates, J.R., 3rd; Liu, Y.C. K33-linked polyubiquitination of T cell receptor-zeta regulates proteolysis-independent T cell signaling. *Immunity* **2010**, *33*, 60–70. [CrossRef]
158. Giamboi-Miraglia, A.; Cianfarani, F.; Cattani, C.; Lena, A.M.; Serra, V.; Campione, E.; Terrinoni, A.; Zambruno, G.; Odorisio, T.; Di Daniele, N.; et al. The E3 ligase Itch knockout mice show hyperproliferation and wound healing alteration. *FEBS J* **2015**, *282*, 4435–4449. [CrossRef]
159. Stermer, A.R.; Myers, J.L.; Murphy, C.J.; Di Bona, K.R.; Matesic, L.; Richburg, J.H. Female mice with loss-of-function ITCH display an altered reproductive phenotype. *Exp. Biol. Med. (Maywood)* **2016**, *241*, 367–374. [CrossRef]

160. Marino, A.; Menghini, R.; Fabrizi, M.; Casagrande, V.; Mavilio, M.; Stoehr, R.; Candi, E.; Mauriello, A.; Moreno-Navarrete, J.M.; Gomez-Serrano, M.; et al. ITCH deficiency protects from diet-induced obesity. *Diabetes* **2014**, *63*, 550–561. [CrossRef]
161. Chang, L.; Kamata, H.; Solinas, G.; Luo, J.L.; Maeda, S.; Venuprasad, K.; Liu, Y.C.; Karin, M. The E3 ubiquitin ligase itch couples JNK activation to TNFalpha-induced cell death by inducing c-FLIP(L) turnover. *Cell* **2006**, *124*, 601–613. [CrossRef] [PubMed]
162. Rathinam, C.; Matesic, L.E.; Flavell, R.A. The E3 ligase Itch is a negative regulator of the homeostasis and function of hematopoietic stem cells. *Nat. Immunol.* **2011**, *12*, 399–407. [CrossRef] [PubMed]
163. Thien, C.B.; Langdon, W.Y. c-Cbl and Cbl-b ubiquitin ligases: Substrate diversity and the negative regulation of signalling responses. *Biochem. J.* **2005**, *391*, 153–166. [CrossRef] [PubMed]
164. Mohapatra, B.; Ahmad, G.; Nadeau, S.; Zutshi, N.; An, W.; Scheffe, S.; Dong, L.; Feng, D.; Goetz, B.; Arya, P.; et al. Protein tyrosine kinase regulation by ubiquitination: Critical roles of Cbl-family ubiquitin ligases. *Biochim. Biophys. Acta* **2013**, *1833*, 122–139. [CrossRef] [PubMed]
165. Tanaka, S.; Neff, L.; Baron, R.; Levy, J.B. Tyrosine phosphorylation and translocation of the c-cbl protein after activation of tyrosine kinase signaling pathways. *J. Biol. Chem.* **1995**, *270*, 14347–14351. [CrossRef] [PubMed]
166. Naramura, M.; Kole, H.K.; Hu, R.J.; Gu, H. Altered thymic positive selection and intracellular signals in Cbl-deficient mice. *Proc. Natl. Acad. Sci. USA* **1998**, *95*, 15547–15552. [CrossRef] [PubMed]
167. Murphy, M.A.; Schnall, R.G.; Venter, D.J.; Barnett, L.; Bertoncello, I.; Thien, C.B.; Langdon, W.Y.; Bowtell, D.D. Tissue hyperplasia and enhanced T-cell signalling via ZAP-70 in c-Cbl-deficient mice. *Mol. Cell. Biol.* **1998**, *18*, 4872–4882. [CrossRef]
168. Naramura, M.; Jang, I.K.; Kole, H.; Huang, F.; Haines, D.; Gu, H. c-Cbl and Cbl-b regulate T cell responsiveness by promoting ligand-induced TCR down-modulation. *Nat. Immunol.* **2002**, *3*, 1192–1199. [CrossRef]
169. Bachmaier, K.; Krawczyk, C.; Kozieradzki, I.; Kong, Y.Y.; Sasaki, T.; Oliveira-dos-Santos, A.; Mariathasan, S.; Bouchard, D.; Wakeham, A.; Itie, A.; et al. Negative regulation of lymphocyte activation and autoimmunity by the molecular adaptor Cbl-b. *Nature* **2000**, *403*, 211–216. [CrossRef]
170. Wang, H.Y.; Altman, Y.; Fang, D.; Elly, C.; Dai, Y.; Shao, Y.; Liu, Y.C. Cbl promotes ubiquitination of the T cell receptor zeta through an adaptor function of Zap-70. *J. Biol. Chem.* **2001**, *276*, 26004–26011. [CrossRef]
171. D'Oro, U.; Munitic, I.; Chacko, G.; Karpova, T.; McNally, J.; Ashwell, J.D. Regulation of constitutive TCR internalization by the zeta-chain. *J. Immunol.* **2002**, *169*, 6269–6278. [CrossRef] [PubMed]
172. Lutz-Nicoladoni, C.; Wolf, D.; Sopper, S. Modulation of Immune Cell Functions by the E3 Ligase Cbl-b. *Front. Oncol.* **2015**, *5*, 58. [CrossRef] [PubMed]
173. Adams, C.O.; Housley, W.J.; Bhowmick, S.; Cone, R.E.; Rajan, T.V.; Forouhar, F.; Clark, R.B. Cbl-b(-/-) T cells demonstrate in vivo resistance to regulatory T cells but a context-dependent resistance to TGF-beta. *J. Immunol.* **2010**, *185*, 2051–2058. [CrossRef] [PubMed]
174. Chiusaroli, R.; Sanjay, A.; Henriksen, K.; Engsig, M.T.; Horne, W.C.; Gu, H.; Baron, R. Deletion of the gene encoding c-Cbl alters the ability of osteoclasts to migrate, delaying resorption and ossification of cartilage during the development of long bones. *Dev. Biol.* **2003**, *261*, 537–547. [CrossRef]
175. Molero, J.C.; Jensen, T.E.; Withers, P.C.; Couzens, M.; Herzog, H.; Thien, C.B.; Langdon, W.Y.; Walder, K.; Murphy, M.A.; Bowtell, D.D.; et al. c-Cbl-deficient mice have reduced adiposity, higher energy expenditure, and improved peripheral insulin action. *J. Clin. Investig.* **2004**, *114*, 1326–1333. [CrossRef]
176. Li, X.; Gadzinsky, A.; Gong, L.; Tong, H.; Calderon, V.; Li, Y.; Kitamura, D.; Klein, U.; Langdon, W.Y.; Hou, F.; et al. Cbl Ubiquitin Ligases Control B Cell Exit from the Germinal-Center Reaction. *Immunity* **2018**, *48*, 530–541.e536. [CrossRef]
177. Gustin, S.E.; Thien, C.B.; Langdon, W.Y. Cbl-b is a negative regulator of inflammatory cytokines produced by IgE-activated mast cells. *J. Immunol.* **2006**, *177*, 5980–5989. [CrossRef]
178. Naramura, M.; Nandwani, N.; Gu, H.; Band, V.; Band, H. Rapidly fatal myeloproliferative disorders in mice with deletion of Casitas B-cell lymphoma (Cbl) and Cbl-b in hematopoietic stem cells. *Proc. Natl. Acad. Sci. USA* **2010**, *107*, 16274–16279. [CrossRef]
179. Mohapatra, B.; Zutshi, N.; An, W.; Goetz, B.; Arya, P.; Bielecki, T.A.; Mushtaq, I.; Storck, M.D.; Meza, J.L.; Band, V.; et al. An essential role of CBL and CBL-B ubiquitin ligases in mammary stem cell maintenance. *Development* **2017**, *144*, 1072–1086. [CrossRef]
180. Meng, X.M.; Nikolic-Paterson, D.J.; Lan, H.Y. TGF-beta: The master regulator of fibrosis. *Nat. Rev. Nephrol.* **2016**, *12*, 325–338. [CrossRef]

181. Taipale, J.; Miyazono, K.; Heldin, C.H.; Keski-Oja, J. Latent transforming growth factor-beta 1 associates to fibroblast extracellular matrix via latent TGF-beta binding protein. *J. Cell Biol.* **1994**, *124*, 171–181. [CrossRef] [PubMed]
182. Massague, J. TGFbeta signalling in context. *Nat. Rev. Mol. Cell Biol.* **2012**, *13*, 616–630. [CrossRef] [PubMed]
183. Itoh, F.; Divecha, N.; Brocks, L.; Oomen, L.; Janssen, H.; Calafat, J.; Itoh, S.; Dijke Pt, P. The FYVE domain in Smad anchor for receptor activation (SARA) is sufficient for localization of SARA in early endosomes and regulates TGF-beta/Smad signalling. *Genes Cells Devoted Mol. Cell. Mech.* **2002**, *7*, 321–331. [CrossRef]
184. Miura, S.; Takeshita, T.; Asao, H.; Kimura, Y.; Murata, K.; Sasaki, Y.; Hanai, J.I.; Beppu, H.; Tsukazaki, T.; Wrana, J.L.; et al. Hgs (Hrs), a FYVE domain protein, is involved in Smad signaling through cooperation with SARA. *Mol. Cell. Biol.* **2000**, *20*, 9346–9355. [CrossRef]
185. Massague, J.; Seoane, J.; Wotton, D. Smad transcription factors. *Genes Dev.* **2005**, *19*, 2783–2810. [CrossRef]
186. Janknecht, R.; Wells, N.J.; Hunter, T. TGF-beta-stimulated cooperation of smad proteins with the coactivators CBP/p300. *Genes Dev.* **1998**, *12*, 2114–2119. [CrossRef]
187. Pei, D.; Shu, X.; Gassama-Diagne, A.; Thiery, J.P. Mesenchymal-epithelial transition in development and reprogramming. *Nat. Cell Biol.* **2019**, *21*, 44–53. [CrossRef]
188. Moustakas, A.; Kardassis, D. Regulation of the human p21/WAF1/Cip1 promoter in hepatic cells by functional interactions between Sp1 and Smad family members. *Proc. Natl. Acad. Sci. USA* **1998**, *95*, 6733–6738. [CrossRef]
189. Nakao, A.; Afrakhte, M.; Moren, A.; Nakayama, T.; Christian, J.L.; Heuchel, R.; Itoh, S.; Kawabata, M.; Heldin, N.E.; Heldin, C.H.; et al. Identification of Smad7, a TGFbeta-inducible antagonist of TGF-beta signalling. *Nature* **1997**, *389*, 631–635. [CrossRef]
190. Chong, P.A.; Lin, H.; Wrana, J.L.; Forman-Kay, J.D. An expanded WW domain recognition motif revealed by the interaction between Smad7 and the E3 ubiquitin ligase Smurf2. *J. Biol. Chem.* **2006**, *281*, 17069–17075. [CrossRef]
191. Kavsak, P.; Rasmussen, R.K.; Causing, C.G.; Bonni, S.; Zhu, H.; Thomsen, G.H.; Wrana, J.L. Smad7 binds to Smurf2 to form an E3 ubiquitin ligase that targets the TGF beta receptor for degradation. *Mol. Cell* **2000**, *6*, 1365–1375. [CrossRef]
192. Zhou, F.; Li, F.; Xie, F.; Zhang, Z.; Huang, H.; Zhang, L. TRAF4 mediates activation of TGF-beta signaling and is a biomarker for oncogenesis in breast cancer. *Sci. China Life Sci.* **2014**, *57*, 1172–1176. [CrossRef] [PubMed]
193. Wang, X.; Jin, C.; Tang, Y.; Tang, L.Y.; Zhang, Y.E. Ubiquitination of tumor necrosis factor receptor-associated factor 4 (TRAF4) by Smad ubiquitination regulatory factor 1 (Smurf1) regulates motility of breast epithelial and cancer cells. *J. Biol. Chem.* **2013**, *288*, 21784–21792. [CrossRef] [PubMed]
194. Zhang, L.; Zhou, F.; Garcia de Vinuesa, A.; de Kruijf, E.M.; Mesker, W.E.; Hui, L.; Drabsch, Y.; Li, Y.; Bauer, A.; Rousseau, A.; et al. TRAF4 promotes TGF-beta receptor signaling and drives breast cancer metastasis. *Mol. Cell* **2013**, *51*, 559–572. [CrossRef] [PubMed]
195. Zhang, Y.; Chang, C.; Gehling, D.J.; Hemmati-Brivanlou, A.; Derynck, R. Regulation of Smad degradation and activity by Smurf2, an E3 ubiquitin ligase. *Proc. Natl. Acad. Sci. USA* **2001**, *98*, 974–979. [CrossRef] [PubMed]
196. Tang, L.Y.; Yamashita, M.; Coussens, N.P.; Tang, Y.; Wang, X.; Li, C.; Deng, C.X.; Cheng, S.Y.; Zhang, Y.E. Ablation of Smurf2 reveals an inhibition in TGF-beta signalling through multiple mono-ubiquitination of Smad3. *EMBO J.* **2011**, *30*, 4777–4789. [CrossRef]
197. Bonni, S.; Wang, H.R.; Causing, C.G.; Kavsak, P.; Stroschein, S.L.; Luo, K.; Wrana, J.L. TGF-beta induces assembly of a Smad2-Smurf2 ubiquitin ligase complex that targets SnoN for degradation. *Nat. Cell Biol.* **2001**, *3*, 587–595. [CrossRef]
198. Alarcon, C.; Zaromytidou, A.I.; Xi, Q.; Gao, S.; Yu, J.; Fujisawa, S.; Barlas, A.; Miller, A.N.; Manova-Todorova, K.; Macias, M.J.; et al. Nuclear CDKs drive Smad transcriptional activation and turnover in BMP and TGF-beta pathways. *Cell* **2009**, *139*, 757–769. [CrossRef]
199. Aragon, E.; Goerner, N.; Zaromytidou, A.I.; Xi, Q.; Escobedo, A.; Massague, J.; Macias, M.J. A Smad action turnover switch operated by WW domain readers of a phosphoserine code. *Genes Dev.* **2011**, *25*, 1275–1288. [CrossRef]
200. Bai, Y.; Yang, C.; Hu, K.; Elly, C.; Liu, Y.C. Itch E3 ligase-mediated regulation of TGF-beta signaling by modulating smad2 phosphorylation. *Mol. Cell* **2004**, *15*, 825–831. [CrossRef]

201. Park, S.H.; Jung, E.H.; Kim, G.Y.; Kim, B.C.; Lim, J.H.; Woo, C.H. Itch E3 ubiquitin ligase positively regulates TGF-beta signaling to EMT via Smad7 ubiquitination. *Mol. Cells* **2015**, *38*, 20–25. [CrossRef] [PubMed]
202. Pefani, D.E.; Pankova, D.; Abraham, A.G.; Grawenda, A.M.; Vlahov, N.; Scrace, S.; O'Neill, E. TGF-beta Targets the Hippo Pathway Scaffold RASSF1A to Facilitate YAP/SMAD2 Nuclear Translocation. *Mol. Cell* **2016**, *63*, 156–166. [CrossRef] [PubMed]
203. Koinuma, D.; Shinozaki, M.; Komuro, A.; Goto, K.; Saitoh, M.; Hanyu, A.; Ebina, M.; Nukiwa, T.; Miyazawa, K.; Imamura, T.; et al. Arkadia amplifies TGF-beta superfamily signalling through degradation of Smad7. *EMBO J.* **2003**, *22*, 6458–6470. [CrossRef] [PubMed]
204. Liu, F.Y.; Li, X.Z.; Peng, Y.M.; Liu, H.; Liu, Y.H. Arkadia-Smad7-mediated positive regulation of TGF-beta signaling in a rat model of tubulointerstitial fibrosis. *Am. J. Nephrol.* **2007**, *27*, 176–183. [CrossRef]
205. Liu, W.; Rui, H.; Wang, J.; Lin, S.; He, Y.; Chen, M.; Li, Q.; Ye, Z.; Zhang, S.; Chan, S.C.; et al. Axin is a scaffold protein in TGF-beta signaling that promotes degradation of Smad7 by Arkadia. *EMBO J.* **2006**, *25*, 1646–1658. [CrossRef]
206. Zhang, L.; Huang, H.; Zhou, F.; Schimmel, J.; Pardo, C.G.; Zhang, T.; Barakat, T.S.; Sheppard, K.A.; Mickanin, C.; Porter, J.A.; et al. RNF12 controls embryonic stem cell fate and morphogenesis in zebrafish embryos by targeting Smad7 for degradation. *Mol. Cell* **2012**, *46*, 650–661. [CrossRef]
207. Nagano, Y.; Mavrakis, K.J.; Lee, K.L.; Fujii, T.; Koinuma, D.; Sase, H.; Yuki, K.; Isogaya, K.; Saitoh, M.; Imamura, T.; et al. Arkadia induces degradation of SnoN and c-Ski to enhance transforming growth factor-beta signaling. *J. Biol. Chem.* **2007**, *282*, 20492–20501. [CrossRef]
208. Inoue, Y.; Imamura, T. Regulation of TGF-beta family signaling by E3 ubiquitin ligases. *Cancer Sci.* **2008**, *99*, 2107–2112. [CrossRef]
209. Le Scolan, E.; Zhu, Q.; Wang, L.; Bandyopadhyay, A.; Javelaud, D.; Mauviel, A.; Sun, L.; Luo, K. Transforming growth factor-beta suppresses the ability of Ski to inhibit tumor metastasis by inducing its degradation. *Cancer Res.* **2008**, *68*, 3277–3285. [CrossRef]
210. Huang, Y.; Yang, Y.; Gao, R.; Yang, X.; Yan, X.; Wang, C.; Jiang, S.; Yu, L. RLIM interacts with Smurf2 and promotes TGF-beta induced U2OS cell migration. *Biochem. Biophys. Res. Commun.* **2011**, *414*, 181–185. [CrossRef]
211. Gruber, T.; Hinterleitner, R.; Hermann-Kleiter, N.; Meisel, M.; Kleiter, I.; Wang, C.M.; Viola, A.; Pfeifhofer-Obermair, C.; Baier, G. Cbl-b mediates TGFbeta sensitivity by downregulating inhibitory SMAD7 in primary T cells. *J. Mol. Cell Biol.* **2013**, *5*, 358–368. [CrossRef] [PubMed]
212. Xie, F.; Jin, K.; Shao, L.; Fan, Y.; Tu, Y.; Li, Y.; Yang, B.; van Dam, H.; Ten Dijke, P.; Weng, H.; et al. FAF1 phosphorylation by AKT accumulates TGF-beta type II receptor and drives breast cancer metastasis. *Nat. Commun.* **2017**, *8*, 15021. [CrossRef] [PubMed]
213. He, W.; Dorn, D.C.; Erdjument-Bromage, H.; Tempst, P.; Moore, M.A.; Massague, J. Hematopoiesis controlled by distinct TIF1gamma and Smad4 branches of the TGFbeta pathway. *Cell* **2006**, *125*, 929–941. [CrossRef] [PubMed]
214. Morsut, L.; Yan, K.P.; Enzo, E.; Aragona, M.; Soligo, S.M.; Wendling, O.; Mark, M.; Khetchoumian, K.; Bressan, G.; Chambon, P.; et al. Negative control of Smad activity by ectodermin/Tif1gamma patterns the mammalian embryo. *Development* **2010**, *137*, 2571–2578. [CrossRef] [PubMed]
215. Xi, Q.; Wang, Z.; Zaromytidou, A.I.; Zhang, X.H.; Chow-Tsang, L.F.; Liu, J.X.; Kim, H.; Barlas, A.; Manova-Todorova, K.; Kaartinen, V.; et al. A poised chromatin platform for TGF-beta access to master regulators. *Cell* **2011**, *147*, 1511–1524. [CrossRef] [PubMed]
216. Agricola, E.; Randall, R.A.; Gaarenstroom, T.; Dupont, S.; Hill, C.S. Recruitment of TIF1gamma to chromatin via its PHD finger-bromodomain activates its ubiquitin ligase and transcriptional repressor activities. *Mol. Cell* **2011**, *43*, 85–96. [CrossRef] [PubMed]
217. Tracy Cai, X.; Li, H.; Safyan, A.; Gawlik, J.; Pyrowolakis, G.; Jasper, H. AWD regulates timed activation of BMP signaling in intestinal stem cells to maintain tissue homeostasis. *Nat. Commun.* **2019**, *10*, 2988. [CrossRef]
218. McCabe, B.D.; Hom, S.; Aberle, H.; Fetter, R.D.; Marques, G.; Haerry, T.E.; Wan, H.; O'Connor, M.B.; Goodman, C.S.; Haghighi, A.P. Highwire regulates presynaptic BMP signaling essential for synaptic growth. *Neuron* **2004**, *41*, 891–905. [CrossRef]

219. Liang, M.; Liang, Y.Y.; Wrighton, K.; Ungermannova, D.; Wang, X.P.; Brunicardi, F.C.; Liu, X.; Feng, X.H.; Lin, X. Ubiquitination and proteolysis of cancer-derived Smad4 mutants by SCFSkp2. *Mol. Cell. Biol.* **2004**, *24*, 7524–7537. [CrossRef]
220. Yang, X.; Li, C.; Xu, X.; Deng, C. The tumor suppressor SMAD4/DPC4 is essential for epiblast proliferation and mesoderm induction in mice. *Proc. Natl. Acad. Sci. USA* **1998**, *95*, 3667–3672. [CrossRef]
221. Shull, M.M.; Ormsby, I.; Kier, A.B.; Pawlowski, S.; Diebold, R.J.; Yin, M.; Allen, R.; Sidman, C.; Proetzel, G.; Calvin, D.; et al. Targeted disruption of the mouse transforming growth factor-beta 1 gene results in multifocal inflammatory disease. *Nature* **1992**, *359*, 693–699. [CrossRef] [PubMed]
222. Mavrakis, K.J.; Andrew, R.L.; Lee, K.L.; Petropoulou, C.; Dixon, J.E.; Navaratnam, N.; Norris, D.P.; Episkopou, V. Arkadia enhances Nodal/TGF-beta signaling by coupling phospho-Smad2/3 activity and turnover. *PLoS Biol.* **2007**, *5*, e67. [CrossRef] [PubMed]
223. Yamashita, M.; Ying, S.X.; Zhang, G.M.; Li, C.; Cheng, S.Y.; Deng, C.X.; Zhang, Y.E. Ubiquitin ligase Smurf1 controls osteoblast activity and bone homeostasis by targeting MEKK2 for degradation. *Cell* **2005**, *121*, 101–113. [CrossRef] [PubMed]
224. Ramkumar, C.; Kong, Y.; Trabucco, S.E.; Gerstein, R.M.; Zhang, H. Smurf2 regulates hematopoietic stem cell self-renewal and aging. *Aging Cell* **2014**, *13*, 478–486. [CrossRef]
225. Zhao, L.; Huang, J.; Guo, R.; Wang, Y.; Chen, D.; Xing, L. Smurf1 inhibits mesenchymal stem cell proliferation and differentiation into osteoblasts through JunB degradation. *J. Bone Min. Res.* **2010**, *25*, 1246–1256. [CrossRef]
226. Guo, R.; Yamashita, M.; Zhang, Q.; Zhou, Q.; Chen, D.; Reynolds, D.G.; Awad, H.A.; Yanoso, L.; Zhao, L.; Schwarz, E.M.; et al. Ubiquitin ligase Smurf1 mediates tumor necrosis factor-induced systemic bone loss by promoting proteasomal degradation of bone morphogenetic signaling proteins. *J. Biol. Chem.* **2008**, *283*, 23084–23092. [CrossRef]
227. Zhu, K.; Tang, Y.; Xu, X.; Dang, H.; Tang, L.Y.; Wang, X.; Wang, X.W.; Zhang, Y.E. Non-proteolytic ubiquitin modification of PPARgamma by Smurf1 protects the liver from steatosis. *PLoS Biol.* **2018**, *16*, e3000091. [CrossRef]
228. Ramkumar, C.; Kong, Y.; Cui, H.; Hao, S.; Jones, S.N.; Gerstein, R.M.; Zhang, H. Smurf2 regulates the senescence response and suppresses tumorigenesis in mice. *Cancer Res.* **2012**, *72*, 2714–2719. [CrossRef]
229. Ramkumar, C.; Cui, H.; Kong, Y.; Jones, S.N.; Gerstein, R.M.; Zhang, H. Smurf2 suppresses B-cell proliferation and lymphomagenesis by mediating ubiquitination and degradation of YY1. *Nat. Commun.* **2013**, *4*, 2598. [CrossRef]
230. Sriramachandran, A.M.; Meyer-Teschendorf, K.; Pabst, S.; Ulrich, H.D.; Gehring, N.H.; Hofmann, K.; Praefcke, G.J.K.; Dohmen, R.J. Arkadia/RNF111 is a SUMO-targeted ubiquitin ligase with preference for substrates marked with SUMO1-capped SUMO2/3 chain. *Nat. Commun.* **2019**, *10*, 3678. [CrossRef]
231. Sharma, V.; Antonacopoulou, A.G.; Tanaka, S.; Panoutsopoulos, A.A.; Bravou, V.; Kalofonos, H.P.; Episkopou, V. Enhancement of TGF-beta signaling responses by the E3 ubiquitin ligase Arkadia provides tumor suppression in colorectal cancer. *Cancer Res.* **2011**, *71*, 6438–6449. [CrossRef] [PubMed]
232. Episkopou, V.; Arkell, R.; Timmons, P.M.; Walsh, J.J.; Andrew, R.L.; Swan, D. Induction of the mammalian node requires Arkadia function in the extraembryonic lineages. *Nature* **2001**, *410*, 825–830. [CrossRef] [PubMed]
233. Carrano, A.C.; Eytan, E.; Hershko, A.; Pagano, M. SKP2 is required for ubiquitin-mediated degradation of the CDK inhibitor p27. *Nat. Cell. Biol.* **1999**, *1*, 193–199. [CrossRef] [PubMed]
234. Tsvetkov, L.M.; Yeh, K.H.; Lee, S.J.; Sun, H.; Zhang, H. p27(Kip1) ubiquitination and degradation is regulated by the SCF(Skp2) complex through phosphorylated Thr187 in p27. *Curr. Biol.* **1999**, *9*, 661–664. [CrossRef]
235. Ganoth, D.; Bornstein, G.; Ko, T.K.; Larsen, B.; Tyers, M.; Pagano, M.; Hershko, A. The cell-cycle regulatory protein Cks1 is required for SCF(Skp2)-mediated ubiquitinylation of p27. *Nat. Cell. Biol.* **2001**, *3*, 321–324. [CrossRef] [PubMed]
236. Nakayama, K.; Nagahama, H.; Minamishima, Y.A.; Matsumoto, M.; Nakamichi, I.; Kitagawa, K.; Shirane, M.; Tsunematsu, R.; Tsukiyama, T.; Ishida, N.; et al. Targeted disruption of Skp2 results in accumulation of cyclin E and p27(Kip1), polyploidy and centrosome overduplication. *EMBO J.* **2000**, *19*, 2069–2081. [CrossRef] [PubMed]
237. Kossatz, U.; Dietrich, N.; Zender, L.; Buer, J.; Manns, M.P.; Malek, N.P. Skp2-dependent degradation of p27kip1 is essential for cell cycle progression. *Genes Dev.* **2004**, *18*, 2602–2607. [CrossRef]

238. Minamishima, Y.A.; Nakayama, K.; Nakayama, K. Recovery of liver mass without proliferation of hepatocytes after partial hepatectomy in Skp2-deficient mice. *Cancer Res.* **2002**, *62*, 995–999.
239. Yoshida, K.; Nakayama, K.; Nagahama, H.; Harada, T.; Harada, C.; Imaki, J.; Matsuda, A.; Yamamoto, K.; Ito, M.; Ohno, S.; et al. Involvement of p27(KIP1) degradation by Skp2 in the regulation of proliferation in response to wounding of corneal epithelium. *Investig. Ophthalmol. Vis. Sci.* **2002**, *43*, 364–370.
240. Ge, Z.; Guo, X.; Li, J.; Hartman, M.; Kawasawa, Y.I.; Dovat, S.; Song, C. Clinical significance of high c-MYC and low MYCBP2 expression and their association with Ikaros dysfunction in adult acute lymphoblastic leukemia. *Oncotarget* **2015**, *6*, 42300–42311. [CrossRef]
241. Lewcock, J.W.; Genoud, N.; Lettieri, K.; Pfaff, S.L. The ubiquitin ligase Phr1 regulates axon outgrowth through modulation of microtubule dynamics. *Neuron* **2007**, *56*, 604–620. [CrossRef] [PubMed]
242. Bloom, A.J.; Miller, B.R.; Sanes, J.R.; DiAntonio, A. The requirement for Phr1 in CNS axon tract formation reveals the corticostriatal boundary as a choice point for cortical axons. *Genes Dev.* **2007**, *21*, 2593–2606. [CrossRef] [PubMed]
243. Han, S.; Kim, S.; Bahl, S.; Li, L.; Burande, C.F.; Smith, N.; James, M.; Beauchamp, R.L.; Bhide, P.; DiAntonio, A.; et al. The E3 ubiquitin ligase protein associated with Myc (Pam) regulates mammalian/mechanistic target of rapamycin complex 1 (mTORC1) signaling in vivo through N- and C-terminal domains. *J. Biol. Chem.* **2012**, *287*, 30063–30072. [CrossRef] [PubMed]
244. Han, S.; Witt, R.M.; Santos, T.M.; Polizzano, C.; Sabatini, B.L.; Ramesh, V. Pam (Protein associated with Myc) functions as an E3 ubiquitin ligase and regulates TSC/mTOR signaling. *Cell Signal* **2008**, *20*, 1084–1091. [CrossRef] [PubMed]
245. Babetto, E.; Beirowski, B.; Russler, E.V.; Milbrandt, J.; DiAntonio, A. The Phr1 ubiquitin ligase promotes injury-induced axon self-destruction. *Cell Rep.* **2013**, *3*, 1422–1429. [CrossRef] [PubMed]
246. Chretien, M.L.; Legouge, C.; Martin, R.Z.; Hammann, A.; Trad, M.; Aucagne, R.; Largeot, A.; Bastie, J.N.; Delva, L.; Quere, R. Trim33/Tif1gamma is involved in late stages of granulomonopoiesis in mice. *Exp. Hematol.* **2016**, *44*, 727–739.e726. [CrossRef]
247. Kim, J.; Kaartinen, V. Generation of mice with a conditional allele for Trim33. *Genesis* **2008**, *46*, 329–333. [CrossRef]
248. Ferri, F.; Parcelier, A.; Petit, V.; Gallouet, A.S.; Lewandowski, D.; Dalloz, M.; van den Heuvel, A.; Kolovos, P.; Soler, E.; Squadrito, M.L.; et al. TRIM33 switches off Ifnb1 gene transcription during the late phase of macrophage activation. *Nat. Commun.* **2015**, *6*, 8900. [CrossRef]
249. Kusy, S.; Gault, N.; Ferri, F.; Lewandowski, D.; Barroca, V.; Jaracz-Ros, A.; Losson, R.; Romeo, P.H. Adult hematopoiesis is regulated by TIF1gamma, a repressor of TAL1 and PU.1 transcriptional activity. *Cell Stem Cell* **2011**, *8*, 412–425. [CrossRef]
250. Bai, X.; Trowbridge, J.J.; Riley, E.; Lee, J.A.; DiBiase, A.; Kaartinen, V.M.; Orkin, S.H.; Zon, L.I. TiF1-gamma plays an essential role in murine hematopoiesis and regulates transcriptional elongation of erythroid genes. *Dev. Biol.* **2013**, *373*, 422–430. [CrossRef]
251. Quere, R.; Saint-Paul, L.; Carmignac, V.; Martin, R.Z.; Chretien, M.L.; Largeot, A.; Hammann, A.; Pais de Barros, J.P.; Bastie, J.N.; Delva, L. Tif1gamma regulates the TGF-beta1 receptor and promotes physiological aging of hematopoietic stem cells. *Proc. Natl. Acad. Sci. USA* **2014**, *111*, 10592–10597. [CrossRef] [PubMed]
252. Gontan, C.; Achame, E.M.; Demmers, J.; Barakat, T.S.; Rentmeester, E.; van, I.W.; Grootegoed, J.A.; Gribnau, J. RNF12 initiates X-chromosome inactivation by targeting REX1 for degradation. *Nature* **2012**, *485*, 386–390. [CrossRef] [PubMed]
253. Goodrich, L.; Panning, B.; Leung, K.N. Activators and repressors: A balancing act for X-inactivation. *Semin. Cell Dev. Biol.* **2016**, *56*, 3–8. [CrossRef] [PubMed]
254. Shin, J.; Bossenz, M.; Chung, Y.; Ma, H.; Byron, M.; Taniguchi-Ishigaki, N.; Zhu, X.; Jiao, B.; Hall, L.L.; Green, M.R.; et al. Maternal Rnf12/RLIM is required for imprinted X-chromosome inactivation in mice. *Nature* **2010**, *467*, 977–981. [CrossRef] [PubMed]
255. Kammoun, M.; Maas, E.; Criem, N.; Gribnau, J.; Zwijsen, A.; Vermeesch, J.R. RLIM enhances BMP signalling mediated fetal lung development in mice. *bioRxiv* **2018**. [CrossRef]
256. Shin, J.; Wallingford, M.C.; Gallant, J.; Marcho, C.; Jiao, B.; Byron, M.; Bossenz, M.; Lawrence, J.B.; Jones, S.N.; Mager, J.; et al. RLIM is dispensable for X-chromosome inactivation in the mouse embryonic epiblast. *Nature* **2014**, *511*, 86–89. [CrossRef]

257. Wang, F.; Shin, J.; Shea, J.M.; Yu, J.; Boskovic, A.; Byron, M.; Zhu, X.; Shalek, A.K.; Regev, A.; Lawrence, J.B.; et al. Regulation of X-linked gene expression during early mouse development by Rlim. *Elife* **2016**, *5*. [CrossRef]
258. Jiao, B.; Ma, H.; Shokhirev, M.N.; Drung, A.; Yang, Q.; Shin, J.; Lu, S.; Byron, M.; Kalantry, S.; Mercurio, A.M.; et al. Paternal RLIM/Rnf12 is a survival factor for milk-producing alveolar cells. *Cell* **2012**, *149*, 630–641. [CrossRef]
259. Chen, W.; Jiang, X.; Luo, Z. WWP2: A multifunctional ubiquitin ligase gene. *Pathol. Oncol. Res.* **2014**, *20*, 799–803. [CrossRef]
260. Zou, W.; Chen, X.; Shim, J.H.; Huang, Z.; Brady, N.; Hu, D.; Drapp, R.; Sigrist, K.; Glimcher, L.H.; Jones, D. The E3 ubiquitin ligase Wwp2 regulates craniofacial development through mono-ubiquitylation of Goosecoid. *Nat. Cell Biol.* **2011**, *13*, 59–65. [CrossRef]
261. Yang, Y.; Liao, B.; Wang, S.; Yan, B.; Jin, Y.; Shu, H.B.; Wang, Y.Y. E3 ligase WWP2 negatively regulates TLR3-mediated innate immune response by targeting TRIF for ubiquitination and degradation. *Proc. Natl. Acad. Sci. USA* **2013**, *110*, 5115–5120. [CrossRef]
262. Li, H.; Zhang, P.; Zhang, Q.; Li, C.; Zou, W.; Chang, Z.; Cui, C.P.; Zhang, L. WWP2 is a physiological ubiquitin ligase for phosphatase and tensin homolog (PTEN) in mice. *J. Biol. Chem.* **2018**, *293*, 8886–8899. [CrossRef]
263. Ambrozkiewicz, M.C.; Schwark, M.; Kishimoto-Suga, M.; Borisova, E.; Hori, K.; Salazar-Lazaro, A.; Rusanova, A.; Altas, B.; Piepkorn, L.; Bessa, P.; et al. Polarity Acquisition in Cortical Neurons Is Driven by Synergistic Action of Sox9-Regulated Wwp1 and Wwp2 E3 Ubiquitin Ligases and Intronic miR-140. *Neuron* **2018**, *100*, 1097–1115.e1015. [CrossRef]
264. Guruharsha, K.G.; Kankel, M.W.; Artavanis-Tsakonas, S. The Notch signalling system: Recent insights into the complexity of a conserved pathway. *Nat. Rev. Genet.* **2012**, *13*, 654–666. [CrossRef]
265. Nowell, C.S.; Radtke, F. Notch as a tumour suppressor. *Nat. Rev. Cancer* **2017**, *17*, 145–159. [CrossRef]
266. Zavadil, J.; Cermak, L.; Soto-Nieves, N.; Bottinger, E.P. Integration of TGF-beta/Smad and Jagged1/Notch signalling in epithelial-to-mesenchymal transition. *EMBO J.* **2004**, *23*, 1155–1165. [CrossRef]
267. Niimi, H.; Pardali, K.; Vanlandewijck, M.; Heldin, C.H.; Moustakas, A. Notch signaling is necessary for epithelial growth arrest by TGF-beta. *J. Cell Biol.* **2007**, *176*, 695–707. [CrossRef]
268. Bray, S.J. Notch signalling in context. *Nat. Rev. Mol. Cell Biol.* **2016**, *17*, 722–735. [CrossRef]
269. Haines, N.; Irvine, K.D. Glycosylation regulates Notch signalling. *Nat. Rev. Mol. Cell Biol.* **2003**, *4*, 786–797. [CrossRef]
270. Logeat, F.; Bessia, C.; Brou, C.; LeBail, O.; Jarriault, S.; Seidah, N.G.; Israel, A. The Notch1 receptor is cleaved constitutively by a furin-like convertase. *Proc. Natl. Acad. Sci. USA* **1998**, *95*, 8108–8112. [CrossRef]
271. Blobel, C.P. Metalloprotease-disintegrins: Links to cell adhesion and cleavage of TNF alpha and Notch. *Cell* **1997**, *90*, 589–592. [CrossRef]
272. Pan, D.; Rubin, G.M. Kuzbanian controls proteolytic processing of Notch and mediates lateral inhibition during Drosophila and vertebrate neurogenesis. *Cell* **1997**, *90*, 271–280. [CrossRef]
273. Itoh, M.; Kim, C.H.; Palardy, G.; Oda, T.; Jiang, Y.J.; Maust, D.; Yeo, S.Y.; Lorick, K.; Wright, G.J.; Ariza-McNaughton, L.; et al. Mind bomb is a ubiquitin ligase that is essential for efficient activation of Notch signaling by Delta. *Dev. Cell* **2003**, *4*, 67–82. [CrossRef]
274. De Strooper, B.; Annaert, W.; Cupers, P.; Saftig, P.; Craessaerts, K.; Mumm, J.S.; Schroeter, E.H.; Schrijvers, V.; Wolfe, M.S.; Ray, W.J.; et al. A presenilin-1-dependent gamma-secretase-like protease mediates release of Notch intracellular domain. *Nature* **1999**, *398*, 518–522. [CrossRef]
275. Wu, L.; Aster, J.C.; Blacklow, S.C.; Lake, R.; Artavanis-Tsakonas, S.; Griffin, J.D. MAML1, a human homologue of Drosophila mastermind, is a transcriptional co-activator for NOTCH receptors. *Nat. Genet.* **2000**, *26*, 484–489. [CrossRef]
276. Tamura, K.; Taniguchi, Y.; Minoguchi, S.; Sakai, T.; Tun, T.; Furukawa, T.; Honjo, T. Physical interaction between a novel domain of the receptor Notch and the transcription factor RBP-J kappa/Su(H). *Curr. Biol.* **1995**, *5*, 1416–1423. [CrossRef]
277. Nagel, A.C.; Krejci, A.; Tenin, G.; Bravo-Patino, A.; Bray, S.; Maier, D.; Preiss, A. Hairless-mediated repression of notch target genes requires the combined activity of Groucho and CtBP corepressors. *Mol. Cell. Biol.* **2005**, *25*, 10433–10441. [CrossRef]

278. Oswald, F.; Winkler, M.; Cao, Y.; Astrahantseff, K.; Bourteele, S.; Knochel, W.; Borggrefe, T. RBP-Jkappa/SHARP recruits CtIP/CtBP corepressors to silence Notch target genes. *Mol. Cell. Biol.* **2005**, *25*, 10379–10390. [CrossRef]
279. Qiu, L.; Joazeiro, C.; Fang, N.; Wang, H.Y.; Elly, C.; Altman, Y.; Fang, D.; Hunter, T.; Liu, Y.C. Recognition and ubiquitination of Notch by Itch, a hect-type E3 ubiquitin ligase. *J. Biol. Chem.* **2000**, *275*, 35734–35737. [CrossRef]
280. Puca, L.; Chastagner, P.; Meas-Yedid, V.; Israel, A.; Brou, C. Alpha-arrestin 1 (ARRDC1) and beta-arrestins cooperate to mediate Notch degradation in mammals. *J. Cell Sci.* **2013**, *126*, 4457–4468. [CrossRef]
281. McGill, M.A.; McGlade, C.J. Mammalian numb proteins promote Notch1 receptor ubiquitination and degradation of the Notch1 intracellular domain. *J. Biol. Chem.* **2003**, *278*, 23196–23203. [CrossRef]
282. Nie, J.; McGill, M.A.; Dermer, M.; Dho, S.E.; Wolting, C.D.; McGlade, C.J. LNX functions as a RING type E3 ubiquitin ligase that targets the cell fate determinant Numb for ubiquitin-dependent degradation. *EMBO J.* **2002**, *21*, 93–102. [CrossRef]
283. Mund, T.; Graeb, M.; Mieszczanek, J.; Gammons, M.; Pelham, H.R.; Bienz, M. Disinhibition of the HECT E3 ubiquitin ligase WWP2 by polymerized Dishevelled. *Open Biol.* **2015**, *5*, 150185. [CrossRef]
284. Jung, J.G.; Stoeck, A.; Guan, B.; Wu, R.C.; Zhu, H.; Blackshaw, S.; Shih Ie, M.; Wang, T.L. Notch3 interactome analysis identified WWP2 as a negative regulator of Notch3 signaling in ovarian cancer. *PLoS Genet.* **2014**, *10*, e1004751. [CrossRef]
285. Sorensen, E.B.; Conner, S.D. gamma-secretase-dependent cleavage initiates notch signaling from the plasma membrane. *Traffic* **2010**, *11*, 1234–1245. [CrossRef]
286. Zheng, L.; Conner, S.D. PI5P4Kgamma functions in DTX1-mediated Notch signaling. *Proc. Natl. Acad. Sci. USA* **2018**, *115*, E1983–E1990. [CrossRef]
287. Fryer, C.J.; White, J.B.; Jones, K.A. Mastermind recruits CycC:CDK8 to phosphorylate the Notch ICD and coordinate activation with turnover. *Mol. Cell* **2004**, *16*, 509–520. [CrossRef]
288. Rallis, C.; Pinchin, S.M.; Ish-Horowicz, D. Cell-autonomous integrin control of Wnt and Notch signalling during somitogenesis. *Development* **2010**, *137*, 3591–3601. [CrossRef]
289. Ruel, L.; Bourouis, M.; Heitzler, P.; Pantesco, V.; Simpson, P. Drosophila shaggy kinase and rat glycogen synthase kinase-3 have conserved activities and act downstream of Notch. *Nature* **1993**, *362*, 557–560. [CrossRef]
290. Espinosa, L.; Ingles-Esteve, J.; Aguilera, C.; Bigas, A. Phosphorylation by glycogen synthase kinase-3 beta down-regulates Notch activity, a link for Notch and Wnt pathways. *J. Biol. Chem.* **2003**, *278*, 32227–32235. [CrossRef]
291. Zhou, T.; Yi, F.; Wang, Z.; Guo, Q.; Liu, J.; Bai, N.; Li, X.; Dong, X.; Ren, L.; Cao, L.; et al. The Functions of DNA Damage Factor RNF8 in the Pathogenesis and Progression of Cancer. *Int. J. Biol. Sci.* **2019**, *15*, 909–918. [CrossRef] [PubMed]
292. Pettersson, S.; Sczaniecka, M.; McLaren, L.; Russell, F.; Gladstone, K.; Hupp, T.; Wallace, M. Non-degradative ubiquitination of the Notch1 receptor by the E3 ligase MDM2 activates the Notch signalling pathway. *Biochem. J.* **2013**, *450*, 523–536. [CrossRef] [PubMed]
293. Kim, H.; Ronai, Z.A. Rewired Notch/p53 by Numb'ing Mdm2. *J. Cell Biol.* **2018**, *217*, 445–446. [CrossRef] [PubMed]
294. Deblandre, G.A.; Lai, E.C.; Kintner, C. Xenopus neuralized is a ubiquitin ligase that interacts with XDelta1 and regulates Notch signaling. *Dev. Cell* **2001**, *1*, 795–806. [CrossRef]
295. Kramer, H. Neuralized: Regulating notch by putting away delta. *Dev. Cell* **2001**, *1*, 725–726. [CrossRef]
296. Fischer, A.; Schumacher, N.; Maier, M.; Sendtner, M.; Gessler, M. The Notch target genes Hey1 and Hey2 are required for embryonic vascular development. *Genes Dev.* **2004**, *18*, 901–911. [CrossRef]
297. Zhang, N.; Gridley, T. Defects in somite formation in lunatic fringe-deficient mice. *Nature* **1998**, *394*, 374–377. [CrossRef]
298. Swiatek, P.J.; Lindsell, C.E.; del Amo, F.F.; Weinmaster, G.; Gridley, T. Notch1 is essential for postimplantation development in mice. *Genes Dev.* **1994**, *8*, 707–719. [CrossRef]
299. Koo, B.K.; Yoon, M.J.; Yoon, K.J.; Im, S.K.; Kim, Y.Y.; Kim, C.H.; Suh, P.G.; Jan, Y.N.; Kong, Y.Y. An obligatory role of mind bomb-1 in notch signaling of mammalian development. *PLoS ONE* **2007**, *2*, e1221. [CrossRef]

300. Koo, B.K.; Lim, H.S.; Song, R.; Yoon, M.J.; Yoon, K.J.; Moon, J.S.; Kim, Y.W.; Kwon, M.C.; Yoo, K.W.; Kong, M.P.; et al. Mind bomb 1 is essential for generating functional Notch ligands to activate Notch. *Development* **2005**, *132*, 3459–3470. [CrossRef]
301. Barsi, J.C.; Rajendra, R.; Wu, J.I.; Artzt, K. Mind bomb1 is a ubiquitin ligase essential for mouse embryonic development and Notch signaling. *Mech. Dev.* **2005**, *122*, 1106–1117. [CrossRef] [PubMed]
302. Yeh, C.H.; Bellon, M.; Nicot, C. FBXW7: A critical tumor suppressor of human cancers. *Mol. Cancer* **2018**, *17*, 115. [CrossRef] [PubMed]
303. Mao, J.H.; Perez-Losada, J.; Wu, D.; Delrosario, R.; Tsunematsu, R.; Nakayama, K.I.; Brown, K.; Bryson, S.; Balmain, A. Fbxw7/Cdc4 is a p53-dependent, haploinsufficient tumour suppressor gene. *Nature* **2004**, *432*, 775–779. [CrossRef] [PubMed]
304. Busino, L.; Millman, S.E.; Scotto, L.; Kyratsous, C.A.; Basrur, V.; O'Connor, O.; Hoffmann, A.; Elenitoba-Johnson, K.S.; Pagano, M. Fbxw7alpha- and GSK3-mediated degradation of p100 is a pro-survival mechanism in multiple myeloma. *Nat. Cell Biol.* **2012**, *14*, 375–385. [CrossRef] [PubMed]
305. Sato, M.; Rodriguez-Barrueco, R.; Yu, J.; Do, C.; Silva, J.M.; Gautier, J. MYC is a critical target of FBXW7. *Oncotarget* **2015**, *6*, 3292–3305. [CrossRef] [PubMed]
306. Tetzlaff, M.T.; Yu, W.; Li, M.; Zhang, P.; Finegold, M.; Mahon, K.; Harper, J.W.; Schwartz, R.J.; Elledge, S.J. Defective cardiovascular development and elevated cyclin E and Notch proteins in mice lacking the Fbw7 F-box protein. *Proc. Natl. Acad. Sci. USA* **2004**, *101*, 3338–3345. [CrossRef]
307. Tsunematsu, R.; Nakayama, K.; Oike, Y.; Nishiyama, M.; Ishida, N.; Hatakeyama, S.; Bessho, Y.; Kageyama, R.; Suda, T.; Nakayama, K.I. Mouse Fbw7/Sel-10/Cdc4 is required for notch degradation during vascular development. *J. Biol. Chem.* **2004**, *279*, 9417–9423. [CrossRef]
308. Onoyama, I.; Tsunematsu, R.; Matsumoto, A.; Kimura, T.; de Alboran, I.M.; Nakayama, K.; Nakayama, K.I. Conditional inactivation of Fbxw7 impairs cell-cycle exit during T cell differentiation and results in lymphomatogenesis. *J. Exp. Med.* **2007**, *204*, 2875–2888. [CrossRef]
309. Matsuoka, S.; Oike, Y.; Onoyama, I.; Iwama, A.; Arai, F.; Takubo, K.; Mashimo, Y.; Oguro, H.; Nitta, E.; Ito, K.; et al. Fbxw7 acts as a critical fail-safe against premature loss of hematopoietic stem cells and development of T-ALL. *Genes Dev.* **2008**, *22*, 986–991. [CrossRef]
310. Sancho, R.; Jandke, A.; Davis, H.; Diefenbacher, M.E.; Tomlinson, I.; Behrens, A. F-box and WD repeat domain-containing 7 regulates intestinal cell lineage commitment and is a haploinsufficient tumor suppressor. *Gastroenterology* **2010**, *139*, 929–941. [CrossRef]
311. Matsumoto, A.; Onoyama, I.; Sunabori, T.; Kageyama, R.; Okano, H.; Nakayama, K.I. Fbxw7-dependent degradation of Notch is required for control of "stemness" and neuronal-glial differentiation in neural stem cells. *J. Biol. Chem.* **2011**, *286*, 13754–13764. [CrossRef] [PubMed]
312. Onoyama, I.; Suzuki, A.; Matsumoto, A.; Tomita, K.; Katagiri, H.; Oike, Y.; Nakayama, K.; Nakayama, K.I. Fbxw7 regulates lipid metabolism and cell fate decisions in the mouse liver. *J. Clin. Investig.* **2011**, *121*, 342–354. [CrossRef] [PubMed]
313. Krebs, L.T.; Iwai, N.; Nonaka, S.; Welsh, I.C.; Lan, Y.; Jiang, R.; Saijoh, Y.; O'Brien, T.P.; Hamada, H.; Gridley, T. Notch signaling regulates left-right asymmetry determination by inducing Nodal expression. *Genes Dev.* **2003**, *17*, 1207–1212. [CrossRef] [PubMed]
314. Yoon, M.J.; Koo, B.K.; Song, R.; Jeong, H.W.; Shin, J.; Kim, Y.W.; Kong, Y.Y.; Suh, P.G. Mind bomb-1 is essential for intraembryonic hematopoiesis in the aortic endothelium and the subaortic patches. *Mol. Cell. Biol.* **2008**, *28*, 4794–4804. [CrossRef] [PubMed]
315. Kang, K.; Lee, D.; Hong, S.; Park, S.G.; Song, M.R. The E3 ligase Mind bomb-1 (Mib1) modulates Delta-Notch signaling to control neurogenesis and gliogenesis in the developing spinal cord. *J. Biol. Chem.* **2013**, *288*, 2580–2592. [CrossRef] [PubMed]
316. Horn, S.; Kobberup, S.; Jorgensen, M.C.; Kalisz, M.; Klein, T.; Kageyama, R.; Gegg, M.; Lickert, H.; Lindner, J.; Magnuson, M.A.; et al. Mind bomb 1 is required for pancreatic beta-cell formation. *Proc. Natl. Acad. Sci. USA* **2012**, *109*, 7356–7361. [CrossRef] [PubMed]

317. Luxan, G.; Casanova, J.C.; Martinez-Poveda, B.; Prados, B.; D'Amato, G.; MacGrogan, D.; Gonzalez-Rajal, A.; Dobarro, D.; Torroja, C.; Martinez, F.; et al. Mutations in the NOTCH pathway regulator MIB1 cause left ventricular noncompaction cardiomyopathy. *Nat. Med.* **2013**, *19*, 193–201. [CrossRef]
318. Kim, Y.W.; Koo, B.K.; Jeong, H.W.; Yoon, M.J.; Song, R.; Shin, J.; Jeong, D.C.; Kim, S.H.; Kong, Y.Y. Defective Notch activation in microenvironment leads to myeloproliferative disease. *Blood* **2008**, *112*, 4628–4638. [CrossRef]
319. Song, R.; Kim, Y.W.; Koo, B.K.; Jeong, H.W.; Yoon, M.J.; Yoon, K.J.; Jun, D.J.; Im, S.K.; Shin, J.; Kong, M.P.; et al. Mind bomb 1 in the lymphopoietic niches is essential for T and marginal zone B cell development. *J. Exp. Med.* **2008**, *205*, 2525–2536. [CrossRef]
320. Hsu, T.S.; Mo, S.T.; Hsu, P.N.; Lai, M.Z. c-FLIP is a target of the E3 ligase deltex1 in gastric cancer. *Cell Death Dis.* **2018**, *9*, 135. [CrossRef]
321. Hsiao, H.W.; Liu, W.H.; Wang, C.J.; Lo, Y.H.; Wu, Y.H.; Jiang, S.T.; Lai, M.Z. Deltex1 is a target of the transcription factor NFAT that promotes T cell anergy. *Immunity* **2009**, *31*, 72–83. [CrossRef] [PubMed]
322. Storck, S.; Delbos, F.; Stadler, N.; Thirion-Delalande, C.; Bernex, F.; Verthuy, C.; Ferrier, P.; Weill, J.C.; Reynaud, C.A. Normal immune system development in mice lacking the Deltex-1 RING finger domain. *Mol. Cell. Biol.* **2005**, *25*, 1437–1445. [CrossRef] [PubMed]
323. Hsiao, H.W.; Hsu, T.S.; Liu, W.H.; Hsieh, W.C.; Chou, T.F.; Wu, Y.J.; Jiang, S.T.; Lai, M.Z. Deltex1 antagonizes HIF-1alpha and sustains the stability of regulatory T cells in vivo. *Nat. Commun.* **2015**, *6*, 6353. [CrossRef] [PubMed]
324. Ou-Yang, H.F.; Zhang, H.W.; Wu, C.G.; Zhang, P.; Zhang, J.; Li, J.C.; Hou, L.H.; He, F.; Ti, X.Y.; Song, L.Q.; et al. Notch signaling regulates the FOXP3 promoter through RBP-J- and Hes1-dependent mechanisms. *Mol. Cell Biochem.* **2009**, *320*, 109–114. [CrossRef]
325. Burghardt, S.; Claass, B.; Erhardt, A.; Karimi, K.; Tiegs, G. Hepatocytes induce Foxp3(+) regulatory T cells by Notch signaling. *J. Leukoc. Biol.* **2014**, *96*, 571–577. [CrossRef]
326. Panier, S.; Durocher, D. Regulatory ubiquitylation in response to DNA double-strand breaks. *DNA Repair.* **2009**, *8*, 436–443. [CrossRef]
327. Kolas, N.K.; Chapman, J.R.; Nakada, S.; Ylanko, J.; Chahwan, R.; Sweeney, F.D.; Panier, S.; Mendez, M.; Wildenhain, J.; Thomson, T.M.; et al. Orchestration of the DNA-damage response by the RNF8 ubiquitin ligase. *Science* **2007**, *318*, 1637–1640. [CrossRef]
328. Li, L.; Halaby, M.J.; Hakem, A.; Cardoso, R.; El Ghamrasni, S.; Harding, S.; Chan, N.; Bristow, R.; Sanchez, O.; Durocher, D.; et al. Rnf8 deficiency impairs class switch recombination, spermatogenesis, and genomic integrity and predisposes for cancer. *J. Exp. Med.* **2010**, *207*, 983–997. [CrossRef]
329. Lu, L.Y.; Wu, J.; Ye, L.; Gavrilina, G.B.; Saunders, T.L.; Yu, X. RNF8-dependent histone modifications regulate nucleosome removal during spermatogenesis. *Dev. Cell* **2010**, *18*, 371–384. [CrossRef]
330. Ouyang, S.; Song, Y.; Tian, Y.; Chen, Y.; Yu, X.; Wang, D. RNF8 deficiency results in neurodegeneration in mice. *Neurobiol. Aging* **2015**, *36*, 2850–2860. [CrossRef]
331. Valnegri, P.; Huang, J.; Yamada, T.; Yang, Y.; Mejia, L.A.; Cho, H.Y.; Oldenborg, A.; Bonni, A. RNF8/UBC13 ubiquitin signaling suppresses synapse formation in the mammalian brain. *Nat. Commun.* **2017**, *8*, 1271. [CrossRef] [PubMed]
332. Senturk, E.; Manfredi, J.J. Mdm2 and tumorigenesis: Evolving theories and unsolved mysteries. *Genes Cancer* **2012**, *3*, 192–198. [CrossRef] [PubMed]
333. Mendrysa, S.M.; McElwee, M.K.; Michalowski, J.; O'Leary, K.A.; Young, K.M.; Perry, M.E. mdm2 Is critical for inhibition of p53 during lymphopoiesis and the response to ionizing irradiation. *Mol. Cell. Biol.* **2003**, *23*, 462–472. [CrossRef] [PubMed]
334. Jones, S.N.; Roe, A.E.; Donehower, L.A.; Bradley, A. Rescue of embryonic lethality in Mdm2-deficient mice by absence of p53. *Nature* **1995**, *378*, 206–208. [CrossRef]
335. Mendrysa, S.M.; O'Leary, K.A.; McElwee, M.K.; Michalowski, J.; Eisenman, R.N.; Powell, D.A.; Perry, M.E. Tumor suppression and normal aging in mice with constitutively high p53 activity. *Genes Dev.* **2006**, *20*, 16–21. [CrossRef]

336. Bult, C.J.; Blake, J.A.; Smith, C.L.; Kadin, J.A.; Richardson, J.E.; Mouse Genome Database, G. Mouse Genome Database (MGD) 2019. *Nucleic Acids Res.* **2019**, *47*, D801–D806. [CrossRef]
337. Amberger, J.S.; Bocchini, C.A.; Schiettecatte, F.; Scott, A.F.; Hamosh, A. OMIM.org: Online Mendelian Inheritance in Man (OMIM(R)), an online catalog of human genes and genetic disorders. *Nucleic Acids Res.* **2015**, *43*, D789–D798. [CrossRef]

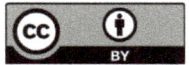

© 2019 by the authors. Licensee MDPI, Basel, Switzerland. This article is an open access article distributed under the terms and conditions of the Creative Commons Attribution (CC BY) license (http://creativecommons.org/licenses/by/4.0/).

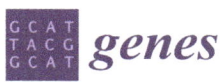 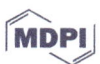

Review

Gut Microbiota Influences Experimental Outcomes in Mouse Models of Colorectal Cancer

Alyssa A. Leystra and Margie L. Clapper *

Cancer Prevention and Control Program, Fox Chase Cancer Center, Philadelphia, PA 19111, USA; alyssa.leystra@fccc.edu
* Correspondence: Margie.Clapper@fccc.edu

Received: 13 September 2019; Accepted: 5 November 2019; Published: 7 November 2019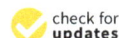

Abstract: Colorectal cancer (CRC) is a leading cause of cancer-related deaths worldwide. Mouse models are a valuable resource for use throughout the development and testing of new therapeutic strategies for CRC. Tumorigenesis and response to therapy in humans and mouse models alike are influenced by the microbial communities that colonize the gut. Differences in the composition of the gut microbiota can confound experimental findings and reduce the replicability and translatability of the resulting data. Despite this, the contribution of resident microbiota to preclinical tumor models is often underappreciated. This review does the following: (1) summarizes evidence that the gut microbiota influence CRC disease phenotypes; (2) outlines factors that can influence the composition of the gut microbiota; and (3) provides strategies that can be incorporated into the experimental design, to account for the influence of the microbiota on intestinal phenotypes in mouse models of CRC. Through careful experimental design and documentation, mouse models can continue to rapidly advance efforts to prevent and treat colon cancer.

Keywords: colorectal cancer; mouse models; microbiota; antitumor immunity

1. Introduction

Colorectal cancer (CRC) remains the second leading cause of cancer-related deaths worldwide [1]. Although research advances during the past decade have led to some of the most exciting breakthroughs in cancer treatment, including immune checkpoint blockade, the majority of CRC cases fail to respond to these new therapies [2,3]. A critical need exists to develop new strategies for the early detection, prevention, and treatment of colorectal cancer, as well as to elucidate the basis for the ineffectiveness of existing therapies. Such studies rely heavily on preclinical in vivo models that recapitulate the biology of human disease.

Studies in both chemically induced and genetically engineered mouse models of CRC have enhanced our understanding of colon tumor initiation, progression, and response to therapy. Such models continue to play an essential role in assessing promising chemopreventive, chemotherapeutic, and immunomodulatory agents for their ability to impact tumor development. However, as in humans, interpretation of the resulting study data is often compromised by significant inter-individual variability in tumor development and response to therapy. This heterogeneity can exist within a single genetically defined strain of mice and is even observed among caged littermates maintained under identical environmental and dietary conditions [4]. Our ability to refine existing in vivo models to more accurately mimic human colon tumor biology is predicated on a more in-depth understanding of the factors that contribute to phenotypic variability and impact therapeutic response.

Tumorigenesis and response to therapy in humans and mice alike are influenced by the microenvironment in which the colon tumor arises. Complex interactions among the commensal microbiota and the tissue-resident immune cells within the colon provide a dynamic microenvironment that is well equipped to rapidly respond to stimuli. Perturbations in the microenvironment directly impact the homeostasis of the colonic epithelium and dictate propensity for disease. Despite mounting evidence for the critical role the resident microbiota play in influencing the frequency of tumor initiation, rate of progression, and response to therapy, there is an underappreciation for these factors when selecting and developing animal models of CRC.

The present review provides mounting evidence that the bacteria that colonize the mammalian gut play a pivotal role in tumorigenesis and the response to therapy in classic mouse models of CRC (Table 1). Numerous environmental and genetic factors are discussed that can impact disease phenotypes in mouse models by altering the composition of the gut microbiota (Figure 1). Finally, strategies are presented that investigators can employ to improve reproducibility and translatability of findings from mouse models of colon tumorigenesis and control factors that influence the composition of the microbiota.

Table 1. Influence of microbiota on disease phenotype in common mouse models of CRC (colorectal cancer).

Tumor Induction	Mouse Model	Impact of Microbiota on Colon Phenotype	References
Sporadic Familial Adenomatous Polyposis	$Apc^{Min/+}$ $Apc^{Min\Delta 716/+}$ $Cdx2\text{-}Cre\ Apc^{flox/+}$	Mice administered continuous broad-spectrum antibiotics develop fewer colon tumors, whereas mice administered intermittent antibiotics develop more tumors. Infection of $Apc^{Min/+}$ mice by *Fusobacterium nucleatum*, or $Apc^{Min716/+}$ mice by enterotoxigenic *Bacteroides fragilis* and/or pks+ *Escherichia coli* increases tumor multiplicity.	[5–9]
Inflammation	$Il10^{-/-}$	Germ-free mice do not develop intestinal inflammation. Differences in the composition of microbiota influence severity of sporadic colitis in mice housed at different institutions. Infection with *E. coli* increases tumorigenesis following azoxymethane (AOM) treatment.	[10–13]
DNA mismatch repair deficiency	$Msh2^{-/-}$	Germ-free and antibiotic (broad-spectrum)-treated $Apc^{Min/+}$ $Msh2^{-/-}$ mice develop fewer colon tumors than 'conventional' untreated mice (bearing natural microbiota).	[14]
Chemical induction	AOM/DSS	Treatment with either AOM or dextran sodium sulfate (DSS) changes the composition of the gut microbiota. Germ-free mice exhibit delayed tissue repair and develop more tumors than conventional mice. Conventional C57BL/6 mice develop more tumors than the genetically identical mice colonized with microbiota from wild-caught mice.	[15–17]
Transplantation	CT26 MC38	*E. coli* modifies the response of tumors to chemotherapy. Depletion of microbiota by broad-spectrum antibiotics attenuates the response of tumors to immunotherapeutics.	[18–20]

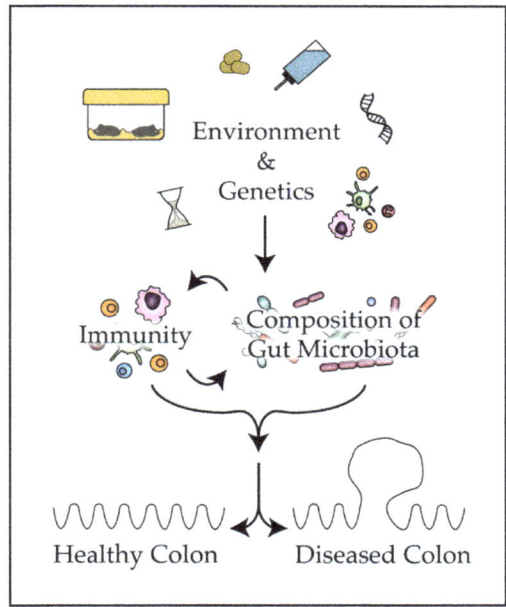

Figure 1. Many aspects of the murine environment can impact the composition of the gut microbiota, activity of the immune system, and ultimately the penetrance of disease phenotypes in mouse models of colon tumorigenesis.

2. Gut Microbiota Modulate Colon Tumorigenesis

The mammalian gut contains trillions of bacteria that coexist to form a complex ecosystem. Many of these microbes live in symbiosis with the host, metabolizing partially digested food, producing vitamins and nutrients, providing protection from opportunistic pathogens, and participating in the maturation, education, and activation of the tissue-resident and systemic immune system [21,22]. In delicate balance with the gut microbiota, the host epithelium and stroma form a tight barrier, consisting of a layer of mucin and antimicrobial products, in an attempt to protect the mucosa and underlying vasculature from invading microbes. Additional protection is afforded by the stroma of the gut, which is heavily infiltrated by tissue-resident immune cells that are poised to do the following: (1) respond rapidly to damage to the intestinal epithelium by producing wound-healing factors; and (2) mount a rapid response to invasion of the mucosal barrier by foreign microbes. The healthy colonic immune system is maintained as a balance of pro-inflammatory cells that are primed to respond to pathogens and danger-associated antigens and anti-inflammatory cells that suppress potentially damaging responses to commensal microbes and their byproducts. Perturbations in the composition of the gut microflora and/or direct contact of the microbes with the intestinal epithelium can skew the balance between pro-inflammatory and anti-inflammatory immune responses. Such alterations promote colon pathogenesis, leading to autoimmune activity, inflammatory bowel disease, and tumorigenesis.

Reduced microbial diversity, due to changes in the identity, richness, and relative abundance of microbial taxa, can be detected within the gut of mice with both spontaneous and chemically induced colon tumorigenesis prior to tumor formation. For example, $Apc^{Min/+}$ mice spontaneously develop intestinal tumors due to a point mutation in codon 850 of the *Apc* tumor-suppressor gene. A reduction in microbial diversity was observed prior to the formation of visible tumors in C57BL/6J $Apc^{Min/+}$ mice as compared to age and strain-matched C57BL/6J mice with wild-type *Apc* [23]. This decrease in diversity was driven primarily by an increase in the relative abundance of *Bacteroidetes* spp. within the colon of $Apc^{Min/+}$ mice [23]. Similar findings have been reported for a murine model of chemically induced colitis-associated neoplasia. The azoxymethane/dextran sodium sulfate (AOM/DSS) mouse model is employed routinely as a prototypic model for the study of inflammatory signaling in a setting that recapitulates inflammation-associated colon tumorigenesis (ulcerative colitis) in humans. In this model, injection of the classic colon carcinogen AOM (single or multiple doses) initiates the colonic epithelium. Subsequent administration of DSS, a tumor-promoting agent, induces ulceration of the colonic mucosa followed by wound healing and proliferation of the epithelium. Interestingly, treatment with AOM/DSS resulted in broad shifts in the composition of the gut microbiota, as compared to that of healthy (untreated) mice, prior to the formation of visible tumors [15]. An increase in the relative abundance of members of the *Bacteroides* genus and a concomitant decrease in members of the *Prevotella* genus and unclassified genera within the Porphyromonadaceae family led to the observed reduction in diversity [15]. Taken together, these findings from spontaneous and chemically induced colon tumor models indicate that differences in the composition of the microbiota can be detected in mice that eventually develop tumors compared to mice that do not.

2.1. Evidence that Microbiota Can Restrain Colon Tumorigenesis

Depletion of microbiota can lead to an increase in the incidence and multiplicity of colon tumors in some mouse models of CRC. Intermittent, long-term administration of broad-spectrum antibiotics to $Apc^{Min/+}$ mice produced shifts in the microbial composition of the gut and increased tumor number over time [5]. Exposure to antibiotics caused a dramatic decrease in the overall abundance and diversity of microbes, as indicated by an increase in the relative abundance of three genera (*Enterococcus*, *Ureaplasma*, and *Peptoclostridium*) and a decrease in many others (including *Bacteroides*, *Lactobacillus*, and *Desulfovibrio*). Antibiotic treatment caused a ~1.5-fold increase in the number of tumors throughout the intestine. Likewise, antibiotic use is associated with an increased risk of colon tumorigenesis in humans [24]. Thus, reduced microbial abundance may lead to an increase in the incidence and multiplicity of colon tumors in humans and mouse models alike.

Animals exhibiting a complete absence of commensal microbiota face an increased risk of developing colon tumors following exposure to an inflammatory stimulus. Germ-free (GF) AOM/DSS mice developed more tumors than conventional AOM/DSS mice that had been colonized with diverse and largely undefined microbiota since birth [16]. Delayed activation of tissue-repair pathways was observed within the gut of AOM/DSS-treated GF animals lacking commensal bacteria. Animals colonized with microbiota exhibited an acute inflammatory response to initial DSS treatment within 12 days, as characterized by increased cytokine signaling and recruitment of inflammatory cells involved in tissue repair. In contrast, GF animals failed to initiate an acute inflammatory response to the epithelial damage induced by DSS; tissue repair did not begin until 3–4 weeks later. The delayed onset of tissue repair in GF mice relative to conventional mice was coupled with dysregulation of repair pathways, resulting in hyperproliferation and formation of microadenomas. Ultimately, GF mice developed more and larger tumors than conventional mice. The increased tumor burden observed in GF mice was partially reversed by administering lipopolysaccharide, a microbial byproduct, in the drinking water. Complete rescue was achieved by colonizing GF mice with microbiota from conventional mice prior to AOM/DSS treatment. Together, these findings suggest that commensal microbes and their byproducts assist in the initiation of appropriate tissue repair and recovery from inflammatory insults.

Laboratory mice colonized with microbiota from wild-caught mice displayed a dramatic increase in gut microbial diversity and a decrease in the number and size of AOM/DSS-induced tumors relative to conventional AOM/DSS-treated laboratory mice [17]. Changes in the phylum-level composition of the gut microbiota included an increased relative abundance of Bacteroidetes and Proteobacteria and a reduction in Firmicutes, Tenericutes, and Verrucomicrobia in wild-caught vs. C57BL/6 mice. Following AOM/DSS treatment, C57BL/6 mice colonized with microbiota from wild-caught mice developed less inflammation and ~3-fold fewer colon tumors than AOM/DSS-treated C57BL/6 mice colonized with microbiota from conventional laboratory C57BL/6 mice. Thus, increased diversity of the gut microbiota was associated with decreased tumorigenesis in the AOM/DSS-treated C57BL/6 model, perhaps due to modulation of the inflammatory response to DSS treatment.

Colonization of mice with mixtures of specific strains of bacteria can reduce tumorigenesis. One such mixture of bacteria, a probiotic called "VSL#3", consists of *Lactobacillus casei, Lactobacillus pantarum, Lactobacillus acidophilus, Lactobacillus delbrueckii* subsp. *Blugaricus, Bifidobacterium longum, Bifidobacterium breve, Bifidobacterium infantis*, and *Streptococcus salivarius*. Administration of VSL#3 to conventional mice resulted in a significant decrease in the number and size of colon tumors per mouse following AOM/DSS treatment [25,26]. These experiments provide proof-of-concept that modulation of the abundance of specific strains of bacteria in the gut can restrain colon tumorigenesis.

2.2. Evidence that Microbiota Can Promote Colon Tumorigenesis

Microbiota likely perform dual roles in tumorigenesis. Many commensal species protect against invasion of the gut epithelium by pathogens, while other species promote inflammation and pro-tumorigenic signaling. Thus, depletion of bacteria can be either harmful or beneficial in a context-dependent manner. In contrast to the above studies where microbial depletion resulted in increased tumorigenesis, other studies have yielded opposing data. Mice treated with broad-spectrum antibiotics prior to and throughout AOM/DSS administration developed ~2-fold fewer tumors than those that didn't receive antibiotics [15]. Similarly, treatment of *Cdx2-Cre Apc*$^{flox/+}$ mice with broad-spectrum antibiotics led to a 2-fold decrease in the number of spontaneous colon tumors, as compared to untreated animals [27]. Furthermore, GF and broad-spectrum antibiotic-treated *Apc*$^{Min/+}$ *Msh2*$^{-/-}$ mice with microsatellite instable disease developed fewer colon tumors than conventional mice [14]. When combined, these studies provide convincing evidence for the pro-tumorigenic role of microbiota in a number of distinct animal models.

Experiments involving the inoculation of mice with microbiota from either healthy or diseased hosts provide direct evidence of the ability of the microbiota to either protect against or promote tumorigenesis. Mice colonized with gut microbiota from tumor-bearing animals prior to treatment with AOM and DSS developed ~2-fold more colon tumors than similarly treated mice colonized with a 'healthy' gut microbiota obtained from tumor-free mice that were not treated with either agent [15]. Similarly, AOM-treated mice colonized with microbiota from CRC patients developed more severe inflammation as well as a higher tumor incidence and grade than mice that received microbiota from healthy donors or no microbiota [28]. These findings demonstrate that the composition of the gut microbiota can impact inflammatory responses and subsequent tumor formation in mouse models of colon tumorigenesis.

2.3. Contribution of Specific Bacteria to Colon Tumorigenesis

Clearly, the composition of the gut microbiota influences the incidence and multiplicity of colon tumors that develop in mouse models. However, only a few individual species of human microbes have been identified that reproducibly promote colon tumorigenesis in immunocompetent mouse models.

2.3.1. *Fusobacterium Nucleatum*

Fusobacterium nucleatum, a commensal microbe that can become pathogenic under conditions of reduced microbial diversity, is enriched within the colon of patients with colonic adenomas and/or cancer as compared to healthy subjects [29]. *Apc*$^{Min/+}$ mice colonized with *F. nucleatum* develop more aberrant crypt foci and tumors in the colon than sham-colonized *Apc*$^{Min/+}$ mice, as well as a greater number of small intestinal adenomas and adenocarcinomas [29]. Tumors from mice colonized with *F. nucleatum* exhibit higher expression of pro-inflammatory genes, including *Ptgs2, Il1b, Il6, Il8, Tnf*, and *Mmp3*, than tumors from sham-colonized controls. These findings suggest that *F. nucleatum* may drive the development and progression of intestinal tumors via activation of inflammatory pathways.

2.3.2. Bacteroides Fragilis

Bacteroides fragilis, another common commensal bacterium, has also been implicated in the development and growth of colon tumors in both humans and mice [6–9]. Enterotoxigenic *B. fragilis* (ETBF) induces colon tumorigenesis in $Apc^{Min/+}$ mice by inducing pro-inflammatory IL-17 and NF-κB signaling throughout the colonic mucosa [6,8]. Prompt clearance of ETBF with the antibiotic cefoxitin can mitigate these effects [7]. Use of a nontoxigenic strain of *B. fragilis* that does not produce BFT upon colonization is insufficient to enhance either inflammatory signaling or tumorigenesis as compared to sham-colonized $Apc^{Min/+}$ mice. Thus, toxin production by EBFT is required for induction of inflammatory signaling and subsequent enhanced tumorigenesis [6].

2.3.3. Escherichia Coli

Strains of *Escherichia coli* that carry the *pks* gene locus and thus produce colibactin, a known genotoxin, enhance tumor formation and growth in both humans and mice. Expression of genes at the *pks* island of *pks+ E. coli* is enhanced in mice during carcinogenesis [30]. Colonization of GF $Il10^{-/-}$ mice, which are susceptible to inflammation due to deletion of the *Il10* gene, with either *pks+* or *pks− E. coli* results in the induction of severe colitis [10]. Colonization of AOM-treated GF $Il10^{-/-}$ [10] or AOM/DSS [31] mice with *pks+ E. coli* increased the number of colon tumors per animal beyond that of mice colonized with *pks− E. coli*. In contrast, *pks+ E. coli* was insufficient to induce either colonic inflammation or tumorigenesis in AOM-treated GF $Il10^{+/+}$ (wild-type) mice [10]. Together, these findings indicate that expression of the *pks* locus in *E. coli* may cooperate with inflammation to promote tumor growth and progression within the colon.

2.4. Activities of the Microbiota that Impact the Homeostasis of the Colonic Mucosa

2.4.1. Biofilm Formation

Under homeostatic conditions, the colonic epithelium produces a layer of mucin that serves as a barrier between the commensal microbiota and the colonic mucosa. Successful invasion of the mucin layer by bacteria results in the formation of a dense, matrix-enclosed aggregation of multiple species of bacteria that adhere tightly to surfaces [32]. Such biofilms perform a potentially pathogenic function within the colon by doing the following: (1) bringing the bacteria in closer proximity with the mucosal surface of the colon; (2) protecting the bacteria from external insults, including antibiotic treatment; and (3) facilitating cooperation between multiple bacterial species through nutrient exchange and horizontal gene transfer, to enhance survival of the community [32]. In humans, bacterial biofilms are frequently detected on adenomas and cancers alike; one study identified biofilms on 50% of the CRCs examined [33]. These biofilms are not restricted to the tumor, but can extend to the nontumor tissue. Normal tissue covered with biofilm displays pro-tumorigenic changes, as depicted by reduced crypt cell expression of E-cadherin, increased epithelial cell expression of IL-6, and increased proliferation relative to biofilm-free tissue [33]. These changes, which occur irrespective of whether the tissue is from a CRC patient or healthy subject, provide evidence that the biofilm may promote tumorigenesis.

Biofilms found in the colons of CRC patients are commonly co-colonized with *E. coli* and ETBF [9]. Co-colonization of $Apc^{Min\Delta716/+}$ mice or AOM-treated wild-type mice with pathogenic strains of both *pks+ E. coli* and ETBF significantly increased colon tumor multiplicity relative to co-colonization with a single pathogenic strain of either *E. coli* or ETBF and the nonpathogenic strain of the other. Co-colonization with both pathogenic strains of bacteria also resulted in enhanced *pks+ E. coli* invasion into the biofilm and tissue relative to colonization with *pks+ E. coli* alone. This observation suggests that ETBF may be required to break down the protective mucus layer, thus allowing *pks+ E. coli* to come in direct contact with epithelial cells. Thus, multiple species of pathogenic bacteria can cooperate within biofilms to promote tumorigenesis.

While colonic biofilms containing pathogenic bacteria promote tumorigenesis, biofilms colonized by beneficial bacteria could hypothetically promote host defense and protect against tumorigenesis.

Bacterial biofilms can promote good health in some tissues, such as the oral cavity [34]. However, the existence of similar health-promoting roles for intestinal biofilms remains controversial [32]. Additional research is required to determine if biofilms containing nonpathogenic bacteria can form and persist in close contact with the healthy colonic mucosa and, if so, what impact (if any) they have on colon cancer risk and treatment response.

2.4.2. Metabolites Produced by Microbiota

Intestinal bacteria participate in the metabolism of carbohydrates, lipids, and amino acids that pass through the gut. Products of this metabolism influence the pH, oxidative environment, energy availability, and presence of carcinogens in the microenvironment of the colonic mucosa [35,36]. Many of these metabolites either promote or restrain colon tumorigenesis. For example, the genotoxin colibactin, produced by pks+ E. coli, promotes tumorigenesis by inducing DNA damage [37]. In contrast, colonization of GF mice with *Butyrivibrio fibrisolvens* increases the amount of the protective short chain fatty acid (SCFA) butyrate within the colon relative to uncolonized GF mice [38]. Butyrate production is inversely correlated with tumor multiplicity in AOM/DSS-treated mice; *B. fibrisolvens*-colonized mice fed a high fiber diet develop 3-fold fewer colon tumors than GF mice maintained on the same diet. This protective effect is lost when mice are colonized with a mutated strain of *B. fibrisolvens* incapable of metabolizing soluble fiber to butyrate, providing strong evidence for the ability of butyrate to inhibit tumor formation in these animals. Butyrate and other SCFAs likely modulate colon tumor formation in part by reducing colonic inflammation [39,40]. Mice deficient in SCFA receptors exhibit more severe colitis in response to repeated DSS treatment relative to wild-type mice [39]. In addition, SCFA receptor-deficient animals develop greater numbers of colonic tumors after AOM/DSS treatment than wild-type mice. Interestingly, SCFAs can induce the activation and expansion of colon-resident immune cells and attenuate colonic inflammation in a T-cell transfer model of colitis [40]. The anti-inflammatory properties of butyrate cooperate with other chemopreventive dietary components including (n-3) polyunsaturated fatty acids (PUFAs) to dramatically reduce severity of inflammation, accumulation of DNA damage, risk of tumor formation, and growth of tumor cells [41]. These findings illustrate that production of metabolites by gut microbial communities may promote or restrain colon tumorigenesis by modulating DNA damage and inflammatory immune responses to harmful stimuli. Thus, evaluating metabolite production by the gut microbiota may provide greater mechanistic insight into how microbiota interact with the colonic mucosa to either promote or restrain colon tumorigenesis.

2.4.3. Interactions with Tissue-Resident Immune Cells

Gut microbiota shape the maturation of the immune system and its activation in mice, starting at a young age. Mice that remain GF throughout development exhibit abnormally organized immune organs, including spleens and lymph nodes, as compared to pups that are colonized with microbes at birth [42]. Although many of these defects can be corrected by microbial colonization later in life, some persist [43]. For example, mice that do not encounter bacterial antigens prior to weaning exhibit immune intolerance to bacterial antigens upon gut-barrier disruption by DSS in early adulthood (30 days of age), resulting in increased expansion of gut mucosal T cells, fewer Tregs, and more severe colitis than mice exposed to bacterial antigens prior to weaning [44].

Gut microbiota regulate the recruitment and activation of pro-inflammatory lymphocytes, including T-helper 17 (Th17) and $\gamma\delta$ T-cells within the colon [45,46]. For example, inoculation of germ-free mice with feces from patients with CRC resulted in increased recruitment of Th17 cells to the colon as compared to mice inoculated with feces from healthy subjects [28]. Invasion of the colonic epithelial layer by gut microbiota also enhanced Th17 cell recruitment and stimulation [27,47,48]. Similarly, mice colonized with bacteria exhibited greater $\gamma\delta$ T-cell recruitment and stimulation in the intestine than antibiotic-treated or GF mice [46]. These lymphocytes in turn produced pro-inflammatory cytokines, including IL-23 and downstream IL-17, upon activation. IL-17 production from tumor-infiltrating Th17 and γδT cells increased colon tumor development in $Apc^{Min/+}$ mice [49]. Conversely, ablation of IL-23 signaling in immune cells resulted in reduced expression of IL-17 and fewer tumors within the colon of $Cdx2$-Cre $Apc^{flox/+}$ mice [27]. Together, these findings indicate that pro-inflammatory signaling by the adaptive immune system can promote colon tumor growth.

Gut microbiota also regulate the recruitment and activation of the immunosuppressive T regulatory cell (Treg) population within the colon. Tregs are common residents of the colon and oppose the activity of pro-inflammatory lymphocytes. Colons of GF mice harbor fewer Tregs than colons of conventional mice, a phenotype which could be rescued by colonization of mice with strains of *Clostridium* but not by colonizing with other bacterial strains [50]. Colonization of GF mice with a mixture of 17 strains of Clostridia, including *Clostridium* species *C. asparagiforme*, *C. bolteae*, *C. scindens*, *C. indolis*, *C. ramosum*, and *C. hathewayi*, substantially increased the number of activated Tregs in the intestines of poly-colonized animals relative to GF and mono-colonized animals [51]. Furthermore, Tregs from GF mice exhibit reduced immunosuppressive function, as measured by IL-10 production, compared to *Clostridium*-colonized and conventional mice [50]. Thus, gut microbiota, including some strains of *Clostridium*, stimulate Tregs and protect against inflammation. Consistent with the finding that pro-inflammatory signaling from the immune system promotes tumorigenesis, ablation of Tregs in the setting of colitis and prior to tumor formation results in more severe colitis and the formation of a greater number of colon tumors in AOM/DSS-treated mice [52]. However, ablation of Tregs after tumor formation results in increased infiltration of the tumor by cytotoxic T cells, and a decrease in the number and size of the colon tumors. These data provide support for two opposing roles for Treg-induced immunosuppression during colon tumorigenesis: (1) protection against colonic inflammation and tumor initiation; and (2) a reduction in antitumor immunity after tumor initiation that promotes tumor growth.

3. Gut Microbiota Modulate the Response of Colon Tumors to Chemotherapy

3.1. Activation of Autophagy in Cancer Cells

In addition to directly modulating tumorigenesis through antitumorigenic and protumorigenic interactions with the colonic epithelium and underlying stroma, bacteria can also modify the response of tumors to therapy. For example, high levels of *F. nucleatum* in tumor tissues are associated with decreased recurrence-free [53] and overall survival [54] in CRC patients, indicating a potential role for *F. nucleatum* in modulating chemotherapy resistance. In vitro, coculture of CRC cell lines with *F. nucleatum* increased autophagy-related gene expression relative to culture in the absence of bacteria or coculture with other bacterial species, including *Prevotella intermedia*, *Parvimonas micra*, and *Peptostreptococcus anaerobius* [53]. Consequently, CRC cells cocultured with *F. nucleatum* exhibited reduced apoptosis in response to treatment with common CRC chemotherapies, such as 5-fluorouracil (5-FU) or oxaliplatin. Similar results were obtained in vivo: injection of xenograft tumors with *F. nucleatum* activated autophagy and in turn attenuated the antitumor activity of 5-FU or oxaliplatin. *F. nucleatum*-dependent chemotherapy resistance could be overcome by treatment of cells or mice with an autophagy inhibitor. Together, these data indicate that tumor-infiltrating *F. nucleatum* can activate autophagy and thus contribute to chemotherapy resistance in CRC. Interestingly, *F. nucleatum* levels predict response to adjuvant chemotherapy in esophageal squamous cell carcinoma, indicating a potential role for tumor-associated bacteria, such as *F. nucleatum*, in modulating the response of CRC, as well as extra-intestinal cancers to therapy [55].

3.2. Metabolism of Chemotherapeutic Agents

Metabolism of some therapeutic agents by specific gut-colonizing bacteria leads to structural alterations and changes in drug efficacy. In one study, 30 different chemotherapeutic agents were incubated for two hours in vitro with *E. coli* prior to filter-sterilization, and then added to cancer cell lines [18]. Preincubation of six agents, including 5-fluorocytosine and CB1954, with *E. coli* enhanced their cytotoxicity. Preincubation decreased the cytotoxicity of 10 other drugs, including Doxorubicin and Gemcitabine, as compared to those that were not preincubated with *E. coli*. Drugs with altered cytotoxicity exhibited changes on HPLC chromatograms indicative of biotransformation. The altered efficacy of some chemotherapeutic agents was further confirmed in vivo, using CT26 colon carcinoma isografts. Flank tumors were injected with *E. coli* or mock-colonized with sterile PBS, and chemotherapeutic efficacy was assessed by monitoring tumor volume over time, following intraperitoneal injection of either Gemcitabine or CB1954. Gemcitabine was less efficacious in decreasing the growth of tumors colonized with *E. coli*. Mice developed larger tumors and exhibited shorter survival times, as compared to mock-colonized mice treated in a similar manner. Conversely, the efficacy of CB1954 was enhanced in mice bearing tumors colonized with *E. coli*, leading to a decrease in tumor size and enhanced survival. When combined, these data indicate that common tumor-invasive bacteria, such as *E. coli*, can alter the biotransformation and efficacy of chemotherapeutic agents in vitro and in vivo. The potential impact of gut-colonizing bacteria on therapeutic efficacy may extend beyond the colon; the therapeutic response of lymphomas, melanomas, and lung carcinomas, as well as other tumor types, has been reported to correlate with changes in the composition of the gut microbiota [56].

3.3. Promotion of Antitumor Immunity

The gut microbiota can indirectly influence tumor response to therapy by modulating the antitumor immune response. Disruption of microbiota with broad-spectrum antibiotics impairs tumor response to CpG-oligonucleotide and anti-CTLA4 immunotherapies [19,20]. These therapies induce tumor cell death in mice bearing MC38 colon carcinoma isografts by promoting production of IL-17 and reactive oxygen species by tumor-infiltrating immune cells [19,20]. However, secretion of cytotoxic species by tumor-infiltrating immune cells was attenuated in mice treated with broad-spectrum antibiotics prior to immunotherapy. Consequently, mice treated with antibiotics and immunotherapies had larger tumors and shorter lifespans than mice treated with immunotherapy alone. Interestingly, the efficacy of anti-CTLA4 treatment in antibiotic-treated MC38-grafted mice could be rescued by colonizing mice with *B. fragilis*, immunizing with *B. fragilis* polysaccharides, or performing adoptive transfer with *B. fragilis*-specific T cells. Thus, activation of the immune system with microbial by-products is required for efficient tumor-cell killing in this model [20]. These effects are not limited to colon cancers; many genera of bacteria, including *Akkermansia*, *Bifidobacterium*, *Collinsella*, and *Enterococcus*, have been implicated in modulating response to immune checkpoint blockade in extra-intestinal cancers (e.g., melanoma, non-small cell lung cancer, and renal cell carcinoma) in both preclinical and clinical settings [57]. Thus, gut microbiota can modulate response to immunotherapy through activation of the immune system.

Given the critical role of the microbiota in shaping the maturation and activation of the immune system, it is likely that they also influence the efficacy of newly developed immunotherapeutics. Interestingly, antibiotic treatment prior to and following vaccination reduced vaccine-induced immune responses in humans, indicating that the microbiota may participate in vaccine-mediated immunity [58]. A recent surge of interest in stimulating antitumor immunity has resulted in the design of vaccines against antigens commonly expressed on CRC cells [59]. Vaccination of mice with antigens that are aberrantly expressed on colon tumor cells has been shown to prevent tumor formation [60], growth [61], and colonization in distant organs [62]. However, despite promising results in preclinical models, clinical trials to test the therapeutic efficacy of vaccines in CRC patients have yielded mixed results [59]. Future studies are needed to assess the similarity of the microbial and immune microenvironment of tumors in preclinical CRC models with that of human tumors, thus dictating the relevance of the observed efficacy of these vaccines in mice to a clinical setting.

4. Factors that Influence the Composition of the Gut Microbiota

Clearly, gut bacteria influence colon tumor formation, progression, and response to therapy in mouse models and humans alike, through interactions with the mucosal epithelium, metabolism of therapeutic compounds, and modulation of tissue-resident immune cells. Thus, variability in the colonic microflora of mouse models of CRC can influence disease penetrance, phenotypes, and experimental outcomes in these animals. These observations underscore the importance of understanding factors that influence the composition of the gut microbiota in mouse models.

4.1. Genetics

Genetic differences between mice may influence the resident gut microbiota [63–65]. Although genetic differences among strains likely influence the composition of the colonic microflora, specific strain influences are difficult to separate from strong environmental pressures, including cohort and litter effects. However, gene mutations and deletions that impact gut epithelial and/or immune homeostasis do appear to influence the resident gut microbiota. For example, when GF $Il10^{-/-}$ mice were acclimated to nonsterile conditions at weaning, the IL-10 deficient mice initially colonized (and maintained) a greater abundance of bacteria from the Enterobacteriaceae family, including *E. coli*, than wild-type mice [30]. Mutations in *Apc* may also drive divergent evolution of microbiota; six-week-old female C57BL/6J $Apc^{Min/+}$ mice possess less diverse gut microbiota but greater relative abundance of *Bacteroidetes* spp than age- and gender-matched C57BL/6J wild-type mice [23]. However, animals in this study were born to dams in separate colonies and housed independently, providing an opportunity for natural drift of the colonizing microbiota in each strain. An evaluation of littermates ($Apc^{Min/+}$ and wild-type) would be the best approach to deciphering the impact of mutations in genetic drivers of colon tumorigenesis on the gut microbiota.

4.2. Birth Mother

The composition of the colonic microbiota of a young mouse is initially dictated at or before birth by the mother [66,67]. Strain-specific differences in the composition of the gut microbiota largely disappear when embryos of multiple strains are implanted into a single mouse; instead, each pup develops the biome of the birth dam irrespective of strain. Thus, littermates tend to be colonized with highly analogous microbiota. Similarities are shared across generations; litters born to dams that are sisters are colonized with similar microbiota, whereas litters born to dams that are not sisters are colonized with divergent microbiota [68]. Importantly, colonization of pups by microbes from the dam can influence disease penetrance: C57BL/6 mice born from dams bearing conventional laboratory microbes developed more and larger tumors in response to AOM/DSS treatment than C57BL/6 mice born from dams bearing microbiota of wild-caught mice [17].

4.3. Age

The composition of gut microbiota changes rapidly in mice prior to weaning. Microbiota in young mice tend to be less diverse than that of older mice [69,70]. After initial colonization by vaginal microbes from the dam, the gut microbiota of pups shift, within the first few days of life, toward a low-diversity composition dominated by *Lactobacillus* [67]. As mice switch from nursing to solid food, the diversity of the gut microbiota increases rapidly to match the composition of the dam's fecal material. After weaning, the microbiota equilibrates with that of co-housed animals, likely due to sharing of microbiota via ingestion of feces [65].

Aging leads to changes in the microbiota that can drive pro-inflammatory processes. Elderly mice (e.g., 18 months of age) exhibit increased systemic inflammation relative to young adult mice (2 months of age), characterized by increased serum levels of proinflammatory cytokines (IL-1β and TNFα) [71]. Age-induced changes in systemic inflammation correlate with decreased integrity of the gut barrier, and the increased relative abundance of specific genera of gut microbiota, including *Odoribacter*, *Butyricimonas*, *Gelria*, *Anaerosporobacter*, *Clostridium*, and *Oxalobacter*. The expression of pro-inflammatory genes was upregulated in the colonic mucosa of GF mice after colonization with microbiota from elderly mice vs. colonization with microbiota from young mice [72].

4.4. Housing

Gut microbiota are dynamic, and changes occur naturally over time. Even mice that start with highly similar and defined gut microbiota, including germ-free mice that are simultaneously acclimated to a nonsterile environment or gavaged with specific bacteria, develop divergent gut microbiota over time [69,70,73]. In one study, GF mice were inoculated with a defined microbiome and then housed either in microisolators or in individual ventilated cages [69]. The microbiota that developed in mice housed in microisolator cages differed from that of mice housed in individual ventilated cages. Irrespective of the type of cage, taxa were identified over time that were not present in the original inoculum. Furthermore, the number of genera detected increased significantly within three months, demonstrating that the composition of the gut microbiota among animals in a single cage can drift rapidly away from that of the original inoculum. Consistent with this observation, animals housed in the same cage exhibit significantly less inter-individual variation in the composition of the gut microbiota than animals housed in independent cages [65]. This natural microbial drift may contribute to variability in disease phenotype and experimental outcomes between cages. For example, the degree of inflammation observed in mice treated with a colitis-inducing agent varies significantly more among mice housed in different cages than in mice housed together in the same cage [70].

4.5. Diet

Diet heavily influences the composition of gut microbiota in the adult host. Shifts in the composition of the microbiota of laboratory mice can be detected within 48 hours following a dietary modification [74]. These shifts may influence disease penetrance. Mice fed a diet high in the milk protein casein harbor gut microbiota with less diversity, characterized in part by decreased relative abundance of Firmicutes and increased Bacteroidetes, and develop more severe DSS-induced colitis than mice fed a diet low in casein. A diet high in psyllium, a soluble plant fiber, increased microbial diversity and decreased severity of DSS-induced colitis in mice compared to a diet high the insoluble fiber cellulose. The aggravating effects of casein protein and protective effects of soluble fiber on DSS-induced colitis are attenuated in GF mice relative to conventional mice, indicating that gut microbiota are responsible in part for modulating disease severity.

The way in which the rodent chow and water are sterilized prior to administration influences the composition of the gut microbiota in recipient mice. The number of bacterial species in the gut of mice maintained on irradiated chow is lower than that of mice maintained on autoclaved or untreated chow [75]. In addition, the relative abundance of microbial phyla, including Firmicutes and Bacteroidetes, are altered. Mice given autoclaved water, as compared to that sterilized by H_2SO_4 acidification, exhibit a reduction in microbial diversity and a change in the abundance of various microbial taxa [76]. Interestingly, NOD mice maintained on acidified drinking water develop Type 1 Diabetes (T1D) more rapidly than NOD mice maintained on neutral pH drinking water [77]. The change in incidence and rate of developing T1D is preceded by differences in the number and relative abundance of specific genera of gut microbes, including a decreased prevalence of *Bacteroides*. In addition, *Parabacteroides* and *Prevotella* are acquired when mice are switched from acidified water to neutral pH water. Thus, the ability of the gut microbiota to impact disease susceptibility in mouse models is influenced by the nutrient composition of the diet, and the manner in which the diet and drinking water are sterilized.

4.6. Institution

The influence of environmental factors on the composition of the gut microbiota is compounded over generations, and thus identical strains of mice housed at different institutions can exhibit dramatic differences in the composition of their gut-resident microflora. Examination of the gut microbiota of C57BL/6J breeding stocks from 21 different animal facilities revealed profound differences [75]. Variability in animal housing, handling, and care likely contributed to this heterogeneity; treatment of the chow (untreated, irradiated, or autoclaved), type of housing (whether using individually ventilated cages or not), the vendor who supplied the mice, and the presence of other mouse strains in the facility all influenced the number of bacterial species identified and their relative abundance.

Importantly, differences in the composition of the microbiota at different institutions has been shown to influence disease susceptibility when utilizing the same mouse model [78]. $Il10^{-/-}$ mice serve as a prototypic example of the impact of institutional-specific microbiota on disease severity. The investigators who initially developed the $Il10^{-/-}$ mouse observed that mice exhibited severe enterocolitis, resulting in anemia, weight loss, and mortality by 4–12 weeks of age. Colitis was attenuated in mice housed under specific pathogen-free (SPF) conditions relative to those housed under conventional conditions [79]. Subsequent studies revealed that SPF $Il10^{-/-}$ mice housed at some institutions readily developed extensive colitis, while $Il10^{-/-}$ mice housed at other institutions fail to develop colitis [11–13]. Furthermore, $Il10^{-/-}$ mice infected with *H. hepaticus* developed more severe colitis than uninfected mice at one institution but not at another; GF mice never developed colitis [12,13]. Thus, the penetrance and severity of disease phenotypes in mouse models can change dramatically when mice are rederived at new institutions, likely due to colonization by different microbiota.

4.7. Immune System

The composition of the gut microbiota is influenced significantly by the immune system of the mouse. Mice that lack functional adaptive immune systems harbor biomes with a modified composition relative to wild-type mice [80–82]. For example, the intestinal microbiota of immunodeficient C57BL/6J $Rag1^{-/-}$ mice that lack mature lymphocytes contain taxa that are significantly different from those of C57BL/6J wild-type ($Rag1^{+/+}$) mice, including decreased relative abundance of Lactobacillales and increased species of Verrucomicrobiales, such as *Akkermansia muciniphila* [80]. However, the abundance of *A. muciniphila* in $Rag1^{-/-}$ mice bearing bone marrow grafted from $Rag1^{+/+}$ mice was similar to that of $Rag1^{+/+}$ mice, indicating that the adaptive immune system may play a role in modulating the abundance of some microbial species within the gut. Inflammation produced as a consequence of immune dysregulation likely also influences gut microbial communities. This may explain the shifts in microbiota observed in mice after DSS treatment, as well as shifts in the gut communities of $Il10^{-/-}$ vs. wild type littermates [15,30]. These data serve as evidence of the ability of the immune system to shape the gut microbial communities.

5. Implications for Model Selection and Experimental Design

Gut microbiota coexist in a delicate balance with the colonic mucosa and have the power to either restrain or promote colon cancer. Unfortunately, factors that influence the microbiota can have unexpected consequences in preclinical tumor models, negatively influencing experimental reproducibility and the broad applicability of findings. Phenotypes initially attributed to specific gene mutations or mouse strains may instead arise as a result of litter or cage effects [63,64]. Mouse models that readily develop colonic inflammation at one institution can remain totally healthy at another center [12,13]. Therapies that appear effective in specific mouse models may lose their potency or have unexpected side effects in other models and/or humans due to differences in gut microbiota and immunity [18,83,84]. Through in-depth characterization of the model to be used and with significant attention to experimental design and systematic reporting, researchers can circumvent major sources of variability that hinder translatability, thus ensuring that their data are accurate and can be used to advance the efforts to prevent and treat colon cancer.

5.1. Characterizing Microbiota to Improve Mouse Models of CRC

As discussed above, variations in the gut microbiota of laboratory mice can influence disease phenotypes and experimental outcomes in mouse models of CRC. Characterization of the gut microflora throughout an experiment allows investigators to do the following: (1) quantify the number and abundance of microbial genera present in the model; (2) determine how the microbiota change over the course of the experiment; and (3) understand how the microbiota interact with the colonic mucosa to influence disease phenotypes in the model. Characterization is routinely accomplished through 16s rRNA gene sequencing, which can identify and quantify the microbial genera present within the gut [85]. Using this approach, the number and identity of each unique genus, as well as its abundance among the total microflora, can be assessed. Importantly, the methods used to collect, store, and analyze microbiota from colon samples can influence the sequencing results [86,87]. For example, sequencing results can vary significantly depending upon which regions of the 16s gene are selected for analysis [87]. Furthermore, the sequencing platform selected can yield different results; the Illumina MiSeq and Ion Torrent PGM sequencing platforms differ in their sensitivity to detect specific microbial species and assessment of overall diversity, as indicated by scores calculated from sequencing data [86]. As an alternative to 16s rRNA targeted sequencing, shotgun whole genome sequencing (WGS) is sometimes used [85]. This approach provides additional information about the gut-resident microbiota, as it allows detection of genes required for the production of toxins and other key metabolites that can influence microbial activity within the gut. Notably, WGS detects more total species, identifies different relative abundances, and yields higher diversity scores than 16s rRNA sequencing of the same samples [88]. Given the dramatic impact that gut-microbiome-sequencing methods can have upon the results obtained, standardization and clear reporting of procedures used throughout an experiment are critical for accurate interpretation and direct comparison of results to those obtained by others.

While knowledge of the overall composition of the gut microbiome represents a step toward greater understanding of how the microflora influence disease phenotypes in mouse models, it provides limited information about the functional activity of the microbes. Emerging technologies, including transcriptomics, proteomics, and metabolomics, allow investigators to examine the activity of members of the resident microbiota [85]. These data should enhance our understanding of how the microbiota interact with the colonic mucosa to either restrain or promote tumorigenesis, and may ultimately inform strategies to improve therapeutic interventions. Furthermore, these data are anticipated to facilitate the more accurate interpretation of variable experimental results obtained from preclinical CRC models.

5.2. Modifying Microbiota to Improve Mouse Models of CRC

Some institutions have tried to standardize the gut microflora of laboratory mice via rederivation using dams colonized with defined microbial inoculum, such as the altered Schaedler flora [75]. Although this results in initial colonization with defined species, it does not prevent rapid drift from the composition of the initial inoculum, based on institutional- and cage-specific environmental factors, such as those described above [65,69,75]. Many institutions maintain their mouse colonies under specific pathogen-free (SPF) conditions; however, 'SPF status' provides no information about the composition of the microbiota and does not imply similarity to SPF mice at other institutions. SPF mice are tested regularly to ensure they remain free of a set of predefined pathogens. Since each institution defines its own criteria for acceptable pathogens and SPF status, the gut microbiota of SPF mice at different institutions and from different vendors can vary dramatically both in the types and relative abundance of microbial species present [75,89].

Manipulation of the gut microbiota may be required to establish mouse models that more accurately mimic human immune responses throughout tumorigenesis and dictate response to therapy. While mouse strains have been used to test immunotherapies alone or in combination with conventional chemotherapeutic agents [60–62,90,91], these models are usually selected without considering whether the tumor immune microenvironment recapitulates that of human cancer patients. In any event, the microenvironment of the tumor clearly impacts the response of the tumor to therapeutic interventions [18,83]. Given the important role of the microbiota in the tumor microenvironment, through direct interactions with both the tumor and resident immune cells, one approach to mimicking the tumor microenvironment in mice may be to 'humanize' the murine gut with microbiota from the human gut. Unfortunately, microbial species from humans colonize mice with variable efficiency, resulting in a bias for certain species (especially members of the *Bacteroides* and *Parabacteroides* genera) over others [92,93]. In addition, immune infiltration and activation within the gut of mice bearing human-derived microbiota is less mature than that within the gut of mice bearing conventional microbiota [44]. Additional research is required to determine whether mice bearing 'humanized' gut microflora accurately model various aspects of human disease progression, including activation of the immune system and response to therapy.

Alternatively, embracing the natural microflora of the mouse may lead to models that better recapitulate human immune responses. The diversity of gut microbiota in wild mice is significantly higher than that of conventional laboratory mice [84]. Rederivation of laboratory mice by transplantation of C57BL/6 embryos into pathogen-free, wild-caught pseudopregnant *Mus musculus domesticus* results in 'wildling' C57BL/6 mice colonized with the diverse microbiota of wild mice. Although genetically identical to conventional C57BL/6 mice, the immune cell landscape of the gut of most wildlings differed from that of conventional mice, including increased numbers of cytotoxic T cells and decreased numbers of NK cells. Interestingly, immune responses of wildling mice more closely mimicked human immune responses to CD28-superagonist therapy and TNF-α blockade than that of conventional laboratory mice. Additional research is required to determine whether wildling mice also phenocopy human immune responses during therapeutic treatment of colon tumors.

5.3. Experimental Design—Correcting for Factors that Influence Gut Microbiota in Experiments

While some factors that influence the colonic microflora can be controlled, such as sterilization of drinking water, other factors, including natural drift within colonies over time, are more elusive. Given the staggering number of subtle environmental factors that can influence gut microbial diversity and composition, many of which are beyond the control of the investigator, it is impossible to perfectly standardize and replicate all conditions performed within a single laboratory, much less across all laboratories worldwide. In fact, controlling and standardizing all variables that influence microbial composition and phenotypic outcomes within mouse models of CRC is not desirable. Lack of heterogeneity between mice, as seen in humans, may contribute to biases in study results. Such findings may be highly specific to the conditions of the experiment instead of broadly applicable and translatable to the inherent heterogeneity of humans [94–96]. Instead, some environmental variability between subjects within an experiment may be ideal, providing it is applied equally across all groups. Heterogeneity can be introduced quite naturally into an experiment by enrolling mice in batches over time, thus ensuring that subtle changes in the environment are introduced over the course of the experiment. Batch-specific effects can then be estimated and accounted for through appropriate statistical modeling approaches.

To correct for factors that strongly influence the microbiota, appropriate randomization of mice to study groups is essential. Block randomization, based on factors that are likely to confound experimental outcomes (e.g., litter), ensures that confounding variables are equally spread across all treatment groups. Housing of animals should be carefully considered and recorded. Co-housing mice from multiple experimental groups will help standardize the microbiota across animals in each group. However, if the outcome of the experiment is dependent in part on the gut microbes, co-housing animals may make it difficult to detect the effect, as mice will participate in coprophagy and thus share microbiota. Regardless of the approach employed, it is important to provide these details so other investigators can understand and replicate the experiments.

5.4. Reporting Experimental Details

In an effort to improve reproducibility in animal research, Kilkenny et al. published a set of comprehensive guidelines for reporting animal research [97]. The ARRIVE guidelines encourage researchers to report strain and environmental factors that might influence the composition of the gut microbiota and immune system in experimental models, including providing international strain nomenclature, genotype, age, sex, and weight, as well as the husbandry conditions, housing type, diet, time of day the experiment was performed, and the pathogen status of the experimental animals. While it is impossible to control and replicate all environmental conditions that contribute to diversity of the gut microbiota and immune system, cataloguing and reporting these factors make it easier for other researchers to replicate studies precisely and identify the basis for results that differ. Thus, thorough and systematic reporting of study variables by following the ARRIVE guidelines could improve replicability and lead to the discovery of unexpected interactions between environmental, microbiological, immunological factors and cancer biology.

New insights into colon tumor biology are continuously arising from the careful study of both well-established and newly designed mouse models. Clearly, interactions between the gut microbiota and the host immune system influence colon-tumor outcomes. Through careful characterization of mouse models, appropriate study design, and clear reporting of environmental and experimental conditions, mouse models can continue to rapidly advance our understanding of the complex biology that contributes to colon cancer initiation, progression, and therapeutic response.

Author Contributions: A.A.L., writing—original draft preparation, writing—review and editing; M.L.C., supervision, writing—review and editing.

Funding: This publication was supported by grant number P30 CA006927 from the National Cancer Institute. Its contents are solely the responsibility of the authors and does not necessarily represent the official views of the National Cancer Institute or the National Institutes of Health.

Acknowledgments: The authors wish to thank Wen-Chi Chang and Mariana Fragoso for invaluable comments and Darlene Curran for assistance in preparing this article for publication.

Conflicts of Interest: The authors declare no conflict of interest.

References

1. Bray, F.; Ferlay, J.; Soerjomataram, I.; Siegel, R.L.; Torre, L.A.; Jemal, A. Global cancer statistics 2018: GLOBOCAN estimates of incidence and mortality worldwide for 36 cancers in 185 countries. *CA Cancer J. Clin.* **2018**, *68*, 394–424. [CrossRef] [PubMed]
2. Ciardiello, D.; Vitiello, P.P.; Cardone, C.; Martini, G.; Troiani, T.; Martinelli, E.; Ciardiello, F. Immunotherapy of colorectal cancer: Challenges for therapeutic efficacy. *Cancer Treat. Rev.* **2019**, *76*, 22–32. [CrossRef] [PubMed]
3. Tintelnot, J.; Stein, A. Immunotherapy in colorectal cancer: Available clinical evidence, challenges and novel approaches. *WJG* **2019**, *25*, 3920–3928. [CrossRef] [PubMed]
4. Chang, W.-C.L.; Jackson, C.; Riel, S.; Cooper, H.S.; Devarajan, K.; Hensley, H.H.; Zhou, Y.; Vanderveer, L.A.; Nguyen, M.T.; Clapper, M.L. Differential preventive activity of sulindac and atorvastatin in Apc +/Min-FCCCmice with or without colorectal adenomas. *Gut* **2018**, *67*, 1290–1298. [CrossRef] [PubMed]
5. Kaur, K.; Saxena, A.; Debnath, I.; O'Brien, J.L.; Ajami, N.J.; Auchtung, T.A.; Petrosino, J.F.; Sougiannis, A.-J.; Depaep, S.; Chumanevich, A.; et al. Antibiotic-mediated bacteriome depletion in Apc Min/+ mice is associated with reduction in mucus-producing goblet cells and increased colorectal cancer progression. *Cancer Med.* **2018**, *7*, 2003–2012. [CrossRef] [PubMed]
6. Wu, S.; Rhee, K.-J.; Albesiano, E.; Rabizadeh, S.; Wu, X.; Yen, H.-R.; Huso, D.L.; Brancati, F.L.; Wick, E.; Mcallister, F.; et al. A human colonic commensal promotes colon tumorigenesis via activation of T helper type 17 T cell responses. *Nat. Med.* **2009**, *15*, 1016–1022. [CrossRef] [PubMed]
7. Destefano Shields, C.E.; Van Meerbeke, S.W.; Housseau, F.; Wang, H.; Huso, D.L.; Casero, R.A.; O'Hagan, H.M.; Sears, C.L. Reduction of Murine Colon Tumorigenesis Driven by Enterotoxigenic Bacteroides fragilis Using Cefoxitin Treatment. *J. Infect. Dis.* **2016**, *214*, 122–129. [CrossRef] [PubMed]
8. Chung, L.; Thiele Orberg, E.; Geis, A.L.; Chan, J.L.; Fu, K.; Destefano Shields, C.E.; Dejea, C.M.; Fathi, P.; Chen, J.; Finard, B.B.; et al. Bacteroides fragilis Toxin Coordinates a Pro-carcinogenic Inflammatory Cascade via Targeting of Colonic Epithelial Cells. *Cell Host Microbe* **2018**, *23*, 203–214.e5. [CrossRef]
9. Dejea, C.M.; Fathi, P.; Craig, J.M.; Boleij, A.; Taddese, R.; Geis, A.L.; Wu, X.; Destefano Shields, C.E.; Hechenbleikner, E.M.; Huso, D.L.; et al. Patients with familial adenomatous polyposis harbor colonic biofilms containing tumorigenic bacteria. *Science* **2018**, *359*, 592–597. [CrossRef]

10. Arthur, J.C.; Perez-Chanona, E.; Muhlbauer, M.; Tomkovich, S.; Uronis, J.M.; Fan, T.J.; Campbell, B.J.; Abujamel, T.; Dogan, B.; Rogers, A.B.; et al. Intestinal Inflammation Targets Cancer-Inducing Activity of the Microbiota. *Science* **2012**, *338*, 120–123. [CrossRef]
11. Yang, I.; Eibach, D.; Kops, F.; Brenneke, B.; Woltemate, S.; Schulze, J.; Bleich, A.; Gruber, A.D.; Muthupalani, S.; Fox, J.G.; et al. Intestinal Microbiota Composition of Interleukin-10 Deficient C57BL/6J Mice and Susceptibility to Helicobacter hepaticus-Induced Colitis. *PLoS ONE* **2013**, *8*, e70783-13. [CrossRef] [PubMed]
12. Kullberg, M.C.; Ward, J.M.; Gorelick, P.L.; Caspar, P.; Hieny, S.; Cheever, A.; Jankovic, D.; Sher, A. Helicobacter hepaticus triggers colitis in specific-pathogen-free interleukin-10 (IL-10)-deficient mice through an IL-12- and gamma interferon-dependent mechanism. *Infect. Immun.* **1998**, *66*, 5157–5166. [PubMed]
13. Dieleman, L.A.; Arends, A.; Tonkonogy, S.L.; Goerres, M.S.; Craft, D.W.; Grenther, W.; Sellon, R.K.; Balish, E.; Sartor, R.B. Helicobacter hepaticus does not induce or potentiate colitis in interleukin-10-deficient mice. *Infect. Immun.* **2000**, *68*, 5107–5113. [CrossRef] [PubMed]
14. Belcheva, A.; Irrazabal, T.; Robertson, S.J.; Streutker, C.; Maughan, H.; Rubino, S.; Moriyama, E.H.; Copeland, J.K.; Surendra, A.; Kumar, S.; et al. Gut Microbial Metabolism Drives Transformation of Msh2-Deficient Colon Epithelial Cells. *Cell* **2014**, *158*, 288–299. [CrossRef]
15. Zackular, J.P.; Baxter, N.T.; Iverson, K.D.; Sadler, W.D.; Petrosino, J.F.; Chen, G.Y.; Schloss, P.D. The Gut Microbiome Modulates Colon Tumorigenesis. *mBio* **2013**, *4*, e00692-13. [CrossRef]
16. Zhan, Y.; Chen, P.-J.; Sadler, W.D.; Wang, F.; Poe, S.; Nunez, G.; Eaton, K.A.; Chen, G.Y. Gut microbiota protects against gastrointestinal tumorigenesis caused by epithelial injury. *Cancer Res.* **2013**, *73*, 7199–7210. [CrossRef]
17. Rosshart, S.P.; Vassallo, B.G.; Angeletti, D.; Hutchinson, D.S.; Morgan, A.P.; Takeda, K.; Hickman, H.D.; Mcculloch, J.A.; Badger, J.H.; Ajami, N.J.; et al. Wild Mouse Gut Microbiota Promotes Host Fitness and Improves Disease Resistance. *Cell* **2017**, *171*, 1015–1028.e13. [CrossRef]
18. Lehouritis, P.; Cummins, J.; Stanton, M.; Murphy, C.T.; McCarthy, F.O.; Reid, G.; Urbaniak, C.; Byrne, W.L.; Tangney, M. Local bacteria affect the efficacy of chemotherapeutic drugs. *Sci. Rep.* **2015**, *5*, 14554. [CrossRef]
19. Iida, N.; Dzutsev, A.; Stewart, C.A.; Smith, L.; Bouladoux, N.; Weingarten, R.A.; Molina, D.A.; Salcedo, R.; Back, T.; Cramer, S.; et al. Commensal Bacteria Control Cancer Response to Therapy by Modulating the Tumor Microenvironment. *Science* **2013**, *342*, 967–970. [CrossRef]
20. Vetizou, M.; Pitt, J.M.; Daillere, R.; Lepage, P.; Waldschmitt, N.; Flament, C.; Rusakiewicz, S.; Routy, B.; Roberti, M.P.; Duong, C.P.M.; et al. Anticancer immunotherapy by CTLA-4 blockade relies on the gut microbiota. *Science* **2015**, *350*, 1079–1084. [CrossRef]
21. Hooper, L.V.; Littman, D.R.; Macpherson, A.J. Interactions Between the Microbiota and the Immune System. *Science* **2012**, *336*, 1268–1273. [CrossRef]
22. Carroll, I.M.; Threadgill, D.W.; Threadgill, D.S. The gastrointestinal microbiome: A malleable, third genome of mammals. *Mamm. Genome* **2009**, *20*, 395–403. [CrossRef] [PubMed]
23. Son, J.S.; Khair, S.; Pettet, D.W.; Ouyang, N.; Tian, X.; Zhang, Y.; Zhu, W.; Mackenzie, G.G.; Robertson, C.E.; Ir, D.; et al. Altered Interactions between the Gut Microbiome and Colonic Mucosa Precede Polyposis in APCMin/+ Mice. *PLoS ONE* **2015**, *10*, e0127985. [CrossRef] [PubMed]
24. Zhang, J.; Haines, C.; Watson, A.J.M.; Hart, A.R.; Platt, M.J.; Pardoll, D.M.; Cosgrove, S.E.; Gebo, K.A.; Sears, C.L. Oral antibiotic use and risk of colorectal cancer in the United Kingdom, 1989–2012: A matched case-control study. *Gut* **2019**, *68*, 1971–1978. [CrossRef] [PubMed]
25. Wang, C.-S.-E.; Li, W.-B.; Wang, H.-Y.; Ma, Y.-M.; Zhao, X.-H.; Yang, H.; Qian, J.-M.; Li, J.-N. VSL#3 can prevent ulcerative colitis-associated carcinogenesis in mice. *WJG* **2018**, *24*, 4254–4262.
26. Do, E.-J.; Hwang, S.W.; Kim, S.-Y.; Ryu, Y.-M.; Cho, E.A.; Chung, E.-J.; Park, S.; Lee, H.J.; Byeon, J.-S.; Ye, B.D.; et al. Suppression of colitis-associated carcinogenesis through modulation of IL-6/STAT3 pathway by balsalazide and VSL#3. *J. Gastroenterol. Hepatol.* **2016**, *31*, 1453–1461.
27. Grivennikov, S.I.; Wang, K.; Mucida, D.; Stewart, C.A.; Schnabl, B.; Jauch, D.; Taniguchi, K.; Yu, G.-Y.; Österreicher, C.H.; Hung, K.E.; et al. Adenoma-linked barrier defects and microbial products drive IL-23/IL-17-mediated tumour growth. *Nature* **2012**, *491*, 254–258. [CrossRef]
28. Wong, S.H.; Zhao, L.; Zhang, X.; Nakatsu, G.; Han, J.; Xu, W.; Xiao, X.; Kwong, T.N.Y.; Tsoi, H.; Wu, W.K.K.; et al. Gavage of Fecal Samples From Patients With Colorectal Cancer Promotes Intestinal Carcinogenesis in Germ-Free and Conventional Mice. *Gastroenterology* **2017**, *153*, 1621–1633. [CrossRef]

29. Kostic, A.D.; Chun, E.; Robertson, L.; Glickman, J.N.; Gallini, C.A.; Michaud, M.; Clancy, T.E.; Chung, D.C.; Lochhead, P.; Hold, G.L.; et al. Fusobacterium nucleatum potentiates intestinal tumorigenesis and modulates the tumor-immune microenvironment. *Cell Host Microbe* **2013**, *14*, 207–215. [CrossRef]
30. Arthur, J.C.; Gharaibeh, R.Z.; Mühlbauer, M.; Perez-Chanona, E.; Uronis, J.M.; Mccafferty, J.; Fodor, A.A.; Jobin, C. Microbial genomic analysis reveals the essential role of inflammation in bacteria-induced colorectal cancer. *Nat. Commun.* **2014**, *5*, 4724. [CrossRef]
31. Cougnoux, A.; Dalmasso, G.; Martinez, R.; Buc, E.; Delmas, J.; Gibold, L.; Sauvanet, P.; Darcha, C.; Déchelotte, P.; Bonnet, M.; et al. Bacterial genotoxin colibactin promotes colon tumour growth by inducing a senescence-associated secretory phenotype. *Gut* **2014**, *63*, 1932–1942. [CrossRef] [PubMed]
32. Tytgat, H.L.P.; Nobrega, F.L.; van der Oost, J.; de Vos, W.M. Bowel Biofilms: Tipping Points between a Healthy and Compromised Gut? *Trends Microbiol.* **2019**, *27*, 17–25. [CrossRef] [PubMed]
33. Dejea, C.M.; Wick, E.C.; Hechenbleikner, E.M.; White, J.R.; Mark Welch, J.L.; Rossetti, B.J.; Peterson, S.N.; Snesrud, E.C.; Borisy, G.G.; Lazarev, M.; et al. Microbiota organization is a distinct feature of proximal colorectal cancers. *Proc. Natl. Acad. Sci. USA* **2014**, *111*, 18321–18326. [CrossRef] [PubMed]
34. Zarco, M.F.; Vess, T.J.; Ginsburg, G.S. The oral microbiome in health and disease and the potential impact on personalized dental medicine. *Oral Dis.* **2012**, *18*, 109–120. [CrossRef]
35. Han, S.; Gao, J.; Zhou, Q.; Liu, S.; Wen, C.; Yang, X. Role of intestinal flora in colorectal cancer from the metabolite perspective: A systematic review. *CMAR* **2018**, *10*, 199–206. [CrossRef]
36. Seidel, D.V.; Azcarate-Peril, M.A.; Chapkin, R.S.; Turner, N.D. Shaping functional gut microbiota using dietary bioactives to reduce colon cancer risk. *Semin. Cancer Biol.* **2017**, *46*, 191–204. [CrossRef]
37. Wilson, M.R.; Jiang, Y.; Villalta, P.W.; Stornetta, A.; Boudreau, P.D.; Carrá, A.; Brennan, C.A.; Chun, E.; Ngo, L.; Samson, L.D.; et al. The human gut bacterial genotoxin colibactin alkylates DNA. *Science* **2019**, *363*, eaar7785. [CrossRef]
38. Donohoe, D.R.; Holley, D.; Collins, L.B.; Montgomery, S.A.; Whitmore, A.C.; Hillhouse, A.; Curry, K.P.; Renner, S.W.; Greenwalt, A.; Ryan, E.P.; et al. A Gnotobiotic Mouse Model Demonstrates That Dietary Fiber Protects against Colorectal Tumorigenesis in a Microbiota- and Butyrate-Dependent Manner. *Cancer Discov.* **2014**, *4*, 1387–1397. [CrossRef]
39. Kim, M.; Friesen, L.; Park, J.; Kim, H.M.; Kim, C.H. Microbial metabolites, short-chain fatty acids, restrain tissue bacterial load, chronic inflammation, and associated cancer in the colon of mice. *Eur. J. Immunol.* **2018**, *48*, 1235–1247. [CrossRef]
40. Smith, P.M.; Howitt, M.R.; Panikov, N.; Michaud, M.; Gallini, C.A.; Bohlooly-Y, M.; Glickman, J.N.; Garrett, W.S. The microbial metabolites, short-chain fatty acids, regulate colonic Treg cell homeostasis. *Science* **2013**, *341*, 569–573. [CrossRef]
41. Chapkin, R.S.; Davidson, L.A.; Ly, L.; Weeks, B.R.; Lupton, J.R.; McMurray, D.N. Immunomodulatory effects of (n-3) fatty acids: Putative link to inflammation and colon cancer. *J. Nutr.* **2007**, *137*, 200S–204S. [CrossRef] [PubMed]
42. Bauer, H.; Horowitz, R.E.; Levenson, S.M.; Popper, H. The response of the lymphatic tissue to the microbial flora. Studies on germfree mice. *Am. J. Pathol.* **1963**, *42*, 471–483. [PubMed]
43. Gensollen, T.; Iyer, S.S.; Kasper, D.L.; Blumberg, R.S. How colonization by microbiota in early life shapes the immune system. *Science* **2016**, *352*, 539–544. [CrossRef]
44. Knoop, K.A.; Gustafsson, J.K.; McDonald, K.G.; Kulkarni, D.H.; Coughlin, P.E.; McCrate, S.; Kim, D.; Hsieh, C.-S.; Hogan, S.P.; Elson, C.O.; et al. Microbial antigen encounter during a preweaning interval is critical for tolerance to gut bacteria. *Sci. Immunol.* **2017**, *2*, eaao1314. [CrossRef] [PubMed]
45. Ivanov, I.I.; Atarashi, K.; Manel, N.; Brodie, E.L.; Shima, T.; Karaoz, U.; Wei, D.; Goldfarb, K.C.; Santee, C.A.; Lynch, S.V.; et al. Induction of Intestinal Th17 Cells by Segmented Filamentous Bacteria. *Cell* **2009**, *139*, 485–498. [CrossRef]
46. Duan, J.; Chung, H.; Troy, E.; Kasper, D.L. Microbial colonization drives expansion of IL-1 receptor 1-expressing and IL-17-producing gamma/delta T cells. *Cell Host Microbe* **2010**, *7*, 140–150. [CrossRef]
47. Bhattacharya, N.; Yuan, R.; Prestwood, T.R.; Penny, H.L.; DiMaio, M.A.; Reticker-Flynn, N.E.; Krois, C.R.; Kenkel, J.A.; Pham, T.D.; Carmi, Y.; et al. Normalizing Microbiota-Induced Retinoic Acid Deficiency Stimulates Protective CD8 + T Cell-Mediated Immunity in Colorectal Cancer. *Immunity* **2016**, *45*, 641–655. [CrossRef]

48. Britton, G.J.; Contijoch, E.J.; Mogno, I.; Vennaro, O.H.; Llewellyn, S.R.; Ng, R.; Li, Z.; Mortha, A.; Merad, M.; Das, A.; et al. Microbiotas from Humans with Inflammatory Bowel Disease Alter the Balance of Gut Th17 and RORγt+ Regulatory T Cells and Exacerbate Colitis in Mice. *Immunity* **2019**, *50*, 212–224.e4. [CrossRef]
49. Housseau, F.; Wu, S.; Wick, E.C.; Fan, H.; Wu, X.; Llosa, N.J.; Smith, K.N.; Tam, A.; Ganguly, S.; Wanyiri, J.W.; et al. Redundant Innate and Adaptive Sources of IL17 Production Drive Colon Tumorigenesis. *Cancer Res.* **2016**, *76*, 2115–2124. [CrossRef]
50. Atarashi, K.; Tanoue, T.; Shima, T.; Imaoka, A.; Kuwahara, T.; Momose, Y.; Cheng, G.; Yamasaki, S.; Saito, T.; Ohba, Y.; et al. Induction of colonic regulatory T cells by indigenous Clostridium species. *Science* **2011**, *331*, 337–341. [CrossRef]
51. Atarashi, K.; Tanoue, T.; Oshima, K.; Suda, W.; Nagano, Y.; Nishikawa, H.; Fukuda, S.; Saito, T.; Narushima, S.; Hase, K.; et al. Treg induction by a rationally selected mixture of Clostridia strains from the human microbiota. *Nature* **2013**, *500*, 232–236. [CrossRef] [PubMed]
52. Pastille, E.; Bardini, K.; Fleissner, D.; Adamczyk, A.; Frede, A.; Wadwa, M.; Von Smolinski, D.; Kasper, S.; Sparwasser, T.; Gruber, A.D.; et al. Transient Ablation of Regulatory T cells Improves Antitumor Immunity in Colitis-Associated Colon Cancer. *Cancer Res.* **2014**, *74*, 4258–4269. [CrossRef] [PubMed]
53. Yu, T.; Guo, F.; Yu, Y.; Sun, T.; Ma, D.; Han, J.; Qian, Y.; Kryczek, I.; Sun, D.; Nagarsheth, N.; et al. Fusobacterium nucleatum Promotes Chemoresistance to Colorectal Cancer by Modulating Autophagy. *Cell* **2017**, *170*, 548–563.e16. [CrossRef] [PubMed]
54. Kunzmann, A.T.; Proença, M.A.; Jordao, H.W.; Jiraskova, K.; Schneiderova, M.; Levy, M.; Liska, V.; Buchler, T.; Vodickova, L.; Vymetalkova, V.; et al. Fusobacterium nucleatum tumor DNA levels are associated with survival in colorectal cancer patients. *Eur. J. Clin. Microbiol. Infect. Dis.* **2019**, *38*, 1891–1899. [CrossRef] [PubMed]
55. Yamamura, K.; Izumi, D.; Kandimalla, R.; Sonohara, F.; Baba, Y.; Yoshida, N.; Kodera, Y.; Baba, H.; Goel, A. Intratumoral Fusobacterium Nucleatum Levels Predict Therapeutic Response to Neoadjuvant Chemotherapy in Esophageal Squamous Cell Carcinoma. *Clin. Cancer Res.* **2019**, *25*, 6170–6179. [CrossRef] [PubMed]
56. Panebianco, C.; Andriulli, A.; Pazienza, V. Pharmacomicrobiomics: Exploiting the drug-microbiota interactions in anticancer therapies. *Microbiome* **2018**, *6*, 92. [CrossRef] [PubMed]
57. Cong, J.; Zhang, X. Roles of intestinal microbiota in response to cancer immunotherapy. *Eur. J. Clin. Microbiol. Infect. Dis.* **2018**, *37*, 2235–2240. [CrossRef]
58. Hagan, T.; Cortese, M.; Rouphael, N.; Boudreau, C.; Linde, C.; Maddur, M.S.; Das, J.; Wang, H.; Guthmiller, J.; Zheng, N.-Y.; et al. Antibiotics-Driven Gut Microbiome Perturbation Alters Immunity to Vaccines in Humans. *Cell* **2019**, *178*, 1313–1328.e13. [CrossRef]
59. Kalyan, A.; Kircher, S.; Shah, H.; Mulcahy, M.; Benson, A. Updates on immunotherapy for colorectal cancer. *J. Gastrointest. Oncol.* **2018**, *9*, 160–169. [CrossRef]
60. Rioux, C.R.; Clapper, M.L.; Cooper, H.S.; Michaud, J.; St Amant, N.; Koohsari, H.; Workman, L.; Kaunga, E.; Hensley, H.; Pilorget, A.; et al. Self-antigen MASH2 combined with the AS15 immunostimulant induces tumor protection in colorectal cancer mouse models. *PLoS ONE* **2019**, *14*, e0210261. [CrossRef]
61. Kwon, S.; Kim, Y.-E.; Park, J.-A.; Kim, D.-S.; Kwon, H.-J.; Lee, Y. Therapeutic effect of a TM4SF5-specific peptide vaccine against colon cancer in a mouse model. *BMB Rep.* **2014**, *47*, 215–220. [CrossRef] [PubMed]
62. Song, C.; Zheng, X.-J.; Liu, C.-C.; Zhou, Y.; Ye, X.-S. A cancer vaccine based on fluorine-modified sialyl-Tn induces robust immune responses in a murine model. *Oncotarget* **2017**, *8*, 47330–47343. [CrossRef] [PubMed]
63. Kurilshikov, A.; Wijmenga, C.; Fu, J.; Zhernakova, A. Host Genetics and Gut Microbiome: Challenges and Perspectives. *Trends Immunol.* **2017**, *38*, 633–647. [CrossRef] [PubMed]
64. Benson, A.K.; Kelly, S.A.; Legge, R.; Ma, F.; Low, S.J.; Kim, J.; Zhang, M.; Oh, P.L.; Nehrenberg, D.; Hua, K.; et al. Individuality in gut microbiota composition is a complex polygenic trait shaped by multiple environmental and host genetic factors. *Proc. Natl. Acad. Sci. USA* **2010**, *107*, 18933–18938. [CrossRef]
65. Deloris Alexander, A.; Orcutt, R.P.; Henry, J.C.; Baker, J.; Bissahoyo, A.C.; Threadgill, D.W. Quantitative PCR assays for mouse enteric flora reveal strain-dependent differences in composition that are influenced by the microenvironment. *Mamm. Genome* **2006**, *17*, 1093–1104. [CrossRef]
66. Friswell, M.K.; Gika, H.; Stratford, I.J.; Theodoridis, G.; Telfer, B.; Wilson, I.D.; Mcbain, A.J. Site and strain-specific variation in gut microbiota profiles and metabolism in experimental mice. *PLoS ONE* **2010**, *5*, e8584. [CrossRef]

67. Pantoja-Feliciano, I.G.; Clemente, J.C.; Costello, E.K.; Perez, M.E.; Blaser, M.J.; Knight, R.; Dominguez-Bello, M.G. Biphasic assembly of the murine intestinal microbiota during early development. *ISME J.* **2013**, *7*, 1112–1115. [CrossRef]
68. Hufeldt, M.R.; Nielsen, D.S.; Vogensen, F.K.; Midtvedt, T.; Hansen, A.K. Family relationship of female breeders reduce the systematic inter-individual variation in the gut microbiota of inbred laboratory mice. *Lab. Anim.* **2010**, *44*, 283–289. [CrossRef]
69. Lundberg, R.; Bahl, M.I.; Licht, T.R.; Toft, M.F.; Hansen, A.K. Microbiota composition of simultaneously colonized mice housed under either a gnotobiotic isolator or individually ventilated cage regime. *Sci. Rep.* **2017**, *7*, 42245. [CrossRef]
70. Mccafferty, J.; Mühlbauer, M.; Gharaibeh, R.Z.; Arthur, J.C.; Perez-Chanona, E.; Sha, W.; Jobin, C.; Fodor, A.A. Stochastic changes over time and not founder effects drive cage effects in microbial community assembly in a mouse model. *ISME J.* **2013**, *7*, 2116–2125. [CrossRef]
71. Scott, K.A.; Ida, M.; Peterson, V.L.; Prenderville, J.A.; Moloney, G.M.; Izumo, T.; Murphy, K.; Murphy, A.; Ross, R.P.; Stanton, C.; et al. Revisiting Metchnikoff: Age-related alterations in microbiota-gut-brain axis in the mouse. *Brain Behav. Immun.* **2017**, *65*, 20–32. [CrossRef] [PubMed]
72. Fransen, F.; van Beek, A.A.; Borghuis, T.; Aidy, S.E.; Hugenholtz, F.; van der Gaast de Jongh, C.; Savelkoul, H.F.J.; De Jonge, M.I.; Boekschoten, M.V.; Smidt, H.; et al. Aged Gut Microbiota Contributes to Systemical Inflammaging after Transfer to Germ-Free Mice. *Front. Immunol.* **2017**, *8*, 1385. [CrossRef] [PubMed]
73. Choo, J.M.; Trim, P.J.; Leong, L.E.X.; Abell, G.C.J.; Brune, C.; Jeffries, N.; Wesselingh, S.; Dear, T.N.; Snel, M.F.; Rogers, G.B. Inbred Mouse Populations Exhibit Intergenerational Changes in Intestinal Microbiota Composition and Function Following Introduction to a Facility. *Front. Microbiol.* **2017**, *8*, 608. [CrossRef] [PubMed]
74. Llewellyn, S.R.; Britton, G.J.; Contijoch, E.J.; Vennaro, O.H.; Mortha, A.; Colombel, J.-F.; Grinspan, A.; Clemente, J.C.; Merad, M.; Faith, J.J. Interactions Between Diet and the Intestinal Microbiota Alter Intestinal Permeability and Colitis Severity in Mice. *Gastroenterology* **2018**, *154*, 1037–1046.e2. [CrossRef] [PubMed]
75. Rausch, P.; Basic, M.; Batra, A.; Bischoff, S.C.; Blaut, M.; Clavel, T.; Gläsner, J.; Gopalakrishnan, S.; Grassl, G.A.; Günther, C.; et al. Analysis of factors contributing to variation in the C57BL/6J fecal microbiota across German animal facilities. *Int. J. Med. Microbiol.* **2016**, *306*, 343–355. [CrossRef] [PubMed]
76. Bidot, W.A.; Ericsson, A.C.; Franklin, C.L. Effects of water decontamination methods and bedding material on the gut microbiota. *PLoS ONE* **2018**, *13*, e0198305. [CrossRef] [PubMed]
77. Sofi, M.H.; Gudi, R.; Karumuthil-Melethil, S.; Perez, N.; Johnson, B.M.; Vasu, C. pH of drinking water influences the composition of gut microbiome and type 1 diabetes incidence. *Diabetes* **2014**, *63*, 632–644. [CrossRef]
78. Franklin, C.L.; Ericsson, A.C. Microbiota and reproducibility of rodent models. *Lab. Anim.* **2017**, *46*, 114–122. [CrossRef] [PubMed]
79. Kühn, R.; Löhler, J.; Rennick, D.; Rajewsky, K.; Muller, W. Interleukin-10-deficient mice develop chronic enterocolitis. *Cell* **1993**, *75*, 263–274. [CrossRef]
80. Zhang, H.; Sparks, J.B.; Karyala, S.V.; Settlage, R.; Luo, X.M. Host adaptive immunity alters gut microbiota. *ISME J.* **2015**, *9*, 770–781. [CrossRef]
81. Larsson, E.; Tremaroli, V.; Lee, Y.S.; Koren, O.; Nookaew, I.; Fricker, A.; Nielsen, J.; Ley, R.E.; Bäckhed, F. Analysis of gut microbial regulation of host gene expression along the length of the gut and regulation of gut microbial ecology through MyD88. *Gut* **2012**, *61*, 1124–1131. [CrossRef]
82. Vijay-Kumar, M.; Aitken, J.D.; Carvalho, F.A.; Cullender, T.C.; Mwangi, S.; Srinivasan, S.; Sitaraman, S.V.; Knight, R.; Ley, R.E.; Gewirtz, A.T. Metabolic Syndrome and Altered Gut Microbiota in Mice Lacking Toll-Like Receptor 5. *Science* **2010**, *328*, 228–231. [CrossRef]
83. Zhao, X.; Li, L.; Starr, T.K.; Subramanian, S. Tumor location impacts immune response in mouse models of colon cancer. *Oncotarget* **2017**, *8*, 54775–54787. [CrossRef]
84. Rosshart, S.P.; Herz, J.; Vassallo, B.G.; Hunter, A.; Wall, M.K.; Badger, J.H.; Mcculloch, J.A.; Anastasakis, D.G.; Sarshad, A.A.; Leonardi, I.; et al. Laboratory mice born to wild mice have natural microbiota and model human immune responses. *Science* **2019**, *365*, eaaw4361. [CrossRef]
85. Arnold, J.W.; Roach, J.; Azcarate-Peril, M.A. Emerging Technologies for Gut Microbiome Research. *Trends Microbiol.* **2016**, *24*, 887–901. [CrossRef] [PubMed]

86. Panek, M.; Čipčić Paljetak, H.; Barešić, A.; Perić, M.; Matijašić, M.; Lojkić, I.; Vranešić Bender, D.; Krznarić, Ž.; Verbanac, D. Methodology challenges in studying human gut microbiota—Effects of collection, storage, DNA extraction and next generation sequencing technologies. *Sci. Rep.* **2018**, *8*, 5143. [CrossRef]
87. Rintala, A.; Pietilä, S.; Munukka, E.; Eerola, E.; Pursiheimo, J.-P.; Laiho, A.; Pekkala, S.; Huovinen, P. Gut Microbiota Analysis Results Are Highly Dependent on the 16S rRNA Gene Target Region, Whereas the Impact of DNA Extraction Is Minor. *J. Biomol. Tech.* **2017**, *28*, 19–30. [CrossRef]
88. Ranjan, R.; Rani, A.; Metwally, A.; McGee, H.S.; Perkins, D.L. Analysis of the microbiome: Advantages of whole genome shotgun versus 16S amplicon sequencing. *Biochem. Biophys. Res. Commun.* **2016**, *469*, 967–977. [CrossRef] [PubMed]
89. Laukens, D.; Brinkman, B.M.; Raes, J.; De Vos, M.; Vandenabeele, P. Heterogeneity of the gut microbiome in mice: Guidelines for optimizing experimental design. *FEMS Microbiol. Rev.* **2016**, *40*, 117–132. [CrossRef] [PubMed]
90. Wu, Y.-G.; Wu, G.-Z.; Wang, L.; Zhang, Y.-Y.; Li, Z.; Li, D.-C. Tumor cell lysate-pulsed dendritic cells induce a T cell response against colon cancer in vitro and in vivo. *Med. Oncol.* **2010**, *27*, 736–742. [CrossRef] [PubMed]
91. Vo, M.-C.; Nguyen-Pham, T.-N.; Lee, H.-J.; Jaya Lakshmi, T.; Yang, S.; Jung, S.-H.; Kim, H.-J.; Lee, J.-J. Combination therapy with dendritic cells and lenalidomide is an effective approach to enhance antitumor immunity in a mouse colon cancer model. *Oncotarget* **2017**, *8*, 27252–27262. [CrossRef] [PubMed]
92. Zhou, W.; Chow, K.-H.; Fleming, E.; Oh, J. Selective colonization ability of human fecal microbes in different mouse gut environments. *ISME J.* **2019**, *13*, 805–823. [CrossRef]
93. Staley, C.; Kaiser, T.; Beura, L.K.; Hamilton, M.J.; Weingarden, A.R.; Bobr, A.; Kang, J.; Masopust, D.; Sadowsky, M.J.; Khoruts, A. Stable engraftment of human microbiota into mice with a single oral gavage following antibiotic conditioning. *Microbiome* **2017**, *5*, 87. [CrossRef] [PubMed]
94. Bailoo, J.D.; Reichlin, T.S.; Wurbel, H. Refinement of Experimental Design and Conduct in Laboratory Animal Research. *ILAR J.* **2014**, *55*, 383–391. [CrossRef]
95. Bodden, C.; von Kortzfleisch, V.T.; Karwinkel, F.; Kaiser, S.; Sachser, N.; Richter, S.H. Heterogenising study samples across testing time improves reproducibility of behavioural data. *Sci. Rep.* **2019**, *9*, 8247. [CrossRef] [PubMed]
96. Voelkl, B.; Vogt, L.; Sena, E.S.; Würbel, H. Reproducibility of preclinical animal research improves with heterogeneity of study samples. *PLoS Biol.* **2018**, *16*, e2003693. [CrossRef] [PubMed]
97. Kilkenny, C.; Browne, W.J.; Cuthill, I.C.; Emerson, M.; Altman, D.G. Improving bioscience research reporting: The ARRIVE guidelines for reporting animal research. *PLoS Biol.* **2010**, *8*, e1000412. [CrossRef]

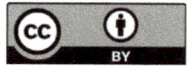

© 2019 by the authors. Licensee MDPI, Basel, Switzerland. This article is an open access article distributed under the terms and conditions of the Creative Commons Attribution (CC BY) license (http://creativecommons.org/licenses/by/4.0/).

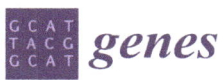 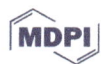

Review

Melanoma-Bearing Libechov Minipig (MeLiM): The Unique Swine Model of Hereditary Metastatic Melanoma

Vratislav Horak, Anna Palanova, Jana Cizkova, Veronika Miltrova, Petr Vodicka and Helena Kupcova Skalnikova *

Czech Academy of Sciences, Institute of Animal Physiology and Genetics, Laboratory of Applied Proteome Analyses and Research Center PIGMOD, 277 21 Libechov, Czech Republic; horakv@iapg.cas.cz (V.H.); palanova@iapg.cas.cz (A.P.); cizkova@iapg.cas.cz (J.C.); miltrova@iapg.cas.cz (V.M.); vodicka@iapg.cas.cz (P.V.)
* Correspondence: skalnikova@iapg.cas.cz; Tel.: +420-315-639-581

Received: 1 October 2019; Accepted: 7 November 2019; Published: 9 November 2019

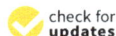

Abstract: National cancer databases document that melanoma is the most aggressive and deadly cutaneous malignancy with worldwide increasing incidence in the Caucasian population. Around 10% of melanomas occur in families. Several germline mutations were identified that might help to indicate individuals at risk for preventive interventions and early disease detection. More than 50% of sporadic melanomas carry mutations in Ras/Raf/mitogen-activated protein kinase (MAPK/MEK) pathway, which may represent aims of novel targeted therapies. Despite advances in targeted therapies and immunotherapies, the outcomes in metastatic tumor are still unsatisfactory. Here, we review animal models that help our understanding of melanoma development and treatment, including non-vertebrate, mouse, swine, and other mammal models, with an emphasis on those with spontaneously developing melanoma. Special attention is paid to the melanoma-bearing Libechov minipig (MeLiM). This original swine model of hereditary metastatic melanoma enables studying biological processes underlying melanoma progression, as well as spontaneous regression. Current histological, immunohistochemical, biochemical, genetic, hematological, immunological, and skin microbiome findings in the MeLiM model are summarized, together with development of new therapeutic approaches based on tumor devitalization. The ongoing study of molecular and immunological base of spontaneous regression in MeLiM model has potential to bring new knowledge of clinical importance.

Keywords: melanoma; mutation; genetics; animal model; swine; MeLiM; progression; spontaneous regression; devitalization

1. Introduction

Skin cancer is a heterogeneous group of oncological diseases that demonstrate worldwide increasing incidence and include cutaneous melanoma (also known as malignant melanoma) and non-melanoma skin cancers (with basal cell carcinoma and squamous cell carcinoma being the most frequent). Non-melanoma skin cancers are more frequent, affect mainly the elderly population, and demonstrate relatively lower aggressiveness, metastatic activity, and mortality. On the contrary, melanoma represents the least frequent but most aggressive skin cancer resulting in 65% of all skin cancer deaths. Skin damage caused by sunlight (ultraviolet radiation) exposure is the main risk factor for development of such skin malignancies [1–4].

Melanoma cells arise from neoplastic transformation of melanocytes, which are pigmented cells originating from melanoblasts. Melanoblasts are non-pigmented precursors derived from multipotent neural crest cells, which migrate during embryonic development to the target tissues. Mature pigmented melanocytes are dispersed in the basal layer of the epidermis and in hair follicles, where they are responsible for skin and hair color. Moreover, melanocytes are naturally present in the iris of the eye, inner ear, nervous system, heart, and other organs [5]. The cutaneous melanoma is the most frequent form. Rarely, neoplastic transformation can arise during fetal development, manifesting as neonatal congenital melanoma [6]. More common is postnatal neoplastic transformation, giving rise to several distinct melanoma variants [7]. In affected humans, long-term monitoring of growing skin lesions and their particular biological analyses are not possible for ethical reasons. Thus, various animal models serve as indispensable objects for detailed research of melanoma and development of new therapeutic procedures. Swine represents an invaluable model with anatomical and physiological resemblance and considerably similar skin architecture to human [8,9].

2. Human Melanoma

2.1. Incidence

The incidence of cutaneous melanoma steadily increased over the last 50 years, particularly in fair-skinned populations in Europe, North America, Australia, and New Zealand [10]. The highest incidence is recorded in Queensland, Australia (approximately 50 cases per 100,000 people per year); in European populations, the incidence reaches 15–20 cases per 100,000 per year [11]. Almost 100,000 new cases are predicted to be diagnosed in 2019 in the United States, making melanoma the fifth most frequently diagnosed cancer [12]. Rising incidence was also reported for young and middle-aged people [10,13]. The increasing incidence is accompanied by increasing mortality from such a disease. However, due to education on melanoma prevention, early diagnosis, and advances in treatment, a descent in mortality is expected in the following years, at least in developed countries.

2.2. Risk Factors

The risk of melanoma development depends mainly on interaction between environmental exposure and susceptibility of the host [13]. The major environmental cause of melanoma is sun exposure, particularly intermittent (short and intense) sun exposure and the number of sunburns [14]. Additional environmental factors, such as exposure to cosmic radiation (e.g., in airway pilots and crew), polycyclic aromatic hydrocarbons, benzene, heavy metals, and other chemicals, were suggested to play a part in the etiology of the disease. However, the information from studies of such factors is not strong [14].

The most important host risk factors are the number and type of melanocytic nevi. Presence of a high number of nevi, large nevi (diameter over 2 mm), and/or dysplastic or atypical nevi, even on body parts not chronically exposed to sunlight, is associated with an increased risk of melanoma [14]. For example, individuals with more than 100 normal nevi are at almost seven-fold higher risk than people with fewer than 15 nevi [14]. Skin, hair, and eye colors, ability to tan, and propensity to burn are additional host factors influencing melanoma development [13,14]. As approximately 10% of cases occur in families, genetic factors contribute to the susceptibility to melanoma. The discovery of melanoma susceptibility genes and their mutations could lead to development of more accurate prediction and screening tools to identify high-risk populations and to identify new therapeutic targets or prevention strategies [14,15].

2.3. Genetic Background in Melanoma

2.3.1. Germline Mutations in Familial Melanoma

In the human population, an increased incidence of melanoma observed in relatives of affected individuals led to the suggestion of a hereditary cause [16]. First genetic studies on melanoma cell lines established from patient metastases identified loss of heterozygosity in several autosomal and X-linked loci [17]. Five years later, deletion within the human chromosome 9p.21 region was identified [18]. The linkage analysis of melanoma prone families from Australia confirmed the existence of a melanoma susceptibility gene in region 9p [19]. Kamb et al. identified a candidate gene in the 9p region as the cyclin-dependent kinase inhibitor 2A (*CDKN2A*) gene, encoding the p16^{INK4A} protein, which is an inhibitor of cyclin-dependent kinase 4 (CDK4). All three identified mutations in the *CDKN2A* gene changed the p16 amino-acid sequence [20]. Many *CDKN2A* gene mutations were later observed in populations of various countries including southern Sweden [21], Massachusetts, United States of America (USA) [22], United Kingdom [23], France [24], and Queensland, Australia, where the mutations were found only in high-risk families [25]. An additional transcript variant of *CDKN2A* gene was discovered in 1995 by Quelle et al., sharing exons 2 and 3 with p16 but having a different exon 1, and was named p19^{ARF} in mouse [26]. The human counterpart (p14^{ARF}) was identified three years later [27]. Currently, germline *CDKN2A* mutations are observed in 20–40% of families with hereditary melanoma across continents [28]. More than 60 different mutations in the *CDKN2A* gene were found in hereditary melanoma families, with the majority of them represented by missense mutations in p16 [29]. In contrast, incidence of somatic *CDKN2A* mutations in sporadic melanomas is very low [30].

In 1995, a mutated *CDK4* was found in cultured melanoma cells and metastatic tissue. This mutation prevented binding of p16^{INK4A} to CDK4, thus obstructing inhibition of the CDK4 enzyme activity [31]. A *CDK4* mutation was later found in two unrelated melanoma families [32], and the role of *CDK4* mutations in melanoma development was confirmed [24]. In 17 familial melanoma pedigrees, two germline mutations in *CDK4* were observed by Puntervol et al. [33]. Both *CDKN2A* and *CDK4* represent high-susceptibility genes for malignant melanoma, i.e., mutation in such genes greatly increases the chance of melanoma development.

Additional gene mutations were identified as causal for predisposition to melanoma itself or in combination with other cancers in the last decade. Germline mutations in the breast cancer 1 (BRCA1)-associated protein-1 (*BAP1*) gene were found in highly metastatic uveal melanoma [34] and later also in familial cutaneous melanoma [35,36]. The *BAP1* mutations frequently lead to loss of BAP1 expression (e.g., due to homozygous deletions, premature stop codon, or missense mutations). Loss of *BAP1* expression was observed in 5% of cutaneous melanomas by immunohistochemistry [37]. The BAP1 functions as part of the DNA damage response proteins promoting repair of DNA double-strand breaks [38]. However, the exact mechanism of *BAP1* mutations that promote melanoma genesis is yet to be elucidated [39].

Germline mutation in telomerase reverse transcriptase (*TERT* gene) [40] and other proteins, which protect the ends of chromosomes from deterioration and the cells from senescence, were also reported in melanoma affected families. Mutations in the protection of telomeres 1 (*POT1*) gene may lead to insufficient capping of telomeres by the shelterin complex and may also regulate telomerase function [39]. Loss-of-function, missense mutations or other *POT1* variants were observed in familial melanoma patients in the United Kingdom, the Netherlands, and Australia [41] and in another study also in Italy, USA, and France [42]. Incidence of pathogenic germline mutations of *POT1* is low (~2–5%) [43]. Mutation in additional shelterin complex genes (adrenocortical dysplasia protein homolog, *ACD*; telomeric repeat-binding factor 2-interacting protein 1, *TERF2IP*) were found in familial melanoma patients [44].

Mutations in the microphthalmia (mi) locus in mice are causative for several defects, including small unpigmented eyes and lack of skin melanocytes [45]. A human homolog, microphthalmia-associated transcription factor (*MITF*) gene codes for a transcription factor activating expression of tyrosinase, a rate-limiting enzyme in melanin biosynthesis [46]. MITF is also a major transcriptional regulator of melanoma inhibitor of apoptosis (ML-IAP) expression in melanoma tissues. This suggests that MITF has pro-survival activity in melanoma progression [47]. *MITF* germline mutations increase risk of cutaneous melanoma development by three- to five-fold [39]. *MITF* amplification is more prevalent in metastatic disease and correlated with decreased patient survival [48]. Mutations in the *MITF* gene are found not only in melanomas but also in other cancers, such as renal cell carcinoma [49].

As mutations in high-susceptibility genes greatly increase risk of melanoma development, individuals carrying *CDKN2A*, *CDK4*, *BAP1*, *POT1*, or *MITF* mutations should be educated on the importance of melanoma prevention and early detection and should undergo regular medical skin examination [15]. Unfortunately, it still remains uncertain how these mutations influence patient phenotypes, as the melanoma risk is influenced by variations in penetrance, environmental exposure, and coinheritance with low-susceptibility genes [29,39].

Low-susceptibility genes are genes with variants increasing risk of melanoma development with lower penetrance. Melanocortin 1 receptor (*MC1R*) gene variants are associated with red hair and fair skin, a skin phototype with higher risk of melanoma development [50,51]. Presence of *MC1R* variants, together with *CDKN2A* mutations, significantly increases melanoma risk [52].

The protective role of calcitriol, a hormonal derivate of vitamin D3, was confirmed in melanoma studies [53,54]. Several polymorphisms of the vitamin D receptor (*VDR*) gene have a supporting effect in melanoma formation and correlate with a negative outcome in affected patients [55].

Epidermal growth factor (EGF) is relevant to wound healing, proliferation of epidermal tissues, and tumorigenesis. Functional polymorphisms of this gene are associated with melanoma development [56].

Many other gene variants may increase melanoma risk. Due to the only partial penetration and combination with other (host, environmental) factors, low-susceptibility genes are difficult to identify. More detailed information and additional gene candidates can be found in several reviews [14,39,57–60]. Genome-wide association studies (GWAS) are used to investigate the entire genomes for single-nucleotide polymorphisms or other gene variants associated with diseases. GWAS allow examination of genes previously not known to be connected to a disease, especially in polygenic diseases with incomplete penetrance, such as many cancers. Results from 11 GWAS in melanoma identified more than 20 loci, including skin pigmentation, epidermal development, telomere maintenance, and cell-cycle progression gene loci, to be associated with melanoma [61]. Pigmentation-related genes, such as *MC1R* (discussed above), oculocutaneous albinism type 2 (*OCA2*), Agouti signaling protein (*ASIP*), tyrosinase (*TYR*), Tyrosinase-related protein 1 (*TYRP1*), solute carrier family 45 member 2 (*SLC45A2*), and a locus encoding interferon regulatory factor 4 (*IRF4*) and exocyst complex component 2 (*EXOC2*), associate with increased risk of melanoma and also other cutaneous malignancies (basal cell carcinoma, squamous cell carcinoma) [62,63].

2.3.2. Somatic Mutations in Sporadic Melanoma

The majority (~90%) of cutaneous melanoma cases occur sporadically without any records in family pedigree. Such tumors result from somatic mutations and other changes accumulated in the pigmented tissues during the life of an individual. In the majority of sporadic human melanomas, mutations activating the mitogen-activated protein kinase (MAPK/MEK) pathway (Figure 1) are present, affecting mainly *BRAF*, *NRAS*, or neurofibromin 1 (*NF1*) genes (see below).

BRAF encodes B-Raf signal transduction serine–threonine kinase regulated by Ras and activating the MAPK signaling cascade [64]. About 50% of cutaneous melanomas carry a mutation in *BRAF* gene, which is in approximately 50% cases represented by V600E substitution, followed by V600K (10–15%) and several less frequent mutations [65]. Interestingly, mutation *BRAF* V600E was detected also in a majority of benign nevi [65].

The Ras proteins are essential regulators the MAPK and the phosphatidylinositol 3-kinase (PI3K) pathways [66]. In 10–15% of melanomas, mutations in *NRAS* occur, predominantly in codon 61. Such *NRAS* mutations are an adverse prognostic factor [67]. Mutations in *KRAS* are rare in cutaneous melanoma (2% of cases), in contrast to other cancers such as colorectal cancer [67]. Interestingly, *KRAS* mutations were detected in several mouse melanoma models and melanoma cell lines [67].

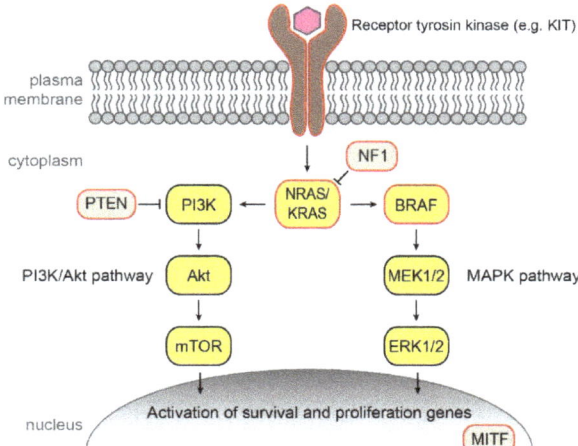

Figure 1. Mitogen-activated protein kinase (MAPK/MEK) and phosphatidylinositol 3-kinase (PI3K)/ protein kinase B (Akt) pathways involved in sporadic melanoma. Mutations frequently present in melanoma tissue are highlighted in red.

Neurofibromin 1 is a negative regulator of Ras. NF1 inactivation leads to the constitutive activation of the MAPK and PI3K pathways. Mutations inactivating NF1 were reported in approximately 50% of melanomas [66].

Increased expression of receptor tyrosine protein kinase erbB-3, also known as human epidermal growth factor receptor 3 (HER3), a member of the EGFR family of receptor tyrosine kinases, was described as a marker of poor prognosis in melanoma [65]. Less than 2% of cutaneous melanomas carry mutation in transmembrane receptor tyrosine kinase *KIT* [11,65].

Amplifications of the *MITF* gene were observed in 20% of metastatic melanomas and are associated with decreased five-year survival. It was suggested that MITF can be activated by the MAPK pathway in malignant melanoma development [66].

Mutation in other molecules and pathways outside of the MAPK pathway were also reported in sporadic melanoma, e.g., mutations and deletions in phosphatase and tensin homolog (*PTEN*), which encodes a phosphatase and a key regulator of the PI3K signaling pathway, as well as mutations in p53, telomerase catalytic subunit *TERT*, cell-cycle regulating proteins, and many others [65,66,68].

According to the most prevalent significantly mutated genes, The Cancer Genome Atlas Network recently provided a schema for cutaneous melanoma genomic classification into four subtypes: mutant *BRAF*, mutant *RAS*, mutant *NF1*, and triple-WT (wild-type) [69]. Elucidation of important mutations in melanoma led in the last decade to the development of targeted therapies that improved survival of melanoma and also other cancer patients. The examples include B-Raf inhibitors that are used in B-Raf V600E and V600K mutated cancers or MEK inhibitors for treatment cancers with activated upper parts of the MAPK cascade [64]. The genetic classification of melanoma represents a significant step toward personalized medicine from both prognostic and treatment points of view [70].

2.4. Regression

Spontaneous regression is a disappearance of the tumor or its part in the absence of any treatment. It occurs more frequently in melanoma than in other human tumors [71]. However, this observation might be biased by easier identification and visualization of cutaneous tumor regression compared to internal cancers such as breast cancer and colon cancer [72]. Signs of depigmentation can develop in local parts of the melanoma lesions. Such partial regression is observed in about 20% of primary human melanomas. The complete melanoma regression is a very rare phenomenon with only 57 described cases in years 1866–2009 [73] or 52 well-documented cases in the literature between 1963 and 2014 [74].

Spontaneous regression is probably related to high immunogenicity of the malignant melanoma, which is able to attract infiltrating immune cells into the tissue. These cells then destroy the tumor and create an inflammatory environment that further activates the immune system [75,76]. The possible triggers of regression may include trauma (including surgery), infection, or immune response of the patient [73,77]. Histopathologically, the early regression involves inflammatory changes with lymphocytic infiltration, as well as the presence of melanophages [73]. Later, dense fibrotic tissue is formed with few or no lymphocytes, and the tissue changes are similar to those observed in a scar [78].

Opinions on the prognostic significance of spontaneous regression remained controversial for years. On the base of current clinical and histological data, the regression of melanoma seems to be a positive prognostic factor associated with a lower possibility of metastases in sentinel lymph nodes [78,79].

2.5. Therapy of Melanoma

Current melanoma therapies rely mainly on surgical excision, chemotherapy, targeted therapy, and immunotherapy. Tumors in situ are treated by surgical excision, which is highly effective for early cancer stages and patients with early diagnosed melanoma (stage 1A or 1B), showing a 10-year survival rate of 94–98% [80]. Surgery may be combined with lymphadenectomy in patients with positive findings in sentinel lymph node biopsy. In specific cases, the surgery may be combined with radiotherapy [70]. Metastatic disease is mostly inaccessible by surgery. Chemotherapy is used in selected late-stage melanoma patients with progressive or relapsed disease [81].

The identification of mutations in the B-Raf kinase constitutively activating the MAPK pathway triggered new targeted therapies with small-molecule inhibitors of B-Raf and/or MEK kinases. These inhibitors initially showed an excellent response with a significant reduction of tumor burden. Unfortunately, MAPK inhibitors frequently face the development of drug resistance within months of application [81,82].

As melanoma is a highly immunogenic tumor, attempts to boost the patient's immune system against the tumor by immunotherapy or vaccines are applied in advanced melanoma stages. Since 1998, interleukin-2 (IL-2) was approved for such a purpose, followed by interferon α-2b (IFNα-2b) in 2011 [81]. Current immunotherapies are aimed at increasing cytotoxic cluster of differentiation 8 (CD8)$^+$ cell number or efficacy, mostly by targeting cytotoxic T-lymphocyte-associated antigen 4 (CTLA-4) and the programmed cell death protein 1 (PD-1)/programmed death-ligand 1 (PDL-1) pathways [70]. Development of such drugs, called immune checkpoint inhibitors, marks a major progress in treatment of several solid tumors including metastatic melanoma [81]. Additional immune checkpoint inhibitors targeting new molecules are in clinical trials [83–85]. Numerous clinical trials are also ongoing to explore efficacy, safety, and tolerability of immunotherapies in combination with chemotherapy, MAPK pathway inhibition, oncolytic viruses, gut microbiota modulation, and other approaches [83,84,86].

3. Animal Models

Direct melanoma research in affected humans is not possible for procedural and ethical reasons. Therefore, various animal models were developed that allow detailed study of cancer development, growth, and metastasis, as well as potential therapy of this life-threatening disease. Selected animal models are introduced in the sections below with an emphasis on those with spontaneously developing melanoma.

3.1. Non-Mammalian Models

Non-mammalian species, particularly *Drosophila melanogaster* and *Danio rerio*, are popular to study the development of various diseases including cancer, mainly because of easy breeding, short generation interval, and the possibility of genetic modification, allowing cell transplantation experiments and drug screening [87–90]. Optical transparency of certain models/developmental stages is advantageous for in vivo imaging [90].

Non-vertebrate species such as fruit fly (*Drosophila melanogaster*) are particularly useful for the study of gene and pathway regulations associated with tumor development or progression [91]. Current transgenic tools allow knockdown or overexpression of any fruit-fly gene in almost any tissue at any stage of development or adulthood [90]. In melanoma, fruit fly was used to study the effect of *Tum1* (tumorous-lethal) mutation on melanotic neoplasm growth [92].

Central American fish *Xiphophorus* was historically among the first fishes in cancerogenesis studies, as, in this fish, various cancers, including melanoma, spontaneously evolve in nature. In 1928, monitoring of *Xiphophorus* offspring led to the discovery of hereditary melanoma transmitted by Mendelian genetics. Such experiments laid a base for existence of cancer-causing genes, currently called "oncogenes" [88,93]. In *Xiphophorus*, melanoma can be also induced by various physical and chemical means, such as ultraviolet (UV) radiation [94,95], X-rays, N-methyl-N-nitrosourea, or N-ethyl-N-nitrosourea [93]. A *Xiphophorus* gene associated with aggressive melanoma formation was identified as Xiphophorus melanoma receptor tyrosine-protein kinase (*Xmrk*). The *Xmrk* gene encodes a membrane tyrosine kinase, which has homology to the epidermal growth factor receptor (*HER* gene) [96].

Zebrafish (*Danio rerio*) was the first fish species used to study chemical cancerogenesis [87]. Availability of genetic manipulation enabled generation of transgenic zebrafish models. Patton et al. generated transgenic zebrafish expressing common V600E mutant *BRAF* under the control of the *MITF* promotor. In p53-deficient fish, activated B-Raf induced development of invasive melanomas [97]. Since that time, many transgenic zebrafish models were created for oncogenesis studies [98–102]. Transplantation experiments revealed that human melanoma cells grafted to zebrafish kept their phenotype, i.e., proliferated, migrated, stimulated angiogenesis, and produced melanin [103]. Transplantation of the ZMEL1 melanoma cell line derived from a transgenic zebrafish into transparent zebrafish strain reliably gives rise to widespread metastases [104].

Medaka (*Oryzias latipes*) represents an additional fish model for melanoma studies. Medaka is easy to breed, produces externally developing transparent embryos, does not have naturally occurring tumors, and transgenic technologies are available to modify its genome. Transgenic medaka was developed to express the *Xmrk* gene under the control of a pigment cell-specific promoter. Several stable transgenic medaka lines with spontaneously developing melanomas at 100% penetrance were created [105]. The transcriptomic comparison of medaka and human melanoma revealed molecular conservation between fish models and human tumors at various levels, including the expression of classical melanoma markers, upregulation of N-cadherin, downregulation of E-cadherin, inhibitors of cell-cycle, growth-promoting genes, and inhibitors of apoptosis [106].

3.2. Mammalian Models

3.2.1. Mouse Models

The first mouse melanoma models were created by the subcutaneous application of melanoma cells [107] or chemical induction [108]. Later, for study of genetically determined melanoma, the transgenic mice were developed by integration of a recombinant gene comprising the tyrosinase promoter and the simian virus 40 early (SV40E) region. Affected animals developed ocular and cutaneous melanomas, which were histopathologically similar to the human ones [109]. These Tyr-SV40E mice were used in a donor–acceptor study, where grafts of full-thickness skin from a high-susceptibility line were transplanted to the host of a low-susceptibility line (of the same inbred strain). Pigment cells persisted as expected; however, at the outermost rim of all the grafts, a blackened edge arose. Later, the hyperpigmentation spread to surrounding skin, and one or more cases of local thickening arose, signaling vertical growth. These tissue areas became early melanomas. It was noteworthy that all melanomas were strictly confined within the grafts. The origin of melanomas from the host grafts was confirmed by Southern blot analysis of DNA [110]. These results indicate that mouse is a useful model for both allograft and xenograft studies [111].

In 1996, spontaneous melanoma formation was observed as a side effect of the construction of a transgenic mouse strain. Such a result showed how uncontrollable the insertion of genetic information can be, affecting areas other than originally intended [112]. Affected animals from this study were used for establishment of a transgenic melanoma-bearing mouse line that allows the detailed study of development and spreading of melanoma lesions in mice [113].

Current melanoma research relies mostly on syngeneic, xenograft, and genetically engineered models. In syngeneic models, mouse melanoma cells are inoculated into inbred animals of the same genetic background. Due to the presence of a fully functional immune system, syngeneic models allow the investigation of melanoma behavior, metastases formation [114], and immune cell role in tumor microenvironment or cancer immunotherapies [115]. The most commonly used model is B16 melanoma cell grafting to C57BL/6 mice [116].

Severe combined immunodeficiency (SCID) mice became one of the most popular animal models of many human diseases including cancer due to the possibility of inoculating different cell lines and even xenografts without rejection. Patient tumor-derived xenografts (PDX) into immunocompromised mice are widely used to study the response to therapeutic agents [117] or metastasis formation [116]. However, PDX mice lack a functional immune system, which hampers the investigation of immunotherapies. Thus, mouse PDX models with partially or completely humanized immune systems were recently developed. The human immune system can be introduced to irradiated or immunodeficient mice by grafting of purified human CD34$^+$ hematopoietic stem cells [118].

Genetically engineered mouse models are extensively used to study the effects of genetic alterations in melanoma initiation, progression, and metastasis, as well as for drug efficacy assessment [116]. Transgenic models were the subject of several recent reviews, where detailed information can be found [116,119,120]. The presence of germline mutations in genetically engineered mouse models may affect developmental and reproductive fitness, as well as lead to the formation of tumors in other tissues [119]. Inducible or tissue-specific gene expression may help to overcome such limitations. For that purpose, RCAS/TVA mouse models were developed. Such systems use an RCAS viral vector, derived from the avian sarcoma-leukosis virus, which can deliver genes up to 3 kb. Mammalian cells to be affected by this vector must be engineered to express receptors allowing avian virus entry (TVA) on their surface, e.g., transgenic mice expressing TVA early in melanocyte development from the tyrosinase-related protein 2 (TRP2) promoter [119]. The RCAS/TVA model allows investigation of the carcinogenic potential of candidate oncogenes in somatic cells in vivo [121]. A different model uses conditional melanocyte-specific expression of *BRAF* V600E mutation combined with conditional *PTEN* tumor suppressor gene silencing under the control of Cre recombinase expression from the tyrosinase promoter (BPT-mouse), leading to metastatic melanoma formation with 100% penetrance [122]. The Cre/LoxP system was later used for spatiotemporal control of other oncogene expression in melanoma development [120].

Interestingly, the induction of cutaneous melanoma with ultraviolet radiation was not very successful in non-transgenic mice. Therefore, several transgenic mice lines were established that are susceptible to melanoma induction by UV [123–125].

Each mouse model system possesses unique advantages and disadvantages [115,116,119]. Moreover, the interpretation of results from mice melanoma models should take into account the different location on melanocytes in skin, which is dermal in mice in contrast to epidermal in human [125,126]. Such a different microenvironment may influence melanoma growth and spreading.

3.2.2. Dog Models

Spontaneously developed pigmented lesions are common in dogs and share some features with human pigmented lesions. In purebred dogs (especially Standard and Miniature Schnauzers, Doberman Pinschers, Scottish Terriers, Irish and Gordon Setters, and Golden Retrievers), the prevalence of this disease is higher, which indicates its genetic basis [127]. Canine dermal melanoma is largely a benign tumor; however, uveal, oral, and mucocutaneous melanomas are aggressive forms frequently metastatic into regional lymph nodes and lungs. They are poorly responsive to conventional therapy [128]. The oral cavity is the most frequent location of canine melanomas (approximately 60% of cases) and such tumors mimic human mucosal melanomas [129]. Results from a study of tumor suppressors in melanoma samples and melanoma cell lines derived from dog tumors indicate that loss of function of certain proteins is a common occurrence that may contribute to the origin of canine melanomas. The most frequent abnormality was significant reduction or loss of p16 protein expression. In the case of p53 tumor suppressor, the exclusion of protein from the nuclear compartment was seen in almost all of the studied samples [130]. Transcriptomic analysis of canine oral melanoma revealed mutations in *NRAS* and *PTEN* genes, but not in *BRAF* [131], as well as upregulation of matrix metalloproteinase 2 (*MMP2*) and downregulation of *MMP7* [132]. Activation of the PI3K/protein kinase B(Akt) pathway was detected in malignant melanomas on distant extremities [133]. In a genomic study of 27 canine malignant melanoma tumors, mutations in genes including *BAP1*, *KIT*, *KRAS*, *NRAS*, *PTEN*, and *TP53* were found, while no mutation in *TERT* promoter, *BRAF*, *CDK4*, *MITF*, or *NF1* genes was detected. In approximately 20% tumors, mutations in *PTPRJ* (protein tyrosine phosphatase, receptor type J), a putative tumor suppressor gene not previously shown to have frequent inactivating point mutations in cancer, was observed [134]. Dog melanomas and their epidemiological, clinical, histological, and genetic comparison to human ones were the subject of a recent excellent review by Prouteau and André, where additional information can be found [129].

3.2.3. Equine Models

Spontaneous occurrence of dermal melanomas was seen in horses with a gray coat color [135]. In Camargue-type gray-skinned horses, multiple melanomas were observed. Most horses had tumor(s) underneath the tail, and less often in the perianal region, on lips, in the eyelids, and in genitals. The skin tumors were rarely seen in other body regions. In some of the strongly affected animals, the metastases developed; however, clinical examination and other observations suggest that melanomas in these horses are clinically different to those in human patients [136]. In graying white horses from the Old Kladruber strain, melanomas usually naturally occur at the age of 5–6 years, and statistically significant differences between the sire lines indicate a possible influence of heritable factors [137]. The 4.6-kb duplication in the intron of the syntaxin 17 (*STX17*) gene was found to cause the graying in horses and is associated with a high incidence of melanoma and vitiligo-like skin depigmentation [138]. Transcription factor MITF is appropriate for the identification of melanocytic cells in horse melanoma. Moreover, the receptor for activated C kinase 1 (RACK1) protein was found as a useful marker to discriminate melanoma cells from healthy skin and melanocytic lesions [139].

4. Swine Melanoma Models

Spontaneous occurrence of melanoma in pigs is generally very low. Skin tumors were occasionally observed in pigmented meat breeds such as Duroc, Bazna, and Iberian pig. Metastases into lymph nodes and visceral organs were found in the affected Duroc pigs [140–143]. An extensive study of 747,014 swine carcasses (without information about breed) revealed 220 cases (i.e., 0.03% only) with cutaneous and lymph node lesions suggestive of melanoma. Histological analysis of samples taken from 176 cutaneous lesions revealed that almost all of them (with the exception of two non-regressing melanomas) were spontaneously regressing [144]. Monitoring offspring from the crossing of Duroc pigs suggested the inherited characteristics of melanocytic tumors [145]. Using selective breeding, three miniature pig models with hereditary melanoma were established: the Sinclair miniature swine, the Munich miniature swine Troll, and the melanoma-bearing Libechov minipig (MeLiM). Melanomas in these three models show similarities such as early postnatal development, histopathology, and spontaneous regression connected with depigmentation.

4.1. Sinclair Miniature Swine

The Sinclair miniature swine was derived from the Hormel miniature pig (also known as the Minnesota miniature pig) that was developed as a small pig model at the Hormel Institute (University of Minnesota, Austin, USA). A portion of the original Sinclair herd was moved to the University of Missouri (Columbia, USA) in 1965 and then to the Sinclair Comparative Medicine Research Farm (Columbia, USA). The first Sinclair swine with cutaneous melanoma observed in this strain appeared in 1967 [146]. The incidence of melanoma changed during development of this pig model. The initial incidence of pigmented cutaneous lesions was 21% [146]. In subsequent generations, the incidence was highly influenced by selective breeding, reaching the highest level around 60% in newborn offspring of both affected parents [147,148]. Black pigs showed multiple primary skin lesions of variable size and appearance (exophytic, flat, ulcerated, locally necrotic) that were often present already at birth (congenital) or developed postnatally. On the contrary, no tumors were found in piglets with the red coat color.

Cutaneous pigmented lesions in the Sinclair miniature swine have a variety of histopathologic forms showing many similarities to human lesions. They were classified as benign nevi, superficial spreading melanoma, or nodular melanoma metastatic to lymph nodes and visceral organs (mainly lungs and liver). Skin tumors spontaneously regressed during postnatal life, and this was often accompanied by a local or generalized depigmentation of skin and bristles. Complete regression of melanoma including metastatic regional lymph nodes was also observed [147,149–152]. The proportion of animals with melanoma regression ranged between 85% and 100%. Detailed histological evaluation of the regressing melanomas revealed a biphasic immunological process. The first phase took place mainly during the second month after birth and was characterized by massive macrophage infiltration. This initial phase displayed tumor mass with less variation and was followed by regrowth of the residual melanoma tissue. The second phase (starting around the beginning of the fourth month of age) showed lymphocyte infiltration and complete elimination of melanomas [153]. Immunophenotyping of tumor-infiltrating lymphocytes in the second regression phase revealed significantly more cytotoxic ($CD4^-/CD8^+$) T-lymphocytes compared to peripheral blood, whereas percentages of the T-helper ($CD4^+/CD8^-$) lymphocytes and double-positive (DP) $CD4^+/CD8^+$ T-lymphocytes were reduced. The percentage of B-lymphocytes ($CD1^+$) was very low [154]. These results demonstrate that the cytotoxic T-lymphocytes play the main role in the final elimination of melanoma cells during the second regression phase. However, role of specific antibodies in the spontaneous regression cannot be excluded, as antibodies against melanoma antigens were found in sera collected from the Sinclair miniature swine with spontaneously regressing melanoma. Their levels increased with the age of the pigs, usually preceding or appearing together with tumor regression and depigmentation. This suggests an antibody-mediated immune response directed against common antigens presented by both malignant and normal swine pigmented cells [155]. Findings in melanoma cells derived from spontaneously regressing Sinclair melanomas suggested that spontaneous regression is associated with higher sensitivity of the melanoma cells to apoptosis [156], the loss of telomerase activity, reduction of telomeric repeats, extensive DNA fragmentation, and formation of apoptotic bodies [157]. Since 1994, the Sinclair miniature swine is produced for research purposes by Sinclair Bio-Resources (Auxvasse, Missouri, USA) as a spontaneously regressing pig melanoma model.

Inheritance of melanoma in the Sinclair miniature swine was intensively studied. However, exact genetic determinants responsible for its development remain to be discovered. A two-locus model was suggested for expression of the exophytic form of melanoma on the basis of complex segregation analysis. One locus lies within the swine major histocompatibility (SLA) complex. The other, yet unidentified, putative dominant tumor-initiator locus segregates independently of the SLA complex. The melanoma-producing allele at this locus is inherited in the heterozygous state and requires a somatic mutation of the normal allele to initiate melanoma development. SLA haplotype B was associated with the expression of Sinclair melanoma. A single dose of the B haplotype is required for full penetrance of the dominant allele at the tumor-initiator locus [158–160]. Cytogenetic analyses of three melanoma cell lines from the Sinclair miniature swine revealed specific common chromosomal abnormalities. Structural alteration in chromosomes 2, 3, 6, 7, and 12 were found that probably represent the initial step of melanoma development. In addition, monosomies of chromosomes 2, 4, 7, 10, and 17 and three marker chromosomes (labeled M1, M2, and M3) resulting from chromosomal translocations were detected [161].

4.2. Munich Miniature Swine Troll

The Munich miniature swine Troll is historically the second swine model with hereditary melanoma. Literature data about this model and its experimental utilization are very limited. It was established at the University of Munich, Germany, in 1986. One melanoma-bearing boar and two unaffected sows were founders of this herd. They were derived from the herd originally developed from the Hanford and the Columbian miniature swine at the Medical Service Munich. Selective breeding of melanoma-affected animals increased the incidence of malignant tumors to 70%. Benign melanocytic lesions were also observed in addition to melanomas in darkly pigmented (black and red) animals. Skin lesions were already present at birth or they mostly developed within the first two months of life. Complete spontaneous regression of melanomas accompanied by hair and skin depigmentation was also observed in the Munich miniature swine Troll; however, the frequency of regressing pigs was not given. Breeding of Munich miniature swine Troll (manifesting cutaneous melanomas) with the German Landrace (white color, without any skin lesions) and analyses of F1-, F2-, and B1-generations showed that the dominant allele I at the I-locus (responsible for white phenotype) suppressed melanoma lesions. This is explained by a mutation of the *KIT* gene, leading to a failure of melanoblast migration and subsequent lack of melanocytes in the skin of white pigs. The segregation data for skin melanomas in this breed are best explained by a three-locus model with two recessive alleles per locus. An influence of SLA haplotypes on the penetrance of melanocytic lesions was not observed in the Munich miniature swine Troll [162,163]. An in vitro study with melanoma cells of Munich miniature swine Troll suggested a low importance (if any) of blood natural killer (NK) cells for spontaneous regression of melanoma in this animal model [164]. Elevated expression of porcine endogenous retroviruses was detected in melanomas and cell cultures derived from pulmonary metastasis in this swine melanoma model [165]. A similar observation of human endogenous retrovirus K was also reported for human melanomas [166]. Endogenous retroviruses can support cancer formation by inducing chromosomal translocations in somatic cells and promoting immunosuppressor pathways [167]. The publication of Dieckhoff et al. in 2007 [165] is the latest that can be found through PubMed about melanoma research on the Munich miniature swine Troll. Thus, it is not clear if this animal melanoma model still exists.

5. The Melanoma-Bearing Libechov Minipig

5.1. Development of the MeLiM Model

Pigs were kept in the Institute of Animal Physiology and Genetics (IAPG) of the Czech Academy of Sciences in Libechov originally for the study of blood groups since 1966. Firstly, two boars and two sows of the Goettingen miniature swine from the University of Goettingen (Institute of Animal Breeding and Genetics, Germany) were imported in December 1966 and another two sows of the same strain in August 1967. The Minnesota miniature pigs from the Hormel Foundation (Austin, USA) and Vietnamese pigs from German zoos were used as foundation stock for development of the Goettingen miniature swine [168]. Then, two imports of the Minnesota miniature pigs (Hormel Foundation, Austin, USA) followed, consisting of two boars and three sows in September 1967 and two boars in February 1969. To maximize genetic variability for the analysis of a wide range of pig blood groups, animals of these two strains of miniature pigs were crossed with pigs of several commercial meat breeds (Canadian Landrace, Cornwall, and Large White) and with Vietnamese pigs. The first few black piglets with cutaneous melanomas were observed in this genetically highly heterogeneous pig population in 1989. They came from mating of two boars (brothers) with four related sows, all without any cutaneous lesions. Selective breeding of melanoma-bearing animals for several generations confirmed genetic predisposition to melanoma with its incidence around 50%. This new pig melanoma model was designated by the acronym MeLiM (melanoma-bearing Libechov minipig; originally melanoblastoma-bearing Libechov minipig) [169,170]. Long-term monitoring of the MeLiM strain showed that values of melanoma incidence varied during individual years depending on tumor burden of parents. For this reason, more affected parental pigs were included in the breeding program, thus increasing melanoma incidence in the MeLiM roughly to 80% in 2018. Tumor devitalization (ischemization) was successfully applied in very affected pigs (see Section 5.8) to increase survival and allow their use in breeding. Currently, eight sows and four boars of the MeLiM line are bred to produce piglets used in experiments.

Extensive cooperation was established between IAPG (Laboratory of Tumor Biology (LTB)) and other research institutions in the Czech Republic (Czech University of Life Sciences Prague; First Faculty of Medicine of the Charles University Prague; Institute of Microbiology and Institute of Molecular Genetics of the Czech Academy of Sciences, Prague; University of Veterinary and Pharmaceutical Sciences, Brno) for characterization of the MeLiM model. The study of melanoma inheritance in the MeLiM strain was carried out in international cooperation with the INRA/CEA (Institute National de la Recherche Agronomic/Commissariat à l'Energie Atomique, Laboratoire de Radiobiologieet Etude du Génome (LREG), Jouy en Josas, France). Repeated exports of MeLiM animals (melanoma-bearing and melanoma-free) of both sexes and various ages were made from LTB to LREG. They included two boars (age one year) with two pregnant sows (age three years) in June 1997, four boars with six sows (all five months old) in October 1998, six sows (age 6–12 months) in November 2002, and three boars with four sows (age 14–18 months) in June 2008. To reveal genes responsible for melanoma susceptibility in the MeLiM strain, the transported animals were crossed with healthy Duroc pigs in LREG. It is not clear whether the offspring of transported pigs at LREG are currently maintained as a pure MeLiM strain or only as MeLiM × Duroc hybrids. Thus, results obtained in the original MeLiM strain kept in IAPG Libechov and in the MeLiM strain derived from the pigs transported into INRA (Jouy en Josas) may differ.

5.2. Histopathological, Biochemical, and Immunohistochemical Characterization

Variability in color coat is observed in the MeLiM animals that reflects the multi-hybrid characteristics of this strain. Pigs are usually black (Figure 2a); however, rusty-red, brown, or white (with black spots) individuals are also rarely found (Figure 2b). Small white spots can infrequently appear in colored animals. Black pigs are the most affected by melanoma. Cutaneous tumors are usually multiple, of deep-black pigmentation, nodular type (with local necrosis in larger tumors), and they are distributed on all body parts (Figure 2c). Rusty-red and brown animals show only one or a few cutaneous melanomas, and white pigs with black spots are without skin lesions. Nevi and superficial spreading melanomas also appear in affected pigs.

Similarly as in the Sinclair miniature swine, skin lesions are found already at birth or they develop shortly thereafter during the first two months of postnatal life. They grow exophytically, reaching sizes of about 15–70 mm, exceptionally up to 150 mm (Figure 2d). Histological observation of cutaneous nodular melanomas revealed variable concentration of brown–black melanoma cells. In the dermis, they formed areas with compact aggregation or were dispersed showing vertical spreading from the basal layer of epidermis into a deeper layer of the dermis (stratum papillare and stratum reticulare) and invading the hypodermis. Thus, these tumors correspond to Clark's level V of human melanoma. The epidermis was considerably reduced or totally destroyed [169,171]. The malignant characteristic of melanoma in the MeLiM strain is confirmed by presence of numerous metastases. They are commonly found in the lymph nodes (Figure 2e), lungs, and spleen (Figure 2f). Heavily affected animals also demonstrate metastases in other visceral organs such as the stomach, liver, small and large intestine, pancreas, kidneys, heart, and thymus [169,172–174].

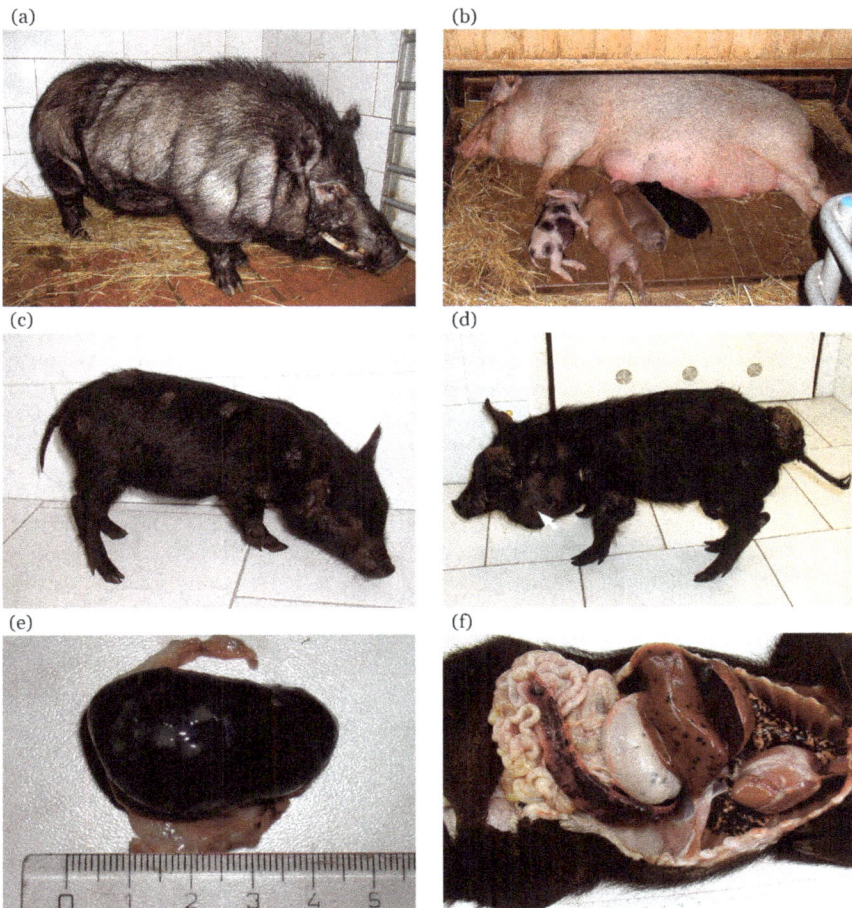

Figure 2. Melanoma-bearing Libechov minipig (MeLiM) swine model of hereditary melanoma: (**a**) black boar of the MeLiM strain after spontaneous regression of melanoma (without any changes in pigmentation) (age three years); (**b**) originally black sow of the MeLiM strain (age four years) after spontaneous regression of melanoma (with almost total depigmentation), together with piglets of different coat color (age three weeks); (**c**) MeLiM piglet with multiple cutaneous nodular melanomas (age six weeks); (**d**) MeLiM piglet showing several large nodular melanomas with local necrosis and beginning cachexia (age seven weeks). Note the vastly increased cervical lymph node (arrow) due to melanoma metastasis; (**e**) very enlarged inguinal lymph node totally infiltrated by metastatic melanoma cells (taken from MeLiM piglet with melanoma progression, age six weeks), scale in cm; (**f**) autopsy of MeLiM piglet that died from melanoma progression (age four weeks). Numerous melanoma metastases (seen as black spots) in visceral organs (lungs, liver, stomach, and spleen) clearly document the malignant characteristic of melanoma in the MeLiM model.

The presence of tyrosinase messenger RNA (mRNA) in the blood is assumed to indicate melanoma metastases [175]. While tyrosinase mRNA was detected by RT-PCR in the blood of MeLiM animals with advanced disease [176], how much this represents the presence of migrating cells contributing to metastasis formation is still unclear. In addition to RT-PCR for the detection of selected pigmented-cell specific mRNAs, novel and more specific techniques are currently being developed for the detection of circulating melanoma cells, applicable for human disease staging, diagnosis, and prognosis [177,178].

Basic biochemical and ultrastructural characterization of the MeLiM melanoma was performed by Borovanský et al. [179]. A very high concentration of melanosomes with a high proportion of melanin (almost 40% of the organelle dry weight) corresponds to deep-black pigmentation of the tumor. Aberrant forms of melanosomes were found by electron microscopy similarly as in the Sinclair miniature swine [180] and human nodular melanoma [181]. Three main melanosome enzymes involved in melanogenesis, biochemical melanoma differentiation, and metastatic activity, i.e., tyrosinase, α-mannosidase, and γ-glutamyltransferase [182–184], were detected in the MeLiM melanoma tissue [179].

Immunohistochemical analyses showed further similarities of the MeLiM melanoma with the human one. High expression of *RACK1* was observed in the cytoplasm of cutaneous and metastatic pig melanoma cells. These tumor cells showed also nuclear staining for MITF, a specific marker of the melanocytic lineage. Because of similar findings in human cutaneous melanomas and melanoma metastases, *RACK1* expression could serve as a potential marker of malignancy of human melanoma [185]. Expression of the S100 protein, used for human melanoma diagnosis [186], was also found in cryosections of progressing MeLiM melanomas and cells derived from them in vitro (V. Horak, unpublished observation). Four extracellular matrix proteins, collagen IV, laminin [187], tenascin C, and fibronectin [188,189], as well as matrix metalloproteinase 2 (the enzyme degrading the extracellular matrix) [189], were immunohistochemically found in extracellular spaces of cutaneous melanomas, suggesting their production by the MeLiM melanoma cells. All these proteins can support tumor cell proliferation, migration, and metastases [190–193]. More than a three-fold increase of tenascin C mRNA in MeLiM melanoma tissue compared to contralateral normal skin was observed, accompanied by elevated protein level [188]. Tenascin C is highly upregulated during wound healing, accompanied by rapid angiogenesis, fibroblast migration to the damaged area, and re-epithelialization by migrating keratinocytes. Elevated tenascin C level is also frequently found in human melanomas, where this protein supports malignant melanocyte survival, invasion, and metastasis [194].

A new computer-supported method for spatial mapping of various metals in tissue sections was developed recently using MeLiM melanomas as a suitable cancer model [195]. The method is based on image registration of digital data obtained from scans of two neighboring cryosections, of which the first one is processed by standard histological staining and the second one is analyzed for metallic content by laser ablation inductively coupled plasma mass spectrometry (LA-ICP-MS). Detailed histological analysis of cutaneous melanomas sampled from MeLiM pigs aged 4–22 weeks revealed four structurally different tissue zones—growing melanoma tissue (GMT), early spontaneous regression (ESR), late spontaneous regression (LSR), and fibrous tissue (FT)—whose presence, size, and proportion in melanoma tissue changed with animal age and advancing melanoma regression. This pilot study showed the highest concentrations of zinc and cooper in growing melanoma tissue, whereas the lowest ones were found in fibrous tissue. Both these metals are important players in various cancer diseases. Zinc level is increased in the majority of human melanomas but copper level is elevated only in some of them [196]. Application of matrix-assisted laser desorption/ionization mass spectrometry imaging (MALDI MSI) revealed four ion peaks, m/z 3044, 6011, 6140, and 10180, which were overexpressed in MeLiM melanoma tissue in comparison to healthy skin. Moreover, the ion peaks at m/z 6011 and 6140 were overexpressed in the GMT region. These findings agree with the high zinc content observed in this region in a previous study, leading to the assumption that both peaks represent metallothioneins [197]. Elevated metallothionein content in the MeLiM melanoma was already detected previously by the adsorptive transfer stripping differential pulse voltammetry Brdicka reaction [198]. Overexpression of metallothioneins was associated with a poor prognosis in human cutaneous melanoma [199]. These recent studies of MeLiM melanoma show the usefulness of this swine model for basic melanoma research and suggest possibilities for its further use in the search for markers of melanoma progression and spontaneous regression that could serve in clinical practice.

5.3. MeLiM Melanoma Progression and Spontaneous Regression

In the MeLiM model, multiple cutaneous melanomas found on various parts of body develop differently over time for each individual. Two main situations may occur—cancer progression and/or spontaneous regression [200]. Small cutaneous tumors (found at birth or developed shortly thereafter) initially grow in all affected piglets.

In a smaller part of affected piglets (about 5–30% depending on disease burden in parents), cancer progression continues. Melanoma progression mainly affects black piglets, while it is very rare in rusty-red and brown ones. Cutaneous melanomas grow further reaching a large size (Figure 3a), with occasional bleeding and local necrosis. These heavily affected piglets initially lag in bodyweight gains behind their less affected (spontaneous regression showing) siblings (Figure 3b). At the later stage, they lose weight and develop strong cachexia with melanoma progression. Extensive metastases are observed in the lungs, lymph nodes, and spleen. Metastases in lymph nodes, mainly in cervical and inguinal areas, are also macroscopically visible in some animals due to their increasing size (Figure 2d, arrow). Additionally, metastases are present in the liver, various parts of the gastrointestinal system (Figure 2f), thymus, heart, and brain [169,173]. The animals with progressive melanoma usually die during the first three months of age. The main cause of death seems to be breathing difficulties and insufficient oxygen supply of the whole organism due to severe damage of lung tissue with a vast number of melanoma metastases.

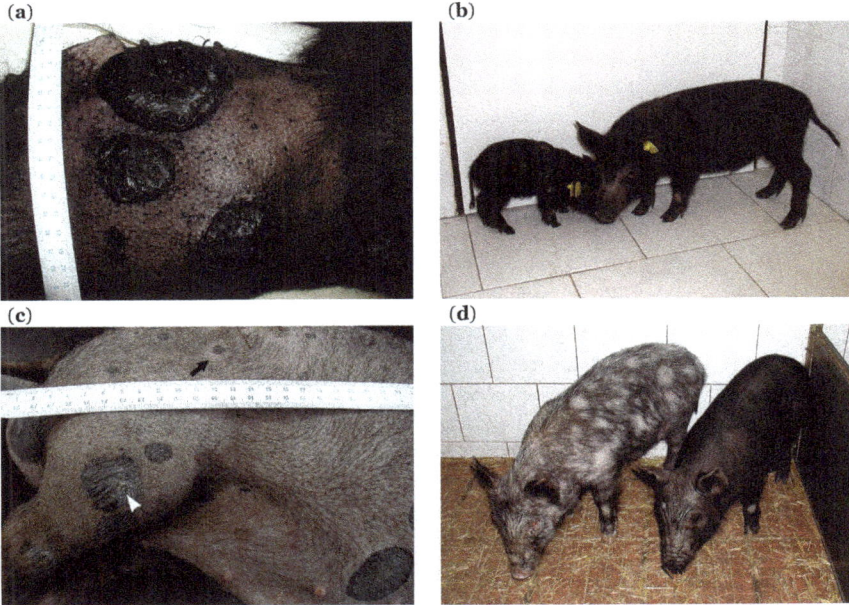

Figure 3. Progression and spontaneous regression in MeLiM model: (**a**) three growing cutaneous nodular melanomas (with local necrosis) are well visible after shaving off the bristles (age 11 weeks); (**b**) comparison of two MeLiM siblings, one with melanoma progression causing heavy cachexia and body size reduction (left side) and one with spontaneous regression and normal body size (right side) (age 10 weeks); (**c**) flattening and graying of originally nodular melanoma (arrowhead) and halo around one smaller melanoma (arrow), together with partial depigmentation of skin and bristles observed in MeLiM pig with ongoing spontaneous regression of melanoma (age four months); (**d**) partial bristle and skin depigmentation versus preserved black pigmentation in two MeLiM siblings with spontaneous regression of melanoma (age 5.5 months); scales in cm.

Spontaneous regression of melanoma is observed in the majority of MeLiM piglets. After the initial period of growth, tumors begin to flatten, reduce in size, and change color from black to gray. Piglet body weight reaches normal or almost normal values. Melanoma regression is usually associated with skin and bristle depigmentation (Figure 3c, white arrowhead). It starts as sparsely dispersed white bristles over the body or localized discoloration around several cutaneous tumors. A halo effect around some melanomas is also observed (Figure 3c, black arrow). Then, depigmentation gradually extends to the surrounding parts of the body. This depigmentation spreads sometimes to almost the entire body leading to the originally black pig becoming nearly white (Figure 2b) [169,171]. A specific CD4 haplotype was observed in T-lymphocytes to be related to the depigmentation during regression [201]. However, the black pigmentation is rarely maintained in MeLiM pigs with spontaneous regression (Figure 3d). Skin depigmentation was also observed in melanoma patients with spontaneous regression and/or treated by immunotherapy [72]. These color changes of the skin suggest the activation of immune cells against an antigen that is common to melanoma cells and normal melanocytes.

The spontaneous regression is a very dynamic process in which melanoma cells are gradually destroyed and tumor tissue is replaced with the fibrous tissue. Vincent-Naulleau et al. monitored spontaneous regression of melanoma in a colony of MeLiM pigs that was derived from the MeLiM animals transported from the Czech Republic to France and in their Duroc crossbreeds. They observed that the time course of spontaneous regression was dependent on tumor growth. In fast-growing tumors, spontaneous regression appeared between the third and fourth month, whereas slow-growing tumors demonstrated it between the fifth and seventh month. Moreover, two regression phases were observed in some exophytic tumors that were present at birth. The early regression (between the second and the third month) was followed by a transitional period of relapse and tumor growth (between the 2.5th and 4.5th month) and finally with the latest regression phase (between the 3.5th and sixth month) [171]. Our time-lapse immunohistochemical study of exophytic melanomas taken from pigs of the original MeLiM strain (from three weeks to eight months of age) showed only one regression phase. Expressions of fibronectin, tenascin C, collagen IV, laminin, and MMP2 increased up to the 10th week of age. In older animals, gradual destruction of melanoma cells and rebuilding of melanoma tissue into the fibrous tissue was observed. In agreement with this process, the expression of collagen IV, laminin, and MMP2 declined, whereas the expression of fibronectin and tenascin C raised in the arising fibrous tissue. The age of 10 weeks seems be a turning point in the transition between the initial melanoma growth phase and subsequent spontaneous regression phase [187,189].

Spontaneous regression does not occur synchronously in all melanoma sites on the body. Its duration depends on the number and size of melanoma deposits. The whole process of spontaneous regression is usually completed around 6–12 months of age.

5.4. Genetic Findings

The development of melanoma in pigs is a polygenic process [202]. The *CDKN2A* locus causative in human familial melanoma was studied in MeLiM pigs; however, haplotype analysis, allelic association, and linkage analysis led to exclusion of this gene from candidates for melanoma susceptibility [203]. Later experiments revealed that MeLiM melanoma is inherited as an autosomal dominant trait with incomplete penetrance. The inheritance of melanoma was seen preferably in black animals. Association of regions harboring *CDK4* and *BRAF* genes was not found; however, another three candidate regions which correspond to human regions with melanoma candidate loci were observed [204]. For the black coat color, a variant allele of the *MC1R* gene was found (marked as *MC1R*2*) to be associated with melanoma development. This is in agreement with the fact that human variant alleles of *MC1R* may increase melanoma risk independently of UV exposure [202]. Comparative expression analysis revealed that the *RACK1* gene is overexpressed in melanoma metastases compared to normal melanocytes. This finding is consistent with results observed in human melanoma patients [185]. Functional studies highlighted that the *MITF* gene has potential involvement in porcine melanoma biology; however, direct association of this gene with melanoma development was not confirmed [205]. A 450-kb duplication in the *KIT* gene was found to be responsible for white or belt coat color in pig, as it prevents migration of embryonic melanoblasts to skin. Diverse *KIT* mutations were found in various human cancers, including melanoma, and one variant showed a significant association with cutaneous invasion, melanoma development, and tumor ulceration in the MeLiM strain [206].

Genome-wide time-dependent profiling was conducted to analyze molecular mechanisms involved in MeLiM spontaneous melanoma regression. Among other results, downregulation of genes involved in cell cycle and DNA replication, recombination, and repair was observed in tumors at the 28th, 49th, and 70th day of age in a piglet with spontaneous regression, suggesting the reduced proliferative capacity of melanoma cells. Moreover, upregulation of monocyte/macrophage-related genes at the same time points was accompanied by tumor-infiltrating macrophage infiltration observed in tumor histological sections. At three months of age, upregulation of different T-cell receptor (TCR) chains, as well as T-cell-associated cytokines, together with dramatic downregulation of genes involved in melanogenesis, confirms T-cell activation and loss of melanoma cells at the later phases of regression [207]. In addition, suppression subtractive hybridization was used to study gene expression in progressive and regressive MeLiM melanoma tissue. Verification by RT-PCR and immunohistochemistry confirmed upregulation of CD9 and retinoic acid responder 1 gene (*RARRES1*) in regressive tumors, while *MITF* was upregulated in progressive melanomas [208].

A genome-wide association study performed on 190 animals of the MeLiM × Duroc pedigree revealed several loci on chromosomes 2, 5, 7, 8, and 16, showing significant associations with melanoma occurrence and progression (i.e., clinical ulceration and presence of metastasis). The most significant region associated with melanoma occurrence was located on chromosome 5 harboring the *NUAK1* gene encoding AMP-activated protein kinase (AMPK)-related protein kinase 5 (ARK5) [209]. ARK5 is known to promote survival and invasion of cancer cells and is probably activated by the Akt kinase [210]. GWAS analysis of tumor ulceration revealed a region on chromosome 16 nearby the *IRX4* gene (iroquois homeobox gene) [209], previously identified as a risk factor in human prostate cancer [211]. Interestingly, *IRX4* is located only 600 kb from the *TERT* gene. Mutations in *TERT* promoter are associated with both familial and sporadic melanoma [40]. Genes associated with metastasis in MeLiM were identified on chromosomes 2 (coding long non-coding RNAs (lncRNAs) with functions in tumor suppression and metastasis formation) and on chromosome 8, harboring the *HERC3* (probable E3 ubiquitin–protein ligase) gene [209]. HERC3 is an endosomal protein with probable ubiquitin–protein ligase function. *HERC3* mutations were observed in gastric and colorectal cancers [212]. In MeLiM melanoma, an additional 12 loci, previously reported to associate with melanoma in human, were identified. Several novel gene candidates associated with MeLiM melanoma, not yet reported in human, were also revealed [209].

MicroRNAs (miRNAs) are in the center of current research because they play important roles in all processes in the cell, and they also participate in melanoma development [213]. Analysis of miRNA in MeLiM tumors revealed significant upregulation of let-7b, miR-193b, miR-21, miR-221, and miR-222 in regressive tumors in contrast to miR-92a, which was upregulated in progressive tumors. The expression of miR-92a, let-7b, and miR-193b in regressive MeLiM tumors was in contrast to previous findings in progressive human tumors, suggesting that such miRNAs could be potential actors in the regression process in MeLiM cutaneous melanoma. MiR-193b could regulate cell-cycle-related genes during regression of cutaneous melanoma [214].

5.5. Hematological Findings

Hematological monitoring is an integral part of the diagnosis of cancer and of the subsequent treatment. Values of various hematological parameters, such as leukocyte and neutrophil counts and their ratios (neutrophil–lymphocyte and platelet–lymphocyte ratios), can be used as prognostic markers in different types of cancer [215–218] including melanoma [219,220]. Elevated leukocyte count with neutrophilia was found in metastatic melanoma patients [221]. A baseline neutrophil–lymphocyte ratio lower than five was associated with improved survival of metastatic melanoma patients treated with ipilimumab [222]. Another study of patients with early-stage (I–III) melanoma showed worse survival with a baseline neutrophil–lymphocyte ratio lower than 2.5 [223]. Thrombocytosis [224] and low concentration of blood hemoglobin [225] predicted metastatic disease and worse survival in melanoma patients. Anemia is commonly found in cancer patients indicating a poor prognosis. It is a multifactorial process that is often connected with iron deficiency as a major causal factor [226], manifesting as decreased erythrocyte count and lower hematocrit. The level of blood iron and iron homeostasis is important for both innate and adaptive immunity response [227,228]. One of the many important functions of iron is the regulation of immune cell distribution [229].

Hematological analyses are also important for monitoring animal cancer models, as shown in our recent study [200]. Basic hematological parameters of MeLiM animals with melanoma progression or spontaneous regression were compared to healthy (white, melanoma-free) animals from 5–18 weeks of age. Iron deficiency and microcytic hypochromic anemia were observed in all MeLiM pigs. The group of pigs with melanoma progression was characterized by the lowest values of red blood cell count, hematocrit, and concentration of hemoglobin, as well as by the highest number of platelets. Moreover, a very high number of neutrophils was found (measuring differential white blood cell counts), driving the high number of white blood cells observed in these animals. In the spontaneous regression group, higher values of red blood cell count, hematocrit, and concentration of hemoglobin, together with a lower number of platelets, were ascertained. Thus, monitoring hematological parameters enables distinguishing (together with macroscopic, histologic, immunological, and immunohistochemical observations) MeLiM piglets with progression and spontaneous regression in early postnatal development. These findings extend the characterization of the MeLiM model and show its further similarities with melanoma patients.

5.6. Immunological Findings

Immune cells infiltrating tumors, including melanoma, are responsible for anti-tumor immunological surveillance. However, some tumor-associated immune cell types (such as macrophages and neutrophils) can also support cancer progression depending on tumor milieu [230,231]. A higher infiltration of cutaneous melanomas with lymphocytes is associated with better prognosis and longer survival of melanoma patients. The cytotoxic $CD8^+$ T-lymphocytes collaborating with the $CD4^+$ T-helper cells were found to be the most important components [232,233]. Promising results of treatment of metastatic melanoma patients with adoptive transfer of tumor-infiltrating lymphocytes (TILs) confirmed their anti-cancer effectiveness [234].

The MeLiM animals with melanoma spontaneous regression represent a promising immunological model for monitoring immune cells participating in anti-melanoma reaction. Flow cytometry revealed two DP T-lymphocyte subpopulations, i.e., melanoma-associated $CD4^+/CD8^{high}$ T-lymphocytes in peripheral blood and $CD4^+/CD8^{high}$ TILs in melanoma tissue (together with $CD4^-/CD8^+$ T-lymphocytes), which expanded during melanoma regression. They showed a similar expression of selected CD markers between different pigs and different melanoma loci among the same pig, suggesting that they are effector/memory $\alpha\beta$ T-cells considerably involved in spontaneous regression of MeLiM melanoma [235]. It is important to mention, that $CD4^+/CD8^+$ cells are more frequent in pigs, reaching up to 60% of total T-cell counts in adult pig blood, in contrast to 3% in human [236]. The number of DP T-cells naturally increases during the life of pigs [237], which may mask the increase caused by MeLiM regression. Nonetheless, MeLiM peripheral DP cells differ in the intensity of CD8 expression, with $CD8^{high}$ expression in the melanoma-bearing animals in later stages of tumor regression compared to $CD8^{low}$ positivity in their melanoma-free littermates (both groups at the age of eight months). Importantly, a unique DP cell subpopulation was identified in the blood of regressive MeLiM animals, representing one T-cell clone carrying a mono-specific $TCR\beta$ receptor, which is supposed to be responsible for melanoma regression [235]. Our unpublished data about cytokine production of DP T-cells suggest that these cells represent a non-naïve (activated, recirculating) lymphocyte subpopulation with immunomodulatory activity. Compared to single-positive T-cell populations, where 30% and 50% of CD4 single-positive and cytotoxic T-cells produced IFNγ and/or tumor necrosis factor α (TNFα), respectively, almost 60% of DP T-cells were cytokine producers.

Although the significance of CD4$^+$/CD8$^+$ DP T-cells in cancer conditions remains unclear, they are mentioned to play an important role at peripheral sites. Their functions are probably the consequence of various microenvironments found across different types of tumors. Anti-tumor actions of DP cells were described in various tumor types [236]. Bagot et al. isolated a clone of DP cells with a CD4$^+$/CD8$^+$ dim phenotype from the cutaneous infiltrate of a patient with T-cell lymphoma. These cells were major histocompatibility complex class I (MHC I) restricted and cytolytic against autologous tumor cells in vitro [238]. Concerning clinical outcomes, De Marchi et al. described the presence of CD4$^+$/CD8$^+$ T-cells in cutaneous lesions in mycosis fungoides. Their presence was associated with a slightly slower progression of the disease [239]. A significant increase of DP cells was also noted in human malignant melanomas and their metastases. Increased numbers of DP cells were observed in about 60% of melanomas compared to peripheral blood. A high proportion of these cells were TNF-α-producing in response to autologous melanoma cells. They were also characterized by higher secretion of IL-13, IL-4, and IL-5 compared to single-positive cells [240].

5.7. Skin Microbiome

Microbiome is a term for the community of microorganisms (bacteria, archaea, fungi, protozoa, viruses) living at a given environment, e.g., on the epithelial surfaces of the mammalian body. The local microbiome affects functions of the epithelial barrier and regulates immunity [241]. In cancer, microorganisms may directly contribute to cancer development (e.g., in gastric, colorectal, cervical, and hepatocellular cancer or lymphoma) and may modify patients' immunity and response to therapy [242]. The gut microbiome is increasingly recognized as a modulator of response to anti-cancer treatment, particularly to immune checkpoint inhibitors [242–244]. The skin microbiome is much less explored. In human, the skin microbiome was analyzed in a search for a diagnostic tool for melanoma and melanocytic nevi. However, no significant differences between melanoma and nevi microbiomes were found [245].

In MeLiM piglets, the possible involvement of skin microbiome in melanoma development was studied. Melanoma surface and healthy skin (5 cm from the melanoma lesion) were compared by matrix-assisted laser desorption/ionization time of flight mass spectrometry (MALDI-TOF MS) of cultured microorganisms [246], as well as 16S ribosomal RNA (rRNA) analysis [247]. Using MALDI-TOF, a clear significant difference between the proportions of bacteria on healthy skin and melanoma was observed, with *Staphylococcus sciuri*, *Lactococcus lactis*, and *Staphylococcus cohnii* being typical for healthy skin, while *Staphylococcus chromogenes*, *Staphylococcus hyicus*, and *Enterococcus faecalis* were abundant on the melanoma surface [246]. To monitor the possible involvement of skin microorganisms in melanoma development, skin and melanoma scrapes were analyzed by 16S rRNA PCR and denaturing gradient gel electrophoresis (PCR-DGGE) in six-, eight-, 10-, and 12-week-old MeLiM piglets, which is the age when the regressive/progressive phenotype develops. Similarly to MALDI-TOF results, the predominance and distribution of bacterial genera were different between skin and melanoma samples. The melanoma surface microbiome showed significantly higher microbial diversity than healthy skin, which might be partially caused by melanoma ulceration. The number of *Fusobacteria* was higher in melanoma samples compared to healthy skin and also in progressing melanomas compared to regressing ones. In addition, the quantity of *Fusobacterium necrophorum* increased with the age of piglets with progressing melanoma [247]. In human, the abundance of *Fusobacterium* (particularly *F. nucleatum*) in the gut is connected with colorectal cancer development and progression [248–250]. Additional studies of the MeLiM model are needed to elucidate the possible effects of the skin microbiome on melanoma development or immune reactions in the skin.

5.8. Experimental Therapy of MeLiM Melanoma by Tumor Devitalization

Tumor devitalization (also called devascularization) was developed by the Czech surgeon Karel Fortýn (1930–2001) and suggested as a surgical operation technique for treatment of solid tumors. The principle of this technique is total closure of blood supply (ischemization) to tissue by ligating all vessels—arteries and veins—with non-absorbable material and leaving the treated tissue in situ. This procedure was firstly experimentally tested in healthy (tumor-free) miniature pigs held in IAPG. Segments of the small or large intestine were devitalized by ligation of the mesenteric arteries and veins. Both ends of the devitalized intestine were also ligated (forming a blind loop), left in situ together with its content, and the intestinal passage was renewed by anastomosis. The experimental minipigs survived without any health complications, and the isolated intestinal segments were gradually destroyed over four weeks without causing sepsis [251]. Based on these promising results, devitalization was successfully applied in several elder patients (age 57–82 years) with inoperable colorectal carcinoma. Revision operations showed a small fibrous residue at the site of the original tumor only, and visceral metastases, ascertained before devitalization, were not found. No cancer recurrence was observed in the patients. They died 4–7 years later of a heart attack or stroke [252]. Recently, another case report of a patient with invasive metastatic colorectal carcinoma who survived more than 14 years after devitalization, with no sign of malignancy revealed on computed tomography (CT) scans at present, was published [253]. Using healthy minipigs in IAPG as an anatomical and physiological model similar to human, devitalization of the kidney [254,255], stomach [256], rectum, and sigmoideum [257] was also carried out to acquire practical skills and experimental knowledge as a prerequisite for possible clinical utilization. In all cases, the devitalized tissues were resorbed and no side effects were observed.

Development of the MeLiM strain with hereditary melanoma gave us a very suitable animal model to experimentally test the effects of tumor devitalization in vivo. Devitalization of cutaneous melanoma is a relatively simple surgical technique. Partially overlapping mattress stitches are conducted around the tumor base and strongly tightened; then, the tumor is left in situ without any excision [174]. More than 40 MeLiM animals of both sexes (age 1–2 months) with progressively growing multiple cutaneous nodular melanomas and metastases in inner organs (lymph nodes, spleen, and liver) were used in the first larger study. Devitalization of single cutaneous melanoma led to a gradual melanoma cell destruction in all other non-treated cutaneous melanomas, as well as inner organ metastases, over 4–6 months. Neither side effects (with the exception of local or generalized depigmentation) nor any health complications were ascertained [169]. Melanoma cell destruction was also well documented biochemically, showing a great reduction in α-mannosidase and tyrosinase activities in non-treated melanomas taken six months after devitalization of another cutaneous melanoma [179].

Increased expression of two heat-shock proteins (HSPs)—HSP70 and gp96—was demonstrated immunohistochemically and by Western blotting in the devitalized melanoma as early as one day after treatment, which persisted for the next two weeks. The growing proportion of tumor-infiltrating lymphocytes (cytotoxic T-lymphocytes and DP T-lymphocytes) was proven thereafter by flow cytometry in non-treated cutaneous melanomas [258]. Both monitored HSPs are able to form complexes with immunogenic peptides derived from cancer cells and, through antigen-presenting cells, they activate cytotoxic T-lymphocyte responses against the HSP-bound peptides [259–261]. Based on these findings, HSP70 and gp96-peptide vaccines derived from autologous tumor lysate were tested as a novel promising approach for the treatment of various malignancies including metastatic melanoma. Vitespen (formerly Oncophage) was the first personalized gp96-peptide cancer vaccine developed by the Antigenics Inc. (New York, NY, USA) and used in randomized clinical trials [262–266]. Our finding from devitalization experiments in the MeLiM model are in accordance with this therapeutic trend. Long-term overexpression of HSPs, followed by significant tumor lymphocyte infiltration, suggests that melanoma devitalization in the MeLiM model elicits a cell-mediated anti-tumor immune response. Thus, devitalization can be considered as an immunotherapeutic technique (auto-vaccination by necrotic tumor tissue from devitalized melanoma). At present, we apply melanoma devitalization for therapy of the MeLiM pigs with progressing melanoma to prolong survival and allow their inclusion as parental animals in the MeLiM herd. Their utilization in breeding schemes increases the incidence and severity of melanoma in this animal model.

6. Concluding Remarks

Enormous work was done in melanoma research, and even more remains to be elucidated. The study of intrinsic tumors and in vitro cultured cells, as well as the employment of animal models, enables us to be closer to understanding the disease etiology. The new genetic discoveries may help us to find new therapeutic targets or molecular reporters to monitor the disease development or therapy efficacy. Understanding the role of the immune system in melanoma control is crucial for immunotherapies.

Animal models are indispensable in melanoma research. Various mouse models are prevailingly utilized; however, swine models seem to be more appropriate due to anatomical, physiological, biochemical, and genetic similarities with human. Using genetic engineering, various transgenic swine models are available for biomedical research [267,268] including cancer [269,270]. However, no transgenic melanoma swine model was developed until now.

Several advantages of pig models highlight their importance in melanoma research. The pig skin structure and melanocyte distribution in pigmented skin more closely resemble the human situation (in contrast to mouse skin). Larger litters enable studying progression and regression by comparing sibling pairs. The long lifespan (12–18 years in miniature pig [271]) enables long-term monitoring of pig breeds and experimental outcomes. Large animal models also allow repeated blood and tissue sampling during the life of the individual to monitor the disease development. For example, repeated sampling in MeLiM model allows us to monitor spontaneous regression course and the involvement of immune cells in the disease control. Outcomes of such studies have the potential to bring new knowledge that would be usable in studies of human melanoma and its treatment.

Two already established and well-characterized swine models with spontaneous, hereditary melanoma—the Sinclair miniature swine and the melanoma-bearing Libechov minipig—showing many similarities with human melanoma, seem to be the best choice for melanoma study. These models closely resemble each other with respect to melanoma development, its spontaneous regression, and histopathological findings. However, genes responsible for predisposition to melanoma remain to be identified in both strains. The Hormel (Minnesota) miniature pig used in the establishment of the Sinclair and MeLiM models could carry susceptibility genes for melanoma. The Sinclair miniature swine is generally usable as a spontaneously regressing melanoma model because this biological process appears in most animals. The advantage of the MeLiM model is that, in addition to the spontaneous regression of melanoma observed in most animals, melanoma progression causing death is regularly observed in about 5–30% of affected pigs (depending on the disease burden in parenting individuals). Using repeated tissue and blood analyses and monitoring the health status of piglets from birth, we are able to distinguish pigs with spontaneously regressing melanoma from those with progressing melanoma and use them separately for studying the regression phenomenon and for the development of new techniques for melanoma treatment. Cooperation with research groups that are interested in large animal model melanoma research is desirable to maintain this unique swine model.

Author Contributions: Conceptualization V.H. and H.K.S.; Writing—Original Draft preparation, V.H., A.P., J.C., V.M., and H.K.S.; Writing—Review and Editing, all authors; supervision, P.V. and H.K.S.; project administration, H.K.S.; funding acquisition, H.K.S.

Funding: This study was supported by the Ministry of Education, Youth, and Sports of the Czech Republic from the Operational Program Research, Development, and Education (project reg. No. CZ.02.1.01/0.0/0.0/16_019/0000785) and the National Sustainability Program I (project reg. No. LO1609).

Conflicts of Interest: The authors declare no conflict of interest.

Abbreviations

BAP1: BRCA1-associated protein-1, **CDK4**: cyclin-dependent kinase 4, **CDKN2A**: cyclin-dependent kinase inhibitor 2A, **CTLA-4**: cytotoxic T-lymphocyte-associated protein 4, **DP**: double-positive, **EGF**: epidermal growth factor, **GWAS**: genome-wide association study, **HER**: human epidermal growth factor receptor, **HSPs**: heat-shock proteins, **IFN**: interferon, **IL**: interleukin, **MALDI-TOF MS**: matrix-assisted laser desorption/ionization time of flight mass spectrometry, **MAPK**: mitogen-activated protein kinase, **MC1R**: melanocortin 1 receptor, **MeLiM**: melanoma-bearing Libechov minipig, **miRNAs**: microRNAs, **MITF**: microphthalmia-associated transcription factor, **NF1**: neurofibromin 1, **PD-1**: programmed cell death protein 1, **PD-L1**: programmed death-ligand 1, **PDX**: patient-derived xenograft, **PI3K**: phosphatidylinositol 3-kinase, **POT1**: protection of telomeres protein 1, **PTEN**: phosphatase and tensin homolog, **RACK1**: receptor for activated C kinase 1, **SCID**: severe combined immunodeficiency, **SLA**: swine leukocyte antigen (swine major histocompatibility complex (MHC)), **TIL**: tumor-infiltrating lymphocytes, **TNF**: tumor necrosis factor, **Xmrk**: *Xiphophorus* melanoma receptor tyrosine-protein kinase.

References

1. Cummins, D.L.; Cummins, J.M.; Pantle, H.; Silverman, M.A.; Leonard, A.L.; Chanmugam, A. Cutaneous Malignant Melanoma. *Mayo Clin. Proc.* **2006**, *81*, 500–507. [CrossRef] [PubMed]
2. Lomas, A.; Leonardi Bee, J.; Bath Hextall, F. A Systematic Review of Worldwide Incidence of Nonmelanoma Skin Cancer. *Br. J. Dermatol.* **2012**, *166*, 1069–1080. [CrossRef] [PubMed]
3. Craythorne, E.; Al Niami, F. Skin Cancer. *Medicine (Baltimore)* **2017**, *45*, 431–434. [CrossRef]
4. Garcovich, S.; Colloca, G.; Sollena, P.; Andrea, B.; Balducci, L.; Cho, W.C.; Bernabei, R.; Peris, K. Skin Cancer Epidemics in the Elderly as An Emerging Issue in Geriatric Oncology. *Aging Dis.* **2017**, *8*, 643–661. [CrossRef]
5. Cichorek, M.; Wachulska, M.; Stasiewicz, A.; Tyminska, A. Skin Melanocytes: Biology and Development. *Postepy Dermatol. Alergol.* **2013**, *30*, 30–41. [CrossRef]
6. McElearney, S.T.; Dengel, L.T.; Vaughters, A.B.R.; Patterson, J.W.; McGahren, E.D.; Slingluff, C.L. Neonatal Congenital Malignant Melanoma with Lymph Node Metastasis. *J. Clin. Oncol. Off. J. Am. Soc. Clin. Oncol.* **2009**, *27*, 2726–2728. [CrossRef]
7. Perniciaro, C. Dermatopathologic Variants of Malignant Melanoma. *Mayo Clin. Proc.* **1997**, *72*, 273–279. [CrossRef]
8. O'Brien, K.; Bhatia, A.; Tsen, F.; Chen, M.; Wong, A.K.; Woodley, D.T.; Li, W. Identification of the Critical Therapeutic Entity in Secreted Hsp90α that Promotes Wound Healing in Newly Re-Standardized Healthy and Diabetic Pig Models. *PLoS ONE* **2014**, *9*, e113956. [CrossRef]
9. Summerfield, A.; Meurens, F.; Ricklin, M.E. The Immunology of the Porcine Skin and its Value as a Model for Human Skin. *Mol. Immunol.* **2015**, *66*, 14–21. [CrossRef] [PubMed]
10. Erdmann, F.; Lortet Tieulent, J.; Schuz, J.; Zeeb, H.; Greinert, R.; Breitbart, E.W.; Bray, F. International Trends in the Incidence of Malignant Melanoma 1953–2008-Are Recent Generations at Higher or Lower Risk? *Int. J. Cancer* **2013**, *132*, 385–400. [CrossRef]
11. Eggermont, A.M.; Spatz, A.; Robert, C. Cutaneous Melanoma. *Lancet* **2014**, *383*, 816–827. [CrossRef]
12. Siegel, R.L.; Miller, K.D.; Jemal, A. Cancer Statistics, 2019. *CA Cancer J. Clin.* **2019**, *69*, 7–34. [CrossRef] [PubMed]
13. Rastrelli, M.; Tropea, S.; Rossi, C.R.; Alaibac, M. Melanoma: Epidemiology, Risk Factors, Pathogenesis, Diagnosis and Classification. *Vivo Athens Greece* **2014**, *28*, 1005–1011.
14. Berwick, M.; Buller, D.B.; Cust, A.; Gallagher, R.; Lee, T.K.; Meyskens, F.; Pandey, S.; Thomas, N.E.; Veierod, M.B.; Ward, S. Melanoma Epidemiology and Prevention. *Cancer Treat. Res.* **2016**, *167*, 17–49. [PubMed]
15. Leachman, S.A.; Lucero, O.M.; Sampson, J.E.; Cassidy, P.; Bruno, W.; Queirolo, P.; Ghiorzo, P. Identification, Genetic Testing, and Management of Hereditary Melanoma. *Cancer Metastasis Rev.* **2017**, *36*, 77–90. [CrossRef]
16. Duggleby, W.F.; Stoll, H.; Priore, R.L.; Greenwald, P.; Graham, S. A Genetic Analysis of Melanoma–Polygenic Inheritance as a Threshold Trait. *Am. J. Epidemiol.* **1981**, *114*, 63–72. [CrossRef]
17. Dracopoli, N.C.; Alhadeff, B.; Houghton, A.N.; Old, L.J. Loss of Heterozygosity at Autosomal and X-Linked Loci During Tumor Progression in a Patient with Melanoma. *Cancer Res.* **1987**, *47*, 3995–4000.
18. Fountain, J.W.; Karayiorgou, M.; Ernstoff, M.S.; Kirkwood, J.M.; Vlock, D.R.; Titus-Ernstoff, L.; Bouchard, B.; Vijayasaradhi, S.; Houghton, A.N.; Lahti, J. Homozygous Deletions within Human Chromosome Band 9p21 in Melanoma. *Proc. Natl. Acad. Sci. USA* **1992**, *89*, 10557–10561. [CrossRef]

19. Nancarrow, D.J.; Mann, G.J.; Holland, E.A.; Walker, G.J.; Beaton, S.C.; Walters, M.K.; Luxford, C.; Palmer, J.M.; Donald, J.A.; Weber, J.L. Confirmation of Chromosome 9p Linkage in Familial Melanoma. *Am. J. Hum. Genet.* **1993**, *53*, 936–942.
20. Kamb, A.; Shattuck Eidens, D.; Eeles, R.; Liu, Q.; Gruis, N.A.; Ding, W.; Hussey, C.; Tran, T.; Miki, Y.; Weaver Feldhaus, J. Analysis of the p16 Gene (CDKN2) as a Candidate for the Chromosome 9p Melanoma Susceptibility Locus. *Nat. Genet.* **1994**, *8*, 23–26. [CrossRef]
21. Borg, A.; Johannsson, U.; Johannsson, O.; Hakansson, S.; Westerdahl, J.; Masback, A.; Olsson, H.; Ingvar, C. Novel Germline p16 Mutation in Familial Malignant Melanoma in Southern Sweden. *Cancer Res.* **1996**, *56*, 2497–2500. [PubMed]
22. FitzGerald, M.G.; Harkin, D.P.; Silva Arrieta, S.; MacDonald, D.J.; Lucchina, L.C.; Unsal, H.; O'Neill, E.; Koh, J.; Finkelstein, D.M.; Isselbacher, K.J.; et al. Prevalence of Germ-Line Mutations in p16, p19ARF, and CDK4 in Familial Melanoma: Analysis of a Clinic-Based Population. *Proc. Natl. Acad. Sci. USA* **1996**, *93*, 8541–8545. [CrossRef]
23. Harland, M.; Meloni, R.; Gruis, N.; Pinney, E.; Brookes, S.; Spurr, N.K.; Frischauf, A.M.; Bataille, V.; Peters, G.; Cuzick, J.; et al. Germline Mutations of the CDKN2 Gene in UK Melanoma Families. *Hum. Mol. Genet.* **1997**, *6*, 2061–2067. [CrossRef] [PubMed]
24. Soufir, N.; Avril, M.F.; Chompret, A.; Demenais, F.; Bombled, J.; Spatz, A.; Stoppa Lyonnet, D.; Benard, J.; Bressac De Paillerets, B. Prevalence of p16 and CDK4 Germline Mutations in 48 Melanoma-Prone Families in France. The French Familial Melanoma Study Group. *Hum. Mol. Genet.* **1998**, *7*, 209–216. [CrossRef]
25. Aitken, J.; Welch, J.; Duffy, D.; Milligan, A.; Green, A.; Martin, N.; Hayward, N. CDKN2A Variants in a Population-Based Sample of Queensland Families with Melanoma. *J. Natl. Cancer Inst.* **1999**, *91*, 446–452. [CrossRef]
26. Quelle, D.E.; Zindy, F.; Ashmun, R.A.; Sherr, C.J. Alternative Reading Frames of the INK4a Tumor Suppressor Gene Encode two Unrelated Proteins Capable of Inducing Cell Cycle Arrest. *Cell* **1995**, *83*, 993–1000. [PubMed]
27. Stott, F.J.; Bates, S.; James, M.C.; McConnell, B.B.; Starborg, M.; Brookes, S.; Palmero, I.; Ryan, K.; Hara, E.; Vousden, K.H.; et al. The Alternative Product from the Human CDKN2A Locus, p14(ARF), Participates in a Regulatory Feedback Loop with p53 and MDM2. *EMBO J.* **1998**, *17*, 5001–5014. [CrossRef]
28. Goldstein, A.M.; Chan, M.; Harland, M.; Hayward, N.K.; Demenais, F.; Bishop, D.T.; Azizi, E.; Bergman, W.; Bianchi Scarra, G.; Bruno, W.; et al. Features Associated with Germline CDKN2A Mutations: A GenoMEL Study of Melanoma-Prone Families from Three Continents. *J. Med. Genet.* **2007**, *44*, 99–106. [CrossRef]
29. Rossi, M.; Pellegrini, C.; Cardelli, L.; Ciciarelli, V.; Di Nardo, L.; Fargnoli, M.C. Familial Melanoma: Diagnostic and Management Implications. *Dermatol. Pract. Concept.* **2019**, *9*, 10–16. [CrossRef]
30. Harland, M.; Cust, A.E.; Badenas, C.; Chang, Y.M.; Holland, E.A.; Aguilera, P.; Aitken, J.F.; Armstrong, B.K.; Barrett, J.H.; Carrera, C.; et al. Prevalence and Predictors of Germline CDKN2A Mutations for Melanoma Cases from Australia, Spain and the United Kingdom. *Hered. Cancer Clin. Pract.* **2014**, *12*, 20. [CrossRef]
31. Wolfel, T.; Hauer, M.; Schneider, J.; Serrano, M.; Wolfel, C.; Klehmann Hieb, E.; De Plaen, E.; Hankeln, T.; Meyer Zum Buschenfelde, K.H.; Beach, D. A p16INK4a-Insensitive CDK4 Mutant Targeted by Cytolytic T Lymphocytes in a Human Melanoma. *Science* **1995**, *269*, 1281–1284. [CrossRef] [PubMed]
32. Zuo, L.; Weger, J.; Yang, Q.; Goldstein, A.M.; Tucker, M.A.; Walker, G.J.; Hayward, N.; Dracopoli, N.C. Germline Mutations in the p16INK4a Binding Domain of cdk4 in Familial Melanoma. *Nat. Genet.* **1996**, *12*, 97–99. [CrossRef]
33. Puntervoll, H.E.; Yang, X.R.; Vetti, H.H.; Bachmann, I.M.; Avril, M.F.; Benfodda, M.; Catricala, C.; Dalle, S.; Duval Modeste, A.B.; Ghiorzo, P.; et al. Melanoma Prone Families with CDK4 Germline Mutation: Phenotypic Profile and Associations with MC1R Variants. *J. Med. Genet.* **2013**, *50*, 264–270. [CrossRef]
34. Harbour, J.W.; Onken, M.D.; Roberson, E.D.O.; Duan, S.; Cao, L.; Worley, L.A.; Council, M.L.; Matatall, K.A.; Helms, C.; Bowcock, A.M. Frequent Mutation of BAP1 in Metastasizing Uveal Melanomas. *Science* **2010**, *330*, 1410–1413. [CrossRef] [PubMed]
35. Wiesner, T.; Obenauf, A.C.; Murali, R.; Fried, I.; Griewank, K.G.; Ulz, P.; Windpassinger, C.; Wackernagel, W.; Loy, S.; Wolf, I.; et al. Germline Mutations in BAP1 Predispose to Melanocytic Tumors. *Nat. Genet.* **2011**, *43*, 1018–1021. [CrossRef] [PubMed]

36. Njauw, C.N.J.; Kim, I.; Piris, A.; Gabree, M.; Taylor, M.; Lane, A.M.; DeAngelis, M.M.; Gragoudas, E.; Duncan, L.M.; Tsao, H. Germline BAP1 Inactivation is Preferentially Associated with Metastatic Ocular Melanoma and Cutaneous-Ocular Melanoma Families. *PLoS ONE* **2012**, *7*, e35295. [CrossRef]
37. Murali, R.; Wilmott, J.S.; Jakrot, V.; Al Ahmadie, H.A.; Wiesner, T.; McCarthy, S.W.; Thompson, J.F.; Scolyer, R.A. BAP1 Expression in Cutaneous Melanoma: A Pilot Study. *Pathol. J. PCPA* **2013**, *45*, 606–609. [CrossRef]
38. Ismail, I.H.; Davidson, R.; Gagne, J.P.; Xu, Z.Z.; Poirier, G.G.; Hendzel, M.J. Germline Mutations in BAP1 Impair its Function in DNA Double-Strand Break Repair. *Cancer Res.* **2014**, *74*, 4282–4294. [CrossRef]
39. Soura, E.; Eliades, P.J.; Shannon, K.; Stratigos, A.J.; Tsao, H. Hereditary Melanoma: Update on Syndromes and Management: Emerging Melanoma Cancer Complexes and Genetic Counseling. *J. Am. Acad. Dermatol.* **2016**, *74*, 411–420. [CrossRef]
40. Horn, S.; Figl, A.; Rachakonda, P.S.; Fischer, C.; Sucker, A.; Gast, A.; Kadel, S.; Moll, I.; Nagore, E.; Hemminki, K.; et al. TERT Promoter Mutations in Familial and Sporadic Melanoma. *Science* **2013**, *339*, 959–961. [CrossRef]
41. Robles Espinoza, C.D.; Harland, M.; Ramsay, A.J.; Aoude, L.G.; Quesada, V.; Ding, Z.; Pooley, K.A.; Pritchard, A.L.; Tiffen, J.C.; Petljak, M.; et al. POT1 Loss-of-Function Variants Predispose to Familial Melanoma. *Nat. Genet.* **2014**, *46*, 478–481. [CrossRef]
42. Shi, J.; Yang, X.R.; Ballew, B.; Rotunno, M.; Calista, D.; Fargnoli, M.C.; Ghiorzo, P.; Bressac De Paillerets, B.; Nagore, E.; Avril, M.F.; et al. Rare Missense Variants in POT1 Predispose to Familial Cutaneous Malignant Melanoma. *Nat. Genet.* **2014**, *46*, 482–486. [CrossRef]
43. Potrony, M.; Puig Butille, J.A.; Ribera Sola, M.; Iyer, V.; Robles Espinoza, C.D.; Aguilera, P.; Carrera, C.; Malvehy, J.; Badenas, C.; Landi, M.T.; et al. POT1 Germline Mutations but Not TERT Promoter Mutations are Implicated in Melanoma Susceptibility in a Large Cohort of Spanish Melanoma Families. *Br. J. Dermatol.* **2019**, *181*, 105–113. [CrossRef]
44. Aoude, L.G.; Pritchard, A.L.; Robles Espinoza, C.D.; Wadt, K.; Harland, M.; Choi, J.; Gartside, M.; Quesada, V.; Johansson, P.; Palmer, J.M.; et al. Nonsense Mutations in the Shelterin Complex Genes ACD and TERF2IP in Familial Melanoma. *J. Natl. Cancer Inst.* **2015**, *107*, dju408. [CrossRef]
45. Hodgkinson, C.A.; Moore, K.J.; Nakayama, A.; Steingrímsson, E.; Copeland, N.G.; Jenkins, N.A.; Arnheiter, H. Mutations at the mouse microphthalmia locus are associated with defects in a gene encoding a novel basic-helix-loop-helix-zipper protein. *Cell* **1993**, *74*, 395–404. [CrossRef]
46. Yasumoto, K.; Yokoyama, K.; Shibata, K.; Tomita, Y.; Shibahara, S. Microphthalmia Associated Transcription Factor as a Regulator for Melanocyte-Specific Transcription of the Human Tyrosinase Gene. *Mol. Cell. Biol.* **1994**, *14*, 8058–8070. [CrossRef] [PubMed]
47. Dynek, J.N.; Chan, S.M.; Liu, J.; Zha, J.; Fairbrother, W.J.; Vucic, D. Microphthalmia-Associated Transcription Factor is a Critical Transcriptional Regulator of Melanoma Inhibitor of Apoptosis in Melanomas. *Cancer Res.* **2008**, *68*, 3124–3132. [CrossRef]
48. Garraway, L.A.; Widlund, H.R.; Rubin, M.A.; Getz, G.; Berger, A.J.; Ramaswamy, S.; Beroukhim, R.; Milner, D.A.; Granter, S.R.; Du, J.; et al. Integrative Genomic Analyses Identify MITF as a Lineage Survival Oncogene Amplified in Malignant Melanoma. *Nature* **2005**, *436*, 117–122. [CrossRef] [PubMed]
49. Bertolotto, C.; Lesueur, F.; Giuliano, S.; Strub, T.; De Lichy, M.; Bille, K.; Dessen, P.; D'Hayer, B.; Mohamdi, H.; Remenieras, A.; et al. A SUMOylation-Defective MITF Germline Mutation Predisposes to Melanoma and Renal Carcinoma. *Nature* **2011**, *480*, 94–98. [CrossRef] [PubMed]
50. Palmer, J.S.; Duffy, D.L.; Box, N.F.; Aitken, J.F.; O'Gorman, L.E.; Green, A.C.; Hayward, N.K.; Martin, N.G.; Sturm, R.A. Melanocortin-1 Receptor Polymorphisms and Risk of Melanoma: Is the Association Explained Solely by Pigmentation Phenotype? *Am. J. Hum. Genet.* **2000**, *66*, 176–186. [CrossRef]
51. Kennedy, C.; Ter Huurne, J.; Berkhout, M.; Gruis, N.; Bastiaens, M.; Bergman, W.; Willemze, R.; Bavinck, J.N. Melanocortin 1 Receptor (MC1R) Gene Variants are Associated with an Increased Risk for Cutaneous Melanoma which is Largely Independent of Skin Type and Hair Color. *J. Invest. Dermatol.* **2001**, *117*, 294–300. [CrossRef] [PubMed]
52. Box, N.F.; Duffy, D.L.; Chen, W.; Stark, M.; Martin, N.G.; Sturm, R.A.; Hayward, N.K. MC1R Genotype Modifies Risk of Melanoma in Families Segregating CDKN2A Mutations. *Am. J. Hum. Genet.* **2001**, *69*, 765–773. [CrossRef] [PubMed]

53. Paolino, G.; Moliterni, E.; Corsetti, P.; Didona, D.; Bottoni, U.; Calvieri, S.; Mattozzi, C. Vitamin D and Melanoma: State of the Art and Possible Therapeutic Uses. *G. Ital. Dermatol. E Venereol. Organo Uff. Soc. Ital. Dermatol. E Sifilogr.* **2019**, *154*, 64–71. [CrossRef] [PubMed]
54. Slominski, A.T.; Brozyna, A.A.; Zmijewski, M.A.; Jozwicki, W.; Jetten, A.M.; Mason, R.S.; Tuckey, R.C.; Elmets, C.A. Vitamin D Signaling and Melanoma: Role of Vitamin D and its Receptors in Melanoma Progression and Management. *Lab. Investig. J. Tech. Methods Pathol.* **2017**, *97*, 706–724. [CrossRef]
55. Hutchinson, P.E.; Osborne, J.E.; Lear, J.T.; Smith, A.G.; Bowers, P.W.; Morris, P.N.; Jones, P.W.; York, C.; Strange, R.C.; Fryer, A.A. Vitamin D Receptor Polymorphisms are Associated with Altered Prognosis in Patients with Malignant Melanoma. *Clin. Cancer Res. Off. J. Am. Assoc. Cancer Res.* **2000**, *6*, 498–504.
56. Shahbazi, M.; Pravica, V.; Nasreen, N.; Fakhoury, H.; Fryer, A.A.; Strange, R.C.; Hutchinson, P.E.; Osborne, J.E.; Lear, J.T.; Smith, A.G.; et al. Association between Functional Polymorphism in EGF Gene and Malignant Melanoma. *Lancet Lond. Engl.* **2002**, *359*, 397–401. [CrossRef]
57. Hayward, N.K. Genetics of Melanoma Predisposition. *Oncogene* **2003**, *22*, 3053–3062. [CrossRef]
58. Fargnoli, M.C.; Argenziano, G.; Zalaudek, I.; Peris, K. High-And Low-Penetrance Cutaneous Melanoma Susceptibility Genes. *Expert Rev. Anticancer Ther.* **2006**, *6*, 657–670. [CrossRef]
59. Aoude, L.G.; Wadt, K.A.W.; Pritchard, A.L.; Hayward, N.K. Genetics of Familial Melanoma: 20 Years after CDKN2A. *Pigment Cell Melanoma Res.* **2015**, *28*, 148–160. [CrossRef]
60. Bennett, D.C. Genetics of Melanoma Progression: The Rise and Fall of Cell Senescence. *Pigment Cell Melanoma Res.* **2016**, *29*, 122–140. [CrossRef]
61. Roberts, M.R.; Asgari, M.M.; Toland, A.E. Genome-Wide Association Studies and Polygenic Risk Scores for Skin Cancer: Clinically Useful Yet? *Br. J. Dermatol.* **2019**. [CrossRef] [PubMed]
62. Pho, L.N.; Leachman, S.A. Genetics of Pigmentation and Melanoma Predisposition. *G. Ital. Dermatol. E Venereol. Organo Uff. Soc. Ital. Dermatol. E Sifilogr.* **2010**, *145*, 37–45.
63. Scherer, D.; Kumar, R. Genetics of Pigmentation in Skin Cancer-A Review. *Mutat. Res.* **2010**, *705*, 141–153. [CrossRef] [PubMed]
64. Ritterhouse, L.L.; Barletta, J.A. BRAF V600E Mutation-Specific Antibody: A Review. *Semin. Diagn. Pathol.* **2015**, *32*, 400–408. [CrossRef] [PubMed]
65. Kunz, M. Oncogenes in Melanoma: An Update. *Eur. J. Cell Biol.* **2014**, *93*, 1–10. [CrossRef] [PubMed]
66. Reddy, B.Y.; Miller, D.M.; Tsao, H. Somatic Driver Mutations in Melanoma. *Cancer* **2017**, *123*, 2104–2117. [CrossRef]
67. Cicenas, J.; Tamosaitis, L.; Kvederaviciute, K.; Tarvydas, R.; Staniute, G.; Kalyan, K.; Meskinyte Kausiliene, E.; Stankevicius, V.; Valius, M. KRAS, NRAS and BRAF Mutations in Colorectal Cancer and Melanoma. *Med. Oncol. Northwood Lond. Engl.* **2017**, *34*, 26. [CrossRef]
68. Rabbie, R.; Ferguson, P.; Molina Aguilar, C.; Adams, D.J.; Robles Espinoza, C.D. Melanoma Subtypes: Genomic Profiles, Prognostic Molecular Markers and Therapeutic Possibilities. *J. Pathol.* **2019**, *247*, 539–551. [CrossRef]
69. Cancer Genome Atlas Network Genomic Classification of Cutaneous Melanoma. *Cell* **2015**, *161*, 1681–1696. [CrossRef]
70. Hartman, R.I.; Lin, J.Y. Cutaneous Melanoma A Review in Detection, Staging, and Management. *Hematol. Oncol. Clin. N. Am.* **2019**, *33*, 25–38. [CrossRef]
71. Everson, T.C. Spontaneous Regression of Cancer. *Ann. N. Y. Acad. Sci.* **1964**, *114*, 721–735. [CrossRef] [PubMed]
72. Maio, M. Melanoma as a Model Tumour for Immuno-Oncology. *Ann. Oncol. Off. J. Eur. Soc. Med. Oncol.* **2012**, *23*, viii10–viii14. [CrossRef] [PubMed]
73. Kalialis, L.V.; Drzewiecki, K.T.; Klyver, H. Spontaneous Regression of Metastases from Melanoma: Review of the Literature. *Melanoma Res.* **2009**, *19*, 275–282. [CrossRef] [PubMed]
74. Margaritescu, I.; Chirița, A.D.; Vasilescu, F. Completely Regressed Primary Cutaneous Melanoma-Difficulties in Diagnosis and Classification. *Rom. J. Morphol. Embryol. Rev. Roum. Morphol. Embryol.* **2014**, *55*, 635–642.
75. Cole, W.H.; Everson, T.C. Spontaneous Regression of Cancer: Preliminary Report. *Ann. Surg.* **1956**, *144*, 366–383. [PubMed]
76. Bourneuf, E. The MeLiM Minipig: An Original Spontaneous Model to Explore Cutaneous Melanoma Genetic Basis. *Front. Genet.* **2017**, *8*, 146. [CrossRef]

77. Cervinkova, M.; Kucerova, P.; Cizkova, J. Spontaneous Regression of Malignant Melanoma-Is it Based on the Interplay between Host Immune System and Melanoma Antigens? *Anticancer. Drugs* **2017**, *28*, 819–830. [CrossRef]
78. Ribero, S.; Moscarella, E.; Ferrara, G.; Piana, S.; Argenziano, G.; Longo, C. Regression in Cutaneous Melanoma: A Comprehensive Review from Diagnosis to Prognosis. *J. Eur. Acad. Dermatol. Venereol. JEADV* **2016**, *30*, 2030–2037. [CrossRef]
79. Kaur, C.; Thomas, R.J.; Desai, N.; Green, M.A.; Lovell, D.; Powell, B.W.E.M.; Cook, M.G. The Correlation of Regression in Primary Melanoma with sentinel Lymph Node Status. *J. Clin. Pathol.* **2008**, *61*, 297–300. [CrossRef]
80. Crompton, J.G.; Gilbert, E.; Brady, M.S. Clinical Implications of the Eighth Edition of the American Joint Committee on Cancer Melanoma Staging. *J. Surg. Oncol.* **2019**, *119*, 168–174. [CrossRef]
81. Kozar, I.; Margue, C.; Rothengatter, S.; Haan, C.; Kreis, S. Many Ways to Resistance: How Melanoma Cells Evade Targeted Therapies. *Biochim. Biophys. Acta Rev. Cancer* **2019**, *1871*, 313–322. [CrossRef] [PubMed]
82. Lorentzen, H.F. Targeted Therapy for Malignant Melanoma. *Curr. Opin. Pharmacol.* **2019**, *46*, 116–121. [CrossRef] [PubMed]
83. Glitza Oliva, I.C.; Alqusairi, R. Immunotherapy for Melanoma. *Adv. Exp. Med. Biol.* **2018**, *995*, 43–63. [PubMed]
84. Margolis, N.; Markovits, E.; Markel, G. Reprogramming Lymphocytes for the Treatment of Melanoma: From Biology to Therapy. *Adv. Drug Deliv. Rev.* **2019**, *141*, 104–124. [CrossRef] [PubMed]
85. Weiss, S.A.; Wolchok, J.D.; Sznol, M. Immunotherapy of Melanoma: Facts and Hopes. *Clin. Cancer Res. Off. J. Am. Assoc. Cancer Res.* **2019**, *25*, 5191–5201. [CrossRef] [PubMed]
86. Yu, C.; Liu, X.; Yang, J.; Zhang, M.; Jin, H.; Ma, X.; Shi, H. Combination of Immunotherapy With Targeted Therapy: Theory and Practice in Metastatic Melanoma. *Front. Immunol.* **2019**, *10*, 990. [CrossRef] [PubMed]
87. Stern, H.M.; Zon, L.I. Cancer Genetics and Drug Discovery in the Zebrafish. *Nat. Rev. Cancer* **2003**, *3*, 533–539. [CrossRef]
88. Schartl, M.; Walter, R.B. Xiphophorus and Medaka Cancer Models. *Adv. Exp. Med. Biol.* **2016**, *916*, 531–552.
89. Bootorabi, F.; Manouchehri, H.; Changizi, R.; Barker, H.; Palazzo, E.; Saltari, A.; Parikka, M.; Pincelli, C.; Aspatwar, A. Zebrafish as a Model Organism for the Development of Drugs for Skin Cancer. *Int. J. Mol. Sci.* **2017**, *18*, 1550. [CrossRef]
90. Cagan, R.L.; Zon, L.I.; White, R.M. Modeling Cancer with Flies and Fish. *Dev. Cell* **2019**, *49*, 317–324. [CrossRef]
91. Bennett, D.; Lyulcheva, E.; Cobbe, N. Drosophila as a Potential Model for Ocular Tumors. *Ocul. Oncol. Pathol.* **2015**, *1*, 190–199. [CrossRef] [PubMed]
92. Hanratty, W.P.; Ryerse, J.S. A Genetic Melanotic Neoplasm of Drosophila Melanogaster. *Dev. Biol.* **1981**, *83*, 238–249. [CrossRef]
93. Anders, F. Contributions of the Gordon-Kosswig Melanoma System to the Present Concept of Neoplasia. *Pigment Cell Res.* **1991**, *4*, 7–29. [CrossRef] [PubMed]
94. Setlow, R.B.; Woodhead, A.D.; Grist, E. Animal Model for Ultraviolet Radiation-Induced Melanoma: Platyfish-Swordtail Hybrid. *Proc. Natl. Acad. Sci. USA* **1989**, *86*, 8922–8926. [CrossRef]
95. Wood, S.R.; Berwick, M.; Ley, R.D.; Walter, R.B.; Setlow, R.B.; Timmins, G.S. UV Causation of Melanoma in Xiphophorus is Dominated by Melanin Photosensitized Oxidant Production. *Proc. Natl. Acad. Sci. USA* **2006**, *103*, 4111–4115. [CrossRef]
96. Wittbrodt, J.; Lammers, R.; Malitschek, B.; Ullrich, A.; Schartl, M. The Xmrk Receptor Tyrosine Kinase is Activated in Xiphophorus Malignant Melanoma. *EMBO J.* **1992**, *11*, 4239–4246. [CrossRef]
97. Patton, E.E.; Widlund, H.R.; Kutok, J.L.; Kopani, K.R.; Amatruda, J.F.; Murphey, R.D.; Berghmans, S.; Mayhall, E.A.; Traver, D.; Fletcher, C.D.M.; et al. BRAF Mutations are Sufficient to Promote Nevi Formation and Cooperate with p53 in the Genesis of Melanoma. *Curr. Biol. CB* **2005**, *15*, 249–254. [CrossRef]
98. Dovey, M.; White, R.M.; Zon, L.I. Oncogenic NRAS Cooperates with p53 Loss to Generate Melanoma in Zebrafish. *Zebrafish* **2009**, *6*, 397–404. [CrossRef]
99. Santoriello, C.; Zon, L.I. Hooked! Modeling Human Disease in Zebrafish. *J. Clin. Invest.* **2012**, *122*, 2337–2343. [CrossRef]
100. Scahill, C.M.; Digby, Z.; Sealy, I.M.; Wojciechowska, S.; White, R.J.; Collins, J.E.; Stemple, D.L.; Bartke, T.; Mathers, M.E.; Patton, E.E.; et al. Loss of the Chromatin Modifier Kdm2aa Causes BrafV600E-Independent Spontaneous Melanoma in Zebrafish. *PLoS Genetics* **2017**, *13*, e1006959. [CrossRef]

101. Stoletov, K.; Klemke, R. Catch of the Day: Zebrafish as a Human Cancer Model. *Oncogene* **2008**, *27*, 4509–4520. [CrossRef] [PubMed]
102. Ablain, J.; Zon, L.I. Of Fish and Men: Using Zebrafish to Fight Human Diseases. *Trends Cell Biol.* **2013**, *23*, 584–586. [CrossRef]
103. Haldi, M.; Ton, C.; Seng, W.L.; McGrath, P. Human Melanoma Cells Transplanted into Zebrafish Proliferate, Migrate, Produce Melanin, form Masses and Stimulate Angiogenesis in Zebrafish. *Angiogenesis* **2006**, *9*, 139–151. [CrossRef] [PubMed]
104. Heilmann, S.; Ratnakumar, K.; Langdon, E.; Kansler, E.; Kim, I.; Campbell, N.R.; Perry, E.; McMahon, A.; Kaufman, C.; Van Rooijen, E.; et al. A Quantitative System for Studying Metastasis Using Transparent Zebrafish. *Cancer Res.* **2015**, *75*, 4272–4282. [CrossRef] [PubMed]
105. Schartl, M.; Wilde, B.; Laisney, J.A.G.C.; Taniguchi, Y.; Takeda, S.; Meierjohann, S. A Mutated EGFR is Sufficient to Induce Malignant Melanoma with Genetic Background-Dependent Histopathologies. *J. Invest. Dermatol.* **2010**, *130*, 249–258. [CrossRef] [PubMed]
106. Schartl, M.; Kneitz, S.; Wilde, B.; Wagner, T.; Henkel, C.V.; Spaink, H.P.; Meierjohann, S. Conserved Expression Signatures between Medaka and Human Pigment Cell Tumors. *PLoS ONE* **2012**, *7*, e37880. [CrossRef]
107. Levine, N.; Queen, L.; Chalom, A.A.; Daniels, L.J. Animal Model of Intracutaneous Melanoma. *J. Invest. Dermatol.* **1982**, *78*, 191–193. [CrossRef]
108. Berkelhammer, J.; Oxenhandler, R.W. Evaluation of Premalignant and Malignant Lesions During the Induction of Mouse Melanomas. *Cancer Res.* **1987**, *47*, 1251–1254.
109. Bradl, M.; Klein Szanto, A.; Porter, S.; Mintz, B. Malignant Melanoma in Transgenic Mice. *Proc. Natl. Acad. Sci. USA* **1991**, *88*, 164–168. [CrossRef]
110. Mintz, B.; Silvers, W.K. Transgenic Mouse Model of Malignant Skin Melanoma. *Proc. Natl. Acad. Sci. USA* **1993**, *90*, 8817–8821. [CrossRef]
111. Gattoni Celli, S.; Byers, R.H.; Calorini, L.; Ferrone, S. Organ-Specific Metastases in Melanoma: Experimental Animal Models. *Pigment Cell Res.* **1993**, *6*, 381–384. [CrossRef] [PubMed]
112. Chen, S.; Zhu, H.; Wetzel, W.J.; Philbert, M.A. Spontaneous Melanocytosis in Transgenic Mice. *J. Invest. Dermatol.* **1996**, *106*, 1145–1151. [CrossRef] [PubMed]
113. Zhu, H.; Reuhl, K.; Zhang, X.; Botha, R.; Ryan, K.; Wei, J.; Chen, S. Development of Heritable Melanoma in Transgenic Mice. *J. Invest. Dermatol.* **1998**, *110*, 247–252. [CrossRef] [PubMed]
114. Bobek, V.; Kolostova, K.; Pinterova, D.; Kacprzak, G.; Adamiak, J.; Kolodziej, J.; Boubelik, M.; Kubecova, M.; Hoffman, R.M. A Clinically Relevant, Syngeneic Model of Spontaneous, Highly Metastatic B16 Mouse Melanoma. *Anticancer Res.* **2010**, *5*, 4799–4803.
115. Saleh, J. Murine Models of Melanoma. *Pathol. Res. Pract.* **2018**, *214*, 1235–1238. [CrossRef]
116. Kuzu, O.F.; Nguyen, F.D.; Noory, M.A.; Sharma, A. Current State of Animal (Mouse) Modeling in Melanoma Research. *Cancer Growth Metastasis* **2015**, *8*, 81–94. [CrossRef]
117. Harris, A.L.; Joseph, R.W.; Copland, J.A. Patient-Derived Tumor Xenograft Models for Melanoma Drug Discovery. *Expert Opin. Drug Discov.* **2016**, *11*, 895–906. [CrossRef]
118. Choi, Y.; Lee, S.; Kim, K.; Kim, S.H.; Chung, Y.J.; Lee, C. Studying Cancer Immunotherapy Using Patient-Derived Xenografts (PDXs) in Humanized Mice. *Exp. Mol. Med.* **2018**, *50*, 1–9. [CrossRef]
119. McKinney, A.J.; Holmen, S.L. Animal Models of Melanoma: A Somatic Cell Gene Delivery Mouse Model Allows Rapid Evaluation of Genes Implicated in Human Melanoma. *Chin. J. Cancer* **2011**, *30*, 153–162. [CrossRef]
120. Perez Guijarro, E.; Day, C.P.; Merlino, G.; Zaidi, M.R. Genetically Engineered Mouse Models of Melanoma. *Cancer* **2017**, *123*, 2089–2103. [CrossRef]
121. Niu, Y.; Liang, S. Mammalian Models Based on RCAS-TVA Technique. *Zool. Res.* **2008**, *29*, 335–345.
122. Dankort, D.; Curley, D.P.; Cartlidge, R.A.; Nelson, B.; Karnezis, A.N.; Damsky, W.E.; You, M.J.; DePinho, R.A.; McMahon, M.; Bosenberg, M. Braf(V600E) Cooperates with Pten Loss to Induce Metastatic Melanoma. *Nat. Genet.* **2009**, *41*, 544–552. [CrossRef] [PubMed]
123. Klein Szanto, A.J.; Silvers, W.K.; Mintz, B. Ultraviolet Radiation-Induced Malignant Skin Melanoma in Melanoma-Susceptible Transgenic Mice. *Cancer Res.* **1994**, *54*, 4569–4572. [PubMed]
124. Broome Powell, M.; Gause, P.R.; Hyman, P.; Gregus, J.; Lluria Prevatt, M.; Nagle, R.; Bowden, G.T. Induction of Melanoma in TPras Transgenic Mice. *Carcinogenesis* **1999**, *20*, 1747–1753. [CrossRef]

125. Ley, R.D. Animal Models of Ultraviolet Radiation (UVR)-Induced Cutaneous Melanoma. *Front. Biosci. J. Virtual Libr.* **2002**, *7*, d1531–d1534.
126. Larue, L. Origin of Mouse Melanomas. *J. Invest. Dermatol.* **2012**, *132*, 2135–2136. [CrossRef]
127. Goldschmidt, M.H. Pigmented Lesions of the Skin. *Clin. Dermatol.* **1994**, *12*, 507–514. [CrossRef]
128. Modiano, J.F.; Ritt, M.G.; Wojcieszyn, J. The Molecular Basis of Canine Melanoma: Pathogenesis and Trends in Diagnosis and Therapy. *J. Vet. Intern. Med.* **1999**, *13*, 163–174. [CrossRef]
129. Prouteau, A.; Andre, C. Canine Melanomas as Models for Human Melanomas: Clinical, Histological, and Genetic Comparison. *Genes* **2019**, *10*, 501. [CrossRef]
130. Koenig, A.; Bianco, S.R.; Fosmire, S.; Wojcieszyn, J.; Modiano, J.F. Expression and Significance of p53, rb, p21/waf-1, p16/ink-4a, and PTEN Tumor Suppressors in Canine Melanoma. *Vet. Pathol.* **2002**, *39*, 458–472. [CrossRef]
131. Gillard, M.; Cadieu, E.; De Brito, C.; Abadie, J.; Vergier, B.; Devauchelle, P.; Degorce, F.; Dreano, S.; Primot, A.; Dorso, L.; et al. Naturally Occurring Melanomas in Dogs as Models for Non-UV Pathways of Human Melanomas. *Pigment Cell Melanoma Res.* **2014**, *27*, 90–102. [CrossRef] [PubMed]
132. Pisamai, S.; Rungsipipat, A.; Kalpravidh, C.; Suriyaphol, G. Gene Expression Profiles of Cell Adhesion Molecules, Matrix Metalloproteinases and Their Tissue Inhibitors in Canine Oral Tumors. *Res. Vet. Sci.* **2017**, *113*, 94–100. [CrossRef] [PubMed]
133. Brachelente, C.; Cappelli, K.; Capomaccio, S.; Porcellato, I.; Silvestri, S.; Bongiovanni, L.; De Maria, R.; Verini Supplizi, A.; Mechelli, L.; Sforna, M. Transcriptome Analysis of Canine Cutaneous Melanoma and Melanocytoma Reveals a Modulation of Genes Regulating Extracellular Matrix Metabolism and Cell Cycle. *Sci. Rep.* **2017**, *7*, 6386. [CrossRef] [PubMed]
134. Hendricks, W.P.D.; Zismann, V.; Sivaprakasam, K.; Legendre, C.; Poorman, K.; Tembe, W.; Perdigones, N.; Kiefer, J.; Liang, W.; DeLuca, V.; et al. Somatic Inactivating PTPRJ Mutations and Dysregulated Pathways Identified in Canine Malignant Melanoma by Integrated Comparative Genomic Analysis. *PLoS Genetics* **2018**, *14*. [CrossRef] [PubMed]
135. Valentine, B.A. Equine Melanocytic Tumors: A Retrospective Study of 53 Horses (1988 to 1991). *J. Vet. Intern. Med.* **1995**, *9*, 291–297. [CrossRef] [PubMed]
136. Fleury, C.; Berard, F.; Balme, B.; Thomas, L. The Study of Cutaneous Melanomas in Camargue-Type Gray-Skinned Horses (1): Clinical-Pathological Characterization. *Pigment Cell Res.* **2000**, *13*, 39–46. [CrossRef] [PubMed]
137. Vostry, L.; Hofmanova, B.; Vydrova, H.; Pribyl, J.; Majzlik, I. Estimation of Genetic Parameters for Melanoma in the Old Kladruber Horse. *Czech J. Anim. Sci.* **2012**, *57*, 75–82. [CrossRef]
138. Curik, I.; Druml, T.; Seltenhammer, M.; Sundstrom, E.; Pielberg, G.R.; Andersson, L.; Solkner, J. Complex Inheritance of Melanoma and Pigmentation of Coat and Skin in Grey Horses. *PLoS Genetics* **2013**, *9*, e1003248. [CrossRef]
139. Campagne, C.; Jule, S.; Bernex, F.; Estrada, M.; Aubin Houzelstein, G.; Panthier, J.J.; Egidy, G. RACK1, a Clue to the Diagnosis of Cutaneous Melanomas in Horses. *BMC Vet. Res.* **2012**, *8*, 95. [CrossRef]
140. Thirloway, L.; Rudolph, R.; Leipold, H.W. Malignant Melanomas in a Duroc Boar. *J. Am. Vet. Med. Assoc.* **1977**, *170*, 345–347.
141. Fisher, L.F.; Olander, H.J. Spontaneous Neoplasms of Pigs-A Study of 31 Cases. *J. Comp. Pathol.* **1978**, *88*, 505–517. [CrossRef]
142. Baba, A.I.; Gaboreanu, M.; Rotaru, O.; Kwieczinsky, R. Malignant Melanomas in Farm Animals. *Morphol. Embryol. (Bucur.)* **1983**, *29*, 191–194. [PubMed]
143. Perez, J.; Garcia, P.M.; Bautista, M.J.; Millan, Y.; Ordas, J.; De Las Mulas, J.M. Immunohistochemical Characterization of Tumor Cells and Inflammatory Infiltrate Associated with Cutaneous Melanocytic Tumors of Duroc and Iberian Swine. *Vet. Pathol.* **2002**, *39*, 445–451. [CrossRef] [PubMed]
144. Bundza, A.; Feltmate, T.E. Melanocytic Cutaneous Lesions and Melanotic Regional Lymph Nodes in Slaughter Swine. *Can. J. Vet. Res. Rev. Can. Rech. Vet.* **1990**, *54*, 301–304.
145. Hordinsky, M.K.; Ruth, G.; King, R. Inheritance of Melanocytic Tumors in Duroc Swine. *J. Hered.* **1985**, *76*, 385–386.
146. Strafuss, A.C.; Dommert, A.R.; Tumbleson, M.E.; Middleton, C.C. Cutaneous Melanoma in Miniature Swine. *Lab. Anim. Care* **1968**, *18*, 165–169.

147. Millikan, L.E.; Boylon, J.L.; Hook, R.R.; Manning, P.J. Melanoma in Sinclair Swine: A New Animal Model. *J. Invest. Dermatol.* **1974**, *62*, 20–30. [CrossRef]
148. Hook, R.R.; Aultman, M.D.; Adelstein, E.H.; Oxenhandler, R.W.; Millikan, L.E.; Middleton, C.C. Influence of Selective Breeding on the Incidence of Melanomas in Sinclair Miniature Swine. *Int. J. Cancer* **1979**, *24*, 668–672. [CrossRef]
149. Manning, P.J.; Millikan, L.E.; Cox, V.S.; Carey, K.D.; Hook, R.R. Congenital Cutaneous and Visceral Melanomas of Sinclair Miniature Swine: Three Case Reports. *J. Natl. Cancer Inst.* **1974**, *52*, 1559–1566. [CrossRef]
150. Oxenhandler, R.W.; Adelstein, E.H.; Haigh, J.P.; Hook, R.R.; Clark, W.H. Malignant Melanoma in the Sinclair Miniature Swine: An Autopsy Study of 60 Cases. *Am. J. Pathol.* **1979**, *96*, 707–720.
151. Hook, R.R.; Berkelhammer, J.; Oxenhandler, R.W. Melanoma: Sinclair Swine Melanoma. *Am. J. Pathol.* **1982**, *108*, 130–133. [PubMed]
152. Misfeldt, M.L.; Grimm, D.R. Sinclair Miniature Swine: An Animal Model of Human Melanoma. *Vet. Immunol. Immunopathol.* **1994**, *43*, 167–175. [CrossRef]
153. Greene, J.F.; Townsend, J.S.; Amoss, M.S. Histopathology of Regression in Sinclair Swine Model of Melanoma. *Lab. Investig. J. Tech. Methods Pathol.* **1994**, *71*, 17–24.
154. Morgan, C.D.; Measel, J.W.; Amoss, M.S.; Rao, A.; Greene, J.F. Immunophenotypic Characterization of Tumor Infiltrating Lymphocytes and Peripheral Blood Lymphocytes Isolated from Melanomatous and Non-Melanomatous Sinclair Miniature Swine. *Vet. Immunol. Immunopathol.* **1996**, *55*, 189–203. [CrossRef]
155. Cui, J.; Chen, D.; Misfeldt, M.L.; Swinfard, R.W.; Bystryn, J.C. Antimelanoma Antibodies in Swine with Spontaneously Regressing Melanoma. *Pigment Cell Res.* **1995**, *8*, 60–63. [CrossRef]
156. Gossett, R.; Kier, A.B.; Schroeder, F.; McConkey, D.; Fadok, V.; Amoss, M.S. Cycloheximide-Induced Apoptosis in Melanoma Cells Derived from Regressing Cutaneous Tumours of SINCLAIR Swine. *J. Comp. Pathol.* **1996**, *115*, 353–372. [CrossRef]
157. Pathak, S.; Multani, A.S.; McConkey, D.J.; Imam, A.S.; Amoss, M.S. Spontaneous Regression of Cutaneous Melanoma in Sinclair Swine is Associated with Defective Telomerase Activity and Extensive Telomere Erosion. *Int. J. Oncol.* **2000**, *17*, 1219–1243. [CrossRef]
158. Tissot, R.G.; Beattie, C.W.; Amoss, M.S. The Swine Leucocyte Antigen (SLA) Complex and Sinclair Swine Cutaneous Malignant Melanoma. *Anim. Genet.* **1989**, *20*, 51–57. [CrossRef]
159. Tissot, R.G.; Beattie, C.W.; Amoss, M.S. Inheritance of Sinclair Swine Cutaneous Malignant Melanoma. *Cancer Res.* **1987**, *47*, 5542–5545.
160. Blangero, J.; Tissot, R.G.; Beattie, C.W.; Amoss, M.S. Genetic Determinants of Cutaneous Malignant Melanoma in Sinclair Swine. *Br. J. Cancer* **1996**, *73*, 667–671. [CrossRef]
161. Pathak, S.; Amoss, M.S. Genetic Predisposition and Specific Chromosomal Defects Associated with Sinclair Swine Malignant Melanomas. *Int. J. Oncol.* **1997**, *11*, 53–57. [CrossRef] [PubMed]
162. Muller, S.; Wanke, R.; Distl, O. Inheritance of Melanocytic Lesions and Their Association with the White Colour Phenotype in Miniature Swine. *J. Anim. Breed. Genet.* **2001**, *118*, 275–283. [CrossRef]
163. Muller, S.; Wanke, R.; Distl, O. Segregation of Pigment Cell Anomalies in Munich Miniature Swine (MMS) Troll Crossed with German Landrace. *DTW Dtsch. Tierarztl. Wochenschr.* **1995**, *102*, 391–394. [PubMed]
164. Buttner, M.; Wanke, R.; Obermann, B. Natural Killer (NK) Activity of Porcine Blood Lymphocytes Against Allogeneic Melanoma Target Cells. *Vet. Immunol. Immunopathol.* **1991**, *29*, 89–103. [CrossRef]
165. Dieckhoff, B.; Puhlmann, J.; Buscher, K.; Hafner Marx, A.; Herbach, N.; Bannert, N.; Buttner, M.; Wanke, R.; Kurth, R.; Denner, J. Expression of Porcine Endogenous Retroviruses (PERVs) in Melanomas of Munich Miniature Swine (MMS) Troll. *Vet. Microbiol.* **2007**, *123*, 53–68. [CrossRef]
166. Buscher, K.; Trefzer, U.; Hofmann, M.; Sterry, W.; Kurth, R.; Denner, J. Expression of Human Endogenous Retrovirus K in Melanomas and Melanoma Cell Lines. *Cancer Res.* **2005**, *65*, 4172–4180. [CrossRef]
167. Gonzalez Cao, M.; Iduma, P.; Karachaliou, N.; Santarpia, M.; Blanco, J.; Rosell, R. Human Endogenous Retroviruses and Cancer. *Cancer Biol. Med.* **2016**, *13*, 483–488.
168. Glodek, P. Breeding Program and Population Standards of the Goettingen Miniature Swine. In *Swine in Biomedical Research*; Tumbleson, M.E., Ed.; Plenum Press: New York, NY, USA, 1986; Volume 1, pp. 23–28.
169. Horak, V.; Fortyn, K.; Hruban, V.; Klaudy, J. Hereditary Melanoblastoma in Miniature Pigs and its Successful Therapy by Devitalization Technique. *Cell. Mol. Biol. Noisy Gd. Fr.* **1999**, *45*, 1119–1129.
170. Hruban, V.; Horak, V.; Fortyn, K.; Hradecky, J.; Klaudy, J.; Smith, D.M.; Reisnerova, H.; Majzlik, I. Inheritance of Malignant Melanoma in the MeLiM Strain of Miniature Pigs. *Vet. Med. (Praha)* **2004**, *49*, 453–459. [CrossRef]

171. Vincent Naulleau, S.; Le Chalony, C.; Leplat, J.J.; Bouet, S.; Bailly, C.; Spatz, A.; Vielh, P.; Avril, M.F.; Tricaud, Y.; Gruand, J.; et al. Clinical and Histopathological Characterization of Cutaneous Melanomas in the Melanoblastoma-Bearing Libechov Minipig Model. *Pigment Cell Melanoma Res.* **2004**, *17*, 24–35. [CrossRef]
172. Fortyn, K.; Hruban, V.; Horak, V. Treatment of Malignant Melanoma. *Br. J. Surg.* **1994**, *81*, 146–147. [CrossRef] [PubMed]
173. Fortyn, K.; Hruban, V.; Horak, V.; Tichy, J. Exceptional Occurrence and Extent of Malignant Melanoma in Pig. *Vet. Med. (Praha)* **1998**, *43*, 87–91.
174. Fortyn, K.; Hruban, V.; Horak, V.; Hradecky, J.; Tichy, J. Melanoblastoma in Laboratory Minipigs: A Model for Studying Human Malignant Melan6oma. *Vet. Med. (Praha)* **1994**, *39*, 597–604.
175. Al Shaer, M.; Gollapudi, D.; Papageorgio, C. Melanoma Biomarkers: Vox Clamantis in Deserto (Review). *Oncol. Lett.* **2010**, *1*, 399–405. [CrossRef] [PubMed]
176. Pohlreich, P.; Stribrna, J.; Kleibl, Z.; Horak, V.; Klaudy, J. Detection of Neoplastic Cells in Blood of Miniature Pigs with Hereditary Melanoma. *Vet. Med. (Praha)* **2001**, *46*, 199–204. [CrossRef]
177. De Souza, L.M.; Robertson, B.M.; Robertson, G.P. Future of Circulating Tumor Cells in the Melanoma Clinical and Research Laboratory Settings. *Cancer Lett.* **2017**, *392*, 60–70. [CrossRef]
178. Rodic, S.; Mihalcioiu, C.; Saleh, R.R. Detection Methods of Circulating Tumor Cells in Cutaneous Melanoma: A Systematic Review. *Crit. Rev. Oncol. Hematol.* **2014**, *91*, 74–92. [CrossRef]
179. Borovansky, J.; Horak, V.; Elleder, M.; Fortyn, K.; Smit, N.P.; Kolb, A.M. Biochemical Characterization of a New Melanoma Model-The Minipig MeLiM Strain. *Melanoma Res.* **2003**, *13*, 543–548. [CrossRef]
180. Millikan, L.E.; Hook, R.R.; Manning, P.J. Immunobiology of Melanoma. Gross and Ultrastructural Studies in a New Melanoma Model: The Sinclair Swine. *Yale J. Biol. Med.* **1973**, *46*, 631–645.
181. Hunter, J.A.; Zaynoun, S.; Paterson, W.D.; Bleehen, S.S.; Mackie, R.; Cochran, A.J. Cellular Fine Structure in the Invasive Nodules of Different Histogenetic Types of Malignant Melanoma. *Br. J. Dermatol.* **1978**, *98*, 255–272. [CrossRef]
182. Borovansky, J. Quantitative Parameters of Melanomas Differentiation. *Neoplasma* **1978**, *25*, 349–352. [PubMed]
183. Ochi, Y.; Atsumi, S.; Aoyagi, T.; Umezawa, K. Inhibition of Tumor Cell Invasion in the Boyden Chamber Assay by a Mannosidase Inhibitor, Mannostatin A. *Anticancer Res.* **1993**, *13*, 1421–1424. [PubMed]
184. Borovansky, J.; Hach, P. Disparate behaviour of Two Melanosomal Enzymes (α-Mannosidase and γ-Glutamyltransferase). *Cell. Mol. Biol. Noisy Gd. Fr.* **1999**, *45*, 1047–1052.
185. Egidy, G.; Jule, S.; Bosse, P.; Bernex, F.; Geffrotin, C.; Vincent Naulleau, S.; Horak, V.; Sastre Garau, X.; Panthier, J.J. Transcription Analysis in the MeLiM Swine Model Identifies RACK1 as a Potential Marker of Malignancy for Human Melanocytic Proliferation. *Mol. Cancer* **2008**, *7*, 34. [CrossRef]
186. Xia, J.; Wang, Y.; Li, F.; Wang, J.; Mu, Y.; Mei, X.; Li, X.; Zhu, W.; Jin, X.; Yu, K. Expression of Microphthalmia Transcription Factor, S100 Protein, and HMB-45 in Malignant Melanoma and Pigmented Nevi. *Biomed. Rep.* **2016**, *5*, 327–331. [CrossRef]
187. Planska, D.; Burocziova, M.; Strnadel, J.; Horak, V. Immunohistochemical Analysis of Collagen IV and Laminin Expression in Spontaneous Melanoma Regression in the Melanoma-Bearing Libechov Minipig. *Acta Histochem. Cytochem.* **2015**, *48*, 15–26. [CrossRef]
188. Geffrotin, C.; Horak, V.; Crechet, F.; Tricaud, Y.; Lethias, C.; Vincent Naulleau, S.; Vielh, P. Opposite Regulation of Tenascin-C and Tenascin-X in MeLiM Swine Heritable Cutaneous Malignant Melanoma. *Biochim. Biophys. Acta BBA Gen. Subj.* **2000**, *1524*, 196–202. [CrossRef]
189. Planska, D.; Kovalska, J.; Cizkova, J.; Horak, V. Tissue Rebuilding During Spontaneous Regression of Melanoma in the Melanoma-bearing Libechov Minipig. *Anticancer Res.* **2018**, *38*, 4629–4636. [CrossRef]
190. Engbring, J.A.; Kleinman, H.K. The Basement Membrane Matrix in Malignancy. *J. Pathol.* **2003**, *200*, 465–470. [CrossRef]
191. Pasco, S.; Ramont, L.; Maquart, F.X.; Monboisse, J.C. Control of Melanoma Progression by Various Matrikines from Basement Membrane Macromolecules. *Crit. Rev. Oncol. Hematol.* **2004**, *49*, 221–233. [CrossRef]
192. Hofmann, U.B.; Houben, R.; Brocker, E.B.; Becker, J.C. Role of Matrix Metalloproteinases in Melanoma Cell Invasion. *Biochimie* **2005**, *87*, 307–314. [CrossRef] [PubMed]
193. Kaariainen, E.; Nummela, P.; Soikkeli, J.; Yin, M.; Lukk, M.; Jahkola, T.; Virolainen, S.; Ora, A.; Ukkonen, E.; Saksela, O.; et al. Switch to an Invasive Growth Phase in Melanoma is Associated with Tenascin-C, Fibronectin, and Procollagen-I Forming Specific Channel Structures for Invasion. *J. Pathol.* **2006**, *210*, 181–191. [CrossRef]

194. Shao, H.; Kirkwood, J.M.; Wells, A. Tenascin-C Signaling in Melanoma. *Cell Adhes. Migr.* **2014**, *9*, 125–130. [CrossRef]
195. Anyz, J.; Vyslouzilova, L.; Vaculovic, T.; Tvrdonova, M.; Kanicky, V.; Haase, H.; Horak, V.; Stepankova, O.; Heger, Z.; Adam, V. Spatial Mapping of Metals in Tissue-Sections Using Combination of Mass-Spectrometry and Histology Through Image Registration. *Sci. Rep.* **2017**, *7*, 40169. [CrossRef] [PubMed]
196. Gorodetsky, R.; Sheskin, J.; Weinreb, A. Iron, Copper, and Zinc Concentrations in Normal Skin and in Various Nonmalignant and Malignant Lesions. *Int. J. Dermatol.* **1986**, *25*, 440–445. [CrossRef]
197. Guran, R.; Vanickova, L.; Horak, V.; Krizkova, S.; Michalek, P.; Heger, Z.; Zitka, O.; Adam, V. MALDI MSI of MeLiM Melanoma: Searching for Differences in Protein Profiles. *PLoS ONE* **2017**, *12*, e0189305. [CrossRef]
198. Krizkova, S.; Fabrik, I.; Adam, V.; Kukacka, J.; Prusa, R.; Chavis, G.J.; Trnkova, L.; Strnadel, J.; Horak, V.; Kizek, R. Utilizing of Adsorptive Transfer Stripping Technique Brdicka Reaction for Determination of Metallothioneins Level in Melanoma Cells, Blood Serum and Tissues. *Sensors* **2008**, *8*, 3106–3122. [CrossRef]
199. Weinlich, G. Metallothionein-Overexpression as a Prognostic Marker in Melanoma. *G. Ital. Dermatol. E Venereol. Organo Uff. Soc. Ital. Dermatol. E Sifilogr.* **2009**, *144*, 27–38.
200. Cizkova, J.; Erbanova, M.; Sochor, J.; Jindrova, A.; Strnadova, K.; Horak, V. Relationship Between Haematological Profile and Progression or Spontaneous Regression of Melanoma in the Melanoma-Bearing Libechov Minipigs. *Vet. J. Lond. Engl. 1997* **2019**, *249*, 1–9.
201. Blanc, F.; Crechet, F.; Bruneau, N.; Piton, G.; Leplat, J.J.; Andreoletti, F.; Egidy, G.; Vincent Naulleau, S.; Bourneuf, E. Impact of a CD4 Gene Haplotype on the Immune Response in Minipigs. *Immunogenetics* **2018**, *70*, 209–222. [CrossRef]
202. Du, Z.Q.; Vincent Naulleau, S.; Gilbert, H.; Vignoles, F.; Crechet, F.; Shimogiri, T.; Yasue, H.; Leplat, J.J.; Bouet, S.; Gruand, J.; et al. Detection of Novel Quantitative Trait Loci for Cutaneous Melanoma by Genome-Wide Scan in the MeLiM Swine Model. *Int. J. Cancer* **2007**, *120*, 303–320. [PubMed]
203. Le Chalony, C.; Renard, C.; Vincent Naulleau, S.; Crechet, F.; Leplat, J.J.; Tricaud, Y.; Horak, V.; Gruand, J.; Le Roy, P.; Frelat, G.; et al. CDKN2A Region Polymorphism and Genetic Susceptibility to Melanoma in the Melim Swine Model of Familial Melanoma. *Int. J. Cancer* **2003**, *103*, 631–635. [CrossRef] [PubMed]
204. Geffrotin, C.; Crechet, F.; Le Roy, P.; Le Chalony, C.; Leplat, J.J.; Iannuccelli, N.; Barbosa, A.; Renard, C.; Gruand, J.; Milan, D.; et al. Identification of Five Chromosomal Regions Involved in Predisposition to Melanoma by Genome-Wide Scan in the MeLiM Swine Model. *Int. J. Cancer* **2004**, *110*, 39–50. [CrossRef] [PubMed]
205. Bourneuf, E.; Du, Z.Q.; Estelle, J.; Gilbert, H.; Crechet, F.; Piton, G.; Milan, D.; Geffrotin, C.; Lathrop, M.; Demenais, F.; et al. Genetic and Functional Evaluation of MITF as a Candidate Gene for Cutaneous Melanoma Predisposition in Pigs. *Mamm. Genome Off. J. Int. Mamm. Genome Soc.* **2011**, *22*, 602–612. [CrossRef]
206. Fernandez Rodriguez, A.; Estelle, J.; Blin, A.; Munoz, M.; Crechet, F.; Demenais, F.; Vincent Naulleau, S.; Bourneuf, E. KIT and Melanoma Predisposition in Pigs: Sequence Variants and Association Analysis. *Anim. Genet.* **2014**, *45*, 445–448. [CrossRef]
207. Rambow, F.; Piton, G.; Bouet, S.; Leplat, J.J.; Baulande, S.; Marrau, A.; Stam, M.; Horak, V.; Vincent Naulleau, S. Gene Expression Signature for Spontaneous Cancer Regression in Melanoma Pigs. *Neoplasia* **2008**, *10*, 714. [CrossRef]
208. Rambow, F.; Malek, O.; Geffrotin, C.; Leplat, J.J.; Bouet, S.; Piton, G.; Hugot, K.; Bevilacqua, C.; Horak, V.; Vincent Naulleau, S. Identification of Differentially Expressed Genes in Spontaneously Regressing Melanoma Using the MeLiM Swine Model. *Pigment Cell Melanoma Res.* **2008**, *21*, 147–161. [CrossRef]
209. Bourneuf, E.; Estelle, J.; Blin, A.; Crechet, F.; del Pilar Schneider, M.; Gilbert, H.; Brossard, M.; Vaysse, A.; Lathrop, M.; Vincent Naulleau, S.; et al. New Susceptibility Loci for Cutaneous Melanoma Risk and Progression Revealed Using a Porcine Model. *Oncotarget* **2018**, *9*, 27682–27697. [CrossRef]
210. Sun, X.; Gao, L.; Chien, H.Y.; Li, W.C.; Zhao, J. The Regulation and Function of the NUAK Family. *J. Mol. Endocrinol.* **2013**, *51*, R15–R22. [CrossRef]
211. Xu, X.; Hussain, W.M.; Vijai, J.; Offit, K.; Rubin, M.A.; Demichelis, F.; Klein, R.J. Variants at IRX4 as Prostate Cancer Expression Quantitative Trait Loci. *Eur. J. Hum. Genet. EJHG* **2014**, *22*, 558–563. [CrossRef]
212. Sanchez Tena, S.; Cubillos Rojas, M.; Schneider, T.; Rosa, J.L. Functional and Pathological Relevance of HERC Family Proteins: A Decade Later. *Cell. Mol. Life Sci.* **2016**, *73*, 1955–1968. [CrossRef] [PubMed]

213. Fattore, L.; Costantini, S.; Malpicci, D.; Ruggiero, C.F.; Ascierto, P.A.; Croce, C.M.; Mancini, R.; Ciliberto, G. MicroRNAs in Melanoma Development and Resistance to Target Therapy. *Oncotarget* **2017**, *8*. [CrossRef] [PubMed]
214. Baco, M.; Chu, C.Y.; Bouet, S.; Rogel Gaillard, C.; Bourneuf, E.; Le Provost, F.; Chu, C.Y.; Vincent Naulleau, S. Analysis of Melanoma-Related microRNAs Expression During the Spontaneous Regression of Cutaneous Melanomas in MeLiM Pigs. *Pigment Cell Melanoma Res.* **2014**, *27*, 668–670. [CrossRef] [PubMed]
215. So, K.A.; Hong, J.H.; Jin, H.M.; Kim, J.W.; Song, J.Y.; Lee, J.K.; Lee, N.W. The Prognostic Significance of Preoperative Leukocytosis in Epithelial Ovarian Carcinoma: A Retrospective Cohort Study. *Gynecol. Oncol.* **2014**, *132*, 551–555. [CrossRef] [PubMed]
216. Azab, B.; Mohammad, F.; Shah, N.; Vonfrolio, S.; Lu, W.; Kedia, S.; Bloom, S.W. The Value of the Pretreatment Neutrophil Lymphocyte Ratio vs. Platelet Lymphocyte Ratio in Predicting the Long-Term Survival in Colorectal Cancer. *Cancer Biomark. Sect. Dis. Markers* **2014**, *14*, 303–312. [CrossRef]
217. Zhang, H.; Xia, H.; Zhang, L.; Zhang, B.; Yue, D.; Wang, C. Clinical Significance of Preoperative Neutrophil-Lymphocyte vs Platelet-Lymphocyte Ratio in Primary Operable Patients with Non-Small Cell Lung Cancer. *Am. J. Surg.* **2015**, *210*, 526–535. [CrossRef]
218. Feng, L.; Gu, S.; Wang, P.; Chen, H.; Chen, Z.; Meng, Z.; Liu, L. White Blood Cell and Granulocyte Counts Are Independent Predictive Factors for Prognosis of Advanced Pancreatic Caner. *Gastroenterol. Res. Pract.* **2018**, *2018*, 8096234. [CrossRef]
219. Cananzi, F.C.M.; Dalgleish, A.; Mudan, S. Surgical Management of Intraabdominal Metastases from Melanoma: Role of the Neutrophil to Lymphocyte Ratio as a Potential Prognostic Factor. *World J. Surg.* **2014**, *38*, 1542–1550. [CrossRef]
220. Cassidy, M.R.; Wolchok, R.E.; Zheng, J.; Panageas, K.S.; Wolchok, J.D.; Coit, D.; Postow, M.A.; Ariyan, C. Neutrophil to Lymphocyte Ratio is Associated With Outcome During Ipilimumab Treatment. *EBioMedicine* **2017**, *18*, 56–61. [CrossRef]
221. Davis, J.L.; Ripley, R.T.; Frankel, T.L.; Maric, I.; Lozier, J.N.; Rosenberg, S.A. Paraneoplastic Granulocytosis in Metastatic Melanoma. *Melanoma Res.* **2010**, *20*, 326–329. [CrossRef]
222. Ferrucci, P.F.; Gandini, S.; Battaglia, A.; Alfieri, S.; Di Giacomo, A.M.; Giannarelli, D.; Cappellini, G.C.A.; De Galitiis, F.; Marchetti, P.; Amato, G.; et al. Baseline Neutrophil-To-Lymphocyte Ratio is Associated with Outcome of Ipilimumab-Treated Metastatic Melanoma Patients. *Br. J. Cancer* **2015**, *112*, 1904–1910. [CrossRef] [PubMed]
223. Wade, R.G.; Robinson, A.V.; Lo, M.C.I.; Keeble, C.; Marples, M.; Dewar, D.J.; Moncrieff, M.D.S.; Peach, H. Baseline Neutrophil-Lymphocyte and Platelet-Lymphocyte Ratios as Biomarkers of Survival in Cutaneous Melanoma: A Multicenter Cohort Study. *Ann. Surg. Oncol.* **2018**, *25*, 3341–3349. [CrossRef] [PubMed]
224. Rachidi, S.; Kaur, M.; Lautenschlaeger, T.; Li, Z. Platelet Count Correlates with Stage and Predicts Survival in Melanoma. *Platelets* **2019**, 1–5. [CrossRef] [PubMed]
225. Tas, F.; Erturk, K. Anemia in Cutaneous Malignant Melanoma: Low Blood Hemoglobin Level is Associated with Nodal Involvement, Metastatic Disease, and Worse Survival. *Nutr. Cancer* **2018**, *70*, 236–240. [CrossRef]
226. Busti, F.; Marchi, G.; Ugolini, S.; Castagna, A.; Girelli, D. Anemia and Iron Deficiency in Cancer Patients: Role of Iron Replacement Therapy. *Pharm. Basel Switz.* **2018**, *11*. [CrossRef]
227. Weinstein, D.A. Inappropriate Expression of Hepcidin is Associated with Iron Refractory Anemia: Implications for the Anemia of Chronic Disease. *Blood* **2002**, *100*, 3776–3781. [CrossRef]
228. Porto, G. Iron Overload and Immunity. *World J. Gastroenterol.* **2007**, *13*, 4707. [CrossRef]
229. Vyoral, D.; Petrak, J. Hepcidin: A Direct Link Between Iron Metabolism and Immunity. *Int. J. Biochem. Cell Biol.* **2005**, *37*, 1768–1773. [CrossRef]
230. Gonzalez, H.; Hagerling, C.; Werb, Z. Roles of the Immune System in Cancer: From Tumor Initiation to Metastatic Progression. *Genes Dev.* **2018**, *32*, 1267–1284. [CrossRef]
231. Antohe, M.; Nedelcu, R.I.; Nichita, L.; Popp, C.G.; Cioplea, M.; Brinzea, A.; Hodorogea, A.; Calinescu, A.; Balaban, M.; Ion, D.A.; et al. Tumor Infiltrating Lymphocytes: The Regulator of Melanoma Evolution. *Oncol. Lett.* **2019**, *17*, 4155–4161. [CrossRef]
232. Clemente, C.G.; Mihm, M.C.; Bufalino, R.; Zurrida, S.; Collini, P.; Cascinelli, N. Prognostic Value of Tumor Infiltrating Lymphocytes in the Vertical Growth Phase of Primary Cutaneous Melanoma. *Cancer* **1996**, *77*, 1303–1310. [CrossRef]

233. Van Houdt, I.S.; Sluijter, B.J.R.; Moesbergen, L.M.; Vos, W.M.; De Gruijl, T.D.; Molenkamp, B.G.; Van Den Eertwegh, A.J.M.; Hooijberg, E.; Van Leeuwen, P.A.M.; Meijer, C.J.L.M.; et al. Favorable Outcome in Clinically Stage II Melanoma Patients is Associated with the Presence of Activated Tumor Infiltrating T-Lymphocytes and Preserved MHC Class I Antigen Expression. *Int. J. Cancer* **2008**, *123*, 609–615. [CrossRef] [PubMed]
234. Rohaan, M.W.; Van Den Berg, J.H.; Kvistborg, P.; Haanen, J.B.A.G. Adoptive Transfer of Tumor-Infiltrating lymphocytes in Melanoma: A Viable Treatment Option. *J. Immunother. Cancer* **2018**, *6*, 102. [CrossRef] [PubMed]
235. Cizkova, J.; Sinkorova, Z.; Strnadova, K.; Cervinkova, M.; Horak, V.; Sinkora, J.; Stepanova, K.; Sinkora, M. The Role of αβ T-Cells in Spontaneous Regression of Melanoma Tumors in Swine. *Dev. Comp. Immunol.* **2019**, *92*, 60–68. [CrossRef]
236. Overgaard, N.H.; Jung, J.W.; Steptoe, R.J.; Wells, J.W. CD4+/CD8+ Double-Positive T Cells: More Than Just a Developmental Stage? *J. Leukoc. Biol.* **2015**, *97*, 31–38. [CrossRef]
237. Pomorska Mol, M.; Markowska Daniel, I. AGE-Dependent Changes in Relative and Absolute Size of Lymphocyte Subsets in the Blood of Pigs from Birth to Slaughter. *Bull. Vet. Inst. Pulawy* **2011**, *55*, 305–310.
238. Bagot, M.; Echchakir, H.; Mami Chouaib, F.; Delfau Larue, M.H.; Charue, D.; Bernheim, A.; Chouaib, S.; Boumsell, L.; Bensussan, A. Isolation of Tumor-Specific Cytotoxic CD4+ and CD4+CD8dim+ T-Cell Clones Infiltrating a Cutaneous T-Cell Lymphoma. *Blood* **1998**, *91*, 4331–4341. [CrossRef]
239. De Marchi, S.U.; Stinco, G.; Errichetti, E.; Bonin, S.; Di Meo, N.; Trevisan, G. The Influence of the Coexpression of CD4 and CD8 in Cutaneous Lesions on Prognosis of Mycosis Fungoides: A Preliminary Study. *J. Skin Cancer* **2014**, *2014*, 624143. [CrossRef]
240. Desfrançois, J.; Moreau Aubry, A.; Vignard, V.; Godet, Y.; Khammari, A.; Dreno, B.; Jotereau, F.; Gervois, N. Double Positive CD4CD8 Alphabeta T Cells: A New Tumor-Reactive Population in Human Melanomas. *PLoS ONE* **2010**, *5*, e8437. [CrossRef]
241. Roy, S.; Trinchieri, G. Microbiota: A Key Orchestrator of Cancer Therapy. *Nat. Rev. Cancer* **2017**, *17*, 271–285. [CrossRef]
242. McQuade, J.L.; Daniel, C.R.; Helmink, B.A.; Wargo, J.A. Modulating the Microbiome to Improve Therapeutic Response in Cancer. *Lancet Oncol.* **2019**, *20*, e77–e91. [CrossRef]
243. Warner, A.B.; McQuade, J.L. Modifiable Host Factors in Melanoma: Emerging Evidence for Obesity, Diet, Exercise, and the Microbiome. *Curr. Oncol. Rep.* **2019**, *21*, 72. [CrossRef] [PubMed]
244. Gopalakrishnan, V.; Spencer, C.N.; Nezi, L.; Reuben, A.; Andrews, M.C.; Karpinets, T.V.; Prieto, P.A.; Vicente, D.; Hoffman, K.; Wei, S.C.; et al. Gut Microbiome Modulates Response to Anti-PD-1 Immunotherapy in Melanoma Patients. *Science* **2018**, *359*, 97–103. [CrossRef] [PubMed]
245. Salava, A.; Aho, V.; Pereira, P.; Koskinen, K.; Paulin, L.; Auvinen, P.; Lauerma, A. Skin Microbiome in Melanomas and Melanocytic Nevi. *Eur. J. Dermatol. EJD* **2016**, *26*, 49–55. [CrossRef] [PubMed]
246. Svejstil, R.; Salmonova, H.; Cizkova, J. Analysis of Cutaneous Microbiota of Piglets with Hereditary Melanoma. *Sci. Agric. Bohem.* **2018**, *49*, 285–290. [CrossRef]
247. Mrazek, J.; Mekadim, C.; Kucerova, P.; Svejstil, R.; Salmonova, H.; Vlasakova, J.; Tarasova, R.; Cizkova, J.; Cervinkova, M. Melanoma-Related Changes in Skin Microbiome. *Folia Microbiol. (Praha)* **2019**, *64*, 435–442. [CrossRef]
248. Zhou, Z.; Chen, J.; Yao, H.; Hu, H. Fusobacterium and Colorectal Cancer. *Front. Oncol.* **2018**, *8*, 371. [CrossRef]
249. Brennan, C.A.; Garrett, W.S. Fusobacterium Nucleatum-Symbiont, Opportunist and Oncobacterium. *Nat. Rev. Microbiol.* **2019**, *17*, 156–166. [CrossRef]
250. Yu, L.C.H.; Wei, S.C.; Ni, Y.H. Impact of Microbiota in Colorectal Carcinogenesis: Lessons from Experimental Models. *Intest. Res.* **2018**, *16*, 346–357. [CrossRef]
251. Fortyn, K.; Hradecky, J.; Pazdera, J.; Klaudy, J.; Hruban, V.; Dvorak, P.; Matousek, J.; Tichy, J.; Kolin, V. Experimental Elimination of Various Intestinal Segments by Means of Devascularization (Devitalization). *Z. Exp. Chir. Transplant. Kunstl. Organe Organ Sekt. Exp. Chir. Ges. Chir. DDR* **1985**, *18*, 34–41.
252. Fortyn, K.; Hradecky, J.; Pazdera, J.; Klaudy, J.; Hruban, V.; Dvorak, P.; Matousek, J.; Tichy, J.; Kolin, V. Small and Large Intestine Devascularization (Devitalization) and Potentials in the Therapeutic Use of this Operative Method. *Z. Exp. Chir. Transplant. Kunstl. Organe Organ Sekt. Exp. Chir. Ges. Chir. DDR* **1985**, *18*, 42–50.
253. Vasek, P.; Krajnik, J.; Kopsky, D.J.; Kalina, V.; Frydrych, M. Autologous Tumor Immunizing Devascularization of an Invasive Colorectal Cancer: A Case Report and Literature Review. *Mol. Clin. Oncol.* **2016**, *5*, 521–526. [CrossRef] [PubMed]

254. Fortyn, K.; Hradecky, J.; Hruban, V.; Horak, V.; Dvorak, P.; Tichy, J. Morphology of Regressive Changes in the Kidney Following Experimental Ischaemia. *Int. Urol. Nephrol.* **1987**, *19*, 9–19. [CrossRef] [PubMed]
255. Fortyn, K.; Hruban, V.; Hradecky, J.; Tichy, J.; Dvorak, P.; Horak, V. A Technique of the Segmental Devitalization of Kidneys in Experiment. *Z. Exp. Chir. Transplant. Kunstl. Organe Organ Sekt. Exp. Chir. Ges. Chir. DDR* **1988**, *21*, 275–280.
256. Fortyn, K.; Hruban, V.; Hradecky, J.; Tichy, J.; Dvorak, P.; Horak, V. The Devitalization of the Stomach by a Devascularization Technique. *Acta Chir. Hung.* **1988**, *29*, 163–172.
257. Fortyn, K.; Hruban, V.; Hradecky, J.; Tichy, J.; Dvorak, P.; Horak, V. Experimental Devascularization (Devitalization) of the Rectum and Sigmoideum. *Z. Exp. Chir. Transplant. Kunstl. Organe Organ Sekt. Exp. Chir. Ges. Chir. DDR* **1989**, *22*, 173–179.
258. Horak, V.; Moravkova, A.; Strnadel, J.; Hradecky, J.; Usvald, D.; Vannucci, L. Devitalization as a Special Surgical Tumour Treatment Inducing Anti-Cancer Response–An Experimental Study in Two Animal Models. In Proceedings of the CIMT Cancer Immunotherapy 6th Annual Meeting, Mainz, Germany, 15–16 May 2008.
259. Srivastava, P.K.; Udono, H.; Blachere, N.E.; Li, Z. Heat Shock Proteins Transfer Peptides During Antigen Processing and CTL Priming. *Immunogenetics* **1994**, *39*, 93–98. [CrossRef]
260. Binder, R.J.; Blachere, N.E.; Srivastava, P.K. Heat Shock Protein-Chaperoned Peptides but not Free Peptides Introduced into the Cytosol are Presented Efficiently by Major Histocompatibility Complex I Molecules. *J. Biol. Chem.* **2001**, *276*, 17163–17171. [CrossRef]
261. Singh Jasuja, H.; Hilf, N.; Arnold Schild, D.; Schild, H. The Role of Heat Shock Proteins and Their Receptors in the Activation of the Immune System. *Biol. Chem.* **2001**, *382*, 629–636. [CrossRef]
262. Hoos, A.; Levey, D.L. Vaccination with Heat Shock Protein-Peptide Complexes: From Basic Science to Clinical Applications. *Expert Rev. Vaccines* **2003**, *2*, 369–379. [CrossRef]
263. Testori, A.; Richards, J.; Whitman, E.; Mann, G.B.; Lutzky, J.; Camacho, L.; Parmiani, G.; Tosti, G.; Kirkwood, J.M.; Hoos, A.; et al. Phase III Comparison of Vitespen, an Autologous Tumor-Derived Heat Shock Protein gp96 Peptide Complex Vaccine, with Physician's Choice of Treatment for Stage IV Melanoma: The C-100-21 Study Group. *J. Clin. Oncol. Off. J. Am. Soc. Clin. Oncol.* **2008**, *26*, 955–962. [CrossRef] [PubMed]
264. Tosti, G.; Di Pietro, A.; Ferrucci, P.F.; Testori, A. HSPPC-96 Vaccine in Metastatic Melanoma Patients: From the State of the Art to a Possible Future. *Expert Rev. Vaccines* **2009**, *8*, 1513–1526. [CrossRef] [PubMed]
265. Di Pietro, A.; Tosti, G.; Ferrucci, P.F.; Testori, A. The Immunological era in Melanoma Treatment: New Challenges for Heat Shock Protein-Based Vaccine in the Advanced Disease. *Expert Opin. Biol. Ther.* **2011**, *11*, 1395–1407. [CrossRef] [PubMed]
266. Shevtsov, M.; Multhoff, G. Heat Shock Protein-Peptide and HSP-Based Immunotherapies for the Treatment of Cancer. *Front. Immunol.* **2016**, *7*, 171. [CrossRef] [PubMed]
267. Prather, R.S.; Shen, M.; Dai, Y. Genetically Modified Pigs for Medicine and Agriculture. *Biotechnol. Genet. Eng. Rev.* **2008**, *25*, 245–265.
268. Flisikowska, T.; Kind, A.; Schnieke, A. Genetically Modified Pigs to Model Human Diseases. *J. Appl. Genet.* **2014**, *55*, 53–64. [CrossRef]
269. Watson, A.L.; Carlson, D.F.; Largaespada, D.A.; Hackett, P.B.; Fahrenkrug, S.C. Engineered Swine Models of Cancer. *Front. Genet.* **2016**, *7*, 78. [CrossRef]
270. Schachtschneider, K.M.; Schwind, R.M.; Newson, J.; Kinachtchouk, N.; Rizko, M.; Mendoza Elias, N.; Grippo, P.; Principe, D.R.; Park, A.; Overgaard, N.H.; et al. The Oncopig Cancer Model: An Innovative Large Animal Translational Oncology Platform. *Front. Oncol.* **2017**, *7*, 190. [CrossRef]
271. Vodicka, P.; Smetana, K.; Dvorankova, B.; Emerick, T.; Xu, Y.Z.; Ourednik, J.; Ourednik, V.; Motlik, J. The Miniature Pig as an Animal Model in Biomedical Research. *Ann. N. Y. Acad. Sci.* **2005**, *1049*, 161–171. [CrossRef]

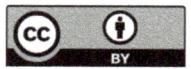

© 2019 by the authors. Licensee MDPI, Basel, Switzerland. This article is an open access article distributed under the terms and conditions of the Creative Commons Attribution (CC BY) license (http://creativecommons.org/licenses/by/4.0/).

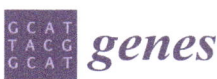

Review

Cdx2 Animal Models Reveal Developmental Origins of Cancers

Kallayanee Chawengsaksophak

Laboratory of Cell Differentiation, Institute of Molecular Genetics of the Czech Academy of Sciences, v.v.i. Vídeňská 1083, 4 14220 Prague, Czech Republic; kchaweng@img.cas.cz

Received: 11 October 2019; Accepted: 13 November 2019; Published: 14 November 2019

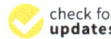

Abstract: The *Cdx2* homeobox gene is important in assigning positional identity during the finely orchestrated process of embryogenesis. In adults, regenerative responses to tissues damage can require a replay of these same developmental pathways. Errors in reassigning positional identity during regeneration can cause metaplasias—normal tissue arising in an abnormal location—and this in turn, is a well-recognized cancer risk factor. In animal models, a gain of *Cdx2* function can elicit a posterior shift in tissue identity, modeling intestinal-type metaplasias of the esophagus (Barrett's esophagus) and stomach. Conversely, loss of *Cdx2* function can elicit an anterior shift in tissue identity, inducing serrated-type lesions expressing gastric markers in the colon. These metaplasias are major risk factors for the later development of esophageal, stomach and colon cancer. Leukemia, another cancer in which *Cdx2* is ectopically expressed, may have mechanistic parallels with epithelial cancers in terms of stress-induced reprogramming. This review will address how animal models have refined our understanding of the role of *Cdx2* in these common human cancers.

Keywords: metaplasia; Cdx; cancer; animal models

---

1. Introduction

During the development of the embryo, the specification of cellular and tissue identity is dictated according to location. This is achieved through a combination of inductive cues and cell-intrinsic genetic factors. Our current understanding of the fundamental molecular mechanisms that underly these processes, referred to as pattern formation, was initially spurred by the study of the fruit fly, *Drosophila melanogaster*, over a century ago [1]. In 1894 William Bateson reported a peculiar mutation in *D. melanogaster*, in which a leg developed in the place of antennae. This he termed "homeosis", developmental anomalies which cause one body part to develop in the likeness of another. Genetic mutations which cause homeosis are called homeotic mutations.

Many homeotic mutations have been identified in *D. melanogaster*. These include the bithorax mutation, where an extra pair of wings are present instead of a pair of halteres, and the aforementioned *Antennapaedia* mutation, where legs developed in the place of antennae. The gene responsible for the *Antennapaedia* mutation would be identified almost 90 years later [2] and others soon followed. Comparative sequence analyses indicated that several homeotic genes, including the *Antennapaedia* gene, contained a conserved 180 nucleotide sequence—the homeobox [3–5]. Although many genes important for pattern formation were found to contain a homeobox sequence, homeotic transformations in *D. melanogaster* were only associated with those genes mapping to a single genetic locus, termed the *HOM-C* locus [6–8].

In human, the *HOM-C* homologues are termed the *HOX* clusters. Duplication events during mammalian evolution have produced four separate *HOX* clusters: *HOXA, HOXB, HOXC* and *HOXD* [9]. The expression of genes within both the *HOX* and *HOM-C* clusters are spatio-temporally regulated;

those located at the 3′-end are expressed earlier and in more anterior regions, while those located at the 5′-end are expressed later and in more posterior regions [10–13].

Mutations in *HOX* genes do not cause the dramatic anatomical transformations observed in *D. melanogaster*, as mammalian development is much less dependent on segmental structures. Only branchial arches, the hindbrain and somites appear to develop on a truly segmental basis, and here the role of *HOX* genes in controlling development of these structures is well documented [13]. In the mouse, loss-of-function mutations of *Hox* genes often cause anterior homeotic transformations—an anterior transformation being when a segmental unit acquires the characteristics of one more rostral. Anterior transformations of the axial skeleton have been reported for several *Hox* null mutants, including *Hoxa2* [14,15], *Hoxb4* [16], *Hoxc8* [17], *Hoxd3* [18] and *Hoxd13* [19].

An additional paralogous *Hox* cluster (*ParaHox*) also exists and, like the *Hox* cluster, also exhibits spatio-temporal co-linearity [20]. Both gene clusters are evolutionarily ancient, splitting from a common ancestral *ProtoHox* cluster prior to the split between Bilaterians and Cnidarians, i.e., before the establishment of body plans with bilateral symmetry [21]. In humans, the *ParaHox* cluster consists of three genes, *GSH, PDX1* and *CDX2*.

As with many of the *Hox* genes, loss-of-function mutation of *Cdx2* in mice is associated with anterior homeotic transformation of the axial skeleton [22]. Similarly, loss-of-function mutation of the related paralogue *Cdx1* also causes anterior homeotic shifts [23] and these patterning defects become further exacerbated in *Cdx1/Cdx2* compound mutants [24]. Null mutants of the third paralogue, *Cdx4*, do not exhibit skeletal defects, but exacerbate the axial patterning defects of both *Cdx1* and *Cdx2* mutants [25]. These findings illustrate not only functional overlap, but show that their collective activity is required to achieve wild-type levels of functional activity—i.e., their functional overlap does not equate to functional redundancy. As such, any genetic or environmental factors that alter Cdx protein levels can have significant effects on establishing positional identity. This is true not only during embryogenesis, but also following regenerative tissue repair in adult tissues, where the reestablishment of positional identity can be required. Incorrect reprogramming of tissue identity in adult tissues is termed metaplasia and metaplasia is increasingly recognized as a major risk factor for developing cancer. This review will focus on the function of *Cdx2* and, less so, its paralogues, *Cdx1* and *Cdx4*, and how genetically engineered mutations of these genes have provided us with animal models that have spurred our understanding of the important links between metaplasia and cancer.

2. Metaplasia is an Important Etiological Factor in Cancer

Metaplasia has long been recognized as a risk factor for cancer development and most often follows a common sequence: an environmental insult will cause tissue damage and, in the course of renewal, this tissue may transdifferentiate into a tissue type inappropriate for its location. An early recognized example is the often observed transition from a normal columnar bronchial epithelium to a squamous epithelium in the lungs of smokers, a metaplastic change that is believed to be the site of origin of lung cancers [26]. In 1985, Jonathan Slack proposed that many of these epithelial metaplasias may be analogous to homeotic transformations [27]. He proposed that epithelial stem cells may sometimes be reprogrammed back to an early ontological state and then, as normal progression proceeds, can acquire a new stable epigenetic state that is phenotypically anteriorized or posteriorized. This hypothesis was bolstered by findings showing an anterior shift in epithelial identity in the focal regions of the large intestine of *Cdx2* mutant mice, occurring concomitant with anterior shifts in the axial skeleton [22,28,29]. Later studies would show that targeted overexpression of *Cdx2* could induce metaplasias in the gut, in which anterior epithelial structures were replaced with posterior structures, i.e., directly analogous to a posterior homeotic shift [30–34] (Table 1, Figure 1). Thus, *Cdx2* insufficiency was associated with shifts in the opposite direction to conditions where *Cdx2* was overexpressed. Nevertheless, in both cases, the shifts were associated with cancer progression pathways. As will be discussed in the following sections, these animal models have been valuable in furthering our understanding of cancers of the esophagus, stomach and colon, as well as its less understood oncogenic role in leukemia.

Table 1. Animal cancer models generated through the genetic manipulation of Cdx genes.

Mutation	Phenotype	Reference
$Cdx2^{KO}$	Homozygotes: preimplantation lethality Heterozygotes: anterior homeotic shift of vertebrae, nondysplastic colonic tumors often containing metaplastic/heterotopic foci with gastric features	[22,28,29]
$Cdx2^{CKO}; Apc^{+/\Delta 14}$	Mixed tumors with adenomatous and serrated features	[35]
Tg(Foxa3–Cdx2)	Metaplasia in stomach	[33]
Tg(Atp4a–Cdx2)	Metaplasia in stomach	[32]
Tg(K14–Cdx2)	Non-intestinal type metaplasia in esophagus	[31]
Tg(Krt7rtTA); Tg(otet-Cdx2)	Intestinal type metaplasia in esophagus	[34]
Tg(krt5:cdx1b–EGFP) [1]	Metaplasia in esophagus	[30]

[1] Transgenic zebrafish model.

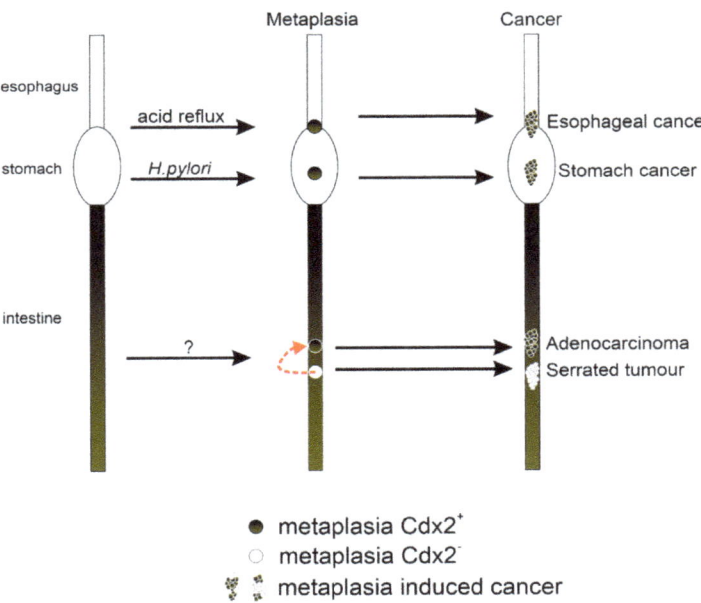

Figure 1. Simplified schematic diagram depicting how metaplasia caused by the alteration of *Cdx2* expression can progress to cancer.

Environmental insults can induce reprogramming of the gut epithelium. These metaplasias and metaplasia-like (i.e., serrated polyps in the colon) alterations can confer risk for subsequent development of cancers of the gastrointestinal tract.

3. Esophageal Cancer

3.1. Barrett's Esophagus is a Major Risk Factor for Human Esophageal Adenocarcinoma

Barrett's esophagus is a metaplastic change of normal squamous esophageal epithelium to an abnormal columnar epithelia with gastric and intestinal features [36,37]. The metaplasia arises as a consequence of the epithelial damage and inflammatory response wrought by chronic acid reflux.

Patients diagnosed with Barrett's esophagus have an approximate 100-fold increased risk of developing esophageal adenocarcinoma [38] and, because this metaplastic transformation appears irreversible, preventative measures have relied on controlling acid reflux, primarily through the use of proton pump inhibitors (PPIs) [39]. A recent clinical trial has shown that patients with existing Barrett's esophagus can still reduce their risk of developing adenocarcinoma by taking PPIs [40].

Not being present in the normal esophagus, *CDX2* expression is a biomarker for Barrett's esophagus [41–44]. Moreover, *CDX2* expression can often be found in esophageal squamous epithelia inflamed by acid reflux, suggesting that its expression precedes the metaplastic transformation [41,45]. *CDX2* is a direct transcriptional target of the key inflammatory mediator NF-κB [46]. Thus, it is likely that the onset of *CDX2* expression is due to activated NF-κB, which has also been shown to be present in pre-metaplastic inflamed squamous epithelia [47,48]. *CDX2* expression is maintained if the metaplasia advances to an adenocarcinoma, but expression diminishes as the cancer loses epithelial morphology [49,50].

3.2. Animal Models Reveal Functional Roles for Cdx2 in Barrett's Esophagus

A *keratin 14* promoter was used to force *Cdx2* overexpression to the squamous epithelia of mouse esophagus [31]. This was sufficient to induce metaplastic changes in the esophagus that resembled Barrett's esophagus, but lacked the intestinal goblet cells that are characteristic of the disease in humans. The transition from squamous to columnar epithelia was also associated with a decrease in barrier function, leading to the hypothesis that the transformed epithelia could, in turn, be more sensitive to reflux esophagitis, reinforcing the transition [31]. A similar model was generated in zebrafish, using a *keratin 5* promoter, to drive expression of *cdx1b* [30]. Like the transgenic mouse model, the zebrafish model exhibited similar metaplastic changes in the esophagus but, once again, without any appearance of goblet cells. More recently, a discrete transitional columnar epithelium was found to exist at the junction of the stomach and esophagus [34] and may represent the true source of Barrett's esophagus. *Keratin 7* was identified as a specific marker of this transitional epithelium and, by employing a *keratin 7* promoter to confine inducible *Cdx2* overexpression to this cell-type, a metaplasia that included goblet cells was observed [34]. Currently, this compound transgenic model (*Krt7rtTA; otet-CDX2-T2A-mCherry*) represents the best animal model for replicating Barrett's esophagus.

4. Stomach Cancer

4.1. CDX2 and the Metaplastic Origins of Human Stomach Cancer

The current model for human gastric carcinogenesis, proposed in 1992 [51], follows a similar course to the model for esophageal carcinogenesis discussed earlier, in that an initial pro-inflammatory stimulus will lead to inflammation (gastritis), followed by intestinal metaplasia, and, ultimately, to adenocarcinoma. In the stomach, the major environmental stimulus initiating this pathway, and thereby conferring the risk of cancer development, is chronic infection with *Helicobacter pylori* [52].

Two major types of metaplastic lineages have been identified adjacent to cancers of the stomach: an intestinal-type metaplasia with the characteristic presence of goblet cells [53] and a spasmolytic polypeptide-expressing metaplasia (SPEM) which expresses trefoil factor 2 (TFF2), then designated as spasmolytic polypeptide [54]. SPEM exhibits similarities to glands of the antrum (the caudal-most region of the stomach) [55,56]. SPEM may represent a reparative response to acute gastritis, while goblet-cell intestinal metaplasia may require a chronic inflammatory environment.

CDX2 expression is detected in gastric intestinal metaplasia but not in normal gastric mucosa [57–59]. *CDX2* could also be detected in chronic gastritis without evidence of metaplasia, suggesting that the onset of *CDX2* expression preceded the metaplastic change [60]. As the metaplasias progresses to carcinoma, *CDX2* levels are often reduced [58].

4.2. Animal Models Reveal Functional Roles for Cdx2 in Stomach Cancer

Cdx2 overexpression in the gastric mucosa of transgenic mice using the parietal cell-specific H^+/K^+-*ATPase subunit b* promoter resulted in gastric intestinal-type metaplasia that spontaneously developed into adenocarcinomas [61,62]. Another line, employing the *Foxa3* promoter to drive *Cdx2* overexpression, also exhibited intestinal-type metaplasia but progression to adenocarcinoma was not observed [33]. The significant overlap in phenotype is somewhat surprising, as *Foxa3* is expressed during embryonic development while the H^+/K^+-*ATPase* promoter is only active postnatally in the acid-producing parietal cells. It is possible that the phenotype may be indirectly influenced by parietal cell loss, as gastrin knockout mice, which exhibit impairment of stomach acid production, also exhibit intestinal-type metaplasia that eventually progresses to stomach cancer [63,64].

Modelling the action of the major risk factor for stomach cancer, *H. pylori* infection, has proven more difficult in mice, as this is heavily mouse strain-dependent [65] and produce SPEM rather than intestinal-type metaplasia [66]. For replicating the human disease, the Mongolian gerbil has been superior, recapitulating upon *H. pylori* infection the progression from gastritis to intestinal metaplasia and, eventually, to gastric cancer [67–69].

5. Colon Cancer

5.1. CDX2 is a Tumour Suppressor in Human Colorectal Cancer

Most colorectal cancers arise from an epithelial-derived adenomatous precursor lesion that, with further mutations in oncogenes and tumor suppressor genes, can clonally progress to carcinoma [70]. This adenoma–carcinoma pathway is most often initiated by activating mutations of the WNT pathway [71]. An alternative pathway, broadly termed the 'serrated pathway', maintains epithelial gland morphology and mucin production in the benign precursor lesions. It has been estimated that 20%–30% of colorectal cancers arise by this alternative pathway, although classification can be difficult as the cancer progresses and loses its serrated morphology [72,73]. This pathway is most often associated with activating mutations in the *BRAF* oncogene [72,74], and is considered to follow a more aggressive course than the conventional pathway [75]. Loss of *CDX2* expression has recently emerged as a biomarker for colon cancers arising via the serrated pathway, often coinciding with activated *BRAF* mutations [76,77]. It also has been identified as a prognostic marker in stage II colon cancer, where it was suggested that patients with CDX-negative cancers would benefit from adjuvant chemotherapy, rather than the common practice of treating all stage II patients with surgery alone [78].

Are serrated pathway cancers derived from metaplastic changes in the colonic epithelium? Suggestive of an anteriorization of epithelial identity is the fact that these cancers often express gastric epithelial markers, including mucin 2 (MUC2), MUC5AC, MUC6 and annexin A10 (ANXA10) [79–81]. Perhaps more compelling is that loss of *CDX2* expression is associated with a gain in *PDX1* expression, the *ParaHox* gene responsible for patterning the midgut [77].

5.2. Animal Models Reveal Functional Roles for Cdx2 in Colorectal Cancer

A possible role for *Cdx2* in colon cancer was initially suggested based on the knockout phenotype in mice; heterozygous mice had numerous tumors, although they never spontaneously advanced to carcinoma [22,29]. Upon closer examination, these tumors consisted of small foci of histologically normal forestomach epithelia that were surrounded in successive order by cardia, corpus, antrum and small intestine epithelia [82]. This observation was ascribed as a heterotopia, analogous to a metaplastic transformation, only with its origins occurring during embryological development instead of as a consequence of mucosal injury and repair. To model the latter, a *Cre-ERT* transgene under the *Cyp1a1* promoter, was used to achieve mosaic inactivation of a $Cdx2^{fl/fl}$ allele, thus allowing the study of *Cdx2* deficient lesions in the context of wild-type mucosa [83]. The *Cdx2* deficient lesions were found to express a number of gastric genes but did not form normal gastric mucosa, presumably because of incompatible mesenchymal signaling [83]. Under current classifications, these lesions could be interpreted as "serrated". Could they therefore be susceptible to transformation via activating mutations of *BRAF*?

Mouse models combining *Cdx2* inactivation and oncogenic *BRAF* ($BRAF^{V600E}$) activation were recently described and indeed, this led to invasive carcinogenesis along the serrated pathway [77,84]. Tamoxifen-regulated Cre protein (CreERT2) was used to inducibly inactivate *loxP*-containing alleles of *Cdx2* ($Cdx2^{fl/fl}$) or to inducibly activate an oncogenic *BRAF* allele ($BRAF^{V600E}$) in the adult intestinal epithelium. Mutation of either allele individually had little to no effect on median survival; however, their combined mutation resulted in progression to carcinoma. Immunohistochemical analyses of tumors revealed ectopic expression of typical serrated pathway markers such as annexin A10 and mucin 5AC [77].

Mouse models have also provided information that loss of *Cdx2* expression can influence not only the serrated pathway, but also the classical adenoma–carcinoma pathway. The classical pathway is associated with activating mutations of the Wnt signaling pathway, most predominantly through loss of function of the Wnt-signaling inhibitor, Apc [71]. Mutations in the human *APC* gene are causative for the cancer syndrome Familial Adenomatous Polyposis (FAP), as well as for sporadic cancers arising predominantly in the distal colon [85]. FAP can be modeled in mice carrying mutations of the *Apc* gene, including the truncated mutant $Apc^{\Delta 716}$ [86], but tumors in mice arise predominantly in the small intestine. When the $Apc^{\Delta 716}$ mutant allele is combined with the $Cdx2^{+/-}$ heterozygous mutation, there is a large increase in the number of adenomatous polyps in the distal colon, more closely reflecting the tumor distribution in human FAP [87].

More recently, it was reported that the tumor-promoting effect of *Cdx2* deficiency on the classical adenoma–carcinoma pathway may be non-cell autonomous [35]. This discovery was enabled by a complex mouse model, where mosaic inactivation of a $Cdx2^{fl/fl}$ allele was combined with a mutant $Apc^{+/\Delta 14}$ allele to drive adenoma formation and a conditionally activated fluorescent reporter allele (*tdTomato*) to trace cells that underwent Cre-mediated recombination. As expected, adenomas contained high levels of nuclear β-catenin, a measure of hyperactive Wnt signaling arising due to the loss of heterozygosity of the *Apc* tumor suppressor allele. However, these cells were never red (Cdx2 negative). The *Cdx2*-negative cells were not contributing to the adenoma, but instead created an environment that promoted neoplasia of *Cdx2*-positive cells—i.e., *Cdx2* was acting as a "non-cell-autonomous tumor suppressor" [35].

Previous studies had shown that $Cdx2^{+/-}$ mice are more susceptible to DSS-induced colitis [88]. Perhaps the permissive environment is pro-inflammatory. Indeed, NF-κB, a key mediator for inflammatory responses, was activated only in the *Cdx2*-positive cells that were adjacent to the regions of incomplete metaplasia [35]. These activated cells also expressed high levels of nitric oxide synthase (iNOS), indicating that these cells were under increased nitrosative and oxidative stress and therefore more susceptible to DNA damage. Supporting this hypothesis, treatment with the iNOS inhibitor aminoguanidine reduced the tumor load in mice carrying a mutant *Cdx2* allele ($Apc^{+/\Delta 14}$; $Cdx2^{+/-}$), while having no effect on mice with only wild-type *Cdx2* alleles ($Apc^{+/\Delta 14}$; $Cdx2^{+/+}$) [35].

6. Leukemia

6.1. CDX2 is a Proto-Oncogene in Human AML

A possible role for *CDX2* in human acute myeloid leukemia (AML) was first suggested following the identification of a novel chromosomal rearrangement, t (12; 13)(p13;q12), in a patient with AML. The rearrangement yielded an ets variant gene 6–CDX2 (*ETV6–CDX2*) fusion protein [89] and, as ETV6 is an important regulator of HSC survival and is frequently affected by translocations [90,91], it was thought that this fusion may be oncogenic. However, when the fusion protein was transduced into murine hematopoietic progenitors, it caused only minor myeloproliferation, and not transplantable AML [92]. It is now accepted that it was the full-length CDX2 protein, driven from an alternative *ETV6* promoter, that was leukemogenic. Indeed, transduction of full-length CDX2 into murine hematopoietic progenitors does result in transplantable lethal AML [92].

Up to 89% of AML cases, and up to 81% of acute lymphoblastic leukemia (ALL) cases, express CDX2 [93–96] and at least for ALL, CDX2 expression levels were directly associated with the aggressiveness of the disease [93,95]. Thus CDX2 is one of the most frequently expressed proto-oncogenes in human leukemia.

Known downstream targets of CDX2, namely the HOX genes, had also been identified as proto-oncogenes in AML [97,98]. Forced expression of Hoxa9 or Hoxa10 are also capable of inducing rapid AML in mice [99,100], and aberrant expression of human HOX genes, including HOXA9, correlates with clinical measures of disease burden [101–104].

During hematopoiesis, HOX genes of the A and B cluster are highly expressed in normal murine and human hematopoietic stem and committed progenitor cells, and become silenced during the course of normal differentiation [105,106]. Bone marrow from Hoxa9 deficient mice has a profound deficiency in the number of hematopoietic stem cells and progenitors [107,108]. On the other hand, CDX2 is not detected in hematopoietic stem or progenitor cells from healthy subjects, neither in human nor in mouse [109]. Also, there were no significant effects on hematopoiesis in knockout mouse models of any of the CDX genes [22,25,109,110]. Thus, although CDX2 and the HOX genes have similar roles in leukemogenesis, the similarities are not readily apparent in regards to the process of normal hematopoiesis. A true functional role would only be revealed as a result of important scientific discoveries in zebrafish.

6.2. Cdx Genes are Required for Normal Hematopoiesis in Zebrafish

The first indication that Cdx genes may have a functional role in hematopoiesis came from studies in zebrafish, when the causative mutation underlying the autosomal recessive mutation kugelig (kgg) was identified in the cdx4 gene [111]. Homozygous kgg embryos die early in development (day 5 to 10 post fertilization) with severe tail defects and a prominent reduction in hemoglobin-staining erythroid cells. This phenotype was consistent with the expression pattern of cdx4, which became restricted to the posterior end of the embryo during early somitogenesis, prior to the emergence of the posterior blood islands. Furthermore, the in vivo injection of cdx4 mRNA was able to rescue hematopoiesis in these kgg mutants [111].

Zebrafish contain a duplication of the Cdx1 gene (cdx1a and cdx1b), while lacking a Cdx2 orthologue. Therefore, although they contain the same number of Cdx genes as in mammals, they lack the prototypical ParaHox cluster. Nevertheless, like in mammals, the zebrafish cohort of Cdx genes does exhibit some degree of functional redundancy. Indeed, morpholino-mediated knockdown of cdx1a in kgg mutant fish exacerbates the phenotype, causing a complete failure to specify blood [112].

The hematopoiesis defect in cdx4 mutant zebrafish is reminiscent of anterior homeotic transformation of the axial skeleton observed in mouse loss of function mutants [22,110], as there appeared to be a posterior shift in the boundary between anteriorly localized hemangioblasts, fated to develop into endothelial cells and the posteriorly localized hemangioblasts, fated to develop both blood and endothelial cells [111]. Both populations are labelled with scl (tal1), which coexpresses with cdx4 in the posterior blood islands [111]. Even though scl overexpression is able to expand hematopoietic cell numbers when overexpressed in wild-type zebrafish embryos [113], it was incapable of rescuing hematopoiesis in cdx4 mutant kgg embryos [111]. Thus, the hematopoietic defect did not seem to be due to an overt lack in the number of scl+ hemangioblast progenitors, but rather a failure to pattern these progenitors to favor differentiation towards the erythrocyte lineage.

An evolutionarily conserved role of Cdx genes in regulating the expression of Hox genes [110,114,115] appears to underly the failure to pattern scl+ hemangioblasts in zebrafish. Indeed, kgg mutants exhibit large alterations in hox expression patterns, which can be restored upon ectopic cdx4 expression [111]. Overexpression of several of the most downregulated hox genes (hoxb6b, hoxb7a and hoxa9a) successfully rescues hematopoiesis in kgg mutants [111], and overexpression of hoxa9a (but not *hoxb7a*) rescues the complete hematopoietic failure observed upon combined *cdx1a* and *cdx4* deficiency [112].

6.3. Cdx Genes Control Mammalian Hematopoiesis

The implications from these studies in zebrafish were that a functional role for mammalian *CDX* genes may be masked by functional redundancies and that the *CDX* genes may exert their function not at the level of hematopoetic stem cells, but by pre-patterning their early mesodermal progenitors during embryogenesis. This possibility could be simply assessed by the in vitro differentiation of embryonic stem cell lines, since differentiation towards hematopoietic lineages involves a transition through a hemangioblast intermediate.

In vitro differentiation of single *Cdx* gene deficient murine embryonic stem cell lines resulted in only minor reductions in the numbers of multipotential blood progenitor colonies [116]. Knockdown of either *Cdx1* or *Cdx2* by RNA interference in a *Cdx4*-deficient background resulted in more severe reductions, while combined knockdown of both *Cdx1* and *Cdx2* in the *Cdx4*-deficient background resulted in an almost complete failure of hematopoiesis [116]. In embryos where *Cdx2* was conditionally inactivated in a $Cdx1^{-/-}$ background, there were defects in primitive hematopoiesis as well as yolk sac vascularization [117]. Thus a previously unrecognized role for *Cdx* genes in hematopoiesis was made evident when all genes in the family were inactivated.

The role of *Cdx* genes in pre-patterning early presomitic mesodermal progenitors, which will later give rise to hematopoietic lineages, can first of all be inferred by their ability to pattern the somitic mesoderm, resulting in the prototypical anterior homeotic transformation of the vertebrae [22,110]. Also, upon in vitro differentiation of human and mouse embryonic stem cells, *Cdx* gene expression peaks at the same time as hemangioblasts are specified and, if inducibly overexpressed during this time window, strongly enhances the production of hematopoietic progenitors [118–120]. The effect on hemangioblast production is likely the result of both a decreased amount of posterior unsegmented mesoderm [121] and an anterior shift in patterning the mesoderm [122]. In zebrafish, the *tbx5a*-expressing anterior cardiogenic mesoderm was expanded in *cdx1a/4* mutants [122]. Similarly, in mice, ectopic *Tbx5* expression was observed in the yolk sac of *Cdx1/2* compound conditional null mutants at the expense of hematopoietic markers [123]. Current evidence supports a mechanism of action for *Cdx* genes in which they stably repress cardiac loci in early Mesp1+ mesoderm by directly recruiting the SWI/SNF epigenetic silencing complex [123]. Thus, the expression of *Cdx* biases these progenitors to hematopoietic lineages at the expense of cardiac lineages.

7. Summary

Metaplasias, long recognized as a cancer risk factor, have been suggested to be analogous to developmental homeosis, where normal tissues develop in an abnormal location [27]. Homeobox genes, including *Cdx2*, are important factors in conferring positional identity to developing tissues, whether during embryogenesis or during the regenerative process following tissue injury. Animal models in which *Cdx2* overexpression is targeted to the esophagus show Barrett's metaplasia (Barrett's esophagus), characterized by the presence of intestinal-type epithelia in place of normal squamous epithelia. [30,31,34]. Similarly, targeted overexpression of *Cdx2* in the stomach also causes metaplasia, with a posteriorization of epithelial identity [32,33]. These tissue alterations model pre-neoplastic metaplasias that are common in humans. Conversely, loss of *Cdx2* in the colon causes metaplasia-like alterations, in which epithelia are misallocated towards an identity characteristic of more anterior structures [22,28,29], and this has provided important insights into understanding the progression of human serrated-type colonic tumors.

It is easy to recognize epithelial metaplasias, as any change in the reacquiring of positional identity in an epithelial stem cell will be conferred as a change in phenotype in its regionally constrained cell progeny. However, this is not the case for another cancer in which *Cdx2* is ectopically expressed—leukemia. Nevertheless, it is possible that the same sequence of events is occurring in leukemia—chronic inflammatory damage triggering a regenerative response, which results in the acquisition of a more "posteriorized" epigenetic state.

While the importance of *CDX2* in human cancer pathology is indisputable, its functional role has been more difficult to define. It has been designated, somewhat contradictorily, as both as an oncogene and a tumor suppressor. But, unlike prototypical oncogenes and tumor suppressor genes, there is no strong statistical evidence for cancer-associated mutations or loss of heterozygosity. The issue is that these terms describe cell-intrinsic functions, while the core function of *CDX2*, as a designator of positional identity, is, by definition, relativistic. Therefore, a true understanding of its role in cancer progression must be context-dependent. Indeed, the conceptual advances in this field, as discussed in this review, have been driven almost exclusively by the judicious use of animal models.

Funding: This work was funded by the Ministry of Education, Youth and Sports of the Czech Republic under the National Sustainability Program I project LO1419 and GACR 17-16959S.

Acknowledgments: I thank Felix Beck and Trevor Epp for helpful comments on this review manuscript and for proofreading.

Conflicts of Interest: The author declares no conflict of interest.

References

1. Bateson, W. *Materials for the Study of Variation: Treated with Especial Regard to Discontinuity in the Origin of Species*; Macmillan: London, UK; New York, NY, USA, 1894; p. 598.
2. Garber, R.L.; Kuroiwa, A.; Gehring, W.J. Genomic and cDNA clones of the homeotic locus Antennapedia in Drosophila. *EMBO J.* **1983**, *2*, 2027–2036. [CrossRef]
3. McGinnis, W.; Garber, R.L.; Wirz, J.; Kuroiwa, A.; Gehring, W.J. A homologous protein-coding sequence in Drosophila homeotic genes and its conservation in other metazoans. *Cell* **1984**, *37*, 403–408. [CrossRef]
4. McGinnis, W.; Hart, C.P.; Gehring, W.J.; Ruddle, F.H. Molecular cloning and chromosome mapping of a mouse DNA sequence homologous to homeotic genes of Drosophila. *Cell* **1984**, *38*, 675–680. [CrossRef]
5. Scott, M.P.; Weiner, A.J. Structural relationships among genes that control development: Sequence homology between the Antennapedia, Ultrabithorax, and fushi tarazu loci of Drosophila. *Proc. Natl. Acad. Sci. USA* **1984**, *81*, 4115–4119. [CrossRef] [PubMed]
6. Lewis, E.B. A gene complex controlling segmentation in Drosophila. *Nature* **1978**, *276*, 565–570. [CrossRef]
7. Nusslein-Volhard, C.; Wieschaus, E. Mutations affecting segment number and polarity in Drosophila. *Nature* **1980**, *287*, 795–801. [CrossRef]
8. Wakimoto, B.T.; Kaufman, T.C. Analysis of larval segmentation in lethal genotypes associated with the antennapedia gene complex in Drosophila melanogaster. *Dev. Biol.* **1981**, *81*, 51–64. [CrossRef]
9. Kappen, C.; Ruddle, F.H. Evolution of a regulatory gene family: HOM/HOX genes. *Curr. Opin. Genet. Dev.* **1993**, *3*, 931–938. [CrossRef]
10. Duboule, D.; Morata, G. Colinearity and functional hierarchy among genes of the homeotic complexes. *Trends Genet.* **1994**, *10*, 358–364. [CrossRef]
11. Graham, A.; Papalopulu, N.; Krumlauf, R. The murine and Drosophila homeobox gene complexes have common features of organization and expression. *Cell* **1989**, *57*, 367–378. [CrossRef]
12. Izpisua-Belmonte, J.C.; Falkenstein, H.; Dolle, P.; Renucci, A.; Duboule, D. Murine genes related to the Drosophila AbdB homeotic genes are sequentially expressed during development of the posterior part of the body. *EMBO J.* **1991**, *10*, 2279–2289. [CrossRef]
13. Krumlauf, R. Hox genes in vertebrate development. *Cell* **1994**, *78*, 191–201. [CrossRef]
14. Gendron-Maguire, M.; Mallo, M.; Zhang, M.; Gridley, T. Hoxa-2 mutant mice exhibit homeotic transformation of skeletal elements derived from cranial neural crest. *Cell* **1993**, *75*, 1317–1331. [CrossRef]
15. Rijli, F.M.; Mark, M.; Lakkaraju, S.; Dierich, A.; Dolle, P.; Chambon, P. A homeotic transformation is generated in the rostral branchial region of the head by disruption of Hoxa-2, which acts as a selector gene. *Cell* **1993**, *75*, 1333–1349. [CrossRef]
16. Ramirez-Solis, R.; Zheng, H.; Whiting, J.; Krumlauf, R.; Bradley, A. Hoxb-4 (Hox-2.6) mutant mice show homeotic transformation of a cervical vertebra and defects in the closure of the sternal rudiments. *Cell* **1993**, *73*, 279–294. [CrossRef]

17. Le Mouellic, H.; Lallemand, Y.; Brulet, P. Homeosis in the mouse induced by a null mutation in the Hox-3.1 gene. *Cell* **1992**, *69*, 251–264. [CrossRef]
18. Condie, B.G.; Capecchi, M.R. Mice homozygous for a targeted disruption of Hoxd-3 (Hox-4.1) exhibit anterior transformations of the first and second cervical vertebrae, the atlas and the axis. *Development* **1993**, *119*, 579–595.
19. Dolle, P.; Dierich, A.; LeMeur, M.; Schimmang, T.; Schuhbaur, B.; Chambon, P.; Duboule, D. Disruption of the Hoxd-13 gene induces localized heterochrony leading to mice with neotenic limbs. *Cell* **1993**, *75*, 431–441. [CrossRef]
20. Brooke, N.M.; Garcia-Fernandez, J.; Holland, P.W. The ParaHox gene cluster is an evolutionary sister of the Hox gene cluster. *Nature* **1998**, *392*, 920–922. [CrossRef]
21. Chourrout, D.; Delsuc, F.; Chourrout, P.; Edvardsen, R.B.; Rentzsch, F.; Renfer, E.; Jensen, M.F.; Zhu, B.; de Jong, P.; Steele, R.E.; et al. Minimal ProtoHox cluster inferred from bilaterian and cnidarian Hox complements. *Nature* **2006**, *442*, 684–687. [CrossRef]
22. Chawengsaksophak, K.; James, R.; Hammond, V.E.; Kontgen, F.; Beck, F. Homeosis and intestinal tumours in Cdx2 mutant mice. *Nature* **1997**, *386*, 84–87. [CrossRef] [PubMed]
23. Subramanian, V.; Meyer, B.; Evans, G.S. The murine Cdx1 gene product localises to the proliferative compartment in the developing and regenerating intestinal epithelium. *Differentiation* **1998**, *64*, 11–18. [CrossRef]
24. Van den Akker, E.; Forlani, S.; Chawengsaksophak, K.; de Graaff, W.; Beck, F.; Meyer, B.I.; Deschamps, J. Cdx1 and Cdx2 have overlapping functions in anteroposterior patterning and posterior axis elongation. *Development* **2002**, *129*, 2181–2193. [PubMed]
25. Van Nes, J.; de Graaff, W.; Lebrin, F.; Gerhard, M.; Beck, F.; Deschamps, J. The Cdx4 mutation affects axial development and reveals an essential role of Cdx genes in the ontogenesis of the placental labyrinth in mice. *Development* **2006**, *133*, 419–428. [CrossRef] [PubMed]
26. Auerbach, O.; Stout, A.P.; Hammond, E.C.; Garfinkel, L. Changes in bronchial epithelium in relation to cigarette smoking and in relation to lung cancer. *N. Engl. J. Med.* **1961**, *265*, 253–267. [CrossRef]
27. Slack, J.M. Homoeotic transformations in man: Implications for the mechanism of embryonic development and for the organization of epithelia. *J. Theor. Biol.* **1985**, *114*, 463–490. [CrossRef]
28. Beck, F.; Chawengsaksophak, K.; Waring, P.; Playford, R.J.; Furness, J.B. Reprogramming of intestinal differentiation and intercalary regeneration in Cdx2 mutant mice. *Proc. Natl. Acad. Sci. USA* **1999**, *96*, 7318–7323. [CrossRef]
29. Tamai, Y.; Nakajima, R.; Ishikawa, T.; Takaku, K.; Seldin, M.F.; Taketo, M.M. Colonic hamartoma development by anomalous duplication in Cdx2 knockout mice. *Cancer Res.* **1999**, *59*, 2965–2970.
30. Hu, B.; Chen, H.; Liu, X.; Zhang, C.; Cole, G.J.; Lee, J.A.; Chen, X. Transgenic overexpression of cdx1b induces metaplastic changes of gene expression in zebrafish esophageal squamous epithelium. *Zebrafish* **2013**, *10*, 218–227. [CrossRef]
31. Kong, J.; Crissey, M.A.; Funakoshi, S.; Kreindler, J.L.; Lynch, J.P. Ectopic Cdx2 expression in murine esophagus models an intermediate stage in the emergence of Barrett's esophagus. *PLoS ONE* **2011**, *6*, e18280. [CrossRef]
32. Mutoh, H.; Satoh, K.; Kita, H.; Sakamoto, H.; Hayakawa, H.; Yamamoto, H.; Isoda, N.; Tamada, K.; Ido, K.; Sugano, K. Cdx2 specifies the differentiation of morphological as well as functional absorptive enterocytes of the small intestine. *Int J. Dev. Biol.* **2005**, *49*, 867–871. [CrossRef] [PubMed]
33. Silberg, D.G.; Sullivan, J.; Kang, E.; Swain, G.P.; Moffett, J.; Sund, N.J.; Sackett, S.D.; Kaestner, K.H. Cdx2 ectopic expression induces gastric intestinal metaplasia in transgenic mice. *Gastroenterology* **2002**, *122*, 689–696. [CrossRef] [PubMed]
34. Jiang, M.; Li, H.; Zhang, Y.; Yang, Y.; Lu, R.; Liu, K.; Lin, S.; Lan, X.; Wang, H.; Wu, H.; et al. Transitional basal cells at the squamous-columnar junction generate Barrett's oesophagus. *Nature* **2017**, *550*, 529–533. [CrossRef] [PubMed]
35. Balbinot, C.; Armant, O.; Elarouci, N.; Marisa, L.; Martin, E.; De Clara, E.; Onea, A.; Deschamps, J.; Beck, F.; Freund, J.N.; et al. The Cdx2 homeobox gene suppresses intestinal tumorigenesis through non-cell-autonomous mechanisms. *J. Exp. Med.* **2018**, *215*, 911–926. [CrossRef]
36. McDonald, S.A.; Lavery, D.; Wright, N.A.; Jansen, M. Barrett oesophagus: Lessons on its origins from the lesion itself. *Nat. Rev. Gastroenterol. Hepatol.* **2015**, *12*, 50–60. [CrossRef]
37. Spechler, S.J.; Souza, R.F. Barrett's esophagus. *N. Engl. J. Med.* **2014**, *371*, 836–845. [CrossRef] [PubMed]

38. Wild, C.P.; Hardie, L.J. Reflux, Barrett's oesophagus and adenocarcinoma: Burning questions. *Nat. Rev. Cancer* **2003**, *3*, 676–684. [CrossRef]
39. El-Serag, H.B.; Aguirre, T.V.; Davis, S.; Kuebeler, M.; Bhattacharyya, A.; Sampliner, R.E. Proton pump inhibitors are associated with reduced incidence of dysplasia in Barrett's esophagus. *Am. J. Gastroenterol.* **2004**, *99*, 1877–1883. [CrossRef]
40. Jankowski, J.A.Z.; de Caestecker, J.; Love, S.B.; Reilly, G.; Watson, P.; Sanders, S.; Ang, Y.; Morris, D.; Bhandari, P.; Brooks, C.; et al. Esomeprazole and aspirin in Barrett's oesophagus (AspECT): A randomised factorial trial. *Lancet* **2018**, *392*, 400–408. [CrossRef]
41. Eda, A.; Osawa, H.; Satoh, K.; Yanaka, I.; Kihira, K.; Ishino, Y.; Mutoh, H.; Sugano, K. Aberrant expression of CDX2 in Barrett's epithelium and inflammatory esophageal mucosa. *J. Gastroenterol.* **2003**, *38*, 14–22. [CrossRef]
42. Groisman, G.M.; Amar, M.; Meir, A. Expression of the intestinal marker Cdx2 in the columnar-lined esophagus with and without intestinal (Barrett's) metaplasia. *Mod. Pathol.* **2004**, *17*, 1282–1288. [CrossRef] [PubMed]
43. Phillips, R.W.; Frierson, H.F., Jr.; Moskaluk, C.A. Cdx2 as a marker of epithelial intestinal differentiation in the esophagus. *Am. J. Surg. Pathol.* **2003**, *27*, 1442–1447. [CrossRef] [PubMed]
44. Vallbohmer, D.; DeMeester, S.R.; Peters, J.H.; Oh, D.S.; Kuramochi, H.; Shimizu, D.; Hagen, J.A.; Danenberg, K.D.; Danenberg, P.V.; DeMeester, T.R.; et al. Cdx-2 expression in squamous and metaplastic columnar epithelia of the esophagus. *Dis Esophagus* **2006**, *19*, 260–266. [CrossRef] [PubMed]
45. Moons, L.M.; Bax, D.A.; Kuipers, E.J.; Van Dekken, H.; Haringsma, J.; Van Vliet, A.H.; Siersema, P.D.; Kusters, J.G. The homeodomain protein CDX2 is an early marker of Barrett's oesophagus. *J. Clin. Pathol.* **2004**, *57*, 1063–1068. [CrossRef]
46. Kim, S.; Domon-Dell, C.; Wang, Q.; Chung, D.H.; Di Cristofano, A.; Pandolfi, P.P.; Freund, J.N.; Evers, B.M. PTEN and TNF-alpha regulation of the intestinal-specific Cdx-2 homeobox gene through a PI3K, PKB/Akt, and NF-kappaB-dependent pathway. *Gastroenterology* **2002**, *123*, 1163–1178. [CrossRef]
47. Huo, X.; Agoston, A.T.; Dunbar, K.B.; Cipher, D.J.; Zhang, X.; Yu, C.; Cheng, E.; Zhang, Q.; Pham, T.H.; Tambar, U.K.; et al. Hypoxia-inducible factor-2alpha plays a role in mediating oesophagitis in GORD. *Gut* **2017**, *66*, 1542–1554. [CrossRef]
48. O'Riordan, J.M.; Abdel-latif, M.M.; Ravi, N.; McNamara, D.; Byrne, P.J.; McDonald, G.S.; Keeling, P.W.; Kelleher, D.; Reynolds, J.V. Proinflammatory cytokine and nuclear factor kappa-B expression along the inflammation-metaplasia-dysplasia-adenocarcinoma sequence in the esophagus. *Am. J. Gastroenterol.* **2005**, *100*, 1257–1264. [CrossRef]
49. Moskaluk, C.A.; Zhang, H.; Powell, S.M.; Cerilli, L.A.; Hampton, G.M.; Frierson, H.F., Jr. Cdx2 protein expression in normal and malignant human tissues: An immunohistochemical survey using tissue microarrays. *Mod. Pathol.* **2003**, *16*, 913–919. [CrossRef]
50. Werling, R.W.; Yaziji, H.; Bacchi, C.E.; Gown, A.M. CDX2, a highly sensitive and specific marker of adenocarcinomas of intestinal origin: An immunohistochemical survey of 476 primary and metastatic carcinomas. *Am. J. Surg. Pathol.* **2003**, *27*, 303–310. [CrossRef]
51. Correa, P. Human gastric carcinogenesis: A multistep and multifactorial process–First American Cancer Society Award Lecture on Cancer Epidemiology and Prevention. *Cancer Res.* **1992**, *52*, 6735–6740.
52. Correa, P.; Houghton, J. Carcinogenesis of Helicobacter pylori. *Gastroenterology* **2007**, *133*, 659–672. [CrossRef] [PubMed]
53. Uemura, N.; Okamoto, S.; Yamamoto, S.; Matsumura, N.; Yamaguchi, S.; Yamakido, M.; Taniyama, K.; Sasaki, N.; Schlemper, R.J. Helicobacter pylori infection and the development of gastric cancer. *N. Engl. J. Med.* **2001**, *345*, 784–789. [CrossRef] [PubMed]
54. Schmidt, P.H.; Lee, J.R.; Joshi, V.; Playford, R.J.; Poulsom, R.; Wright, N.A.; Goldenring, J.R. Identification of a metaplastic cell lineage associated with human gastric adenocarcinoma. *Lab. Investig.* **1999**, *79*, 639–646.
55. Nomura, S.; Baxter, T.; Yamaguchi, H.; Leys, C.; Vartapetian, A.B.; Fox, J.G.; Lee, J.R.; Wang, T.C.; Goldenring, J.R. Spasmolytic polypeptide expressing metaplasia to preneoplasia in H. felis-infected mice. *Gastroenterology* **2004**, *127*, 582–594. [CrossRef] [PubMed]
56. Nomura, S.; Yamaguchi, H.; Ogawa, M.; Wang, T.C.; Lee, J.R.; Goldenring, J.R. Alterations in gastric mucosal lineages induced by acute oxyntic atrophy in wild-type and gastrin-deficient mice. *Am. J. Physiol. Gastrointest. Liver Physiol.* **2005**, *288*, G362–G375. [CrossRef] [PubMed]

57. Almeida, R.; Silva, E.; Santos-Silva, F.; Silberg, D.G.; Wang, J.; De Bolos, C.; David, L. Expression of intestine-specific transcription factors, CDX1 and CDX2, in intestinal metaplasia and gastric carcinomas. *J. Pathol.* **2003**, *199*, 36–40. [CrossRef] [PubMed]
58. Bai, Y.Q.; Yamamoto, H.; Akiyama, Y.; Tanaka, H.; Takizawa, T.; Koike, M.; Kenji Yagi, O.; Saitoh, K.; Takeshita, K.; Iwai, T.; et al. Ectopic expression of homeodomain protein CDX2 in intestinal metaplasia and carcinomas of the stomach. *Cancer Lett.* **2002**, *176*, 47–55. [CrossRef]
59. Mizoshita, T.; Inada, K.; Tsukamoto, T.; Kodera, Y.; Yamamura, Y.; Hirai, T.; Kato, T.; Joh, T.; Itoh, M.; Tatematsu, M. Expression of Cdx1 and Cdx2 mRNAs and relevance of this expression to differentiation in human gastrointestinal mucosa—with special emphasis on participation in intestinal metaplasia of the human stomach. *Gastric Cancer* **2001**, *4*, 185–191. [CrossRef]
60. Eda, A.; Osawa, H.; Yanaka, I.; Satoh, K.; Mutoh, H.; Kihira, K.; Sugano, K. Expression of homeobox gene CDX2 precedes that of CDX1 during the progression of intestinal metaplasia. *J. Gastroenterol.* **2002**, *37*, 94–100. [CrossRef]
61. Mutoh, H.; Hakamata, Y.; Sato, K.; Eda, A.; Yanaka, I.; Honda, S.; Osawa, H.; Kaneko, Y.; Sugano, K. Conversion of gastric mucosa to intestinal metaplasia in Cdx2-expressing transgenic mice. *Biochem. Biophys. Res. Commun.* **2002**, *294*, 470–479. [CrossRef]
62. Mutoh, H.; Sakurai, S.; Satoh, K.; Osawa, H.; Hakamata, Y.; Takeuchi, T.; Sugano, K. Cdx1 induced intestinal metaplasia in the transgenic mouse stomach: Comparative study with Cdx2 transgenic mice. *Gut* **2004**, *53*, 1416–1423. [CrossRef] [PubMed]
63. Friis-Hansen, L.; Rieneck, K.; Nilsson, H.O.; Wadstrom, T.; Rehfeld, J.F. Gastric inflammation, metaplasia, and tumor development in gastrin-deficient mice. *Gastroenterology* **2006**, *131*, 246–258. [CrossRef]
64. Zavros, Y.; Eaton, K.A.; Kang, W.; Rathinavelu, S.; Katukuri, V.; Kao, J.Y.; Samuelson, L.C.; Merchant, J.L. Chronic gastritis in the hypochlorhydric gastrin-deficient mouse progresses to adenocarcinoma. *Oncogene* **2005**, *24*, 2354–2366. [CrossRef] [PubMed]
65. Sakagami, T.; Dixon, M.; O'Rourke, J.; Howlett, R.; Alderuccio, F.; Vella, J.; Shimoyama, T.; Lee, A. Atrophic gastric changes in both Helicobacter felis and Helicobacter pylori infected mice are host dependent and separate from antral gastritis. *Gut* **1996**, *39*, 639–648. [CrossRef] [PubMed]
66. Wang, T.C.; Goldenring, J.R.; Dangler, C.; Ito, S.; Mueller, A.; Jeon, W.K.; Koh, T.J.; Fox, J.G. Mice lacking secretory phospholipase A2 show altered apoptosis and differentiation with Helicobacter felis infection. *Gastroenterology* **1998**, *114*, 675–689. [CrossRef]
67. Honda, S.; Fujioka, T.; Tokieda, M.; Satoh, R.; Nishizono, A.; Nasu, M. Development of Helicobacter pylori-induced gastric carcinoma in Mongolian gerbils. *Cancer Res.* **1998**, *58*, 4255–4259.
68. Watanabe, H.; Fujii, I.; Terada, Y. Induction of intestinal metaplasia in the rat gastric mucosa by local X-irradiation. *Pathol. Res. Pract* **1980**, *170*, 104–114. [CrossRef]
69. Zheng, Q.; Chen, X.Y.; Shi, Y.; Xiao, S.D. Development of gastric adenocarcinoma in Mongolian gerbils after long-term infection with Helicobacter pylori. *J. Gastroenterol. Hepatol.* **2004**, *19*, 1192–1198. [CrossRef]
70. Fearon, E.R.; Vogelstein, B. A genetic model for colorectal tumorigenesis. *Cell* **1990**, *61*, 759–767. [CrossRef]
71. Powell, S.M.; Zilz, N.; Beazer-Barclay, Y.; Bryan, T.M.; Hamilton, S.R.; Thibodeau, S.N.; Vogelstein, B.; Kinzler, K.W. APC mutations occur early during colorectal tumorigenesis. *Nature* **1992**, *359*, 235–237. [CrossRef]
72. Bettington, M.; Walker, N.; Clouston, A.; Brown, I.; Leggett, B.; Whitehall, V. The serrated pathway to colorectal carcinoma: Current concepts and challenges. *Histopathology* **2013**, *62*, 367–386. [CrossRef] [PubMed]
73. Langner, C. Serrated and non-serrated precursor lesions of colorectal cancer. *Dig. Dis.* **2015**, *33*, 28–37. [CrossRef] [PubMed]
74. De Sousa, E.M.F.; Wang, X.; Jansen, M.; Fessler, E.; Trinh, A.; de Rooij, L.P.; de Jong, J.H.; de Boer, O.J.; van Leersum, R.; Bijlsma, M.F.; et al. Poor-prognosis colon cancer is defined by a molecularly distinct subtype and develops from serrated precursor lesions. *Nat. Med.* **2013**, *19*, 614–618. [CrossRef] [PubMed]
75. Garcia-Solano, J.; Conesa-Zamora, P.; Trujillo-Santos, J.; Makinen, M.J.; Perez-Guillermo, M. Tumour budding and other prognostic pathological features at invasive margins in serrated colorectal adenocarcinoma: A comparative study with conventional carcinoma. *Histopathology* **2011**, *59*, 1046–1056. [CrossRef] [PubMed]

76. Landau, M.S.; Kuan, S.F.; Chiosea, S.; Pai, R.K. BRAF-mutated microsatellite stable colorectal carcinoma: An aggressive adenocarcinoma with reduced CDX2 and increased cytokeratin 7 immunohistochemical expression. *Hum. Pathol.* **2014**, *45*, 1704–1712. [CrossRef]
77. Sakamoto, N.; Feng, Y.; Stolfi, C.; Kurosu, Y.; Green, M.; Lin, J.; Green, M.E.; Sentani, K.; Yasui, W.; McMahon, M.; et al. BRAF(V600E) cooperates with CDX2 inactivation to promote serrated colorectal tumorigenesis. *Elife* **2017**, *6*. [CrossRef]
78. Dalerba, P.; Sahoo, D.; Paik, S.; Guo, X.; Yothers, G.; Song, N.; Wilcox-Fogel, N.; Forgo, E.; Rajendran, P.S.; Miranda, S.P.; et al. CDX2 as a Prognostic Biomarker in Stage II and Stage III Colon Cancer. *N. Engl. J. Med.* **2016**, *374*, 211–222. [CrossRef]
79. Kim, J.H.; Kim, K.J.; Rhee, Y.Y.; Bae, J.M.; Cho, N.Y.; Lee, H.S.; Kang, G.H. Gastric-type expression signature in serrated pathway-associated colorectal tumors. *Hum. Pathol.* **2015**, *46*, 643–656. [CrossRef]
80. Tsai, J.H.; Lin, Y.L.; Cheng, Y.C.; Chen, C.C.; Lin, L.I.; Tseng, L.H.; Cheng, M.L.; Liau, J.Y.; Jeng, Y.M. Aberrant expression of annexin A10 is closely related to gastric phenotype in serrated pathway to colorectal carcinoma. *Mod. Pathol.* **2015**, *28*, 268–278. [CrossRef]
81. Walsh, M.D.; Clendenning, M.; Williamson, E.; Pearson, S.A.; Walters, R.J.; Nagler, B.; Packenas, D.; Win, A.K.; Hopper, J.L.; Jenkins, M.A.; et al. Expression of MUC2, MUC5AC, MUC5B, and MUC6 mucins in colorectal cancers and their association with the CpG island methylator phenotype. *Mod. Pathol.* **2013**, *26*, 1642–1656. [CrossRef]
82. Beck, F.; Chawengsaksophak, K.; Luckett, J.; Giblett, S.; Tucci, J.; Brown, J.; Poulsom, R.; Jeffery, R.; Wright, N.A. A study of regional gut endoderm potency by analysis of Cdx2 null mutant chimaeric mice. *Dev. Biol.* **2003**, *255*, 399–406. [CrossRef]
83. Stringer, E.J.; Duluc, I.; Saandi, T.; Davidson, I.; Bialecka, M.; Sato, T.; Barker, N.; Clevers, H.; Pritchard, C.A.; Winton, D.J.; et al. Cdx2 determines the fate of postnatal intestinal endoderm. *Development* **2012**, *139*, 465–474. [CrossRef] [PubMed]
84. Tong, K.; Pellon-Cardenas, O.; Sirihorachai, V.R.; Warder, B.N.; Kothari, O.A.; Perekatt, A.O.; Fokas, E.E.; Fullem, R.L.; Zhou, A.; Thackray, J.K.; et al. Degree of Tissue Differentiation Dictates Susceptibility to BRAF-Driven Colorectal Cancer. *Cell Rep.* **2017**, *21*, 3833–3845. [CrossRef] [PubMed]
85. Groden, J.; Thliveris, A.; Samowitz, W.; Carlson, M.; Gelbert, L.; Albertsen, H.; Joslyn, G.; Stevens, J.; Spirio, L.; Robertson, M.; et al. Identification and characterization of the familial adenomatous polyposis coli gene. *Cell* **1991**, *66*, 589–600. [CrossRef]
86. Fodde, R.; Edelmann, W.; Yang, K.; van Leeuwen, C.; Carlson, C.; Renault, B.; Breukel, C.; Alt, E.; Lipkin, M.; Khan, P.M.; et al. A targeted chain-termination mutation in the mouse Apc gene results in multiple intestinal tumors. *Proc. Natl. Acad. Sci. USA* **1994**, *91*, 8969–8973. [CrossRef]
87. Aoki, K.; Tamai, Y.; Horiike, S.; Oshima, M.; Taketo, M.M. Colonic polyposis caused by mTOR-mediated chromosomal instability in Apc+/Delta716 Cdx2+/− compound mutant mice. *Nat. Genet.* **2003**, *35*, 323–330. [CrossRef]
88. Calon, A.; Gross, I.; Lhermitte, B.; Martin, E.; Beck, F.; Duclos, B.; Kedinger, M.; Duluc, I.; Domon-Dell, C.; Freund, J.N. Different effects of the Cdx1 and Cdx2 homeobox genes in a murine model of intestinal inflammation. *Gut* **2007**, *56*, 1688–1695. [CrossRef]
89. Chase, A.; Reiter, A.; Burci, L.; Cazzaniga, G.; Biondi, A.; Pickard, J.; Roberts, I.A.; Goldman, J.M.; Cross, N.C. Fusion of ETV6 to the caudal-related homeobox gene CDX2 in acute myeloid leukemia with the t(12;13)(p13;q12). *Blood* **1999**, *93*, 1025–1031. [CrossRef]
90. Bohlander, S.K. ETV6: A versatile player in leukemogenesis. *Semin Cancer Biol.* **2005**, *15*, 162–174. [CrossRef]
91. Hock, H.; Meade, E.; Medeiros, S.; Schindler, J.W.; Valk, P.J.; Fujiwara, Y.; Orkin, S.H. Tel/Etv6 is an essential and selective regulator of adult hematopoietic stem cell survival. *Genes Dev.* **2004**, *18*, 2336–2341. [CrossRef]
92. Rawat, V.P.; Cusan, M.; Deshpande, A.; Hiddemann, W.; Quintanilla-Martinez, L.; Humphries, R.K.; Bohlander, S.K.; Feuring-Buske, M.; Buske, C. Ectopic expression of the homeobox gene Cdx2 is the transforming event in a mouse model of t(12;13)(p13;q12) acute myeloid leukemia. *Proc. Natl. Acad. Sci. USA* **2004**, *101*, 817–822. [CrossRef] [PubMed]
93. Thoene, S.; Rawat, V.P.; Heilmeier, B.; Hoster, E.; Metzeler, K.H.; Herold, T.; Hiddemann, W.; Gokbuget, N.; Hoelzer, D.; Bohlander, S.K.; et al. The homeobox gene CDX2 is aberrantly expressed and associated with an inferior prognosis in patients with acute lymphoblastic leukemia. *Leukemia* **2009**, *23*, 649–655. [CrossRef] [PubMed]

94. Scholl, C.; Bansal, D.; Dohner, K.; Eiwen, K.; Huntly, B.J.; Lee, B.H.; Rucker, F.G.; Schlenk, R.F.; Bullinger, L.; Dohner, H.; et al. The homeobox gene CDX2 is aberrantly expressed in most cases of acute myeloid leukemia and promotes leukemogenesis. *J. Clin. Invest.* **2007**, *117*, 1037–1048. [CrossRef] [PubMed]
95. Riedt, T.; Ebinger, M.; Salih, H.R.; Tomiuk, J.; Handgretinger, R.; Kanz, L.; Grunebach, F.; Lengerke, C. Aberrant expression of the homeobox gene CDX2 in pediatric acute lymphoblastic leukemia. *Blood* **2009**, *113*, 4049–4051. [CrossRef] [PubMed]
96. Rawat, V.P.; Thoene, S.; Naidu, V.M.; Arseni, N.; Heilmeier, B.; Metzeler, K.; Petropoulos, K.; Deshpande, A.; Quintanilla-Martinez, L.; Bohlander, S.K.; et al. Overexpression of CDX2 perturbs HOX gene expression in murine progenitors depending on its N-terminal domain and is closely correlated with deregulated HOX gene expression in human acute myeloid leukemia. *Blood* **2008**, *111*, 309–319. [CrossRef] [PubMed]
97. Lawrence, H.J.; Largman, C. Homeobox genes in normal hematopoiesis and leukemia. *Blood* **1992**, *80*, 2445–2453. [CrossRef]
98. Lawrence, H.J.; Sauvageau, G.; Ahmadi, N.; Lopez, A.R.; LeBeau, M.M.; Link, M.; Humphries, K.; Largman, C. Stage-and lineage-specific expression of the HOXA10 homeobox gene in normal and leukemic hematopoietic cells. *Exp. Hematol.* **1995**, *23*, 1160–1166.
99. Thorsteinsdottir, U.; Kroon, E.; Jerome, L.; Blasi, F.; Sauvageau, G. Defining roles for HOX and MEIS1 genes in induction of acute myeloid leukemia. *Mol. Cell Biol.* **2001**, *21*, 224–234. [CrossRef]
100. Thorsteinsdottir, U.; Sauvageau, G.; Humphries, R.K. Hox homeobox genes as regulators of normal and leukemic hematopoiesis. *Hematol. Oncol. Clin. N. Am.* **1997**, *11*, 1221–1237. [CrossRef]
101. Golub, T.R.; Slonim, D.K.; Tamayo, P.; Huard, C.; Gaasenbeek, M.; Mesirov, J.P.; Coller, H.; Loh, M.L.; Downing, J.R.; Caligiuri, M.A.; et al. Molecular classification of cancer: Class discovery and class prediction by gene expression monitoring. *Science* **1999**, *286*, 531–537. [CrossRef]
102. Haferlach, C.; Mecucci, C.; Schnittger, S.; Kohlmann, A.; Mancini, M.; Cuneo, A.; Testoni, N.; Rege-Cambrin, G.; Santucci, A.; Vignetti, M.; et al. AML with mutated NPM1 carrying a normal or aberrant karyotype show overlapping biologic, pathologic, immunophenotypic, and prognostic features. *Blood* **2009**, *114*, 3024–3032. [CrossRef] [PubMed]
103. Krivtsov, A.V.; Armstrong, S.A. MLL translocations, histone modifications and leukaemia stem-cell development. *Nat. Rev. Cancer* **2007**, *7*, 823–833. [CrossRef] [PubMed]
104. Rice, K.L.; Licht, J.D. HOX deregulation in acute myeloid leukemia. *J. Clin. Investig.* **2007**, *117*, 865–868. [CrossRef] [PubMed]
105. Pineault, N.; Helgason, C.D.; Lawrence, H.J.; Humphries, R.K. Differential expression of Hox, Meis1, and Pbx1 genes in primitive cells throughout murine hematopoietic ontogeny. *Exp. Hematol.* **2002**, *30*, 49–57. [CrossRef]
106. Sauvageau, G.; Lansdorp, P.M.; Eaves, C.J.; Hogge, D.E.; Dragowska, W.H.; Reid, D.S.; Largman, C.; Lawrence, H.J.; Humphries, R.K. Differential expression of homeobox genes in functionally distinct CD34+ subpopulations of human bone marrow cells. *Proc. Natl. Acad. Sci. USA* **1994**, *91*, 12223–12227. [CrossRef]
107. Lawrence, H.J.; Christensen, J.; Fong, S.; Hu, Y.L.; Weissman, I.; Sauvageau, G.; Humphries, R.K.; Largman, C. Loss of expression of the Hoxa-9 homeobox gene impairs the proliferation and repopulating ability of hematopoietic stem cells. *Blood* **2005**, *106*, 3988–3994. [CrossRef]
108. Lawrence, H.J.; Helgason, C.D.; Sauvageau, G.; Fong, S.; Izon, D.J.; Humphries, R.K.; Largman, C. Mice bearing a targeted interruption of the homeobox gene HOXA9 have defects in myeloid, erythroid, and lymphoid hematopoiesis. *Blood* **1997**, *89*, 1922–1930. [CrossRef]
109. Lengerke, C.; Daley, G.Q. Patterning definitive hematopoietic stem cells from embryonic stem cells. *Exp. Hematol.* **2005**, *33*, 971–979. [CrossRef]
110. Subramanian, V.; Meyer, B.I.; Gruss, P. Disruption of the murine homeobox gene Cdx1 affects axial skeletal identities by altering the mesodermal expression domains of Hox genes. *Cell* **1995**, *83*, 641–653. [CrossRef]
111. Davidson, A.J.; Ernst, P.; Wang, Y.; Dekens, M.P.; Kingsley, P.D.; Palis, J.; Korsmeyer, S.J.; Daley, G.Q.; Zon, L.I. cdx4 mutants fail to specify blood progenitors and can be rescued by multiple hox genes. *Nature* **2003**, *425*, 300–306. [CrossRef]
112. Davidson, A.J.; Zon, L.I. The caudal-related homeobox genes cdx1a and cdx4 act redundantly to regulate hox gene expression and the formation of putative hematopoietic stem cells during zebrafish embryogenesis. *Dev. Biol.* **2006**, *292*, 506–518. [CrossRef] [PubMed]

113. Gering, M.; Rodaway, A.R.; Gottgens, B.; Patient, R.K.; Green, A.R. The SCL gene specifies haemangioblast development from early mesoderm. *EMBO J.* **1998**, *17*, 4029–4045. [CrossRef] [PubMed]
114. Charite, J.; de Graaff, W.; Consten, D.; Reijnen, M.J.; Korving, J.; Deschamps, J. Transducing positional information to the Hox genes: Critical interaction of cdx gene products with position-sensitive regulatory elements. *Development* **1998**, *125*, 4349–4358.
115. Hunter, C.P.; Harris, J.M.; Maloof, J.N.; Kenyon, C. Hox gene expression in a single Caenorhabditis elegans cell is regulated by a caudal homolog and intercellular signals that inhibit wnt signaling. *Development* **1999**, *126*, 805–814. [PubMed]
116. Wang, Y.; Yabuuchi, A.; McKinney-Freeman, S.; Ducharme, D.M.; Ray, M.K.; Chawengsaksophak, K.; Archer, T.K.; Daley, G.Q. Cdx gene deficiency compromises embryonic hematopoiesis in the mouse. *Proc. Natl. Acad. Sci. USA* **2008**, *105*, 7756–7761. [CrossRef] [PubMed]
117. Brooke-Bisschop, T.; Savory, J.G.A.; Foley, T.; Ringuette, R.; Lohnes, D. Essential roles for Cdx in murine primitive hematopoiesis. *Dev. Biol.* **2017**, *422*, 115–124. [CrossRef] [PubMed]
118. Lengerke, C.; Grauer, M.; Niebuhr, N.I.; Riedt, T.; Kanz, L.; Park, I.H.; Daley, G.Q. Hematopoietic development from human induced pluripotent stem cells. *Ann. N. Y. Acad. Sci.* **2009**, *1176*, 219–227. [CrossRef] [PubMed]
119. Lengerke, C.; McKinney-Freeman, S.; Naveiras, O.; Yates, F.; Wang, Y.; Bansal, D.; Daley, G.Q. The cdx-hox pathway in hematopoietic stem cell formation from embryonic stem cells. *Ann. N. Y. Acad. Sci.* **2007**, *1106*, 197–208. [CrossRef]
120. Lengerke, C.; Schmitt, S.; Bowman, T.V.; Jang, I.H.; Maouche-Chretien, L.; McKinney-Freeman, S.; Davidson, A.J.; Hammerschmidt, M.; Rentzsch, F.; Green, J.B.; et al. BMP and Wnt specify hematopoietic fate by activation of the Cdx-Hox pathway. *Cell Stem Cell* **2008**, *2*, 72–82. [CrossRef]
121. Chawengsaksophak, K.; de Graaff, W.; Rossant, J.; Deschamps, J.; Beck, F. Cdx2 is essential for axial elongation in mouse development. *Proc. Natl. Acad. Sci. USA* **2004**, *101*, 7641–7645. [CrossRef]
122. Lengerke, C.; Wingert, R.; Beeretz, M.; Grauer, M.; Schmidt, A.G.; Konantz, M.; Daley, G.Q.; Davidson, A.J. Interactions between Cdx genes and retinoic acid modulate early cardiogenesis. *Dev. Biol.* **2011**, *354*, 134–142. [CrossRef] [PubMed]
123. Foley, T.E.; Hess, B.; Savory, J.G.A.; Ringuette, R.; Lohnes, D. Role of Cdx factors in early mesodermal fate decisions. *Development* **2019**, *146*. [CrossRef] [PubMed]

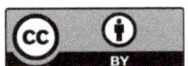

© 2019 by the author. Licensee MDPI, Basel, Switzerland. This article is an open access article distributed under the terms and conditions of the Creative Commons Attribution (CC BY) license (http://creativecommons.org/licenses/by/4.0/).

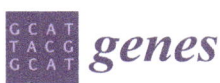 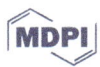

Review

Zebrafish Models of Cancer—New Insights on Modeling Human Cancer in a Non-Mammalian Vertebrate

Martina Hason and Petr Bartůněk *

Institute of Molecular Genetics of the Czech Academy of Sciences, v. v. i. Vídeňská 1083, 142 20 Prague 4, Czech Republic; martina.hason@img.cas.cz
* Correspondence: bartunek@img.cas.cz

Received: 25 July 2019; Accepted: 11 November 2019; Published: 15 November 2019

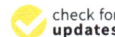

Abstract: Zebrafish (*Danio rerio*) is a valuable non-mammalian vertebrate model widely used to study development and disease, including more recently cancer. The evolutionary conservation of cancer-related programs between human and zebrafish is striking and allows extrapolation of research outcomes obtained in fish back to humans. Zebrafish has gained attention as a robust model for cancer research mainly because of its high fecundity, cost-effective maintenance, dynamic visualization of tumor growth in vivo, and the possibility of chemical screening in large numbers of animals at reasonable costs. Novel approaches in modeling tumor growth, such as using transgene electroporation in adult zebrafish, could improve our knowledge about the spatial and temporal control of cancer formation and progression in vivo. Looking at genetic as well as epigenetic alterations could be important to explain the pathogenesis of a disease as complex as cancer. In this review, we highlight classic genetic and transplantation models of cancer in zebrafish as well as provide new insights on advances in cancer modeling. Recent progress in zebrafish xenotransplantation studies and drug screening has shown that zebrafish is a reliable model to study human cancer and could be suitable for evaluating patient-derived xenograft cell invasiveness. Rapid, large-scale evaluation of in vivo drug responses and kinetics in zebrafish could undoubtedly lead to new applications in personalized medicine and combination therapy. For all of the above-mentioned reasons, zebrafish is approaching a future of being a pre-clinical cancer model, alongside the mouse. However, the mouse will continue to be valuable in the last steps of pre-clinical drug screening, mostly because of the highly conserved mammalian genome and biological processes.

Keywords: zebrafish; epigenetics; xenotransplantation; drug screen; pre-clinical cancer model

1. Introduction

In the last four decades, a significant amount of time and money have been invested into the investigation of cancer. Cancer is a collective term for a large number of genetically diverse diseases that share common hallmarks at the cellular and molecular level. The diversity of tumors seems to be one of the biggest challenges for treating cancer patients as the inter-individual differences are enhanced by intratumor heterogeneity. Intratumor heterogeneity is the cellular variability of cancerous tissue and has been found in the vast majority of cancer types. Tumor cells differ in their genomes, transcriptomes, proteomes as well as their epigenomes. Further, cancer cells undergo subclonal evolution during tumor growth. In consequence, cancer cell metabolism, as well as its proliferative and metastatic potential, rapidly changes in time [1–3]. Until now, there is no easy way to address the great diversity of cancer malignancies, nor in approaching cancer therapy. Usually, the identification and the targeting of frequent driver mutations is a rational approach to cancer treatment. The field of current cancer research has been innovative in the last years by focusing on tumor cell growth, evolution, and heterogeneity, especially by looking into these processes in live animals. A trend towards targeted therapy and combination therapy has been facilitated by testing in various animal models in vivo [4]. The murine model has been routinely used in cancer research mostly because of the physiological as well as the genetic similarities to human. However, the main disadvantage of mice for cancer research is that it is basically impossible to study early tumor dissemination and changes in the tumor microenvironment at the cellular level. Further, the mouse is not suitable for large-scale small molecule screening. Many of the hurdles posed by unknown tumor driver mutations or treatment resistance could be partially overcome by patient-derived cancer cell xenotransplantation (PDX) followed by whole-animal high-throughput small molecule screening. Another drawback of the murine model, specifically for PDX, is the fact that the tumor graft needs to be transplanted into an immunocompromised adult recipient [5–7]. Human cancer research is not limited only to mammalian models [4,8,9].

Fish, as non-mammalian vertebrate models of cancer, are not new to the field. Their advantages for biomedical research are the relatively low-cost maintenance at high numbers of animals, the external development which allows in vivo imaging, and the large number of progeny. The first model of melanoma in fish was established in platyfish (*Xiphophorus*). It was shown that the genetic hybrids of the pigmented platyfish (*Xiphophorus maculatus*) and the non-pigmented swordtails (*Xiphophorus helleri*) spontaneously develop melanoma. This model is one of the earliest animal cancer models [10,11]. Another example is medaka (*Oryzias latipes*), a small freshwater fish which has helped to uncover new aspects of cancerogenesis, again mostly in melanoma pathogenesis [10,12]. Zebrafish (*Danio rerio*) has gained the most attention as a robust animal for studying development and disease. Due to its cost-effective maintenance, high fecundity, fast external development, optical clarity, and small size of the embryos as well as adults, this little fish has become a popular model organism for developmental biology [4,8,9,13,14]. Thanks to the transparency of zebrafish embryos and larvae it is possible to visualize tumor cell growth and dynamics at early stages of cancer development in vivo [15]. A zebrafish genetic strain that maintains much of its transparency throughout adulthood, known as *casper*, has been created as well [16]. Further, the efficiency and relative ease of genetic manipulation for mutant and transgene production makes zebrafish a versatile animal for disease modeling. Major players of human cancer-related pathways have their homologs in the zebrafish genome [17–19]. There are well-established zebrafish transgenic lines with fluorescently labeled tissues available that can add new insights into cancer cell growth, dissemination, and tumor microenvironment in real-time [20–22]. Aspects of human disease can be recapitulated and followed in vivo in zebrafish at the molecular level because of its highly evolutionarily conserved genes and signaling pathways [23]. In the last decade, human cancer cell xenotransplantation into zebrafish has been developed as well. Thus, zebrafish has joined the mouse as a new model for xenograft assays. The possibility to maintain high numbers of larvae at one place and time makes zebrafish a convenient model for small molecule screening in drug discovery [24–26]. This is of high importance in the emerging field of PDX small molecule screening. Zebrafish accelerates the pre-clinical development process as its embryos are suitable for large-scale whole animal screening [19,27,28].

Zebrafish is a poikilothermic fish with a preferred temperature around 28 °C. This might be adverse in studies where the mammalian homeostatic temperature would be important. However, in short time periods, zebrafish can tolerate temperatures ranging from 6 to 38 °C [29]. Another drawback of zebrafish is the teleost genome duplication, where there are genes in more than one copy (paralogs). This means that some genes could be redundant in function or that their function could be sub-divided from the ancestral genes' function. This fact might complicate molecular genetic studies in zebrafish [30,31]. Additionally, there is a lack of commercially available antibodies against zebrafish proteins. This disadvantage is at least partially compensated by the availability of reporter transgenic zebrafish lines [15].

In this review we will provide an insight into zebrafish models of cancer, focusing on genetic modeling of cancer in zebrafish, on recent research progress in transplantation studies, and small molecule drug screening models; and on novel approaches in modeling tumor growth in zebrafish, for example by using transgene electroporation in adult zebrafish (TEAZ) [32]. We will further discuss the use of zebrafish in following cancer metastasis real-time in vivo. Metastasis is a process critical in cancer malignancy, therefore we will further look at the role of tumor microenvironment on influencing cancer cells spreading out of the site of primary tumors [33] which was shown in zebrafish xenograft studies [33]. Another issue, which we want to address in this review, is the importance of epigenetic machinery in such a complex matter as tumor biology. Human whole-genome sequencing has revealed recurrent somatic mutations in many genes encoding epigenetic regulators, several of them were found to be associated with specific cancer types [34–36].

2. Genetic Models of Cancer in Zebrafish

Disease-modeling in zebrafish is versatile and can be approached from many angles, either by creating gene-targeted mutations and stable transgenes or by creating a fish with transient overexpression or downregulation of certain genes. First, forward genetic screens done in zebrafish revealed that the use of common mutagens, such as ethylnitrosourea (ENU) or N-methyl-nitrosoguanidine (MNNG), cause the development of various neoplasms, for example, adenoma or rhabdomyosarcoma (RMS) [37,38]. One of the first models of cancer in zebrafish which was found in an ENU screen was the fish with a mutation in the *tumor suppressor 53* ($tp53^{M214K}$). TP53 is the most frequently mutated tumor suppressor gene found in human cancers. These mutant $tp53^{-/-}$ animals develop malignant peripheral nerve sheath tumor (PNST) which are often recognized as a subtype of sarcoma. PNST was rarely seen in wild-type (WT) fish. The zebrafish phenotype partially recapitulates the situation observed in *TP53* inactivated human patients. They, however, develop a wide array of cancer types in addition to sarcomas, such as breast cancer, brain tumor, or leukemia [39]. A newer zebrafish model with $tp53^{del/del}$ loss-of-function deletion allele created in the CG1 syngeneic zebrafish strain was described more recently. These zebrafish develop various types of tumors besides PNST, such as leukemia or germ cell tumors, which is more akin to the situation in human patients [40].

In consecutive years, many new techniques have emerged for gene manipulation and transgene introduction into the zebrafish genome. All these reverse genetic approaches aim to generate a loss-of-function phenotype or they aim to transfer genes found mutated in human cancer patients into the fish. This could also mean creating a zebrafish model with a mutation in an orthologous gene to a human cancer-related phenotype [41]. It has been shown that zebrafish can develop lymphoma, resembling acute T-cell lymphoblastic leukemia (T-ALL), with lymphoid tissue-specific overexpression (under *rag2* promoter) of the mouse *mMyc* oncogene. This was another implication for the field that zebrafish can indeed acquire tumors similar to mammals [42,43]. Tumor induction was observed also in a $rag2:KRAS^{G12D}$ overexpressing zebrafish which developed RMS in time [44]. The tumorigenesis followed by Langenau et al. was even more pronounced when initiated in $tp53^{-/-}$ deficient zebrafish. The developing tumors were transplantable into other zebrafish recipients [42,43]. These studies were the first ones to describe that tumor suppressor genes and oncogenes can recapitulate cancer phenotypes as we know them from patients, in zebrafish. Together with the evidence for evolutionarily conserved drivers of tumorigenesis, this led to the establishment of zebrafish as a model for human cancer pathogenesis. A contemporary model of melanoma in zebrafish has demonstrated the cooperative function of $tp53^{-/-}$ mutation with the activating mutation in the serine/threonine kinase BRAF [45,46]. This transgenic zebrafish expresses the mutated form of $BRAF^{V600E}$ most commonly found in human melanoma under the control of the melanocyte-specific *mitfa* promoter. $BRAF^{V600E}$ on its own is not sufficient to evoke melanoma in zebrafish. Transgenic animals without $tp53^{-/-}$ mutation form nevi. Nevi are sites with high melanocyte proliferation which do not advance into malignant melanoma [45]. Many transplantation studies have used cancer cells derived from $BRAF^{V600E}$-$tp53^{-/-}$ zebrafish and we will review them further in Section 3 of this paper.

TP53 is often concurrently mutated in human cancers bearing *BRCA2* mutations. The tumor suppressor gene *BRCA2* affects both the meiotic and mitotic cell cycle. Recently, *brca2* mutant zebrafish in a *tp53*$^{-/-}$ background were examined for cell cycle arrest and genomic stability. This model, as it is not embryonically lethal compared to many BRCA2 mouse models, allows for in vivo studies in adult animals [47]. In *brca2* mutant zebrafish, it was previously shown that there is an increased incidence of benign testicular tumors [48]. Concurrent mutations of *brca2/tp53* led to soft tissue sarcomas, predominantly to PNSTs. Surprisingly, *brca2* mutation in females significantly reduced the survival rate after they have developed tumors compared to males with the same genotype. This study further supports the link between *brca2* mutation and cancer aneuploidy with poor survival prognosis [47].

Melanoma has been extensively studied in zebrafish since the first description of the *BRAF*^{V600E} model. Melanoma emerges in a form of transformed melanocytes, which are cells derived from the embryonic neural crest and produce pigment. This disease is commonly driven by mutations in *BRAF* and *RAS* in human patients [49]. Melanomic lesion initiation and the mechanism of sporadic melanoma formation was evaluated in zebrafish *crestin:EGFP* expressing embryos and in adults. In embryos, *crestin* is expressed in neural crest cell progenitors and it is re-expressed in melanoma tumors of adult fish. Neural crest cells were shown to be a key element in melanoma initiation in the *BRAF*^{V600E}-*tp53*$^{-/-}$ zebrafish. [50]. RAS signaling is extensively studied in zebrafish as well. There is a zebrafish model of Costello syndrome driven by *HRAS* mutation derived from human patients (*HRAS*^{G12V}). These fish develop craniofacial and spinal abnormalities. Older fish harboring this mutation were prone to tumor formation, including lymphoma, melanoma, or sarcoma [51]. This model has been further upgraded by the Gal4–UAS system and by the melanocyte-specific expression of *HRAS*^{G12V} under the *kita* promoter. The transgenic fish start to develop tumor masses by 2–4 weeks of life so the progress of the disease is relatively fast. Adult tumors show similarities to human melanoma and they are transplantable. This is in contrast to *mitfa* expressing melanocyte progenitors which form melanoma less efficiently in the same Gal4–UAS setup [52]. Another type of *BRAF*^{V600E} driven cancer was characterized more recently in zebrafish. This model of thyroid carcinoma was described in transgenic fish expressing *BRAF*^{V600E} in thyrocytes, under the expression of *thyroglobulin promoter* (*tg*) [53]. Treatment with MEK and BRAF inhibitors suppressed the oncogenesis and restored normal thyroid morphology. The authors propose in this study a novel potential target responsible for *BRAF*^{V600E} driven thyroid follicle transformation in a *TWIST2* zebrafish orthologue—*twist3*. *twist3* is an important transcriptional regulator of epithelial-to-mesenchymal transition (EMT)—a critical process in tumorigenesis, in the acquisition of tumor resistance, and in metastatic spread of tumor cells out of the primary tumor site [33]. Inactivation of this gene led to the suppression of *BRAF*^{V600E}-induced effects and led to thyroid morphology restoration and rescued hormone production [53]. Previously, MITF, a melanocyte-specific transcription factor, has been found to be important in melanoma pathogenesis. The inhibition of its activity leads to a dramatic regression in melanoma growth [54]. Recently, the effect of constitutively activated *HRAS*^{G12V} on microRNAs (miRNAs) expression level was studied. The transgenic *HRAS*^{G12V} zebrafish develops different types of cancer, however, the authors focused on melanoma onset and progression. Activated RAS signaling was found to promote the expression of six different miRNAs. Among them, the most interesting miRNAs are targeting the *jmjd6* gene. *jmjd6* was found to be a critical player in zebrafish melanoma pathogenesis as its increased expression was correlated to more aggressive phenotypes [55]. Zebrafish has also been used to evaluate the effects of mutated *RAS* in the induction of RMS. A mosaic transgenic zebrafish over-expressing the human mutated version of *KRAS*^{G12D} under the *rag2* promoter developed RMS in nearly 50% of cases until adulthood [44]. However, mutation of *KRAS* in human patients leads most often to pancreatic adenocarcinomas. *ptf1a:KRAS*^{G12V} expressing zebrafish was shown to develop invasive exocrine pancreatic cancer which partially resembled the carcinoma found in human [56]. Recently, there has been an update to this study which presents a zebrafish model with inducible expression of *KRAS*^{G12V} that highly recapitulates human pancreatic neoplasia leading to pancreatic adenocarcinoma [57].

Zebrafish has proven to be a good model for the study of hepatocellular carcinoma (HCC). HCC is the prevailing type of liver cancer worldwide. It has been shown in zebrafish that the liver-specific expression of the human ribose-5-phosphate isomerase A (*RPIA*) under the expression of *fabp10a* promoter can mediate hepatocarcinogenesis. These transgenic zebrafish develop HCC. Further, β-catenin signaling is activated which in the end elevated the expression of downstream target genes. Levels of phosphorylated ERK were also elevated in the livers of RPIA transgenic fish. Combination therapy with β-catenin and ERK inhibitors synergistically reduced RPIA-induced cellular proliferation in zebrafish. [58] *RPIA* was found to be a valuable therapeutic target [58]. Many recent studies are looking at the pathogenesis of *KRAS*-driven cancer. A zebrafish model with inducible expression of a mutated version of $KRAS^{V12}$ in the intestine (under the *ifabp* promoter) developed tubular adenoma of the intestine until adulthood [59]. The effects of cancer cachexia, a syndrome affecting cancer patients, which can result in weight loss, muscle wasting, and is predictive of low survival, was studied in an inducible $KRAS^{G12V}$-driven HCC zebrafish model [60]. The effects of overfeeding in these zebrafish were striking. Overfeeding accelerated cancer progress and in the end leptin, an obesity hormone, was found to be upregulated in the hepatocytes of overfed groups with carcinoma. Knockout fish lacking the leptin receptor had better survival rates in HCC as their WT siblings. Chemical targeting of the leptin receptor also increased the survival rate of tumor-bearing fish [60]. Another interesting study has shown that sex hormones have an effect on HCC pathogenesis with males being more susceptible to HCC development as well as having a higher mortality rate than females [61]. A transgenic zebrafish expressing the double oncogene *Myc/xmrk* developed a severe HCC with different progression in males and females. The effects of androgen and estrogen treatment were tested. Androgen could promote cell proliferation and estrogen had an inhibitory effect on cancer cell growth and therefore might have a protective role in HCC [61]. The role of *cyp7a1* in tumor-liver cross-talk was studied in a $kras^{G12D}$-induced zebrafish model of intestinal cancer. $kras^{G12D}$ expression in the posterior intestine resulted in the formation of intestinal tumors which led to liver inflammation, hepatomegaly, and death. This was the result of defective metabolism as anomalies in *cyp7a1* expression can lead to altered cholesterol–bile alcohol flux in zebrafish. This is an illustration of the importance of tumor–organ interactions and generally of the importance of metabolic homeostasis in tumorigenesis [62]. From all of the above-mentioned studies, it is evident that RAS signaling defects are common in various types of cancer and the oncogenic activity of RAS is not limited only to melanoma or sarcoma. BRAF and RAS mutations seem to be mutually exclusive in cancer, however, there are rare cases when these players of the same signaling pathway coincide, which might be interesting for further studies [63,64]. The above-mentioned studies have shown that zebrafish is indeed a reliable model to describe cellular as well as molecular mechanisms of malignancies caused by recognized tumor suppressors and proto-oncogenes such as TP53, BRAF, or RAS.

Hematopoietic programs are strikingly well conserved between human and zebrafish, making it possible to study hematopoietic diseases in fish. Many models of leukemia have already been established in zebrafish. Most of them are based on known human mutations, deletions, or translocations [17,65]. The individual types of leukemia are so diverse, that many of the factors affecting the onset and progression of these types of cancer are still unknown. There have been many studies done in zebrafish since the first model of *Myc*-induced T-ALL [42]. A Cre-lox regulated conditional model of zebrafish T-ALL was developed because the original *rag2-mMyc* expressing zebrafish developed severe disease phenotypes and typically died around three months of age [66]. The underlying causes of myeloid and lymphoid malignancies are very diverse and our understanding of their disease mechanisms is incomplete. Therefore, it is of high interest to have reliable animal models which would allow to better understand the molecular pathogenesis of hematopoietic malignancies. There are classic models of myeloid leukemia in zebrafish, based on chromosomal rearrangements known from humans as well as murine models, based on oncogene mutations or oncogene overexpression [67]. The fusion of *AML1* with *ETO* is one of the most commonly found fusions in acute myeloid leukemia (AML). A zebrafish model with inducible embryonic overexpression of *AML1-ETO* recapitulates the phenotype observed in human patients [68]. Myelo-erythroid progenitor cells are re-programmed and the accumulation of granulocytic cells is observed in this model of AML. The phenotype was treatable and reverted to normal state after the use of Trichostatin A, a histone deacetylase inhibitor [68]. Looking at the classic fusion protein of *AML1-ETO* in another zebrafish study revealed the functional effect of *TLE1* and *TLE4* loss in AML. The authors have found out that *TLE* proteins might have a tumor-suppressive role in the development of myeloid leukemia [69]. In another transgenic zebrafish model of AML, the fusion protein of *MYST3-NCOA2* is expressed under the myeloid cell-specific promoter *spi1*. Only a small amount of fish, about 1%, developed myeloid leukemia until adulthood. Immature myeloid blast cells were accumulating in the kidney of diseased animals [70]. All of the above-mentioned studies were among the first ones to describe AML in the zebrafish model.

Various fusions of *TEL-JAK2* were found in human patients of myeloid or lymphoblastic leukemia. The expression of *tel-jak2a* fusion protein can disrupt normal embryonic hematopoiesis in zebrafish [71]. Different forms of the zebrafish *tel-jak2a* fusion protein were overexpressed in zebrafish myeloid cells. The authors were able to distinguish two phenotypes when they used two distinct versions of *tel-jak2a* fusions in zebrafish. One phenotype was similar to T-ALL and the other one to atypical chronic myelogenous leukemia (CML). The effects of two different types of *TEL-JAK2* fusions generally found in human patients were compared in the zebrafish *tel-jak2a* model. This study has shown that different types of fusions of the same genes can lead to corresponding phenotypes in zebrafish (ALL and CML respectively), as observed in human patients [72].

Receptor tyrosine kinases are important players in hematopoiesis. FMS-like tyrosine kinase 3 (*FLT3*) is crucial in hematopoietic stem and progenitor cells and it plays a role in the development and differentiation of hematopoietic stem cells, dendritic cell progenitors, B-cell progenitors, and natural killer (NK) cells. An internal tandem duplication (ITD) of *FLT3* is found in about 30% of AML patients [73]. The overexpression of human *FLT3*-ITD and *FLT3*-TKD in zebrafish leads to a leukemic phenotype with expanded myelopoiesis during early embryogenesis. The main cell type expanded was monocyte-like, which is typical for AML [74]. A model of myelodysplastic syndrome (MDS) where zebrafish *tet2* (ten-eleven translocation methylcytosine dioxygenase 2) was disrupted, mimics a frequently observed loss-of-function mutation found in humans. These zebrafish developed normally but progressive dysplasia of myeloid progenitors appeared with age [75]. *TET2* encodes a member of the *TET* family of DNA methylcytosine oxidases which mediate demethylation of DNA within genomic CpG islands. The disease developed from pre-myelodysplasia to MDS in adult kidney marrows. The fish had first decreased numbers of erythrocytes and expanded numbers of myelomonocytes and progenitor cells in the marrow but normal peripheral blood counts. With age, they progressed to full MDS with decreased counts of erythrocytes in blood [75]. All the discussed genetic models of cancer with their exact genotypes are summarized in Table 1. A representation of cancer types discussed in this section is depicted in Figure 1 with individual sites of tumors within an adult zebrafish. Further models of tumorigenesis [8,19,76] and leukemia in zebrafish are compiled in other review papers [65,67,77–79].

With this extensive list of transgenic and mutant zebrafish models of cancer, we are not aiming to be fully comprehensive. It is merely a broad demonstration of the fact that nearly any cancer type, from carcinomas through melanoma to leukemia, could be studied in zebrafish. All in all, with properly combining tumor suppressors/oncogenes or their mutated version with tissue-specific promoter expression it is possible to generate cancer in zebrafish which is often closely resembling human cancer phenotypes at the histological and molecular level.

Table 1. Genetic models of cancer in the zebrafish.

Cancer	Genotype	Zebrafish Background	Reference
Peripheral nerve sheath tumor (PNST)	$tp53^{M214K}$ $brca2^{Q658X}$ $tp53^{M214K}$	WT WT or $tp53^{M214K}$	[39] [47]
PNST, angiosarcoma, leukemia, germ cell tumor	$tp53^{del/del}$	CG1 syngeneic zebrafish strain	[40]
Rhabdomyosarcoma (RMS)	$rag2:KRAS^{G12D}$ $rag2:dsRed2$	WT; α-actin:GFP; $tp53^{M214K}$	[43,44]
Melanoma	$BRAF^{V600E}$ $tp53^{M214K}$ $BRAF^{V600E}$ $tp53^{M214K}$ $BRAF^{V600E}$ $mitfa^{vc7}$ $hsp70I:GFP-HRAS^{G12V}$ $kita:GalTA4,UAS:mCherry$ $UAS:eGFP-HRAS^{GV12}$	$tp53^{M214K}$ crestin:EGFP; $tp53^{M214K}$ $mitfa^{vc7}$ N.A. N.A.	[45] [50] [54] [51,55] [52,55]
	$kita:Gal4TA, UAS:mCherry$ $UAS:eGFP-HRAS^{GV12}$ $UAS:eGFP-jmjd6$	WT or $tp53^{M214K}$	[55]
Thyroid cancer	$tg:BRAF^{V600E}$-pA;tg:TdTomato-pA	WT	[53]
Pancreatic cancer	$ptf1a:eGFP-KRAS^{G12V}$ $ptf1a:CRE^{ERT2}$ $ubb:lox-Nuc-eCFP-stop-lox-GAL4-VP16$ $UAS:eGFP-KRAS^{G12V}$	WT N.A.	[56] [57]
Hepatocellular cancer (HCC)	fabp10a: RPIA; myl7:GFP $fabp10:rtTA2s-M2;TRE2:eGFP-kras^{G12V}$ fabp10:TA; TRE:Myc; krt4:GFP fabp10:TA; TRE:xmrk; krt4:GFP	N.A. WT or $lepr^{+/-}$ WT	[58] [60] [61]
Intestinal tumors	$pDs-ifabp:LexPR-Lexop:eGFP-kras^{V12}$ $5\times UAS:EGFP-P2A-kras^{G12D}$ fabp10a:mCherry fabp10a:mCherry-P2A-cyp7a1 + various Gal4 lines	N.A. WT or $cyp7a1^{-5}$	[59] [62]
Testicular tumor	$brca2^{Q658X}$	WT	[48]
T-cell acute lymphoid leukemia (T-ALL)	rag2:mMyc rag2:GFP rag2:dsRed2 rag2:loxP-dsRED2-loxP-eGFP-mMyc spi1:tel-jak2a	WT WT WT	[42,43] [66] [72]
Acute lymphoid leukemia (AML)	hsp70:AML1-ETO spi1:MYST3/NCOA2-eGFP pHsFLT3-WT-T2a-eGFP pHsFLT3-ITD-T2a-eGFP FLT3-ITD-T2a-mRFP	WT N.A. WT	[68,69] [70] [74]
Chronic myeloid leukemia (CML)	spi1:tel-jak2a	WT	[71,72]
Myelodysplastic syndrome (MDS)	$tet2^{-/-}$	cmyb:eGFP; cd41:eGFP	[75]

WT: Wild type; N.A: Not Available.

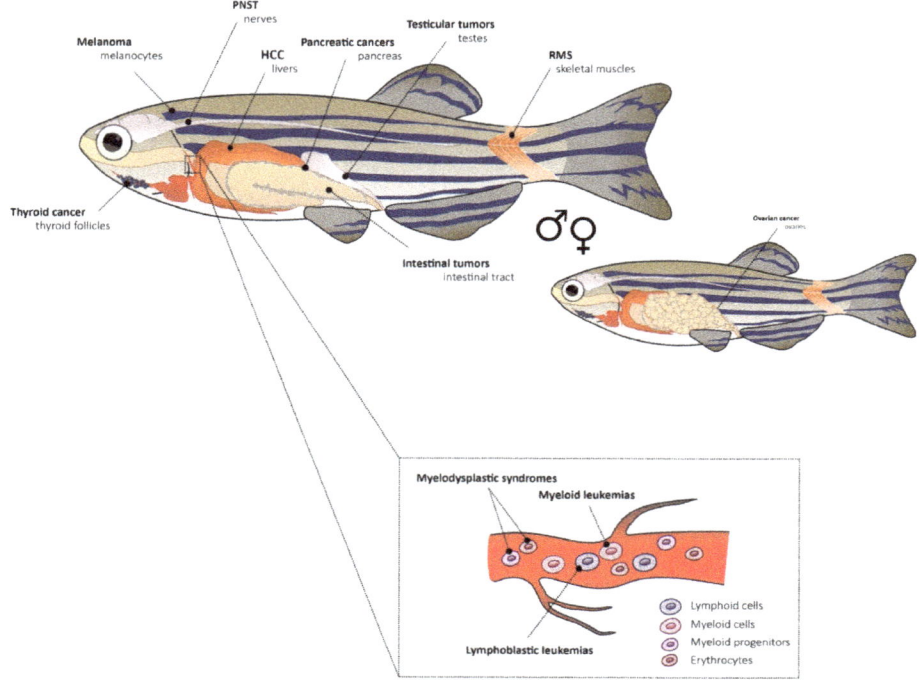

Figure 1. Zebrafish models of cancer. Zebrafish develops cancer phenotypes similar to human cancer in different tissues and organs. All of these cancer types and their zebrafish models are discussed in Section 2. Genetic models of cancer. PNST—peripheral nerve sheath tumor; HCC—hepatocellular carcinoma; RMS—rhabdomyosarcoma; ♂—male; ♀—female.

2.1. Zebrafish and New Methods for Cancer Modelling

In this section, we will discuss in more detail the most popular and widely used gene manipulation techniques which were engaged in the majority of above-discussed zebrafish cancer-modeling studies [80–86]. In zebrafish it is possible to perform forward and reverse genetic screens and directly assess the role of various genes in cancer related phenotypes [87]. Currently, the most widely used techniques for zebrafish gene manipulation are antisense morpholino oligonucleotides (MOs) [83], ZFNs (zinc finger nucleases) [84], TALENs (transcription activator-like effector nucleases), [85] and the CRISPR (clustered regularly interspaced short palindromic repeats) system [86].

MOs are small synthetic oligonucleotides which are able to block mRNA translation in vivo. Zebrafish MO gene knockdown phenotypes were extensively compared to knockout phenotypes over the years. There is a discussion about off-target effects of MOs [88,89] and the fact that they often do not fully copy phenotypes of genome-edited mutants generated by TALENs [90] or CRISPRs [88,91] is concerning. Despite these challenges, MOs are still used in the zebrafish community and with proper validation and with the utilization of appropriate controls they can facilitate the generation of large numbers of experimental embryos really fast. The accepted rule today is to confirm the MO specificity by either repeating the knockdown in $tp53^{-/-}$ mutant embryos or to simultaneously knockdown $tp53$ in morphants [92]. Another substantial drawback of MOs, however, is that they are active only in a short time frame of early embryonic development until they get diluted out [83].

The use of site-directed nucleases is convenient for multiplex gene targeting. This way, the often-complicated disease genotypes could be created in one round of genome editing. Further, it is possible to create not only knock-outs and loss-of-function alleles but also knock-ins, where whole open reading frames can be inserted into the zebrafish genome [93]. As the first tool for targeted mutagenesis in zebrafish ZFN was successfully used in the example of the *golden* gene disruption. The resulting homozygous mutant embryos lacked pigmentation. This study showed that ZFN may be applicable to general gene disruption in zebrafish [84]. There were consequent studies which successfully employed ZFN in targeted mutagenesis. A zebrafish model of neurofibromatosis 1 (NF1) was generated by ZFN targeting of *nf1a* and *nf1b* genes. The mutant embryos exhibited similar phenotypes to the ones observed in NF1 patients, as oligodendrocyte hyperplasia and melanophore hypoplasia [94]. Another example of ZFN utilization in zebrafish is the model of MDS generated by mutating *Tet2* discussed above in Section 2 [75].

TALEN has been overly popular for almost a decade. It was actually in zebrafish where it was shown for the first time that TALENs are able to produce heritable gene disruptions in the vertebrate genome [85]. Bedell et al. [95] updated the TALEN system and created and tested its capabilities to effectively edit the zebrafish genome. *cadherin 5* (*cdh5*) mutant zebrafish was created. It had vascular defects, cardiac edema, and loss of circulating blood cells [95]. An important fact is that TALENs can create mutations in somatic tissues at a high success rate, including bi-allelic mutations. This fact was utilized in a proof of principle study which aimed to analyze the role of somatic mutations of the retinoblastoma (*rb1*) tumor suppressor gene. Genetically mosaic adult mutants developed tumors mostly in the brain. Homozygous germline mutants of *rb1* are embryonically lethal, therefore it is desirable to study the aspects of its somatic inactivation [96]. Brain tumor models, including PNST and medulloblastoma, a type of frequently occurring pediatric brain cancer, were created with the TALEN technology. The *cdkn2a/b* gene was inactivated in the zebrafish $tp53^{-/-}$ background which led to an acceleration in PNST development. The authors also further examined the role of *rb1* somatic inactivation in $tp53^{-/-}$ background. Interestingly, these mutants developed medulloblastoma-like brain tumors specifically [97]. A complete loss-of-function $tp53^{del/del}$ zebrafish deletion mutant was created by TALEN. These animals develop various types of tumors, including PNST, angiosarcoma, leukemia, or germ cell tumors. This is in contrast to the established $tp53^{-/-}$ mutant with the $tp53^{M214K}$ point mutation and it could be explained by the different nature of these two mutations. Tumor onset and pathogenesis might differ based on the nature of *tp53* mutation [40].

The CRISPR/Cas9 technique has evolved quite rapidly in the last five years and has been widely used in the field of zebrafish disease modeling. The Cas9 endonuclease recognizes specific DNA sequences in an RNA-dependent manner. The guide RNA (gRNA) is engineered in a way that it interacts both with the Cas9 enzyme as well as it binds and targets specific parts of genomic DNA [86,98]. A comprehensive study called CRISPRscan provided insight into the mutagenic activity of the CRISPR/Cas9 system in vivo in zebrafish. The study looks at the stability of sgRNAs (single gRNAs), at the specificity of recognized genomic target sequence, and finally at the use of truncated sgRNAs as an efficient alternative to regular sgRNAs [99]. Zebrafish disease models created by CRISPR-based approaches are numerous and widely used today. It is possible to target multiple genes simultaneously with high efficiency. However, the possibility of off-target activity has to be always considered [100]. A recent study of Ablain et al. [101] focused on the identification of cancer driver genes in melanoma. There are still some incompletely described genetic subtypes of melanoma. Specifically, for example, the "triple wild-type" melanoma which lacks mutations in either of the genes usually found mutated - *BRAF*, *NRAS*, and *NF1* genes. Mucosal melanoma, which is discussed in this study, is characterized by genomic instability and a heterogeneous set of mutated genes found in patient samples. *SPRED1* (sprouty-related, EVH1 domain containing protein 1) loss was found as a new driver in mucosal melanoma and the majority of cases with *SPRED1* loss were genetically "triple wild-type" tumors. To evaluate the function of SPRED1 in vivo, zebrafish was used and a new CRISPR-based platform, termed MAZERATI (Modeling Approach in Zebrafish for Rapid Tumor Initiation), was utilized. This system uses two MiniCoopR vectors, one with Cas9 and gRNA expression and the other one expressing the oncogene of interest [101]. One of the main drawbacks of CRISPR/Cas9, and also of the other site-directed nucleases mediated mutagenesis, is the time needed for breeding germline mutants to get a stable line. To be able to screen for loss-of-function phenotypes in F0 founder animals the mutagenesis efficiency would have to be close to 100%. Scientists have tried to overcome this hurdle by assembling Cas9 protein with sgRNA into a ribonucleoprotein complex (RNP) in vitro before injecting it into the cell of zebrafish embryos. This approach led to high mutagenesis rates in target genes with no significant off-target mutagenesis detected. The so-called crispants maintain highly specific mutant phenotypes, however, unpredictable mosaic allele combinations could occur which can hinder phenotype readouts [102]. There is another study which described a similar approach of creating F0 knockout mutants with Cas9 RNP complexes. The authors injected redundant sets of RNPs targeting a single gene and have screened 50 transcription factor genes with this system. In around 90% of F0 embryos, knockout phenotypes were observed. Around 17% of the embryos had morphologic defects indicating toxicity and possible off-target effects but these levels of toxicity were claimed to be acceptable [103].

Novel types of Cas enzymes have been recently discovered in bacterial strains, such as the Cas12a (Cpf1) enzyme. The benefit of Cpf1 is its greater specificity, that it can process a guide RNA array (crRNA) and that a single targeting guide RNA is shorter, compared to Cas9 sgRNAs [104,105]. Cpf1 from *Lachnospiraceae bacterium* (LbCpf1) has been successfully used in zebrafish for genome editing. This enzyme is fully active at 28 °C [106]. New versions of Cas have been developed in vitro, for example the dead version of Cas (dCas). dCas is not enzymatically active but it can be coupled with transcriptional activators (VP64, a synthetic tetramer of the Herpes Simplex Viral Protein) or repressors (KRAB, Kruppel-associated box protein domain). This way it is possible to use CRISPR/Cas for gene up-regulation or down-regulation [100,107].

The conventional zebrafish cancer models, created by either of the above-mentioned techniques, are done by injecting nucleic acids into one-cell stage embryos. There are certain difficulties with addressing cancer development and pathogenesis in these transgenic and mutant animals. In some cases, the onset and localization of developing tumors are not biologically accurate. Furthermore, tumor spread and evaluation of metastases could be difficult. Some of these drawbacks of the genetically engineered models could be addressed with the technique of cancer cell transplantation into zebrafish embryos and adults [19]. We will discuss these approaches in Section 3 of this article. There is, however, a new exciting method, referred to as transgene electroporation in adult zebrafish (TEAZ), which has been recently developed and used for site-specific de novo tumor initiation in zebrafish adults [32]. With this technique it is possible to inject DNA constructs, containing tissue-specific promoters and genes of interest, into adult tissue. The authors have created a model of aggressive melanoma where the tumor onset took only about seven weeks, compared to four months in conventional models. The versatility of TEAZ has been tested in other tissues such as the heart or the brain. This technique is invaluable, as it is rapid and the expression of genes of interest can be spatially and temporally controlled in adult zebrafish [32].

2.2. Zebrafish Cancer Models and Epigenetics

Epigenetic regulators are important factors in development and disease as they regulate gene activation and inhibition. Epigenetic information is reversibly written in the chemical modifications of DNA bases as well as in histone proteins in nucleosomes. The epigenetic machinery consists of transcription factors and chromatin modifiers which regulate gene expression. The disruption of epigenetic mechanisms was shown to be among key drivers of various types of cancer. This dysfunction can be caused by mutations of genes encoding epigenetic regulators. Misbalance can also be caused by exposure to external or internal factors, such as nutrition or inflammation, which can further affect the stability of epigenetic marks [108,109]. Human whole-genome sequencing has revealed recurrent somatic mutations in genes encoding epigenetic regulators, many of them were found to be associated with cancer. In many cases, mutations of epigenetic regulators are the so-called driver mutations which are often present in a specific cancer type. These drivers contribute to cancer pathogenesis to a great extent. In other cases, somatic mutations of epigenetic regulators can represent an additional hit in tumorigenesis which is primarily caused by a mutation of a proto-oncogene or a tumor suppressor [34,110].

Many of the classical models of leukemia, comprising fusion genes, involve an epigenetic regulator as one of the fused genes. This causes deregulation of hematopoiesis and the consequent malignant transformation of cells. For myeloid malignancies, the most prevalent mutations in epigenetic regulators are in *TET2*, isocitrate dehydrogenase 1 and 2 (*IDH1*, *IDH2*), additional sex combs-like 1 (*ASXL1*), enhancer of zeste homolog 2 (*EZH2*), and DNA methyltransferase 3A (*DNMT3A*) [111,112]. As most downstream actions of epigenetic regulators are in theory, reversible, they represent a priority target for therapeutic screens. In the case of solid tumors, there is also evidence about the role of epigenetic regulators in their pathogenesis. There are many cases where the dysfunction of the same epigenetic regulator has a different role in a wide variety of cancers. The development and implementation of a wide array of epigenetic regulator enzyme inhibitors progressed quite fast in the last years. However, it is still a long way to find specificity and selectivity as well as to overcome the pleiotropic effect of these inhibitors outside of the tumor tissue [113–115].

The function of epigenetic regulators is usually not exclusive for a specific tissue, nor cancer type, as mentioned above. Ectopic overexpression of *EZH2* in a benign prostate cancer cell line was shown to act as an oncogene and is correlated with poor prognosis of the disease [116]. On the other hand, the role of EZH2 in myeloid and lymphoid disorders seems to be tumor suppressive. *EZH2* mutations were associated with poor prognosis. EZH2 interacts with other proteins which together form the polycomb repressive complex 2 (PRC2). This suggests that diverse mutations can have different effects on the function of the whole complex, hence the broad number of phenotypes caused by *EZH2* mutations [117]. Interestingly, it has been shown that gain-of-function mutations in the *TP53* tumor suppressor led to a broad upregulation of chromatin remodeling enzymes, for example members of the COMPASS methyltransferase pathway, resulting in an increase of histone acetylation and methylation [118]. A genetic screen done in zebrafish identified the histone H3 lysine 9 histone methyltransferase, *SUV39H1*, out of other chromatin-modifying factors, as a tumor suppressor. This methyltransferase was shown to be important in suppressing RMS formation in *rag2-hKRAS*^{G12D}-induced tumors [80]. The tumor-suppressive role of *SUV39H1* has been shown before in a mouse model of retinoblastoma [119] and this tumor-suppressive role is recapitulated in zebrafish, supporting its importance and evolutionary conservation [80]. The importance of the histone methyltransferase *SETDB1* was shown in a zebrafish model of *BRAF*^{V600E} *tp53*$^{-/-}$ melanoma. The zebrafish used in this study had an additional mutation in *mitfa* and therefore was lacking melanocytes as well as melanoma. The growth of melanocytes in *mitfa:BRAF*^{V600E}; *tp53*$^{-/-}$; *mitfa*$^{-/-}$ fish was rescued with the miniCoopR vector system which simultaneously expressed candidate human genes of interest [81]. *SETDB1* significantly enhanced the aggressiveness of melanoma and accelerated tumor onset. HOX genes were shown to be dysregulated in the presence of upregulated *SETDB1* so *SETDB1* acts as an oncogene in melanoma pathogenesis [81]. Novel epigenetic drug targets have been found thanks to a transgenic zebrafish model of AML expressing the human *NUP98-HOXA9* (*NHA9*) fusion oncogene. These embryos are anemic with myeloid cell expansion and adult animals develop myeloproliferative neoplasms. *NHA9* function depends on downstream activation of *meis1* (*myeloid ecotropic integration site 1*), of the COX (cyclooxygenase) pathway, and of *dnmt1* (*DNA (cytosine-5)-methyltransferase 1*) [82]. The authors used a combination of inhibitors targeting DNMT or COX together with HDAC (histone deacetylase). A strategy for an alternative epigenetic-based treatment of aggressive AML is suggested in this study with zebrafish as a prospective pre-clinical disease model [82]. A study about oncogene drivers in the *rb1* zebrafish model of embryonal brain tumors has found new epigenetic drivers of oncogenesis. Specifically, the authors found more than 170 chromatin regulating genes to be differentially expressed in *rb1* tumors, for example, *histone deacetylase 1* (*hdac1*) and *retinoblastoma binding protein 4* (*rbbp4*) [36]. Zebrafish models of epigenetic regulators involved in cancer are summarized in Table 2.

Table 2. Epigenetic regulators in zebrafish cancer.

Cancer	Zebrafish Genotype	Epigenetic Regulator	Function	Reference
RMS	rag2-hKRAS^{G12D}	SUV39H1	Tumor suppressor	[80]
Melanoma	BRAF^{V600E} tp53^{M214K}	SETDB1	Oncogene	[81]
AML	NUP98-HOXA9	dnmt1	Oncogene	[82]
Retinoblastoma	rb1/rb1	more than 170 tested e.g., hdac1, rbbp4	Oncogenes	[36]

3. Transplantation Models—Allografts and Xenografts

Tumor cell transplantation is a relevant method for tumor invasiveness assessment. Tumor cells from a donor can be grown in a recipient of the same species (allograft) or another species (xenograft). Zebrafish develops cancer, which is invasive and transplantable, in a similar way to humans. Thanks to the natural transparency of zebrafish embryos, and the transparent *casper* strain, it is possible to track and image cancer cell growth in vivo [16]. Zebrafish embryos can engraft transplanted cancer cells until the onset of the adaptive immune system at around seven days post fertilization (dpf). Further maturation of cells leading to immune competence can last until two to four weeks post fertilization [24,28,120]. After surpassing this time window, there are a couple of ways how to deal with the high frequency of transplant rejection when introducing foreign cells into a host organism. The first technique, still widely used, is the sub-lethal irradiation of recipient animals to deplete immune cells in zebrafish [121,122] and mouse [123]. The second way how to introduce and transplant cells from a donor to recipient is to use genetically immunocompromised animals as recipients. This approach has been successfully used for a long time in mouse [5] and the first immunodeficient zebrafish was used for the first time by Tang et al. [124]. These models will be further discussed in the following sections.

3.1. Zebrafish as a Model for Allogeneic Transplantation

The first study describing *mMyc*-induced T-cell leukemia in zebrafish has also shown the possibility to transplant zebrafish leukemic cells into γ-irradiated adult WT zebrafish [42]. Apart from γ-irradiation, it is also possible to decrease the immune response of zebrafish by dexamethasone treatment [125] and there is also a clonal syngeneic zebrafish strain (CG1) which was published as a model for allogeneic tissue and cell engraftment [126]. Transplantation of T-ALL derived cells into syngeneic zebrafish revealed that up to 16% of the transplanted cells are self-renewing and have tumor-initiating potential [127].

Another approach to graft introduction is to employ genetically immunocompromised animals, which lack some or all of the functional cells of the adaptive immune system. Typically, the murine severe combined immunodeficiency (SCID) model has been used for these purposes [5] and other immune-deficient murine models as well [128]. In zebrafish, there are few published immunodeficient strains. The first established immunocompromised zebrafish model harbors a frameshift mutation at amino acid E450 of the *recombination activating gene 2* (*rag2*) gene, resulting in a premature stop codon (*rag2^{E450fs}*). These fish lack mature T-cells and have a reduced number of B cells. The authors used this mutant fish for allograft transplantations into adult fish [124]. Later, a comprehensive study was published about allografts of T-ALL, embryonal RMS, and melanoma in *rag2^{E450fs}* zebrafish in the transparent *casper* background. The authors optimized cell transplantation and were able to follow fluorescently labeled cancer cell growth, tumor formation, and metastasis in adult recipients [129]. A further study published new zebrafish immunodeficient models with affected T-cells, B-cells, and presumptive NK cells. Two zebrafish strains were created in this study. The first, containing a frameshift at aspartic acid residue 3612 resulting in a premature stop codon of the *DNA-dependent protein kinase* (*prkdc^{D3612fs}*), resulted in a lack of T- and B-cells. The other, containing a frameshift at proline residue 369 which leads to a premature stop codon in *janus kinase 3* (*jak3^{P369fs}*), resulted in a lack of T-cells and NK cells [130]. Both mutants were crossed into the *casper* background to allow better options for in vivo imaging of single cells. However, low survival rates were observed after transplantation to the *jak3*^{P369fs} mutant zebrafish. On the contrary, *prkdc*^{D3612fs} mutants are able to engraft allogeneic transplants with high efficiency and survive at high numbers. Unfortunately, probably due to still functional NK cells in this mutant, xenografts of human melanoma, breast cancer nor pancreatic adenocarcinoma cells were able to survive, and their growth in the adult mutant fish regressed a week post-transplantation [130].

In recent years a zebrafish melanoma cancer cell line ZMEL has been widely used to rapidly study melanoma pathogenesis and inhibition. ZMEL was derived from melanomas of the *mitfa-BRAF*^{V600E} *tp53*$^{-/-}$ transgenic fish [131]. ZMELs have been since used for transplantation studies to assess melanoma pathology and metastatic behavior in zebrafish [132]. Hyenne et al. have recently published a paper focusing on the fate of tumor extracellular vesicles (EVs) derived from ZMELs. They show that EVs can be tracked in vivo in zebrafish and that they activate macrophages and promote metastases [133]. Zebrafish models of allogeneic transplantation are summarized in Table 3.

Table 3. Cancer allograft transplantation models in zebrafish.

	Transplanted Cancer Type	Developmental Stage	Injection Site	Reference
Primary cells	T-ALL	Adult	Intraperitoneal cavity	[42,66,124,127]
	RMS	Adult	Intraperitoneal cavity	[124,127]
	Melanoma	Adult	Intraperitoneal cavity	[124]
	T-ALL, RMS, melanoma, neuroblastoma	Adult	Intraperitoneal cavity, retro-orbital, intramuscular	[129,130]
	Melanoma	Adult	N.A.	[131]
ZMELs	Melanoma	Adult	Subcutaneous	[131]
		48 h post-fertilization (hpf)	Circulation (duct of Cuvier)	
		Adult	Retro-orbital Intravenous (cardinal vein)	[132]
		48 hpf	Circulation	[133]

3.2. Zebrafish Xenotransplantation Model for the Evaluation of Cancer Progress and Metastasis

Zebrafish as a tool in human cancer xenotransplantation studies could overcome some of the drawbacks of the murine model. The main benefits of zebrafish are most prominent when using embryonal stages for xenotransplantation. With the small-sized transparent embryos lacking a mature immune system, it is possible to transplant and track high numbers of animals. This fact is a powerful reason for the utilization of zebrafish as a pre-clinical screening model which could lead to patient-derived cancer cell xenotransplantation and to new options for personalized medicine [19]. Most of the recent transplantation studies in zebrafish use embryonal stages of 48 hours post fertilization (hpf) as the stage for transplantation. However, some of the first zebrafish xenograft studies were done in the blastula stage of the embryo. Transplanted melanoma cells survived, divided, stayed in de-differentiated stage but did not form tumors in zebrafish embryos. This was the first observation of human melanoma cells in zebrafish [134]. In a study utilizing the same type of melanoma xenotransplantation into zebrafish blastula, the authors compared different types of human cutaneous and uveal melanoma cancer cell lines. They found out that aggressive melanoma cells secrete Nodal. The expression of Nodal correlated with melanoma aggressiveness and progression, and caused developmental defects of the zebrafish embryo [135]. Haldi et al. optimized the parameters for zebrafish xenotransplantation where they propose the 48 hpf developmental stage as the best for transplantation. At this stage, developmental cell migration is finished, therefore cancer cell migration after injection is likely to be an active process. Human melanoma cells together with other types of cancer cell lines, which they transplanted into zebrafish, were able to survive and formed tumors in the embryo [136]. The site of transplantation might be variable but usually it is the yolk sac, cardinal vein,

Duct of Cuvier, or the hindbrain. Depending on the site of transplantation different phenotypes of tumorigenesis could be followed, for example, cancer cell invasion, extravasation, and metastasis [137], or the interaction of cells with the tumor microenvironment [138]. The importance of increased incubation temperature of zebrafish embryos after xenotransplantation should not be discounted as temperature was shown to be critical for achieving efficient cancer cell proliferation rates [139]. The first study which showed that zebrafish could be used for human PDX provided a simple and fast method for testing the metastatic behavior of primary cancer cells. The authors used a whole set of cancer cell lines as well as primary human cancer cells from pancreas, colon, and stomach carcinomas. Tumor cell invasion and micrometastasis were evaluated and followed in vivo also thanks to the *fli1:eGFP* zebrafish strain with fluorescently labeled vasculature [140]. It is obvious from the studies mentioned above, that zebrafish embryos can engraft human cancer cells and recapitulate disease pathogenesis. Therefore, PDX studies in zebrafish are emerging more often and they can be valuable in accelerating the design of personalized cancer therapy.

Zebrafish has been used to study the tumor microenvironment from the point of tumor-induced angiogenesis. Tumor neovascularization is an important element in tumor growth and metastatic spread. Cancer cells are releasing angiogenic growth factors into the tumor environment which promote neovascularization. Zebrafish embryos enable real-time in vivo visualization of the first steps of tumor neovascularization. *VEGFR2:G-RCFP* transgenic zebrafish embryos with green endothelial cells were transplanted with tumorigenic FGF2-overexpressing mouse aortic endothelial cells and various human cancer cells. The authors showed neovascularization at the tumor site and were able to discriminate between highly and poorly angiogenic tumor cells. The site of transplantation was by the yolk sac, close to the subintestinal veins (SIVs) which originate from the duct of Cuvier. These results were comparable to the effects seen in mouse [141,142]. The contribution of $VEGFR2^+$ individual endothelial cells to the formation of the tumor vascular network was assessed in the *flk1:EGFP* transgenic zebrafish with fluorescently labeled blood vessels. SU5416, a VEGFR2 inhibitor, significantly inhibited the growth and vascularization of murine melanoma xenografts in zebrafish. There was almost no effect on normal vessel formation [143]. Angiogenesis and anti-angiogenic miRNAs have been studied in a zebrafish prostate cancer cell xenograft [144]. Recently, stellettin B, a naturally occurring marine triterpenoid, was tested in a zebrafish xenograft model of glioblastoma. Stellettin B was shown to significantly inhibit angiogenesis in vitro as well as in vivo in zebrafish [145]. There is a recent paper focusing on human melanoma xenotransplantation and the role of interleukin 8 (*CXCL8*) together with *bcl-xL* on cancer cell dissemination and angiogenesis in the zebrafish. The authors suggest that the autocrine CXCL8/CXCR2 signaling pathway can escalate melanoma aggressiveness [146]. These studies have shown that zebrafish is a good in vivo model for rapid identification of inhibitors which could have significance in the development of antiangiogenic cancer therapy.

As we have already discussed in Section 2 of this review, the conservation of hematopoietic programs between human and zebrafish is remarkable. Corkery et al. transplanted human leukemic cancer cell lines into *casper*. The cells, circulating in the embryonic vasculature, were able to proliferate in vivo and survived until 7 dpf in the embryos. The authors have tested treatment with known inhibitors of leukemic cell growth, such as imatinib mesylate, in vivo. There was a significant decrease in the number of leukemic cells in treated groups compared to controls [147]. Another study looked into pathogenesis and inhibition of human leukemic cell growth but added $CD34^+$ leukemic blast cells sorted from blood of AML patients. The xenografted cancer cells were able to survive in zebrafish and were inhibited by imatinib and other antileukemic drugs [148]. Patient-derived T-ALL was successfully engrafted in zebrafish where specific drug response was determined in vivo. The authors identified a gain-of-function *NOTCH1* mutation in patient derived T-ALL primary cells. These cells were sensitive to γ-secretase inhibition [149]. Multiple myeloma (MM) has been studied in zebrafish where the authors evaluated various therapeutic agents after transplanting human MM cell lines as well as primary $CD138^+$ MM cells derived from patients. The cells were able to survive, grow, and disseminate in *casper* and they responded to inhibitors. Furthermore, patient-derived cells responded well to the same drugs such as the ones used in patients. This way it might be possible to use zebrafish PDX to assess drug efficacy and sensitivity [150]. Cancer progress is often characterized by cell dissemination and subsequent homing to the bone marrow. Sacco et al. xenotransplanted human bone marrow-derived MM cells or MM cell lines. The authors then followed cell homing into the area of caudal hematopoietic tissue (CHT), which is the region of zebrafish embryonal hematopoiesis and could represent a bone marrow-like niche. The cells homing to CHT had differentially expressed genes, regulating for example cell adhesion or angiogenesis [151].

Zebrafish has proven to be a good model for the study of human breast and prostate cancer tumorigenesis and invasion. The lack of genetic models of de novo cancers of this type in zebrafish, because of missing mammary glands and prostate tissue, are compensated by xenotransplantation studies. Many of the following studies use seemingly unrelated types of cancer cell lines, however, the authors are usually trying to find correlations between in vitro and in vivo invasion abilities and general pathogenesis as well as the potential of cancer cells to metastasize in vivo. In the last decade, the most commonly studied types of solid tumors in zebrafish are melanoma [152], breast, prostate, colon, and pancreatic cancers [153] and glioblastoma [154]. Here, we will walk through the course of time and illustrate on the diversity of xenograft studies how zebrafish contributed to our understanding of tumorigenesis and helped to describe new potential therapeutics.

Eguiara et al. have developed a rapid assay for cancer stem-like cell identification in a zebrafish breast cancer xenograft model. Cells, which were first grown in culture in mammospheres, were more invasive in zebrafish embryos than cells grown in a monolayer. Curcumin treated cells showed significantly decreased migration and tumor formation in vivo [25]. It has been shown that the zebrafish genome contains estrogen-responsive genes and that estrogen-related signaling pathways are relevant compared to humans. Therefore, zebrafish can be a model for estrogen-dependent cancer research, and estrogen responsiveness is highly conserved between zebrafish and humans [155]. Ghotra et al. developed a whole animal imaging assay for following cancer metastasis and dissemination in vivo in zebrafish. The behavior of xenografted cancer cells corresponded to findings from rodent models. The authors compared highly and low malignant cell lines of breast, colorectal, and prostate cancer. Their results suggest that E-cadherin silencing by shRNA boosted breast carcinoma cell dissemination. [156]. Breast cancer invasiveness is known to be controlled by the transforming growth factor beta (TGF-β) signaling pathway. Metastatic properties of different breast cancer cell lines were assessed for their invasiveness and malignity after xenotransplantation into zebrafish. Inhibition of TGF-β signaling with TGF-β receptor kinase inhibitors prevented the invasion of cancer cells, which correlated with findings from a mouse metastasis model [157]. TGF-β induced EMT was further investigated in a zebrafish model of breast cancer metastasis. The transcription factors Snail and Slug have been found to be important in the process of EMT regulation. The authors claim that overexpression of Snail and Slug could promote metastasis and the invasion of single cancer cells in vivo [158]. However, this signaling pathway and its effects on cancer cell migration seem to be more complicated. Integrins represent a class of receptor proteins promoting adhesion and cell proliferation. Integrins are interesting therapeutic targets in breast cancer treatment. Disruption of $β_1$ integrin mediates cell adhesion, triggers TGF-β signaling, and EMT. It was revealed that the loss of the $β_1$ integrin subunit can block breast tumor growth but also enhance the dissemination of tumor cells [159]. A specific prometastatic switch has been described in E-cadherin positive triple-negative breast cancer (TNBC) cells. The balance between miR-200 microRNAs and the transcription factor zinc finger E-box-binding homeobox 2 (ZEB2) appears to be important for TGF-β signaling and modulates cell survival, proliferation, and migration. The authors suggested reconsidering the use of drugs targeting $β_1$ integrins in TNBC [159]. The role of bone morphogene proteins (BMP) in breast cancer pathogenesis is less well described than that of TGF-β. BMP signaling is regulated by different Smad proteins located downstream in the signaling pathway. BMP signaling was shown to exert anti-metastatic signals in breast cancer cells. [160].

The CXCR4-CXCL12 signaling axis has also been studied in a zebrafish TNBC xenograft model. As TNBC is a highly aggressive type of breast cancer with limited treatment option it is essential to explore new treatment alternatives. The authors have shown that human cancer cells expressing CXCR4 could recognize zebrafish ligands and as a result, they initiate early metastasis. Chemical inhibition by IT1t, a CXCR4 antagonist, blocked TNBC metastasis and thus CXCR4 was proposed as a new pharmacological target in TNBC [161]. Recently, a further role of CXCR4 signaling was described in tumor–immune cell communication. Specifically, the role of neutrophil motility in the onset of micrometastasis formation was shown to be dependent on CXCR4 signaling [162].

It is widely accepted that the ability of cancer cells for self-renewal, also termed stemness, is a marker of highly proliferative, aggressive, dedifferentiated tumor cells. These cells often overexpress marker genes typically found active in embryonic stem cells, such as SOX2 and OCT4 [163,164]. The role of AKT and SOX2 in breast carcinoma was evaluated in zebrafish. AKT can stabilize SOX2 in breast carcinoma cells and CSCs seem to be dependent on AKT signaling. Therefore, inhibiting AKT might provide a new way of targeting SOX2 positive breast carcinoma cells [165].

Mercatali et al. used PDX from bone metastasis of a breast cancer patient and compared the behavior of PDX to established breast cancer cell lines. Primary cells from patients extravasated from vessels and invaded into the CHT of zebrafish. Therefore, zebrafish might be a good preclinical model to identify breast cancer prognostic markers as well as to predict response to therapy [166].

The most commonly found cancer type in males is prostate cancer. To achieve the best results in prostate cancer treatment, it is desirable to detect it in early stages, when it is prostate-confined. The effect of a nonreceptor spleen tyrosine kinase *SYK* on the dissemination of prostate cancer cells has been studied in a zebrafish and mouse xenograft model. The role of *SYK* in epithelial cancer is divergent. Silencing of *SYK* prevented cancer cell dissemination in vitro and in vivo and pharmacological inhibition of *SYK* led to a similar decrease in cancer invasiveness [167]. In another study, the androgen-dependent LNCaP prostate cancer cell line was xenotransplanted into zebrafish. Administration of exogenous testosterone to LNCaP xenografted zebrafish increased cancer cell proliferation compared to controls. This effect was reversed by the anti-androgen receptor drug, enzalutamide. In contrast, the proliferation of a non-androgen-dependent prostate cancer cell line was not affected by testosterone or enzalutamide treatment. The authors suggested that testosterone administration should be considered in zebrafish xenograft studies of prostate cancer [168]. The invasiveness of the PC3 prostate cancer cell line in zebrafish was recently evaluated and it was suggested as a good model for drug targeted screening for prostate cancer. PC3 cells in this study overexpressed calcitonin receptor (CTR), which led to overall enhanced aggressiveness. The authors have looked for prostate cancer-specific markers to better describe and to detect prostate cancer in patients early [169].

Zebrafish as a model for retinoblastoma [170] and glioblastoma [154,171–174] has been popular in the last couple of years. Many of these studies highlight the significance of zebrafish in finding novel treatment targets and evaluating cancer inhibitor efficacy in vivo. Glioblastoma is a very heterogeneous and complex type of cancer and is invasive. Despite surgical resection, radiotherapy, and aggressive treatment survival rates are low and the prognosis often negative [175].

Zebrafish has been also recently used as a model of colorectal carcinoma in search of new treatment methods. Marine guanidine alkaloids [176], clinically standard combinatorial therapy [27] as well as bromelain, a pineapple extract [177], have been tested in zebrafish colorectal cancer xenografts. Despite gastric cancers being among the leading cancer types in terms of death rates worldwide, there are not many models of gastric cancer in zebrafish. Recently, two studies described the possibilities to search for a potential treatment of gastric cancer in zebrafish xenografts. Wu et al. have tested chemotherapeutic treatments on primary cancer cells derived from gastric cancer patients in zebrafish. Their PDX model was shown to be reliable and looks promising in searching for personalized treatment [178]. In another study concerning gastric carcinoma Triphala, a traditional medicinal formulation was tested. Triphala has inhibited the growth of xenografted cells and their metastasis, probably through inhibiting the phosphorylation of EGFR/Akt/ERK signaling cascade proteins [179]. Human oral squamous cell carcinoma has also been studied in the zebrafish xenograft model. The authors have investigated the effects of sandensolide, extracted from the herb *Sinularia flexibilis*. Sandensolide can induce apoptosis and could be used as a supporting agent in the treatment of oral cancer [180].

Although zebrafish do not have lungs it can recapitulate cancer-tumor microenvironment interactions reliably. A human non-small-cell lung cancer (NSCLC) xenograft model has been used to study the efficacy as well as the toxicity of three anti-angiogenic drugs. All tested compounds showed anti-angiogenic effects and the inhibition of tumor growth in zebrafish. [181]. Another study revealed the role of autophagy in zebrafish NSCLC xenografts. The authors demonstrated that the combined use of a sub-lethal dose of C2-ceramide and autophagy inhibitors could be promising in NSCLC treatment [182].

The zebrafish model is a good platform for studying rare cancer pathogenesis, for example, Ewing sarcoma (EWS). EWS is rare aggressive childhood cancer. The most commonly found gene fusion in this cancer is *EWSR1–ETS*. New combination therapy was proposed in a zebrafish xenograft model of EWS. Nutlin-3, a *tp53* activator, and YK-4-279, a EWSR1–ETS inhibitor, were shown to be a promising combination therapy for a subset of EWS patients [183].

Transplantation of human cancer cells into zebrafish is an established technique which provides in vivo environment for real-time visualization of cell–cell interactions. Furthermore, zebrafish PDX can support the discovery of potential targeted anti-cancer treatments. Recent successes in zebrafish PDX might help pre-clinical research to significantly shorten the time needed for drug approval, mostly by drug repurposing. Zebrafish models of human cancer xenotransplantation are summarized in Table 4.

Table 4. Human cancer xenograft transplantation models in zebrafish.

	Transplanted Cancer Type	Developmental Stage	Injection Site	Reference
Cell lines	Melanoma	Blastula	Blastodisc	[134]
	Melanoma (uveal and cutaneous)	Blastula	N.A.	[135]
	Melanoma and colorectal cancer	48 h post-fertilization (hpf)	Yolk sac; hindbrain ventricle; circulation	[136]
	Uveal melanoma	48 hpf	Yolk sac	[152]
	Melanoma	48 hpf	Yolk sac	[146]
	Colorectal cancer	48 hpf	Yolk sac	[139]
	Colorectal cancer	48 hpf	Yolk sac	[27,176,177]
	Pancreatic cancer	48 hpf	Yolk sac	[140]
	Melanoma, adenocarcinoma, triple negative breast cancer (TNBC) and ovarian cancer	48 hpf	Yolk sac, proximity of subintestinal veins (SIV)	[141,142]
	Colorectal cancer, melanoma (both murine)	48 hpf	Yolk sac	[143]
	Prostate cancer	48 hpf	Yolk sac	[144,167]
	Prostate cancer, androgen dependent and independent	48 hpf	Yolk sac	[168]
	Prostate cancer	48 hpf	Subcutaneous, above yol sack	[169]
	Breast, prostate, colon, pancreatic cancer, fibrosarcoma	48 hpf	Yolk sac	[153]
	Breast cancer	48 hpf	Yolk sac	[25]
	Breast, prostate, colorectal cancer	48 hpf	Yolk sac	[156]
	Breast cancer, non-invasive and metastatic	48 hpf	Duct of Cuvier	[157]
	Breast cancer	48 hpf	Duct of Cuvier	[158]
	Breast cancer	48 hpf	Yolk sac	[159]
	Breast adenocarcinoma and TNBC	48 hpf	Duct of Cuvier	[161]
	TNBC and prostate cancer	48 hpf	Duct of Cuvier	[162]
	Breast cancer	48 hpf	Yolk sac	[165]
	Breast cancer and TNBC	48 hpf	Duct of Cuvier	[166]
	TNBC	48 hpf	Duct of Cuvier	[165]
	AML, CML	48 hpf	Yolk sac	[147]

Table 4. Cont.

	Transplanted Cancer Type	Developmental Stage	Injection Site	Reference
Cell lines	AML, T-ALL	48 hpf	Posterior cardinal vein (PCV)	[148]
	T-ALL	48 hpf	Yolk sac	[149]
	Multiple myeloma (MM)	48 hpf	Yolk sac	[150]
	MM, Waldenstrom's macroglobulinemia, TNBC	48 hpf	Pericardium	[151]
	CML, HCC, prostate cancer (sorted for cancer stem cells)	48 hpf / Adult	Yolk sac / Trunk near dorsal aorta	[184]
	AML, HCC	48 hpf / Adult	Yolk sac / Trunk near dorsal aorta; heart	[185]
	Retinoblastoma	48 hpf	Vitreous cavity	[170]
	Glioblastoma	52 hpf	Yolk sack; brain	[154]
	Glioblastoma	36 hpf	Hindbrain	[171]
	Glioblastoma	72 hpf	Brain	[172]
	Glioblastoma and colon cancer	Blastula	Blastoderm	[174]
	Gastrointestinal tumors – pancreas, stomach, colon	48 hpf	Yolk sac; liver	[140]
	Gastric cancer	48 hpf	Yolk sac	[178,179]
	Oral squamous cell carcinoma	48 hpf	Yolk sac	[180]
	Non-small-cell lung cancer (NSCLC)	48 hpf	Yolk sac	[181]
	NCSLC	48 hpf	N.A.	[182]
	Ewing sarcoma (EWS)	48 hpf / Juvenile (35 dpf)	Yolk sac / Eye vessels	[183]
	Various types of human cancer	Adult	Intraperitoneal cavity Peri-ocular muscle	[186]
PDX	AML blast cells	48 hpf	PCV	[148]
	T-ALL from bone marrow	48 hpf	Yolk sac	[149]
	MM cells from plasma	48 hpf	Yolk sac	[150]
	MM cells from bone marrow	48 hpf	Pericardium	[151]
	Glioblastoma	36 hpf	Brain	[173]
	Glioblastoma	blastula	Blastoderm	[174]
	Gastric cancer	48 hpf	Yolk sac	[178]
	Glioblastoma, melanoma, breast cancer, RMS	Adult	Peri-ocular muscle	[186]

3.3. Drug Screening in Zebrafish and Its Future as a Pre-clinical Model

Drug screening in zebrafish has become highly popular over the last 10 years. Previously, high-throughput screening for new drugs was basically conducted in vitro in cultured cells and the hits were taken to rodent models where they often failed, proving to be either ineffective or toxic. It is not trivial to assess all biological properties and characteristics of a compound in vitro without having information from the whole animal [19]. Zebrafish embryonal screens can be carried out at a medium (manual cancer cell transplantation) to high throughput (automated yolk sac cancer cell transplantation, de novo cancer, or cancer-related biological pathways) rates, however, the limiting factor is that not all of the steps could be easily automated. Therefore, compound screens exceeding 1000 compounds have not been done on xenograft zebrafish models, but they were focused more on targeting specific cancer biology related pathways in zebrafish embryos [28,187]. For example, a library of 2000 compounds was tested for inhibition of angiogenesis in zebrafish embryos. Among seven hit compounds, rosuvastatin was further characterized for its antiangiogenic and antineoplastic effects in vitro as well as in vivo in mouse prostate cancer xenografts [188]. In a similar screening study, zebrafish was used to look for neural crest cell growth inhibitors. Leflunomide, an inhibitor of dihydroorotate dehydrogenase, was found as a hit inhibiting also the growth of human melanoma cells, which are originally derived from the embryonic neural crest [189]. Ridges et al. performed a drug screen focused on compounds which are able to eliminate immature T-cells and therefore, prospective for eradicating T-ALL cells as well. For this purpose, they used the *lck:eGFP* transgenic zebrafish line with fluorescently labeled thymic T-cells. After finding primary compound hits which reduced the number of T-cells significantly, these compounds were tested in a human T-ALL cell line. Lenaldekar, a compound with previously unknown biological activity, was identified. Further, its activity was validated in adult T-ALL zebrafish and in a murine xenograft model [190]. A further study looking for potential T-ALL inhibitors in the zebrafish *Myc*-induced T-ALL model was based on hits found in cell culture. An antipsychotic drug targeting protein phosphatase 2A (PP2A), perphenazine, was found to be highly effective in suppressing T-ALL cell growth [191]. Recently, clotrimazol has been discovered as a potential cure for melanoma. The authors further described the effects of clotrimazole co-treatment with other oncogene-specific inhibitors, as Lonafarnib, in vivo in zebrafish [192].

In this way, further potential inhibitors for cancer treatment were identified in zebrafish compound screens, with suggested antineoplastic features mediated by cell cycle delay [193], anti-angiogenic [145,194,195], or anti-lymphangiogenic [196] effects. This approach to compound screening, however, usually requires detailed knowledge about the exact disease pathogenesis and about the target pathway or at least about the biological process which is disordered. Drug treatment is usually done easily by dispensing chemotherapeutics into the fish water as embryos can absorb small molecules dissolved in water. However, it might be difficult to treat zebrafish with water-insoluble drugs, because the carrier solvents for efficient administration may be toxic. For long-term administration of therapeutics in adult zebrafish, a specific protocol for oral gavage has been published [197] and successfully used [186]. Measurement of cancer cell growth can be partially automated as well, by using an automated fluorescent microscopy strategy [156,184]. Using compound libraries containing FDA approved drugs leads to drug repurposing and could accelerate the translation of hits from zebrafish screens to the clinic as in the case of perphenazine [191,198]. Zebrafish has been used as a preclinical model for characterization of nanomedicines as well [199].

The zebrafish cancer xenograft model is an excellent alternative for studying tumor progression and for testing novel therapeutics even in the absence of appropriate transgenic models. Despite lacking tissues such as lung, prostate, or mammary gland, many xenotransplantation studies have proved that zebrafish can recapitulate tumor phenotypes seen in humans, as discussed in the previous section. The effects on tumor microenvironment, as well as the process of metastasis, can be followed real-time and in vivo in zebrafish. The only hurdle which had to be overcome was finding a way for reliable xenotransplantation into adult zebrafish, where the previous immunocompromised models have failed [124,130] and γ-irradiation can be demanding. Cancer stem-like cells (CSCs) have been used for xenotransplantation in adult *casper* immunocompromised by ionizing radiation [184]. In this study, leukemic cells, human prostate cancer cells, as well as liver cancer cells were sorted for high aldehyde dehydrogenase (ALDH) expression. ALDH expression is one of the markers widely used for sorting CSCs from bulk populations of cancer cells. These CSCs were able to rapidly grow in recipients and it was possible to re-transplant them. The authors have established a CSC xenotransplantation model in zebrafish which they suggested as suitable for drug screening purposes [184]. Khan et al. have used busulfan treatment in a recent study and were able to successfully xenograft AML cells and HCC cells into adult zebrafish. The cancer cells survived in the fish for up to 15 days post transplantation [185]. A new double mutant immunodeficient zebrafish model suitable for cancer xenotransplantation was published only recently. This fish has the $prkdc^{D3612fs/D3612fs}$ mutation together with the mutated $l2rga^{Y91fs/Y91fs}$ gene [186]. This combination of mutations is currently widely used also in murine xenograft models [200]. Yan et al. have developed specific procedures for adult immunodeficient zebrafish xenotransplantation, maintenance, treatment, and tumor growth evaluation. They have transplanted a wide variety of cancer cell lines as well as patient-derived primary cancer cells and compared their results from xenografted adult fish to results from xenografted mice. Their results seem to be very promising and this model of adult zebrafish xenografts, mainly PDX, might be valuable in the future of cancer research as a reliable pre-clinical model comparable to the mouse [186]. Altogether, the significance of zebrafish as a preclinical model for cancer research is undoubtful. The high reproductive rate of zebrafish and the relatively low-cost maintenance enables high-throughput whole animal screening. There are other papers extensively reviewing zebrafish as a model for cancer cell transplantation [26,33,76] and as a pre-clinical model in drug discovery [28,201].

4. Conclusions

Zebrafish has proven to be reliable for modeling and visualizing human cancer cell biology and dynamics, including metastases or tumor tissue neo-angiogenesis, in vivo. Further, the involvement of epigenetic modulators in tumor biology could improve our understanding of such complex diseases as cancer. The availability of transgenic and mutant models, as well as the possibility to transplant cancer cells into zebrafish, provides a wide array of options for studying human cancer. Although zebrafish is a non-mammalian model organism, it has striking evolutionary conservation of disease-related genes and pathways with humans. Searching for novel drugs could be done in vitro at large scale but the effects on the whole living organism might be markedly different. Screening for targeted treatment in zebrafish xenografts could provide new opportunities for anticancer personalized therapy in the future as recent research has shown that zebrafish studies are reliable in modeling human cancer.

Funding: This research was funded by the Czech Science Foundation, grant number 18-18363S, Ministry of Education, Youth and Sports, grant number LO1419, MH was partially funded by the Grant Agency of the Charles University, grant number 1380217.

Acknowledgments: We would like to thank Ivana Dobiášovská for her work on the figure for this review paper. Further, we would like to thank Dr. Trevor Epp for his comments and proofreading of the manuscript.

Conflicts of Interest: The authors declare no conflict of interest.

References

1. Hanahan, D.; Weinberg, R.A. Hallmarks of cancer: The next generation. *Cell* **2011**, *144*, 646–674. [CrossRef] [PubMed]
2. Mroz, E.A.; Rocco, J.W. The challenges of tumor genetic diversity. *Cancer* **2017**, *123*, 917–927. [CrossRef] [PubMed]
3. Grzywa, T.M.; Paskal, W.; Wlodarski, P.K. Intratumor and Intertumor Heterogeneity in Melanoma. *Transl. Oncol.* **2017**, *10*, 956–975. [CrossRef] [PubMed]
4. Cagan, R.L.; Zon, L.I.; White, R.M. Modeling Cancer with Flies and Fish. *Dev. Cell* **2019**, *49*, 317–324. [CrossRef] [PubMed]
5. McCune, J.M.; Namikawa, R.; Kaneshima, H.; Shultz, L.D.; Lieberman, M.; Weissman, I.L. The SCID-hu mouse: Murine model for the analysis of human hematolymphoid differentiation and function. *Science* **1988**, *241*, 1632–1639. [CrossRef] [PubMed]
6. Bock, B.C.; Stein, U.; Schmitt, C.A.; Augustin, H.G. Mouse models of human cancer. *Cancer Res.* **2014**, *74*, 4671–4675. [CrossRef]
7. Capasso, A.; Lang, J.; Pitts, T.M.; Jordan, K.R.; Lieu, C.H.; Davis, S.L.; Diamond, J.R.; Kopetz, S.; Barbee, J.; Peterson, J.; et al. Characterization of immune responses to anti-PD-1 mono and combination immunotherapy in hematopoietic humanized mice implanted with tumor xenografts. *J. Immunother. Cancer* **2019**, *7*, 37. [CrossRef]
8. van der Weyden, L.; Patton, E.E.; Wood, G.A.; Foote, A.K.; Brenn, T.; Arends, M.J.; Adams, D.J. Cross-species models of human melanoma. *J. Pathol.* **2016**, *238*, 152–165. [CrossRef]
9. Kucinska, M.; Murias, M.; Nowak-Sliwinska, P. Beyond mouse cancer models: Three-dimensional human-relevant in vitro and non-mammalian in vivo models for photodynamic therapy. *Mutat. Res.* **2017**, *773*, 242–262. [CrossRef]
10. Sarasamma, S.; Lai, Y.H.; Liang, S.T.; Liu, K.; Hsiao, C.D. The Power of Fish Models to Elucidate Skin Cancer Pathogenesis and Impact the Discovery of New Therapeutic Opportunities. *Int. J. Mol. Sci.* **2018**, *19*, 3929. [CrossRef]
11. Schartl, M.; Walter, R.B. Xiphophorus and Medaka Cancer Models. *Adv. Exp. Med. Biol.* **2016**, *916*, 531–552. [PubMed]
12. Hyodo-Taguchi, Y.; Matsudaira, H. Induction of transplantable melanoma by treatment with N-methyl-N'-nitro-N-nitrosoguanidine in an inbred strain of the teleost *Oryzias latipes*. *J. Natl. Cancer Inst.* **1984**, *73*, 1219–1227. [PubMed]
13. Kimmel, C.B.; Ballard, W.W.; Kimmel, S.R.; Ullmann, B.; Schilling, T.F. Stages of embryonic development of the zebrafish. *Dev. Dyn.* **1995**, *203*, 253–310. [CrossRef] [PubMed]

14. Haffter, P.; Granato, M.; Brand, M.; Mullins, M.C.; Hammerschmidt, M.; Kane, D.A.; Odenthal, J.; van Eeden, F.J.; Jiang, Y.J.; Heisenberg, C.P.; et al. The identification of genes with unique and essential functions in the development of the zebrafish, *Danio rerio. Development* **1996**, *123*, 1–36. [PubMed]
15. White, R.; Rose, K.; Zon, L. Zebrafish cancer: The state of the art and the path forward. *Nat. Rev. Cancer* **2013**, *13*, 624–636. [CrossRef]
16. White, R.M.; Sessa, A.; Burke, C.; Bowman, T.; LeBlanc, J.; Ceol, C.; Bourque, C.; Dovey, M.; Goessling, W.; Burns, C.E.; et al. Transparent adult zebrafish as a tool for in vivo transplantation analysis. *Cell Stem Cell* **2008**, *2*, 183–189. [CrossRef]
17. Payne, E.; Look, T. Zebrafish modelling of leukaemias. *Br. J. Haematol.* **2009**, *146*, 247–256. [CrossRef]
18. Veinotte, C.J.; Dellaire, G.; Berman, J.N. Hooking the big one: The potential of zebrafish xenotransplantation to reform cancer drug screening in the genomic era. *Dis. Models Mech.* **2014**, *7*, 745–754. [CrossRef]
19. Kirchberger, S.; Sturtzel, C.; Pascoal, S.; Distel, M. Quo natas, Danio?-Recent Progress in Modeling Cancer in Zebrafish. *Front. Oncol.* **2017**, *7*, 186. [CrossRef]
20. Mathias, J.R.; Dodd, M.E.; Walters, K.B.; Yoo, S.K.; Ranheim, E.A.; Huttenlocher, A. Characterization of zebrafish larval inflammatory macrophages. *Dev. Comp. Immunol.* **2009**, *33*, 1212–1217. [CrossRef]
21. Ellett, F.; Pase, L.; Hayman, J.W.; Andrianopoulos, A.; Lieschke, G.J. mpeg1 promoter transgenes direct macrophage-lineage expression in zebrafish. *Blood* **2011**, *117*, E49–E56. [CrossRef] [PubMed]
22. He, S.; Lamers, G.E.; Beenakker, J.W.; Cui, C.; Ghotra, V.P.; Danen, E.H.; Meijer, A.H.; Spaink, H.P.; Snaar-Jagalska, B.E. Neutrophil-mediated experimental metastasis is enhanced by VEGFR inhibition in a zebrafish xenograft model. *J. Pathol.* **2012**, *227*, 431–445. [CrossRef] [PubMed]
23. Howe, K.; Clark, M.D.; Torroja, C.F.; Torrance, J.; Berthelot, C.; Muffato, M.; Collins, J.E.; Humphray, S.; McLaren, K.; Matthews, L.; et al. The zebrafish reference genome sequence and its relationship to the human genome. *Nature* **2013**, *496*, 498–503. [CrossRef] [PubMed]
24. Taylor, A.M.; Zon, L.I. Zebrafish tumor assays: The state of transplantation. *Zebrafish* **2009**, *6*, 339–346. [CrossRef] [PubMed]
25. Eguiara, A.; Holgado, O.; Beloqui, I.; Abalde, L.; Sanchez, Y.; Callol, C.; Martin, A.G. Xenografts in zebrafish embryos as a rapid functional assay for breast cancer stem-like cell identification. *Cell Cycle* **2011**, *10*, 3751–3757. [CrossRef] [PubMed]
26. Brown, H.K.; Schiavone, K.; Tazzyman, S.; Heymann, D.; Chico, T.J. Zebrafish xenograft models of cancer and metastasis for drug discovery. *Expert Opin. Drug Discov.* **2017**, *12*, 379–389. [CrossRef] [PubMed]
27. Fior, R.; Póvoa, V.; Mendes, R.V.; Carvalho, T.; Gomes, A.; Figueiredo, N.; Ferreira, M.G. Single-cell functional and chemosensitive profiling of combinatorial colorectal therapy in zebrafish xenografts. *Proc. Natl. Acad. Sci. USA* **2017**, *114*, E8234–E8243. [CrossRef] [PubMed]
28. Letrado, P.; de Miguel, I.; Lamberto, I.; Diez-Martinez, R.; Oyarzabal, J. Zebrafish: Speeding Up the Cancer Drug Discovery Process. *Cancer Res.* **2018**, *78*, 6048–6058. [CrossRef]
29. Spence, R.; Gerlach, G.; Lawrence, C.; Smith, C. The behaviour and ecology of the zebrafish, *Danio rerio*. *Biol. Rev.* **2008**, *83*, 13–34. [CrossRef]
30. Force, A.; Lynch, M.; Pickett, F.B.; Amores, A.; Yan, Y.L.; Postlethwait, J. Preservation of duplicate genes by complementary, degenerative mutations. *Genetics* **1999**, *151*, 1531–1545.
31. Taylor, J.S.; Braasch, I.; Frickey, T.; Meyer, A.; Van de Peer, Y. Genome duplication, a trait shared by 22,000 species of ray-finned fish. *Genome Res.* **2003**, *13*, 382–390. [CrossRef] [PubMed]
32. Callahan, S.J.; Tepan, S.; Zhang, Y.M.; Lindsay, H.; Burger, A.; Campbell, N.R.; Kim, I.S.; Hollmann, T.J.; Studer, L.; Mosimann, C.; et al. Cancer modeling by Transgene Electroporation in Adult Zebrafish (TEAZ). *Dis. Models Mech.* **2018**, *11*, dmm034561. [CrossRef] [PubMed]
33. Stuelten, C.H.; Parent, C.A.; Montell, D.J. Cell motility in cancer invasion and metastasis: Insights from simple model organisms. *Nat. Rev. Cancer* **2018**, *18*, 296–312. [CrossRef]
34. Dawson, M.A.; Kouzarides, T. Cancer Epigenetics: From Mechanism to Therapy. *Cell* **2012**, *150*, 12–27. [CrossRef] [PubMed]
35. Chernyavskaya, Y.; Kent, B.; Sadler, K.C. Zebrafish Discoveries in Cancer Epigenetics. *Adv. Exp. Med. Biol.* **2016**, *916*, 169–197. [PubMed]
36. Schultz, L.E.; Haltom, J.A.; Almeida, M.P.; Wierson, W.A.; Solin, S.L.; Weiss, T.J.; Helmer, J.A.; Sandquist, E.J.; Shive, H.R.; McGrail, M. Epigenetic regulators Rbbp4 and Hdac1 are overexpressed in a zebrafish model of

RB1 embryonal brain tumor, and are required for neural progenitor survival and proliferation. *Dis. Models Mech.* **2018**, *11*, dmm034124. [CrossRef]

37. Beckwith, L.G.; Moore, J.L.; Tsao-Wu, G.S.; Harshbarger, J.C.; Cheng, K.C. Ethylnitrosourea induces neoplasia in zebrafish (*Danio rerio*). *Labor. Investig.* **2000**, *80*, 379–385. [CrossRef]
38. Spitsbergen, J.M.; Tsai, H.W.; Reddy, A.; Miller, T.; Arbogast, D.; Hendricks, J.D.; Bailey, G.S. Neoplasia in zebrafish (*Danio rerio*) treated with N-methyl-N'-nitro-N-nitrosoguanidine by three exposure routes at different developmental stages. *Toxicol. Pathol.* **2000**, *28*, 716–725. [CrossRef]
39. Berghmans, S.; Murphey, R.D.; Wienholds, E.; Neuberg, D.; Kutok, J.L.; Fletcher, C.D.; Morris, J.P.; Liu, T.X.; Schulte-Merker, S.; Kanki, J.P.; et al. tp53 mutant zebrafish develop malignant peripheral nerve sheath tumors. *Proc. Natl. Acad. Sci. USA* **2005**, *102*, 407–412. [CrossRef]
40. Ignatius, M.S.; Hayes, M.N.; Moore, F.E.; Tang, Q.; Garcia, S.P.; Blackburn, P.R.; Baxi, K.; Wang, L.; Jin, A.; Ramakrishnan, A.; et al. tp53 deficiency causes a wide tumor spectrum and increases embryonal rhabdomyosarcoma metastasis in zebrafish. *Elife* **2018**, *7*, e37202. [CrossRef]
41. Koster, R.; Sassen, W.A. A molecular toolbox for genetic manipulation of zebrafish. *Adv. Genom. Genet.* **2015**, *5*, 151. [CrossRef]
42. Langenau, D.M.; Traver, D.; Ferrando, A.A.; Kutok, J.L.; Aster, J.C.; Kanki, J.P.; Lin, S.; Prochownik, E.; Trede, N.S.; Zon, L.I.; et al. Myc-induced T cell leukemia in transgenic zebrafish. *Science* **2003**, *299*, 887–890. [CrossRef] [PubMed]
43. Langenau, D.M.; Keefe, M.D.; Storer, N.Y.; Jette, C.A.; Smith, A.C.; Ceol, C.J.; Bourque, C.; Look, A.T.; Zon, L.I. Co-injection strategies to modify radiation sensitivity and tumor initiation in transgenic Zebrafish. *Oncogene* **2008**, *27*, 4242–4248. [CrossRef] [PubMed]
44. Langenau, D.M.; Keefe, M.D.; Storer, N.Y.; Guyon, J.R.; Kutok, J.L.; Le, X.; Goessling, W.; Neuberg, D.S.; Kunkel, L.M.; Zon, L.I. Effects of RAS on the genesis of embryonal rhabdomyosarcoma. *Genes Dev.* **2007**, *21*, 1382–1395. [CrossRef]
45. Patton, E.E.; Widlund, H.R.; Kutok, J.L.; Kopani, K.R.; Amatruda, J.F.; Murphey, R.D.; Berghmans, S.; Mayhall, E.A.; Traver, D.; Fletcher, C.D.; et al. BRAF mutations are sufficient to promote nevi formation and cooperate with p53 in the genesis of melanoma. *Curr. Biol.* **2005**, *15*, 249–254. [CrossRef]
46. Patton, E.E.; Zon, L.I. Taking human cancer genes to the fish: A transgenic model of melanoma in zebrafish. *Zebrafish* **2005**, *1*, 363–368. [CrossRef]
47. Mensah, L.; Ferguson, J.L.; Shive, H.R. Genotypic and Phenotypic Variables Affect Meiotic Cell Cycle Progression, Tumor Ploidy, and Cancer-Associated Mortality in a *brca2*-Mutant Zebrafish Model. *J. Oncol.* **2019**, *2019*, 9218251. [CrossRef]
48. Shive, H.R.; West, R.R.; Embree, L.J.; Azuma, M.; Sood, R.; Liu, P.; Hickstein, D.D. *brca2* in zebrafish ovarian development, spermatogenesis, and tumorigenesis. *Proc. Natl. Acad. Sci. USA* **2010**, *107*, 19350–19355. [CrossRef]
49. Mort, R.L.; Jackson, I.J.; Patton, E.E. The melanocyte lineage in development and disease. *Development* **2015**, *142*, 1387. [CrossRef]
50. Kaufman, C.K.; Mosimann, C.; Fan, Z.P.; Yang, S.; Thomas, A.J.; Ablain, J.; Tan, J.L.; Fogley, R.D.; van Rooijen, E.; Hagedorn, E.J.; et al. A zebrafish melanoma model reveals emergence of neural crest identity during melanoma initiation. *Science* **2016**, *351*, aad2197. [CrossRef]
51. Santoriello, C.; Deflorian, G.; Pezzimenti, F.; Kawakami, K.; Lanfrancone, L.; d'Adda di Fagagna, F.; Mione, M. Expression of H-RASV12 in a zebrafish model of Costello syndrome causes cellular senescence in adult proliferating cells. *Dis. Models Mech.* **2009**, *2*, 56–67. [CrossRef] [PubMed]
52. Santoriello, C.; Gennaro, E.; Anelli, V.; Distel, M.; Kelly, A.; Köster, R.W.; Hurlstone, A.; Mione, M. Kita Driven Expression of Oncogenic HRAS Leads to Early Onset and Highly Penetrant Melanoma in Zebrafish. *PLoS ONE* **2010**, *5*, e15170. [CrossRef] [PubMed]
53. Anelli, V.; Villefranc, J.A.; Chhangawala, S.; Martinez-McFaline, R.; Riva, E.; Nguyen, A.; Verma, A.; Bareja, R.; Chen, Z.; Scognamiglio, T.; et al. Oncogenic BRAF disrupts thyroid morphogenesis and function via twist expression. *Elife* **2017**, *6*, e20728. [CrossRef] [PubMed]
54. Lister, J.A.; Capper, A.; Zeng, Z.; Mathers, M.E.; Richardson, J.; Paranthaman, K.; Jackson, I.J.; Patton, E.E. A conditional zebrafish MITF mutation reveals MITF levels are critical for melanoma promotion vs. regression in vivo. *J. Investig. Dermatol.* **2014**, *134*, 133–140. [CrossRef] [PubMed]

55. Anelli, V.; Ordas, A.; Kneitz, S.; Sagredo, L.M.; Gourain, V.; Schartl, M.; Meijer, A.H.; Mione, M. Ras-Induced miR-146a and 193a Target Jmjd6 to Regulate Melanoma Progression. *Front. Genet.* **2018**, *9*, 675. [CrossRef]
56. Park, S.W.; Davison, J.M.; Rhee, J.; Hruban, R.H.; Maitra, A.; Leach, S.D. Oncogenic KRAS Induces Progenitor Cell Expansion and Malignant Transformation in Zebrafish Exocrine Pancreas. *Gastroenterology* **2008**, *134*, 2080–2090. [CrossRef]
57. Park, J.T.; Leach, S.D. Zebrafish model of KRAS-initiated pancreatic cancer. *Anim. Cells Syst.* **2018**, *22*, 353–359. [CrossRef]
58. Chou, Y.T.; Chen, L.Y.; Tsai, S.L.; Tu, H.C.; Lu, J.W.; Ciou, S.C.; Wang, H.D.; Yuh, C.H. Ribose-5-Phosphate Isomerase a Overexpression Promotes Liver Cancer Development in Transgenic Zebrafish via Activation of ERK and beta-catenin Pathways. *Carcinogenesis* **2018**, *40*, 461–473. [CrossRef]
59. Lu, J.W.; Raghuram, D.; Fong, P.A.; Gong, Z. Inducible Intestine-Specific Expression of kras(V12) Triggers Intestinal Tumorigenesis in Transgenic Zebrafish. *Neoplasia* **2018**, *20*, 1187–1197. [CrossRef]
60. Yang, Q.; Yan, C.; Wang, X.; Gong, Z. Leptin induces muscle wasting in a zebrafish *kras*-driven hepatocellular carcinoma (HCC) model. *Dis. Models Mech.* **2019**, *12*, dmm038240. [CrossRef]
61. Li, H.; Lu, J.W.; Huo, X.; Li, Y.; Li, Z.; Gong, Z. Effects of sex hormones on liver tumor progression and regression in Myc/xmrk double oncogene transgenic zebrafish. *Gen. Comp. Endocrinol.* **2019**, *277*, 112–121. [CrossRef] [PubMed]
62. Enya, S.; Kawakami, K.; Suzuki, Y.; Kawaoka, S. A novel zebrafish intestinal tumor model reveals a role for cyp7a1-dependent tumor-liver crosstalk in causing adverse effects on the host. *Dis. Models Mech.* **2018**, *11*, dmm032383. [CrossRef] [PubMed]
63. Ceol, C.J.; Houvras, Y.; White, R.M.; Zon, L.I. Melanoma biology and the promise of zebrafish. *Zebrafish* **2008**, *5*, 247–255. [CrossRef] [PubMed]
64. Davies, H.; Bignell, G.R.; Cox, C.; Stephens, P.; Edkins, S.; Clegg, S.; Teague, J.; Woffendin, H.; Garnett, M.J.; Bottomley, W.; et al. Mutations of the BRAF gene in human cancer. *Nature* **2002**, *417*, 949–954. [CrossRef]
65. He, S.; Jing, C.B.; Look, A.T. Zebrafish models of leukemia. *Methods Cell Biol.* **2017**, *138*, 563–592.
66. Langenau, D.M.; Feng, H.; Berghmans, S.; Kanki, J.P.; Kutok, J.L.; Look, A.T. Cre/lox-regulated transgenic zebrafish model with conditional myc-induced T cell acute lymphoblastic leukemia. *Proc. Natl. Acad. Sci. USA* **2005**, *102*, 6068–6073. [CrossRef]
67. Potts, K.S.; Bowman, T.V. Modeling Myeloid Malignancies Using Zebrafish. *Front. Oncol.* **2017**, *7*, 297. [CrossRef]
68. Yeh, J.R.; Munson, K.M.; Chao, Y.L.; Peterson, Q.P.; Macrae, C.A.; Peterson, R.T. AML1-ETO reprograms hematopoietic cell fate by downregulating scl expression. *Development* **2008**, *135*, 401–410. [CrossRef]
69. Dayyani, F.; Wang, J.; Yeh, J.R.; Ahn, E.Y.; Tobey, E.; Zhang, D.E.; Bernstein, I.D.; Peterson, R.T.; Sweetser, D.A. Loss of TLE1 and TLE4 from the del(9q) commonly deleted region in AML cooperates with AML1-ETO to affect myeloid cell proliferation and survival. *Blood* **2008**, *111*, 4338–4347. [CrossRef]
70. Zhuravleva, J.; Paggetti, J.; Martin, L.; Hammann, A.; Solary, E.; Bastie, J.N.; Delva, L. MOZ/TIF2-induced acute myeloid leukaemia in transgenic fish. *Br. J. Haematol.* **2008**, *143*, 378–382. [CrossRef]
71. Onnebo, S.M.; Condron, M.M.; McPhee, D.O.; Lieschke, G.J.; Ward, A.C. Hematopoietic perturbation in zebrafish expressing a tel-jak2a fusion. *Exp. Hematol.* **2005**, *33*, 182–188. [CrossRef] [PubMed]
72. Onnebo, S.M.; Rasighaemi, P.; Kumar, J.; Liongue, C.; Ward, A.C. Alternative TEL-JAK2 fusions associated with T-cell acute lymphoblastic leukemia and atypical chronic myelogenous leukemia dissected in zebrafish. *Haematologica* **2012**, *97*, 1895–1903. [CrossRef] [PubMed]
73. Chen, Y.; Pan, Y.; Guo, Y.; Zhao, W.; Ho, W.T.; Wang, J.; Xu, M.; Yang, F.C.; Zhao, Z.J. Tyrosine kinase inhibitors targeting FLT3 in the treatment of acute myeloid leukemia. *Stem Cell Investig.* **2017**, *4*, 48. [CrossRef] [PubMed]
74. He, B.L.; Shi, X.; Man, C.H.; Ma, A.C.; Ekker, S.C.; Chow, H.C.; So, C.W.; Choi, W.W.; Zhang, W.; Zhang, Y.; et al. Functions of flt3 in zebrafish hematopoiesis and its relevance to human acute myeloid leukemia. *Blood* **2014**, *123*, 2518–2529. [CrossRef] [PubMed]
75. Gjini, E.; Mansour, M.R.; Sander, J.D.; Moritz, N.; Nguyen, A.T.; Kesarsing, M.; Gans, E.; He, S.; Chen, S.; Ko, M.; et al. A zebrafish model of myelodysplastic syndrome produced through tet2 genomic editing. *Mol. Cell. Biol.* **2015**, *35*, 789–804. [CrossRef]
76. Idilli, A.I.; Precazzini, F.; Mione, M.C.; Anelli, V. Zebrafish in Translational Cancer Research: Insight into Leukemia, Melanoma, Glioma and Endocrine Tumor Biology. *Genes* **2017**, *8*, 236. [CrossRef]

77. Lu, J.W.; Hsieh, M.S.; Liao, H.A.; Yang, Y.J.; Ho, Y.J.; Lin, L.I. Zebrafish as a Model for the Study of Human Myeloid Malignancies. *BioMed Res. Int.* **2015**, *2015*, 641475. [CrossRef]
78. Rasighaemi, P.; Basheer, F.; Liongue, C.; Ward, A.C. Zebrafish as a model for leukemia and other hematopoietic disorders. *J. Hematol. Oncol.* **2015**, *8*, 29. [CrossRef]
79. Baeten, J.T.; de Jong, J.L.O. Genetic Models of Leukemia in Zebrafish. *Front. Cell Dev. Biol.* **2018**, *6*, 115. [CrossRef]
80. Albacker, C.E.; Storer, N.Y.; Langdon, E.M.; Dibiase, A.; Zhou, Y.; Langenau, D.M.; Zon, L.I. The histone methyltransferase SUV39H1 suppresses embryonal rhabdomyosarcoma formation in zebrafish. *PLoS ONE* **2013**, *8*, e64969. [CrossRef]
81. Ceol, C.J.; Houvras, Y.; Jane-Valbuena, J.; Bilodeau, S.; Orlando, D.A.; Battisti, V.; Fritsch, L.; Lin, W.M.; Hollmann, T.J.; Ferre, F.; et al. The histone methyltransferase SETDB1 is recurrently amplified in melanoma and accelerates its onset. *Nature* **2011**, *471*, 513–517. [CrossRef] [PubMed]
82. Deveau, A.P.; Forrester, A.M.; Coombs, A.J.; Wagner, G.S.; Grabher, C.; Chute, I.C.; Leger, D.; Mingay, M.; Alexe, G.; Rajan, V.; et al. Epigenetic therapy restores normal hematopoiesis in a zebrafish model of NUP98-HOXA9-induced myeloid disease. *Leukemia* **2015**, *29*, 2086–2097. [CrossRef] [PubMed]
83. Nasevicius, A.; Ekker, S.C. Effective targeted gene 'knockdown' in zebrafish. *Nat. Genet.* **2000**, *26*, 216–220. [CrossRef] [PubMed]
84. Doyon, Y.; McCammon, J.M.; Miller, J.C.; Faraji, F.; Ngo, C.; Katibah, G.E.; Amora, R.; Hocking, T.D.; Zhang, L.; Rebar, E.J.; et al. Heritable targeted gene disruption in zebrafish using designed zinc-finger nucleases. *Nat. Biotechnol.* **2008**, *26*, 702–708. [CrossRef]
85. Huang, P.; Xiao, A.; Zhou, M.; Zhu, Z.; Lin, S.; Zhang, B. Heritable gene targeting in zebrafish using customized TALENs. *Nat. Biotechnol.* **2011**, *29*, 699–700. [CrossRef]
86. Ablain, J.; Durand, E.M.; Yang, S.; Zhou, Y.; Zon, L.I. A CRISPR/Cas9 vector system for tissue-specific gene disruption in zebrafish. *Dev. Cell* **2015**, *32*, 756–764. [CrossRef]
87. Amatruda, J.F.; Shepard, J.L.; Stern, H.M.; Zon, L.I. Zebrafish as a cancer model system. *Cancer Cell* **2002**, *1*, 229–231. [CrossRef]
88. Kok, F.O.; Shin, M.; Ni, C.W.; Gupta, A.; Grosse, A.S.; van Impel, A.; Kirchmaier, B.C.; Peterson-Maduro, J.; Kourkoulis, G.; Male, I.; et al. Reverse Genetic Screening Reveals Poor Correlation between Morpholino-Induced and Mutant Phenotypes in Zebrafish. *Dev. Cell* **2015**, *32*, 97–108. [CrossRef]
89. Stainier, D.Y.; Kontarakis, Z.; Rossi, A. Making sense of anti-sense data. *Dev. Cell* **2015**, *32*, 7–8. [CrossRef]
90. Eve, A.M.; Place, E.S.; Smith, J.C. Comparison of Zebrafish *tmem88a* mutant and morpholino knockdown phenotypes. *PLoS ONE* **2017**, *12*, e0172227. [CrossRef]
91. Rossi, A.; Kontarakis, Z.; Gerri, C.; Nolte, H.; Holper, S.; Kruger, M.; Stainier, D.Y. Genetic compensation induced by deleterious mutations but not gene knockdowns. *Nature* **2015**, *524*, 230–233. [CrossRef] [PubMed]
92. Bolli, N.; Payne, E.M.; Grabher, C.; Lee, J.S.; Johnston, A.B.; Falini, B.; Kanki, J.P.; Look, A.T. Expression of the cytoplasmic NPM1 mutant (NPMc+) causes the expansion of hematopoietic cells in zebrafish. *Blood* **2010**, *115*, 3329–3340. [CrossRef] [PubMed]
93. Auer, T.O.; Del Bene, F. CRISPR/Cas9 and TALEN-mediated knock-in approaches in zebrafish. *Methods* **2014**, *69*, 142–150. [CrossRef]
94. Shin, J.; Padmanabhan, A.; de Groh, E.D.; Lee, J.S.; Haidar, S.; Dahlberg, S.; Guo, F.; He, S.; Wolman, M.A.; Granato, M.; et al. Zebrafish neurofibromatosis type 1 genes have redundant functions in tumorigenesis and embryonic development. *Dis. Models Mech.* **2012**, *5*, 881–894. [CrossRef] [PubMed]
95. Bedell, V.M.; Wang, Y.; Campbell, J.M.; Poshusta, T.L.; Starker, C.G.; Krug, R.G., 2nd; Tan, W.; Penheiter, S.G.; Ma, A.C.; Leung, A.Y.; et al. In vivo genome editing using a high-efficiency TALEN system. *Nature* **2012**, *491*, 114–118. [CrossRef]
96. Solin, S.L.; Shive, H.R.; Woolard, K.D.; Essner, J.J.; McGrail, M. Rapid tumor induction in zebrafish by TALEN-mediated somatic inactivation of the *retinoblastoma1* tumor suppressor rb1. *Sci. Rep.* **2015**, *5*, 13745. [CrossRef]
97. Shim, J.; Choi, J.H.; Park, M.H.; Kim, H.; Kim, J.H.; Kim, S.Y.; Hong, D.; Kim, S.; Lee, J.E.; Kim, C.H.; et al. Development of zebrafish medulloblastoma-like PNET model by TALEN-mediated somatic gene inactivation. *Oncotarget* **2017**, *8*, 55280–55297. [CrossRef]
98. Yin, L.; Maddison, L.A.; Chen, W. Multiplex conditional mutagenesis in zebrafish using the CRISPR/Cas system. *Methods Cell Biol.* **2016**, *135*, 3–17.

99. Moreno-Mateos, M.A.; Vejnar, C.E.; Beaudoin, J.D.; Fernandez, J.P.; Mis, E.K.; Khokha, M.K.; Giraldez, A.J. CRISPRscan: Designing highly efficient sgRNAs for CRISPR-Cas9 targeting in vivo. *Nat. Methods* **2015**, *12*, 982–988. [CrossRef]
100. Liu, K.; Petree, C.; Requena, T.; Varshney, P.; Varshney, G.K. Expanding the CRISPR Toolbox in Zebrafish for Studying Development and Disease. *Front. Cell Dev. Biol.* **2019**, *7*, 13. [CrossRef]
101. Ablain, J.; Xu, M.; Rothschild, H.; Jordan, R.C.; Mito, J.K.; Daniels, B.H.; Bell, C.F.; Joseph, N.M.; Wu, H.; Bastian, B.C.; et al. Human tumor genomics and zebrafish modeling identify SPRED1 loss as a driver of mucosal melanoma. *Science* **2018**, *362*, 1055–1060. [CrossRef]
102. Burger, A.; Lindsay, H.; Felker, A.; Hess, C.; Anders, C.; Chiavacci, E.; Zaugg, J.; Weber, L.M.; Catena, R.; Jinek, M.; et al. Maximizing mutagenesis with solubilized CRISPR-Cas9 ribonucleoprotein complexes. *Development* **2016**, *143*, 2025–2037. [CrossRef]
103. Wu, W.Y.; Lebbink, J.H.G.; Kanaar, R.; Geijsen, N.; van der Oost, J. Genome editing by natural and engineered CRISPR-associated nucleases. *Nat. Chem. Biol.* **2018**, *14*, 642–651. [CrossRef]
104. Kleinstiver, B.P.; Sousa, A.A.; Walton, R.T.; Tak, Y.E.; Hsu, J.Y.; Clement, K.; Welch, M.M.; Horng, J.E.; Malagon-Lopez, J.; Scarfo, I.; et al. Engineered CRISPR-Cas12a variants with increased activities and improved targeting ranges for gene, epigenetic and base editing. *Nat. Biotechnol.* **2019**, *37*, 276–282. [CrossRef]
105. Liu, P.; Luk, K.; Shin, M.; Idrizi, F.; Kwok, S.; Roscoe, B.; Mintzer, E.; Suresh, S.; Morrison, K.; Frazao, J.B.; et al. Enhanced Cas12a editing in mammalian cells and zebrafish. *Nucleic Acids Res.* **2019**, *47*, 4169–4180. [CrossRef]
106. Fernandez, J.P.; Vejnar, C.E.; Giraldez, A.J.; Rouet, R.; Moreno-Mateos, M.A. Optimized CRISPR-Cpf1 system for genome editing in zebrafish. *Methods* **2018**, *150*, 11–18. [CrossRef]
107. Liao, H.K.; Hatanaka, F.; Araoka, T.; Reddy, P.; Wu, M.Z.; Sui, Y.; Yamauchi, T.; Sakurai, M.; O'Keefe, D.D.; Nunez-Delicado, E.; et al. In Vivo Target Gene Activation via CRISPR/Cas9-Mediated Trans-epigenetic Modulation. *Cell* **2017**, *171*, 1495–1507. [CrossRef]
108. Plass, C.; Pfister, S.M.; Lindroth, A.M.; Bogatyrova, O.; Claus, R.; Lichter, P. Mutations in regulators of the epigenome and their connections to global chromatin patterns in cancer. *Nat. Rev. Genet.* **2013**, *14*, 765–780. [CrossRef]
109. Herceg, Z.; Ghantous, A.; Wild, C.P.; Sklias, A.; Casati, L.; Duthie, S.J.; Fry, R.; Issa, J.P.; Kellermayer, R.; Koturbash, I.; et al. Roadmap for investigating epigenome deregulation and environmental origins of cancer. *Int. J. Cancer* **2018**, *142*, 874–882. [CrossRef]
110. Wee, S.; Dhanak, D.; Li, H.; Armstrong, S.A.; Copeland, R.A.; Sims, R.; Baylin, S.B.; Liu, X.S.; Schweizer, L. Targeting epigenetic regulators for cancer therapy. *Ann. N. Y. Acad. Sci.* **2014**, *1309*, 30–36. [CrossRef]
111. Grimwade, D.; Ivey, A.; Huntly, B.J. Molecular landscape of acute myeloid leukemia in younger adults and its clinical relevance. *Blood* **2016**, *127*, 29–41. [CrossRef]
112. Shih, A.H.; Meydan, C.; Shank, K.; Garrett-Bakelman, F.E.; Ward, P.S.; Intlekofer, A.; Nazir, A.; Stein, E.; Knapp, K.; Glass, J.; et al. Combination Targeted Therapy to Disrupt Aberrant Oncogenic Signaling and Reverse Epigenetic Dysfunction in *IDH2*- and *TET2*-Mutant Acute Myeloid Leukemia. *Cancer Discov.* **2017**, *7*, 494–505. [CrossRef]
113. Kelly, A.D.; Issa, J.J. The promise of epigenetic therapy: Reprogramming the cancer epigenome. *Curr. Opin. Genet. Dev.* **2017**, *42*, 68–77. [CrossRef]
114. Aspeslagh, S.; Morel, D.; Soria, J.C.; Postel-Vinay, S. Epigenetic modifiers as new immunomodulatory therapies in solid tumours. *Ann. Oncol.* **2018**, *29*, 812–824. [CrossRef]
115. Wang, L.; Zhao, Z.; Ozark, P.A.; Fantini, D.; Marshall, S.A.; Rendleman, E.J.; Cozzolino, K.A.; Louis, N.; He, X.; Morgan, M.A.; et al. Resetting the epigenetic balance of Polycomb and COMPASS function at enhancers for cancer therapy. *Nat. Med.* **2018**, *24*, 758–769. [CrossRef]
116. Karanikolas, B.D.; Figueiredo, M.L.; Wu, L. Polycomb group protein enhancer of zeste 2 is an oncogene that promotes the neoplastic transformation of a benign prostatic epithelial cell line. *Mol. Cancer Res. MCR* **2009**, *7*, 1456–1465. [CrossRef]
117. Ernst, T.; Chase, A.J.; Score, J.; Hidalgo-Curtis, C.E.; Bryant, C.; Jones, A.V.; Waghorn, K.; Zoi, K.; Ross, F.M.; Reiter, A.; et al. Inactivating mutations of the histone methyltransferase gene EZH2 in myeloid disorders. *Nat. Genet.* **2010**, *42*, 722–726. [CrossRef]

118. Zhu, J.; Sammons, M.A.; Donahue, G.; Dou, Z.; Vedadi, M.; Getlik, M.; Barsyte-Lovejoy, D.; Al-awar, R.; Katona, B.W.; Shilatifard, A.; et al. Gain-of-function p53 mutants co-opt chromatin pathways to drive cancer growth. *Nature* **2015**, *525*, 206–211. [CrossRef]
119. Shamma, A.; Takegami, Y.; Miki, T.; Kitajima, S.; Noda, M.; Obara, T.; Okamoto, T.; Takahashi, C. Rb Regulates DNA damage response and cellular senescence through E2F-dependent suppression of N-ras isoprenylation. *Cancer Cell* **2009**, *15*, 255–269. [CrossRef]
120. Lam, S.H.; Chua, H.L.; Gong, Z.; Lam, T.J.; Sin, Y.M. Development and maturation of the immune system in zebrafish, Danio rerio: A gene expression profiling, in situ hybridization and immunological study. *Dev. Comp. Immunol.* **2004**, *28*, 9–28. [CrossRef]
121. Traver, D.; Winzeler, A.; Stern, H.M.; Mayhall, E.A.; Langenau, D.M.; Kutok, J.L.; Look, A.T.; Zon, L.I. Effects of lethal irradiation in zebrafish and rescue by hematopoietic cell transplantation. *Blood* **2004**, *104*, 1298–1305. [CrossRef]
122. Langenau, D.M.; Ferrando, A.A.; Traver, D.; Kutok, J.L.; Hezel, J.P.; Kanki, J.P.; Zon, L.I.; Look, A.T.; Trede, N.S. In vivo tracking of T cell development, ablation, and engraftment in transgenic zebrafish. *Proc. Natl. Acad. Sci. USA* **2004**, *101*, 7369–7374. [CrossRef]
123. King, M.A.; Covassin, L.; Brehm, M.A.; Racki, W.; Pearson, T.; Leif, J.; Laning, J.; Fodor, W.; Foreman, O.; Burzenski, L.; et al. Human peripheral blood leucocyte non-obese diabetic-severe combined immunodeficiency interleukin-2 receptor gamma chain gene mouse model of xenogeneic graft-versus-host-like disease and the role of host major histocompatibility complex. *Clin. Exp. Immunol.* **2009**, *157*, 104–118. [CrossRef]
124. Tang, Q.; Abdelfattah, N.S.; Blackburn, J.S.; Moore, J.C.; Martinez, S.A.; Moore, F.E.; Lobbardi, R.; Tenente, I.M.; Ignatius, M.S.; Berman, J.N.; et al. Optimized cell transplantation using adult rag2 mutant zebrafish. *Nat. Meth.* **2014**, *11*, 821–824. [CrossRef]
125. Stoletov, K.; Montel, V.; Lester, R.D.; Gonias, S.L.; Klemke, R. High-resolution imaging of the dynamic tumor cell vascular interface in transparent zebrafish. *Proc. Natl. Acad. Sci. USA* **2007**, *104*, 17406–17411. [CrossRef]
126. Mizgireuv, I.V.; Revskoy, S.Y. Transplantable tumor lines generated in clonal zebrafish. *Cancer Res.* **2006**, *66*, 3120–3125. [CrossRef]
127. Smith, A.C.; Raimondi, A.R.; Salthouse, C.D.; Ignatius, M.S.; Blackburn, J.S.; Mizgirev, I.V.; Storer, N.Y.; de Jong, J.L.; Chen, A.T.; Zhou, Y.; et al. High-throughput cell transplantation establishes that tumor-initiating cells are abundant in zebrafish T-cell acute lymphoblastic leukemia. *Blood* **2010**, *115*, 3296–3303. [CrossRef]
128. De La Rochere, P.; Guil-Luna, S.; Decaudin, D.; Azar, G.; Sidhu, S.S.; Piaggio, E. Humanized Mice for the Study of Immuno-Oncology. *Trends Immunol.* **2018**, *39*, 748–763. [CrossRef]
129. Tang, Q.; Moore, J.C.; Ignatius, M.S.; Tenente, I.M.; Hayes, M.N.; Garcia, E.G.; Torres Yordan, N.; Bourque, C.; He, S.; Blackburn, J.S.; et al. Imaging tumour cell heterogeneity following cell transplantation into optically clear immune-deficient zebrafish. *Nat. Commun.* **2016**, *7*, 10358. [CrossRef]
130. Moore, J.C.; Tang, Q.; Yordan, N.T.; Moore, F.E.; Garcia, E.G.; Lobbardi, R.; Ramakrishnan, A.; Marvin, D.L.; Anselmo, A.; Sadreyev, R.I.; et al. Single-cell imaging of normal and malignant cell engraftment into optically clear prkdc-null SCID zebrafish. *J. Exp. Med.* **2016**, *213*, 2575–2589. [CrossRef]
131. Heilmann, S.; Ratnakumar, K.; Langdon, E.M.; Kansler, E.R.; Kim, I.S.; Campbell, N.R.; Perry, E.B.; McMahon, A.J.; Kaufman, C.K.; van Rooijen, E.; et al. A Quantitative System for Studying Metastasis Using Transparent Zebrafish. *Cancer Res.* **2015**, *75*, 4272–4282. [CrossRef]
132. Benjamin, D.C.; Hynes, R.O. Intravital imaging of metastasis in adult Zebrafish. *BMC Cancer* **2017**, *17*, 660. [CrossRef]
133. Hyenne, V.; Ghoroghi, S.; Collot, M.; Bons, J.; Follain, G.; Harlepp, S.; Mary, B.; Bauer, J.; Mercier, L.; Busnelli, I.; et al. Studying the Fate of Tumor Extracellular Vesicles at High Spatiotemporal Resolution Using the Zebrafish Embryo. *Dev. Cell* **2019**, *48*, 554–572. [CrossRef]
134. Lee, L.M.; Seftor, E.A.; Bonde, G.; Cornell, R.A.; Hendrix, M.J. The fate of human malignant melanoma cells transplanted into zebrafish embryos: Assessment of migration and cell division in the absence of tumor formation. *Dev. Dyn.* **2005**, *233*, 1560–1570. [CrossRef]
135. Topczewska, J.M.; Postovit, L.M.; Margaryan, N.V.; Sam, A.; Hess, A.R.; Wheaton, W.W.; Nickoloff, B.J.; Topczewski, J.; Hendrix, M.J. Embryonic and tumorigenic pathways converge via Nodal signaling: Role in melanoma aggressiveness. *Nat. Med.* **2006**, *12*, 925–932. [CrossRef]

136. Haldi, M.; Ton, C.; Seng, W.L.; McGrath, P. Human melanoma cells transplanted into zebrafish proliferate, migrate, produce melanin, form masses and stimulate angiogenesis in zebrafish. *Angiogenesis* **2006**, *9*, 139–151. [CrossRef]
137. Olszewski, M.B.; Pruszko, M.; Snaar-Jagalska, E.; Zylicz, A.; Zylicz, M. Diverse and cancer typespecific roles of the p53 R248Q gainoffunction mutation in cancer migration and invasiveness. *Int. J. Oncol.* **2019**, *54*, 1168–1182.
138. Zhang, B.; Xuan, C.; Ji, Y.; Zhang, W.; Wang, D. Zebrafish xenotransplantation as a tool for in vivo cancer study. *Fam. Cancer* **2015**, *14*, 487–493. [CrossRef]
139. Cabezas-Sainz, P.; Guerra-Varela, J.; Carreira, M.J.; Mariscal, J.; Roel, M.; Rubiolo, J.A.; Sciara, A.A.; Abal, M.; Botana, L.M.; Lopez, R.; et al. Improving zebrafish embryo xenotransplantation conditions by increasing incubation temperature and establishing a proliferation index with ZFtool. *BMC Cancer* **2018**, *18*, 3. [CrossRef]
140. Marques, I.J.; Weiss, F.U.; Vlecken, D.H.; Nitsche, C.; Bakkers, J.; Lagendijk, A.K.; Partecke, L.I.; Heidecke, C.D.; Lerch, M.M.; Bagowski, C.P. Metastatic behaviour of primary human tumours in a zebrafish xenotransplantation model. *BMC Cancer* **2009**, *9*, 14. [CrossRef]
141. Nicoli, S.; Presta, M. The zebrafish/tumor xenograft angiogenesis assay. *Nat. Protoc.* **2007**, *2*, 2918–2923. [CrossRef]
142. Nicoli, S.; Ribatti, D.; Cotelli, F.; Presta, M. Mammalian tumor xenografts induce neovascularization in zebrafish embryos. *Cancer Res.* **2007**, *67*, 2927–2931.
143. Zhao, C.; Wang, X.; Zhao, Y.; Li, Z.; Lin, S.; Wei, Y.; Yang, H. A novel xenograft model in zebrafish for high-resolution investigating dynamics of neovascularization in tumors. *PLoS ONE* **2011**, *6*, e21768. [CrossRef]
144. Chiavacci, E.; Rizzo, M.; Pitto, L.; Patella, F.; Evangelista, M.; Mariani, L.; Rainaldi, G. The zebrafish/tumor xenograft angiogenesis assay as a tool for screening anti-angiogenic miRNAs. *Cytotechnology* **2015**, *67*, 969–975. [CrossRef]
145. Cheng, S.Y.; Chen, N.F.; Lin, P.Y.; Su, J.H.; Chen, B.H.; Kuo, H.M.; Sung, C.S.; Sung, P.J.; Wen, Z.H.; Chen, W.F. Anti-Invasion and Antiangiogenic Effects of Stellettin B through Inhibition of the Akt/Girdin Signaling Pathway and VEGF in Glioblastoma Cells. *Cancers* **2019**, *11*, 220. [CrossRef]
146. Gabellini, C.; Gomez-Abenza, E.; Ibanez-Molero, S.; Tupone, M.G.; Perez-Oliva, A.B.; de Oliveira, S.; Del Bufalo, D.; Mulero, V. Interleukin 8 mediates bcl-xL-induced enhancement of human melanoma cell dissemination and angiogenesis in a zebrafish xenograft model. *Int. J. Cancer* **2018**, *142*, 584–596. [CrossRef]
147. Corkery, D.P.; Dellaire, G.; Berman, J.N. Leukaemia xenotransplantation in zebrafish–chemotherapy response assay in vivo. *Br. J. Haematol.* **2011**, *153*, 786–789. [CrossRef]
148. Pruvot, B.; Jacquel, A.; Droin, N.; Auberger, P.; Bouscary, D.; Tamburini, J.; Muller, M.; Fontenay, M.; Chluba, J.; Solary, E. Leukemic cell xenograft in zebrafish embryo for investigating drug efficacy. *Haematologica* **2011**, *96*, 612–616. [CrossRef]
149. Bentley, V.L.; Veinotte, C.J.; Corkery, D.P.; Pinder, J.B.; LeBlanc, M.A.; Bedard, K.; Weng, A.P.; Berman, J.N.; Dellaire, G. Focused chemical genomics using zebrafish xenotransplantation as a preclinical therapeutic platform for T-cell acute lymphoblastic leukemia. *Haematologica* **2015**, *100*, 70–76. [CrossRef]
150. Lin, J.; Zhang, W.; Zhao, J.J.; Kwart, A.H.; Yang, C.; Ma, D.; Ren, X.; Tai, Y.T.; Anderson, K.C.; Handin, R.I.; et al. A clinically relevant in vivo zebrafish model of human multiple myeloma to study preclinical therapeutic efficacy. *Blood* **2016**, *128*, 249–252. [CrossRef]
151. Sacco, A.; Roccaro, A.M.; Ma, D.; Shi, J.; Mishima, Y.; Moschetta, M.; Chiarini, M.; Munshi, N.; Handin, R.I.; Ghobrial, I.M. Cancer Cell Dissemination and Homing to the Bone Marrow in a Zebrafish Model. *Cancer Res.* **2016**, *76*, 463–471. [CrossRef]
152. van der Ent, W.; Burrello, C.; Teunisse, A.F.; Ksander, B.R.; van der Velden, P.A.; Jager, M.J.; Jochemsen, A.G.; Snaar-Jagalska, B.E. Modeling of human uveal melanoma in zebrafish xenograft embryos. *Investig. Ophthalmol. Vis. Sci.* **2014**, *55*, 6612–6622. [CrossRef]
153. Teng, Y.; Xie, X.; Walker, S.; White, D.T.; Mumm, J.S.; Cowell, J.K. Evaluating human cancer cell metastasis in zebrafish. *BMC Cancer* **2013**, *13*, 453. [CrossRef]
154. Vittori, M.; Breznik, B.; Hrovat, K.; Kenig, S.; Lah, T.T. RECQ1 Helicase Silencing Decreases the Tumour Growth Rate of U87 Glioblastoma Cell Xenografts in Zebrafish Embryos. *Genes* **2017**, *8*, 222. [CrossRef]
155. Lam, S.H.; Lee, S.G.; Lin, C.Y.; Thomsen, J.S.; Fu, P.Y.; Murthy, K.R.; Li, H.; Govindarajan, K.R.; Nick, L.C.; Bourque, G.; et al. Molecular conservation of estrogen-response associated with cell cycle regulation,

hormonal carcinogenesis and cancer in zebrafish and human cancer cell lines. *BMC Med. Genom.* **2011**, *4*, 41. [CrossRef]
156. Ghotra, V.P.; He, S.; de Bont, H.; van der Ent, W.; Spaink, H.P.; van de Water, B.; Snaar-Jagalska, B.E.; Danen, E.H. Automated whole animal bio-imaging assay for human cancer dissemination. *PLoS ONE* **2012**, *7*, e31281. [CrossRef]
157. Drabsch, Y.; He, S.; Zhang, L.; Snaar-Jagalska, B.E.; ten Dijke, P. Transforming growth factor-beta signalling controls human breast cancer metastasis in a zebrafish xenograft model. *Breast Cancer Res. BCR* **2013**, *15*, R106. [CrossRef]
158. Naber, H.P.; Drabsch, Y.; Snaar-Jagalska, B.E.; ten Dijke, P.; van Laar, T. Snail and Slug, key regulators of TGF-beta-induced EMT, are sufficient for the induction of single-cell invasion. *Biochem. Biophys. Res. Commun.* **2013**, *435*, 58–63. [CrossRef]
159. Truong, H.H.; Xiong, J.; Ghotra, V.P.; Nirmala, E.; Haazen, L.; Le Devedec, S.E.; Balcioglu, H.E.; He, S.; Snaar-Jagalska, B.E.; Vreugdenhil, E.; et al. beta1 integrin inhibition elicits a prometastatic switch through the TGFbeta-miR-200-ZEB network in E-cadherin-positive triple-negative breast cancer. *Sci. Signal.* **2014**, *7*, ra15. [CrossRef]
160. de Boeck, M.; Cui, C.; Mulder, A.A.; Jost, C.R.; Ikeno, S.; Ten Dijke, P. Smad6 determines BMP-regulated invasive behaviour of breast cancer cells in a zebrafish xenograft model. *Sci. Rep.* **2016**, *6*, 24968. [CrossRef]
161. Tulotta, C.; Stefanescu, C.; Beletkaia, E.; Bussmann, J.; Tarbashevich, K.; Schmidt, T.; Snaar-Jagalska, B.E. Inhibition of signaling between human CXCR4 and zebrafish ligands by the small molecule IT1t impairs the formation of triple-negative breast cancer early metastases in a zebrafish xenograft model. *Dis. Models Mech.* **2016**, *9*, 141–153. [CrossRef]
162. Tulotta, C.; Stefanescu, C.; Chen, Q.; Torraca, V.; Meijer, A.H.; Snaar-Jagalska, B.E. CXCR4 signaling regulates metastatic onset by controlling neutrophil motility and response to malignant cells. *Sci. Rep.* **2019**, *9*, 2399. [CrossRef]
163. Ben-Porath, I.; Thomson, M.W.; Carey, V.J.; Ge, R.; Bell, G.W.; Regev, A.; Weinberg, R.A. An embryonic stem cell-like gene expression signature in poorly differentiated aggressive human tumors. *Nat. Genet.* **2008**, *40*, 499–507. [CrossRef]
164. Finicelli, M.; Benedetti, G.; Squillaro, T.; Pistilli, B.; Marcellusi, A.; Mariani, P.; Santinelli, A.; Latini, L.; Galderisi, U.; Giordano, A. Expression of stemness genes in primary breast cancer tissues: The role of SOX2 as a prognostic marker for detection of early recurrence. *Oncotarget* **2014**, *5*, 9678–9688. [CrossRef]
165. Schaefer, T.; Wang, H.; Mir, P.; Konantz, M.; Pereboom, T.C.; Paczulla, A.M.; Merz, B.; Fehm, T.; Perner, S.; Rothfuss, O.C.; et al. Molecular and functional interactions between AKT and SOX2 in breast carcinoma. *Oncotarget* **2015**, *6*, 43540–43556. [CrossRef]
166. Mercatali, L.; La Manna, F.; Groenewoud, A.; Casadei, R.; Recine, F.; Miserocchi, G.; Pieri, F.; Liverani, C.; Bongiovanni, A.; Spadazzi, C.; et al. Development of a Patient-Derived Xenograft (PDX) of Breast Cancer Bone Metastasis in a Zebrafish Model. *Int. J. Mol. Sci.* **2016**, *17*, 1375. [CrossRef]
167. Ghotra, V.P.; He, S.; van der Horst, G.; Nijhoff, S.; de Bont, H.; Lekkerkerker, A.; Janssen, R.; Jenster, G.; van Leenders, G.J.; Hoogland, A.M.; et al. SYK Is a Candidate Kinase Target for the Treatment of Advanced Prostate Cancer. *Cancer Res.* **2015**, *75*, 230–240. [CrossRef]
168. Melong, N.; Steele, S.; MacDonald, M.; Holly, A.; Collins, C.C.; Zoubeidi, A.; Berman, J.N.; Dellaire, G. Enzalutamide inhibits testosterone-induced growth of human prostate cancer xenografts in zebrafish and can induce bradycardia. *Sci. Rep.* **2017**, *7*, 14698. [CrossRef]
169. Xu, W.; Foster, B.A.; Richards, M.; Bondioli, K.R.; Shah, G.; Green, C.C. Characterization of prostate cancer cell progression in zebrafish xenograft model. *Int. J. Oncol.* **2018**, *52*, 252–260. [CrossRef]
170. Chen, X.; Wang, J.; Cao, Z.; Hosaka, K.; Jensen, L.; Yang, H.; Sun, Y.; Zhuang, R.; Liu, Y.; Cao, Y. Invasiveness and metastasis of retinoblastoma in an orthotopic zebrafish tumor model. *Sci. Rep.* **2015**, *5*, 10351. [CrossRef]
171. Welker, A.M.; Jaros, B.D.; An, M.; Beattie, C.E. Changes in tumor cell heterogeneity after chemotherapy treatment in a xenograft model of glioblastoma. *Neuroscience* **2017**, *356*, 35–43. [CrossRef]
172. Zeng, A.; Ye, T.; Cao, D.; Huang, X.; Yang, Y.; Chen, X.; Xie, Y.; Yao, S.; Zhao, C. Identify a Blood-Brain Barrier Penetrating Drug-TNB using Zebrafish Orthotopic Glioblastoma Xenograft Model. *Sci. Rep.* **2017**, *7*, 14372. [CrossRef]

173. Banasavadi-Siddegowda, Y.K.; Welker, A.M.; An, M.; Yang, X.; Zhou, W.; Shi, G.; Imitola, J.; Li, C.; Hsu, S.; Wang, J.; et al. PRMT5 as a druggable target for glioblastoma therapy. *Neuro Oncol.* **2018**, *20*, 753–763. [CrossRef]
174. Pudelko, L.; Edwards, S.; Balan, M.; Nyqvist, D.; Al-Saadi, J.; Dittmer, J.; Almlof, I.; Helleday, T.; Brautigam, L. An orthotopic glioblastoma animal model suitable for high-throughput screenings. *Neuro Oncol.* **2018**, *20*, 1475–1484. [CrossRef]
175. Ellis, H.P.; Greenslade, M.; Powell, B.; Spiteri, I.; Sottoriva, A.; Kurian, K.M. Current Challenges in Glioblastoma: Intratumour Heterogeneity, Residual Disease, and Models to Predict Disease Recurrence. *Front. Oncol.* **2015**, *5*, 251. [CrossRef]
176. Roel, M.; Rubiolo, J.A.; Guerra-Varela, J.; Silva, S.B.; Thomas, O.P.; Cabezas-Sainz, P.; Sanchez, L.; Lopez, R.; Botana, L.M. Marine guanidine alkaloids crambescidins inhibit tumor growth and activate intrinsic apoptotic signaling inducing tumor regression in a colorectal carcinoma zebrafish xenograft model. *Oncotarget* **2016**, *7*, 83071–83087. [CrossRef]
177. Chang, T.C.; Wei, P.L.; Makondi, P.T.; Chen, W.T.; Huang, C.Y.; Chang, Y.J. Bromelain inhibits the ability of colorectal cancer cells to proliferate via activation of ROS production and autophagy. *PLoS ONE* **2019**, *14*, e0210274. [CrossRef]
178. Wu, J.Q.; Zhai, J.; Li, C.Y.; Tan, A.M.; Wei, P.; Shen, L.Z.; He, M.F. Patient-derived xenograft in zebrafish embryos: A new platform for translational research in gastric cancer. *J. Exp. Clin. Cancer Res. CR* **2017**, *36*, 160. [CrossRef]
179. Tsering, J.; Hu, X. Triphala Suppresses Growth and Migration of Human Gastric Carcinoma Cells In Vitro and in a Zebrafish Xenograft Model. *BioMed Res. Int.* **2018**, *2018*, 7046927. [CrossRef]
180. Yu, C.I.; Chen, C.Y.; Liu, W.; Chang, P.C.; Huang, C.W.; Han, K.F.; Lin, I.P.; Lin, M.Y.; Lee, C.H. Sandensolide Induces Oxidative Stress-Mediated Apoptosis in Oral Cancer Cells and in Zebrafish Xenograft Model. *Mar. Drugs* **2018**, *16*, 387. [CrossRef]
181. Jin, Y.; Wei, L.; Jiang, Q.; Song, X.; Teng, C.; Fan, C.; Lv, Y.; Liu, Y.; Shen, W.; Li, L.; et al. Comparison of efficacy and toxicity of bevacizumab, endostar and apatinib in transgenic and human lung cancer xenograftzebrafish model. *Sci. Rep.* **2018**, *8*, 15837. [CrossRef]
182. Chou, H.L.; Lin, Y.H.; Liu, W.; Wu, C.Y.; Li, R.N.; Huang, H.W.; Chou, C.H.; Chiou, S.J.; Chiu, C.C. Combination Therapy of Chloroquine and C(2)-Ceramide Enhances Cytotoxicity in Lung Cancer H460 and H1299 Cells. *Cancers* **2019**, *11*, 370. [CrossRef]
183. van der Ent, W.; Jochemsen, A.G.; Teunisse, A.F.; Krens, S.F.; Szuhai, K.; Spaink, H.P.; Hogendoorn, P.C.; Snaar-Jagalska, B.E. Ewing sarcoma inhibition by disruption of EWSR1-FLI1 transcriptional activity and reactivation of p53. *J. Pathol.* **2014**, *233*, 415–424. [CrossRef]
184. Zhang, B.; Shimada, Y.; Kuroyanagi, J.; Nishimura, Y.; Umemoto, N.; Nomoto, T.; Shintou, T.; Miyazaki, T.; Tanaka, T. Zebrafish xenotransplantation model for cancer stem-like cell study and high-throughput screening of inhibitors. *Tumor Biol.* **2014**, *35*, 11861–11869. [CrossRef]
185. Khan, N.; Mahajan, N.K.; Sinha, P.; Jayandharan, G.R. An efficient method to generate xenograft tumor models of acute myeloid leukemia and hepatocellular carcinoma in adult zebrafish. *Blood Cells Mol. Dis.* **2019**, *75*, 48–55. [CrossRef]
186. Yan, C.; Brunson, D.C.; Tang, Q.; Do, D.; Iftimia, N.A.; Moore, J.C.; Hayes, M.N.; Welker, A.M.; Garcia, E.G.; Dubash, T.D.; et al. Visualizing Engrafted Human Cancer and Therapy Responses in Immunodeficient Zebrafish. *Cell* **2019**, *177*, 1903–1914. [CrossRef]
187. Zhao, S.; Huang, J.; Ye, J. A fresh look at zebrafish from the perspective of cancer research. *J. Exp. Clin. Cancer Res. CR* **2015**, *34*, 80. [CrossRef]
188. Wang, C.; Tao, W.; Wang, Y.; Bikow, J.; Lu, B.; Keating, A.; Verma, S.; Parker, T.G.; Han, R.; Wen, X.Y. Rosuvastatin, identified from a zebrafish chemical genetic screen for antiangiogenic compounds, suppresses the growth of prostate cancer. *Eur. Urol.* **2010**, *58*, 418–426. [CrossRef]
189. White, R.M.; Cech, J.; Ratanasirintrawoot, S.; Lin, C.Y.; Rahl, P.B.; Burke, C.J.; Langdon, E.; Tomlinson, M.L.; Mosher, J.; Kaufman, C.; et al. DHODH modulates transcriptional elongation in the neural crest and melanoma. *Nature* **2011**, *471*, 518–522. [CrossRef]
190. Ridges, S.; Heaton, W.L.; Joshi, D.; Choi, H.; Eiring, A.; Batchelor, L.; Choudhry, P.; Manos, E.J.; Sofla, H.; Sanati, A.; et al. Zebrafish screen identifies novel compound with selective toxicity against leukemia. *Blood* **2012**, *119*, 5621–5631. [CrossRef]

191. Gutierrez, A.; Pan, L.; Groen, R.W.; Baleydier, F.; Kentsis, A.; Marineau, J.; Grebliunaite, R.; Kozakewich, E.; Reed, C.; Pflumio, F.; et al. Phenothiazines induce PP2A-mediated apoptosis in T cell acute lymphoblastic leukemia. *J. Clin. Investig.* **2014**, *124*, 644–655. [CrossRef] [PubMed]
192. Precazzini, F.; Pancher, M.; Gatto, P.; Tushe, A.; Adami, V.; Anelli, V.; Mione, M.C. Automated in vivo screen in zebrafish identifies Clotrimazole as targeting a metabolic vulnerability in a melanoma model. *Dev. Biol.* **2019**, in press. [CrossRef] [PubMed]
193. Stern, H.M.; Murphey, R.D.; Shepard, J.L.; Amatruda, J.F.; Straub, C.T.; Pfaff, K.L.; Weber, G.; Tallarico, J.A.; King, R.W.; Zon, L.I. Small molecules that delay S phase suppress a zebrafish bmyb mutant. *Nat. Chem. Biol.* **2005**, *1*, 366–370. [CrossRef] [PubMed]
194. Camus, S.; Quevedo, C.; Menendez, S.; Paramonov, I.; Stouten, P.F.; Janssen, R.A.; Rueb, S.; He, S.; Snaar-Jagalska, B.E.; Laricchia-Robbio, L.; et al. Identification of phosphorylase kinase as a novel therapeutic target through high-throughput screening for anti-angiogenesis compounds in zebrafish. *Oncogene* **2012**, *31*, 4333–4342. [CrossRef] [PubMed]
195. Murphy, A.G.; Casey, R.; Maguire, A.; Tosetto, M.; Butler, C.T.; Conroy, E.; Reynolds, A.L.; Sheahan, K.; O'Donoghue, D.; Gallagher, W.M.; et al. Preclinical validation of the small molecule drug quininib as a novel therapeutic for colorectal cancer. *Sci. Rep.* **2016**, *6*, 34523. [CrossRef]
196. Astin, J.W.; Jamieson, S.M.; Eng, T.C.; Flores, M.V.; Misa, J.P.; Chien, A.; Crosier, K.E.; Crosier, P.S. An in vivo antilymphatic screen in zebrafish identifies novel inhibitors of mammalian lymphangiogenesis and lymphatic-mediated metastasis. *Mol. Cancer* **2014**, *13*, 2450–2462. [CrossRef]
197. Dang, M.; Henderson, R.E.; Garraway, L.A.; Zon, L.I. Long-term drug administration in the adult zebrafish using oral gavage for cancer preclinical studies. *Dis. Models Mech.* **2016**, *9*, 811–820. [CrossRef]
198. Tamplin, O.J.; White, R.M.; Jing, L.; Kaufman, C.K.; Lacadie, S.A.; Li, P.; Taylor, A.M.; Zon, L.I. Small molecule screening in zebrafish: Swimming in potential drug therapies. *Wiley Interdiscip. Rev. Dev. Biol.* **2012**, *1*, 459–468. [CrossRef]
199. Gutierrez-Lovera, C.; Vazquez-Rios, A.J.; Guerra-Varela, J.; Sanchez, L.; de la Fuente, M. The Potential of Zebrafish as a Model Organism for Improving the Translation of Genetic Anticancer Nanomedicines. *Genes* **2017**, *8*, 349. [CrossRef]
200. Ito, M.; Hiramatsu, H.; Kobayashi, K.; Suzue, K.; Kawahata, M.; Hioki, K.; Ueyama, Y.; Koyanagi, Y.; Sugamura, K.; Tsuji, K.; et al. NOD/SCID/gamma(c)(null) mouse: An excellent recipient mouse model for engraftment of human cells. *Blood* **2002**, *100*, 3175–3182. [CrossRef]
201. Murphey, R.D.; Zon, L.I. Small molecule screening in the zebrafish. *Methods* **2006**, *39*, 255–261. [CrossRef] [PubMed]

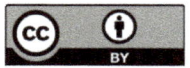

© 2019 by the authors. Licensee MDPI, Basel, Switzerland. This article is an open access article distributed under the terms and conditions of the Creative Commons Attribution (CC BY) license (http://creativecommons.org/licenses/by/4.0/).

MDPI
St. Alban-Anlage 66
4052 Basel
Switzerland
Tel. +41 61 683 77 34
Fax +41 61 302 89 18
www.mdpi.com

Actuators Editorial Office
E-mail: actuators@mdpi.com
www.mdpi.com/journal/genes

www.ingramcontent.com/pod-product-compliance
Lightning Source LLC
LaVergne TN
LVHW070506100526
838202LV00014B/1800